# UROGYNECOLOGY AND RECONSTRUCTIVE PELVIC SURGERY

*Visit our website at www.mosby.com*

# UROGYNECOLOGY
# AND
# RECONSTRUCTIVE
# PELVIC SURGERY

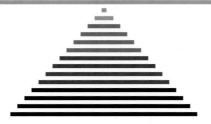

*Edited by*

## MARK D. WALTERS, M.D.

Vice-Chairman and Head
Section of General Gynecology and Urogynecology/Reconstructive Pelvic Surgery
Department of Gynecology and Obstetrics
The Cleveland Clinic Foundation
Cleveland, Ohio

## MICKEY M. KARRAM, M.D.

Associate Director, Department of Obstetrics and Gynecology
Director, Division of Urogynecology and Reconstructive Pelvic Surgery
Good Samaritan Hospital
Assistant Professor of Obstetrics and Gynecology
University of Cincinnati
Cincinnati, Ohio

**SECOND EDITION**

*With 270 illustrations and 5 color plates*

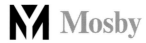 Mosby

St. Louis  Baltimore  Boston  Carlsbad  Chicago  Minneapolis  New York  Philadelphia  Portland
London  Milan  Sydney  Tokyo  Toronto

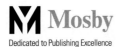

Project Managers: Patricia Tannian and Deborah L. Vogel
Project Specialist: Ann E. Rogers
Design Manager: Gail Morey Hudson
Cover Design: Teresa Breckwoldt

Editing, composition, and lithography by Graphic World, Inc.
Printing and binding by Maple-Vail Book Mfg Group

Mosby, Inc.
11830 Westline Industrial Drive
St. Louis, Missouri 63146

**Library of Congress Cataloging in Publication Data**

Urogynecology and reconstructive pelvic surgery/edited by Mark D.
   Walters, Mickey M. Karram.—2nd ed.
         p.     cm.
      Includes bibliographical references and index.
      ISBN 0-8151-3671-4—ISBN 0-8151-3671-4 (alk. paper)
      1. Urogynecology.    2. Pelvis—Surgery.    3. Generative organs,
   Female—Surgery.    I. Walters, Mark D.    II. Walters, Mark D.
   Clinical urogynecology.
      [DNLM:    1. Genital Diseases, Female.    2. Urinary Incontinence.
   3. Urodynamics.    4. Uterine Prolapse.    5. Fecal Incontinence.
   6. Urogenital Surgical Procedures.    WJ  190  U775u 1999]
   RG484.W35   1999
   616.6—dc21
   DNLM/DLC
   for Library of Congress                                        99-10976
                                                                      CIP

99   00   01   02   03  /  9 8 7 6 5 4 3 2 1

*To my teachers*

with my warmest and most sincere respect and appreciation.

**Mark D. Walters**


The second edition of this book is dedicated to
my wife and best friend

*Mona*

for her love and her support of my academic pursuits
and to my daughters

*Tamara* and *Lena*

who are a continuing source of motivation as I watch them grow.

**Mickey M. Karram**

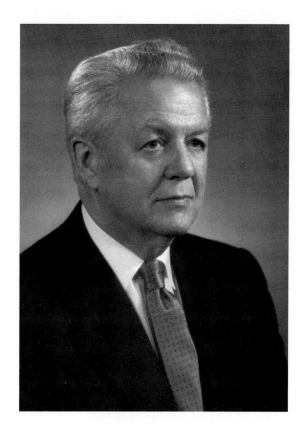

We wish to dedicate the second edition of this textbook to the late

**David H. Nichols, M.D.**

*(1925-1998)*

Dr. Nichols was our mentor, role model, and friend.
He dedicated his life to his patients and to
conveying his extensive knowledge and vast experience to his
students with particular clarity and high energy.
We will greatly miss him.

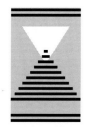

# Contributors

**CLAUDIA G. BACHOFEN, M.D.**
Resident Physician
Department of Obstetrics and Gynecology
Texas A&M University Health Science Center
Scott and White Clinic and Hospital
Temple, Texas

**J. THOMAS BENSON, M.D.**
Clinical Professor, Department of Obstetrics and Gynecology
Indiana University Medical Center
Director of Obstetrics and Gynecology Education
Methodist Hospital of Indiana
Indianapolis, Indiana

**ALFRED E. BENT, M.D.**
Clinical Associate Professor and Program Director of Residency
   Training
Department of Obstetrics and Gynecology
University of Maryland School of Medicine
Head, Division of Urogynecology and Reconstructive Pelvic
   Surgery
Greater Baltimore Medical Center
Baltimore, Maryland

**RAYMOND A. BOLOGNA, M.D.**
Fellow, Pelvic Floor Center
Allegheny University Hospitals
Philadelphia, Pennsylvania

**GEOFFREY W. CUNDIFF, M.D.**
Chief of Urogynecology and Reconstructive Pelvic Surgery
Johns Hopkins School of Medicine
Baltimore, Maryland

**MOLLY C. DOUGHERTY, Ph.D., R.N.**
Frances Hill Fox Professor of Nursing
University of North Carolina
Chapel Hill, North Carolina

**THOMAS E. ELKINS, M.D.†**
Professor and Chief of Gynecology
Director of Reconstructive Pelvic Surgery
Johns Hopkins School of Medicine
Baltimore, Maryland

**TOMMASO FALCONE, M.D.**
Head, Section of Reproductive Endocrinology
Department of Gynecology and Obstetrics
The Cleveland Clinic Foundation
Cleveland, Ohio

**TRACY L. HULL, M.D.**
Assistant Professor of the Cleveland Clinic Health Services
   Center
Ohio State University
Staff Surgeon, Department of Colorectal Surgery
The Cleveland Clinic Foundation
Cleveland, Ohio

**W. GLENN HURT, M.D.**
Professor, Department of Obstetrics and Gynecology
Medical College of Virginia
Richmond, Virginia

**NEERAJ KOHLI, M.D.**
Clinical Instructor
Division of Urogynecology and Reconstructive Pelvic Surgery
Good Samaritan Hospital
Cincinnati, Ohio

**PAUL P. KOONINGS, M.D.**
Oncologic Gynecology
Department of Obstetrics and Gynecology
Kaiser Permanente Medical Center
San Diego, California

**PADMA K. MALLIPEDDI, M.D.**
Clinical Instructor
Division of Urogynecology and Reconstructive Pelvic Surgery
Good Samaritan Hospital
Cincinnati, Ohio

**JOHN R. MIKLOS, M.D.**
Director, Urogynecology and Reconstructive Pelvic Surgery
Department of Obstetrics and Gynecology
Georgia Baptist Medical Center
Marietta, Georgia

---

†Deceased.

**EDWARD R. NEWTON, M.D.**
Professor and Chairman
Department of Obstetrics and Gynecology
East Carolina University School of Medicine
Greenville, North Carolina

**INGRID NYGAARD, M.D.**
Associate Professor
Head, General Women's Health Division
Department of Obstetrics and Gynecology
University of Iowa College of Medicine
Iowa City, Iowa

**MARIE FIDELA R. PARAISO, M.D.**
Staff Physician, Department of Gynecology and Obstetrics
The Cleveland Clinic Foundation
Cleveland, Ohio

**LINDA M. PARTOLL, M.D.**
Assistant Professor, Department of Obstetrics and Gynecology
University of Washington School of Medicine
Seattle, Washington

**JANICE F. RAFFERTY, M.D.**
Assistant Professor, Department of Surgery
University of Cincinnati School of Medicine
Cincinnati, Ohio

**FEZA H. REMZI, M.D.**
Clinical Associate, Department of Colorectal Surgery
The Cleveland Clinic Foundation
Cleveland, Ohio

**BOB L. SHULL, M.D.**
Professor of Obstetrics and Gynecology
Chief, Section of Urogynecology and Pelvic Reconstructive
  Surgery
Department of Obstetrics and Gynecology
Texas A&M University Health Science Center
Scott and White Clinic and Hospital
Temple, Texas

**LASZLO SOGOR, M.D., Ph.D.**
Associate Professor, Department of Reproductive Biology
Case Western Reserve University School of Medicine
Chief, Division of Gynecology
University Hospitals of Cleveland
Cleveland, Ohio

**ANDREW C. STEELE, M.D.**
Clinical Instructor
Division of Urogynecology and Reconstructive Pelvic Surgery
Good Samaritan Hospital
Cincinnati, Ohio

**CARMEN J. SULTANA, M.D.**
Assistant Professor, Department of Obstetrics and Gynecology
Jefferson Medical College
Philadelphia, Pennsylvania

**EDDIE H.M. SZE, M.D.**
Assistant Professor, Department of Obstetrics and Gynecology
East Carolina University School of Medicine
Greenville, North Carolina

**JASON R. THOMPSON, M.D.**
Instructor, Department of Obstetrics and Gynecology
Johns Hopkins School of Medicine
Baltimore, Maryland

**LE MAI TU, M.D.**
Division of Urology, Sherbrooke University
Quebec, Canada

**ANNE M. WEBER, M.D.**
Director of Clinical Research, Department of Gynecology and
  Obstetrics
The Cleveland Clinic Foundation
Cleveland, Ohio

**KRISTENE E. WHITMORE, M.D.**
Associate Professor of Urology
Chief, Division of Urology
Allegheny University Hospitals
Philadelphia, Pennsylvania

We would like to specially acknowledge the following physicians who we believe represent some of the true experts in the fields of urogynecology/reconstructive pelvic surgery and urology and who reviewed the case presentations in Chapter 34 and provided their opinions.

**W. Allen Addison, M.D.,** *Durham, North Carolina*
**Rodney A. Appell, M.D.,** *Cleveland, Ohio*
**Michael P. Aronson, M.D.,** *Boston, Massachusetts*
**Lester A. Ballard, M.D.,** *Cleveland, Ohio*
**J. Thomas Benson, M.D.,** *Indianapolis, Indiana*
**Alfred E. Bent, M.D.,** *Baltimore, Maryland*
**Jerry G. Blaivas, M.D.,** *New York, New York*
**Richard C. Bump, M.D.,** *Durham, North Carolina*
**Jeffrey L. Cornella, M.D.,** *Scottsdale, Arizona*
**Geoffrey W. Cundiff, M.D.,** *Baltimore, Maryland*
**Marvin H. Terry Grody, M.D.,** *Philadelphia, Pennsylvania*
**Nicolette S. Horbach, M.D.,** *Annandale, Virginia*
**W. Glenn Hurt, M.D.,** *Richmond, Virginia*
**Neil D. Jackson, M.D.,** *Providence, Rhode Island*
**Neeraj Kohli, M.D.,** *Cincinnati, Ohio*
**Raymond A. Lee, M.D.,** *Rochester, Minnesota*
**Edward J. McGuire, M.D.,** *Houston, Texas*
**G. Rodney Meeks, M.D.,** *Jackson, Mississippi*
**Fred Miyazaki, M.D.,** *Los Angeles, California*
**David H. Nichols, M.D.,**[†] *Providence, Rhode Island*
**Ingrid Nygaard, M.D.,** *Iowa City, Iowa*
**Donald R. Ostergard, M.D.,** *Long Beach, California*
**Janice F. Rafferty, M.D.,** *Cincinnati, Ohio*
**David R. Staskin, M.D.,** *Boston, Massachusetts*
**Robert L. Summitt, Jr., M.D.,** *Memphis, Tennessee*
**R. Edward Varner, M.D.,** *Birmingham, Alabama*
**O. Lenaine Westney, M.D.,** *Houston, Texas*

[†]Deceased.

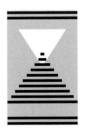

# Foreword

*"The glory of medicine is it is always moving forward, that there is more to learn."*

**W.J. Mayo**

I am honored and pleased to be asked to write the foreword to this stellar textbook in urogynecology. During the first half of the twentieth century, little scientific attention was given to understanding the pathophysiology of urinary and fecal continence and incontinence or pelvic organ prolapse, let alone their alternative operative approaches. Medicine has undergone rapid change and continues to do so. The last half of this century began with a few clinicians calling attention to the different types of urinary incontinence, the importance of an accurate diagnosis, and the advantages of medical and specific surgical approaches to pelvic organ prolapse. There were also suggestive methods to reduce surgical complications to the urinary and intestinal tracts. Imaging, urodynamic, and electromyographic studies have greatly enhanced the understanding of the researcher and the clinician, underscoring the importance of precision of the diagnosis. This interest continues and has resulted in research and clinical efforts that have led to better care for our patients. The first edition of *Clinical Urogynecology* has become well established as a significant reference in the well-rounded surgical library. With the second edition, the time has come to introduce a new spectrum of diagnostic and therapeutic procedures performed with newer techniques—most prominently laparoscopy, which has brought about a significant change in gynecology. The authors have widened the scope to include more conditions of the colon and rectum. A new and unique section is devoted to interesting cases with accompanying discussion from authorities around the country. Updated guidelines from the International Continence Society will prove advantageous. Although these extensive additions have been made, the major goal of the text remains unchanged.

While medicine is changing every day, this multi-authored text is an effort to accumulate and present information as it exists today. It is important that the new knowledge in urogynecology and reconstructive pelvic surgery becomes the knowledge for the next generation of physicians.

This textbook is not written to dictate or advocate a certain mode of diagnosis or treatment, but rather to report advances that have been made and emphasize their appreciation according to the authors' experience. This book is not a comprehensive text of gynecology or a surgical atlas; it has elements of both, but it focuses on urogynecology. The major contribution and effort is provided by two authors, Mark Walters and Mickey Karram—thoughtful educators, experienced clinicians, and consummate urogynecologists, both held in high esteem by their colleagues and students. I know the editors through personal interaction and am pleased they are continuing to emphasize accurate, thorough evaluation of the patient. Many of the contributing authors are the young stars of the future, yet their expertise is apparent throughout each of their informative reviews. I know it is the hope of the authors that those who read this book will apply the knowledge of patient and research studies for the ultimate benefit of the patient.

This new edition should be of interest to the gynecologist and urogynecologist, whether at resident, fellow, or consultant level.

**Raymond A. Lee, M.D.**

*Professor of Obstetrics and Gynecology*
*Mayo Clinic*
*Rochester, Minnesota*

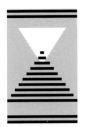

# Foreword to the First Edition

It is a privilege and an honor to prepare this foreword for *Clinical Urogynecology*. Old friends will understand and new colleagues perhaps will be surprised by this brief reentry into the field of urology.

My interest in this field covers a span of more than 40 years, initially stimulated by my experience as a pediatric surgical resident, utilizing (by present standards) primitive urodynamic recording instrumentation to evaluate bladder and urethral function. In those days, a careful clinical evaluation was supplemented by measurements often suspect because of lack of comparative data. Today, regrettably, sophisticated urodynamic testing frequently promises more than it can deliver, often in the absence of a thorough clinical evaluation. Fortunately for our patients, there is increasing recognition that disorders of micturition and symptomatic alterations in pelvic anatomy require an expertise that can best be evaluated and treated by the gynecologist appropriately trained in urogynecology.

The authors have approached this problem from the clinical standpoint but have wisely assumed that a review of anatomy and the basic principles of neurophysiology is essential for a contemporary understanding of the diagnosis and treatment of urinary incontinence and genital prolapse. This text will appeal to the gynecologist interested in disorders of micturition and the diagnosis and treatment of pelvic relaxation. It also provides sufficient information to encourage further inquiry and training in this subspecialty now available through a number of fellowship programs.

The student will be stimulated, the practicing gynecologist challenged, and the expert pleasantly surprised by the completeness and logic of the presentation. I congratulate the authors on their achievement.

**Douglas J. Marchant, M.D.**

*Professor of Obstetrics and Gynecology*
*Professor of Surgery*
*Tufts University School of Medicine*
*Adjunct Professor of Obstetrics and Gynecology*
*Brown University School of Medicine*
*Providence, Rhode Island*

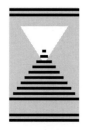

# *Preface*

As the population lives longer and has improved health, the prevalence of certain conditions, such as urinary incontinence, is increasing. Women desire and are able to remain active longer and are less interested in tolerating the lower quality of life that accompanies incontinence and related disorders. This is leading to a greater number of otherwise healthy women presenting to their physicians with various pelvic floor disorders.

National interest in diseases of women and older persons in general has helped to increase awareness of the high prevalence of urinary and fecal incontinence in women. Clinical care guidelines were developed by the Consensus Development Conference on Urinary Incontinence in Adults, sponsored by the National Institute on Aging and the Office of Medical Applications of Research of the National Institutes of Health in conjunction with other agencies. This was followed by expanded national research funding. The demographics of incontinence have also stimulated corporate interest, and many new products for evaluation and treatment (non-surgical and surgical) of incontinence have been and are being developed.

There continues to be a widespread need for education and training in urogynecology and pelvic surgery for practicing generalists and residents in obstetrics and gynecology. More physicians with special expertise in urogynecology are needed to meet the increasing patient volume and the additional training needs within this specialty. Over the last five years, the specialty of urogynecology—renamed urogynecology and reconstructive pelvic surgery—expanded from a special interest to the fourth subspecialty approved by the American Board of Obstetrics and Gynecology. Formal fellowships were extended to three years to conform with the other subspecialties and to allow for more advanced training and research. This expanded textbook is an effort to address the educational needs of physicians and advanced-care practitioners interested in this subspecialty and to serve as a core reference text in urogynecology and reconstructive pelvic surgery.

This second edition, *Urogynecology and Reconstructive Pelvic Surgery,* is a clinically oriented yet comprehensive textbook addressing the new subspecialty. We believe that this subject fundamentally encompasses four main topics: female urinary incontinence and voiding dysfunction, uro-dynamic testing, pelvic organ prolapse, and disorders of defecation. This textbook is separated into six sections. Chapters 1 through 4 describe in detail basic principles and subjects that are needed to understand and treat disorders of the lower urinary tract and pelvic floor. Chapters 5 through 11 outline basic and advanced concepts of the evaluation of lower urinary tract and pelvic floor disorders in women. Chapters 12 through 19 present management guidelines for women with genuine stress incontinence and pelvic organ prolapse. Chapters 20 through 23 address disorders of defecation. Chapters 24 through 33 discuss specific conditions and special subjects that are occasionally encountered by physicians treating patients with pelvic floor disorders. Finally, using an innovative format, Chapter 34 presents a series of interesting and difficult cases with opinions from experts in urogynecology and urology.

The second edition been expanded to include sections on defecation disorders, operative laparoscopy, and hyper-sensitivity disorders of the lower urinary tract. The sections on urodynamic testing, non-surgical treatment of incontinence and prolapse, and vaginal surgery for incontinence and prolapse have been updated and revised. Many of the original drawings from the first edition are retained, and a large number of surgical drawings were added. The new and up-to-date chapter on laparoscopic surgery for genuine stress incontinence and pelvic organ prolapse includes five color plates to help illustrate the surgical anatomy involved. Using computer-generated graphic techniques, the urodynamic illustrations were created from actual drawings of patients with various voiding disorders. This allows for enhanced learning free of the artifacts that are common in actual urodynamic tracings. Because female incontinence is best managed in a multidisciplinary fashion, recognized authorities in nursing, urology, maternal-fetal medicine, colorectal surgery, and gynecologic oncology have contributed chapters related to their particular areas of expertise.

We hope this book will meet the training needs of residents in obstetrics and gynecology and other specialties and can be used by fellows in urogynecology and reconstructive pelvic surgery as an important reference text. We also hope that generalists and urogynecologic experts alike will find it interesting and useful as they strive to take better care of their patients.

**xiii**

## ACKNOWLEDGMENTS

We would like to acknowledge the indispensable and exemplary work of Annette Gholston and Kathy Frye for performing the huge volume of secretarial and transcribing work involved in this book and Joe Chovan for his creation of particularly clear surgical and urodynamic drawings. We also wish to thank Dr. Anne M. Weber for her invaluable medical editing of our manuscripts.

**Mark D. Walters**
**Mickey M. Karram**

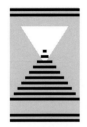

# Contents

# Urogynecology and Reconstructive Pelvic Surgery

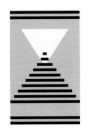

PART I
*Basic Science*

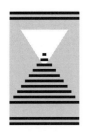

CHAPTER **1**

# Anatomy of the Lower Urinary Tract, Rectum, and Pelvic Floor

Mark D. Walters and Anne M. Weber

## EMBRYOLOGY
### Lower Urinary Tract
#### Formation of Intraembryonic Mesoderm

At approximately 15 days after fertilization, invagination and lateral migration of mesodermal cells occur between the ectodermal and endodermal layers of the presomite embryo. These migrating cells form the intraembryonic mesoderm or mesodermal germ layer. By the seventeenth day of development, the endoderm and ectoderm layers are separated entirely by the mesoderm layer, with the exception of the prochordal plate cephalically and the cloacal plate caudally. The cloacal plate consists of tightly adherent endodermal and ectodermal layers.

#### Formation of Allantois and Cloaca

Concomitantly, at about the sixteenth day of development, the posterior wall of the yolk sac forms a small diverticulum, the allantois, which extends into the connecting stalk. With ventral bending of the embryo cranially and caudally during somite development, the connecting stalk and contained allantois, as well as the cloacal membrane, are displaced onto the ventral aspect of the embryo.

The hindgut undergoes slight dilation to form the cloaca; it receives the allantois ventrally and the two mesonephric ducts laterally. Ventral mesodermal elevations occur, forming the urethral folds (primordia of the labia minora) and genital tubercle (primordium of the clitoris).

#### Partitioning of Cloaca into Urogenital Sinus and Rectum

A spur of mesodermal tissue migrates from the base of the allantois toward the cloacal membrane around 28 days after fertilization, forming the urorectal septum (Fig. 1-1). This structure partitions the cloaca into a ventral urogenital sinus and a dorsal rectum. The urogenital opening (future vestibule) is formed by the independent involution of the urogenital membrane. The point at which the urorectal septum intersects with the cloacal membrane will become the perineal body.

#### Formation of Ureteric Bud and Induction of Future Kidney

By 28 days of development, the mesonephric ducts have reached and fused with the urogenital sinus. At this time, the ureteric bud appears as a diverticulum from the posteromedial aspect of the mesonephric duct at the point where the terminus of the duct bends to enter the cloaca. The free cranial end of the ureter grows dorsally, then cranially, and induces the formation of the metanephrogenic blastema (future kidney; see Fig. 1-1). The presence of the developing ureter is essential for this differentiation; absence of the ureteric bud is invariably associated with renal agenesis. The ureteric bud branches and dilates to create the renal pelvis, major and minor calyces, and collecting ducts. The remaining parts of each are derived from the mesoderm of the metanephrogenic blastema. At this time in the female, the mesonephric system is undergoing degeneration.

The renal blastema originates at the level of the upper sacral segments. The final position of the kidney at the level of the upper lumbar vertebrae is attributed to ascent of the renal blastema. According to Maizels (1986), the four mechanisms that lead to normal renal ascent are caudal growth of the spine, active elongation of the ureter into the metanephrogenic blastema, intrinsic growth and molding of

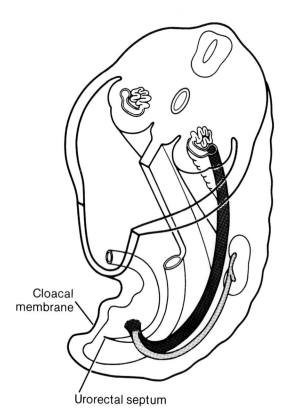

Cloacal
membrane

Urorectal septum

**Fig. 1-1** Embryo approximately 32 days (8 mm crown-rump length) after fertilization. The urorectal septum is shown dividing the cloaca into a ventral urogenital sinus and dorsal rectum. Definitive ureter and mesonephric duct share a common opening into partially divided cloaca. Note that the ureter has induced formation of a kidney from metanephrogenic blastema.

From Gosling JA, Dixon J, Humpherson JR: *Functional anatomy of the urinary tract,* London, 1982, Gower.

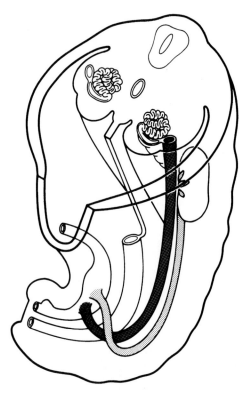

**Fig. 1-2** By thirty-seventh day (14 mm crown-rump length), kidney has continued to ascend and undergo medial rotation, and the mesonephric duct and future ureter have separated. In addition, cloaca has been divided into ventral urogenital and dorsal alimentary parts.

From Gosling JA, Dixon J, Humpherson JR: *Functional anatomy of the urinary tract,* London, 1982, Gower.

the renal parenchyma, and axial growth of the spine after fixing of the kidney to the retroperitoneum.

### Formation of Bladder, Trigone, and Urethra

At the point of its connection with the mesonephric ducts, the urogenital sinus is divided into the vesicourethral canal cranially and the definitive urogenital sinus caudally. Dilation of the cranial portion of the vesicourethral canal forms the definitive bladder, which is of endodermal origin. The vesicourethral canal communicates at its cranial end with the allantois, which becomes obliterated at about 12 weeks of fetal life, forming the urachus. This structure runs from the bladder dome to the umbilicus and is called the median umbilical ligament in the adult.

The ureteric bud begins as an outgrowth of the mesonephric duct, but with positional changes of the embryo during growth, the mesonephric duct and the ureteric bud shift positions so that the ureter comes to lie posterolaterally to the duct (Fig. 1-2). The segment of the mesonephric duct distal to the site of origin of the ureteric bud dilates and is absorbed into the urogenital sinus, forming

the bladder trigone. This structure effectively gives the endodermal wall of the vesicourethral canal a mesodermal contribution. At about 42 days after fertilization, the trigone may be defined as the region of the vesicourethral canal lying between the ureteric orifices and the termination of the mesonephric ducts (Fig. 1-3). The caudal portion of the vesicourethral canal remains narrow and forms the entire urethra. A small portion of the posterior proximal urethra may be derived, like the trigone, from mesoderm of the mesonephric duct, although this theory is controversial. A timetable and schematic representation of the embryologic contributions of the various structures of the urogenital system are shown in Table 1-1 and Fig. 1-4, respectively.

The separate development of the trigone and bladder may explain why the muscle laminae of the trigone are contiguous with the muscle of the ureter, but not with the detrusor muscle of the bladder. This separate development also may account for pharmacologic responses of the musculature of the bladder neck and trigone, which differ partially from those of the detrusor.

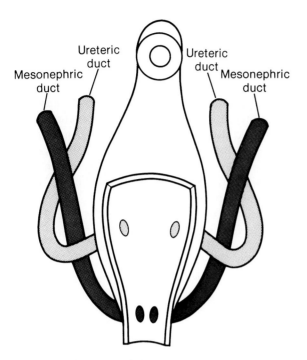

**Fig. 1-3** Urogenital sinus and associated ducts approximately 40 days (17 mm crown-rump length) after fertilization. Trigone lies between separated ureteric and mesonephric ducts.

From Gosling JA, Dixon J, Humpherson JR: *Functional anatomy of the urinary tract,* London, 1982, Gower.

### Congenital Anomalies of the Urinary Tract

Knowledge of the embryology of the genitourinary system is necessary for understanding the causes of the multiple congenital anomalies of the upper and lower urinary tracts. Selected congenital anomalies of the urinary tract and their embryologic causes are shown in Table 1-2.

## Rectum and Anal Sphincters
### Normal Development of the Hindgut

The hindgut, which in the embryo extends from the posterior intestinal portal to the cloacal membrane, gives rise to the distal third of the transverse colon, the descending colon, the sigmoid, the rectum, and the upper part of the anal canal. The terminal portion of the hindgut enters into the cloaca, an endoderm-lined cavity that is in direct contact with the surface ectoderm. In the contact area between the endoderm and ectoderm, the cloacal membrane is formed.

During further development a transverse ridge, the urorectal septum, arises in the angle between the allantois and the hindgut. This septum gradually grows caudad, thereby dividing the cloaca into an anterior portion, the primitive urogenital sinus, and a posterior portion, the anorectal canal. The primitive perineum is formed when the urorectal septum reaches the cloacal membrane when the embryo is 7 weeks old. The cloacal membrane is thus divided into the anal membrane posteriorly and the urogenital membrane anteriorly.

**Table 1-1** Timetable of Events in the Development of the Lower Urinary Tract

| Time after fertilization | Event |
|---|---|
| 15 days | Ingrowth of intraembryonic mesoderm |
| 16-17 days | Allantois appears |
| 17 days | Cloacal plate forms |
| 28-38 days | Partitioning of cloaca by urorectal septum |
| 28 days | Mesonephric duct reaches cloaca; ureteric bud appears |
| 30-37 days | Ureteric bud initiates formation of metanephros (permanent kidney) |
| 41 days | Lumen of urethra is discrete; genital tubercles prominent |
| 42-44 days | Urogenital sinus separates from rectum; mesonephric ducts and ureters drain separately into urogenital sinus, defining boundaries of trigone |
| 51-52 days | Kidneys in lumbar region; glomeruli appear in kidney |
| 9 weeks | First likelihood of renal function |
| 12 weeks | External genitalia become distinctive for sex |
| 13 weeks | Bladder becomes muscularized |
| 20-40 weeks | Further growth and development complete the urogenital organs |

The anal membrane is then surrounded by mesenchymal swellings, and in the ninth week it is found at the bottom of an ectodermal depression, known as the anal pit. The surrounding swellings are the anal folds. Soon thereafter the anal membrane ruptures and an open pathway is formed between the rectum and the outside, which at this stage of development is the amniotic cavity. The upper part of the anal canal is thus endodermal in origin; the lower third of the anal canal is ectodermal.

The external anal sphincter appears in human embryos at approximately 8 weeks or perhaps 7 weeks. This sphincter, together with the levator ani, is believed to originate from hypaxial myotomes. Although the anal sphincter and levator ani may arise from distinct primordia, their relationship is very close.

### Congenital Malformations of the Hindgut

Imperforate anus is one of the more common abnormalities of the hindgut. In simple cases, the anal canal ends blindly at the anal membrane, which then forms a diaphragm between the endodermal and ectodermal portions of the anal canal. In more severe cases, a thick layer of connective tissue may be found between the terminal end of the rectum and the surface because of either a failure of the anal pit to develop or atresia of the ampullar part of the rectum (rectal atresia). A slight deviation of the urorectal septum in the dorsal direction probably causes many rectal and anal abnormalities.

Rectal fistulas are often observed in association with an imperforate anus and may be found between the rectum and vagina, urinary bladder, or urethra. Fistulas may also open to the surface of the perineal region.

## ANATOMY
### Bladder

The bladder is a hollow, muscular organ that is the reservoir for the urinary system. The bladder is flat when empty and globular when distended. The superior surface and upper 1 or 2 cm of the posterior aspect of the bladder are covered by peritoneum, which sweeps off the bladder into the vesicouterine pouch. The anterior bladder is extraperitoneal and adjacent to the retropubic space. Between the bladder and pubic bones lie adipose tissue, pubovesical ligaments and muscle, and a prominent venous plexus. Inferiorly, the bladder rests on the anterior vagina and lower uterine segment, separated by an envelope of adventitia (endopelvic fascia).

The epithelium lining the bladder lumen is loosely attached to the underlying musculature, except at the trigone, where it is firmly adherent. The bladder lining consists of transitional epithelium (urothelium) supported by a layer of loose connective tissue, the lamina propria. The internal surface of the bladder has a rugose appearance formed by mucosal folds in the contracted state. In the distended state, a variably prominent meshlike appearance is formed by mucosa-covered detrusor musculature.

The bladder wall musculature is often described as having three layers: inner longitudinal, middle circular, and outer longitudinal. However, this layering occurs only at the bladder neck; the remainder of the bladder musculature is composed of fibers that run in many directions, both within and between layers. This plexiform arrangement of detrusor muscle bundles is ideally suited to reduce all dimensions of the bladder lumen on contraction.

The inner longitudinal layer has widely separated muscle fibers that course multidirectionally. Near the bladder neck, these muscle fibers assume a longitudinal pattern that is contiguous through the trigone and, according to Tanagho (1986), into the inner longitudinal muscular layer of the urethra. The middle circular layer is prominent at the bladder neck, where it fuses with the deep trigonal muscle, forming a muscular ring. This layer does not continue into the urethra. The outer longitudinal layer forms a sheet of muscle bundles around the bladder wall above the level of the bladder neck. Anteriorly, these fibers continue past the

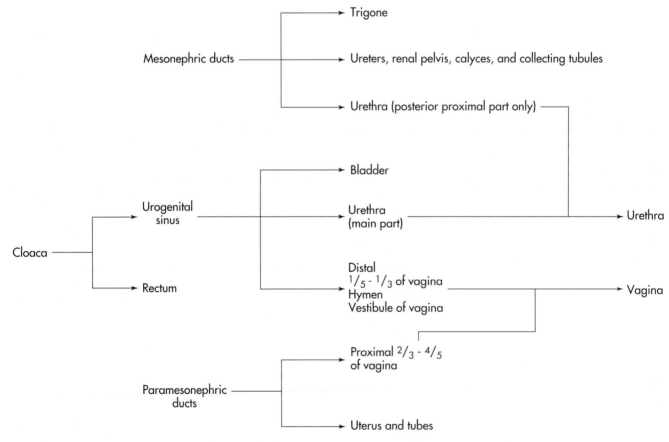

**Fig. 1-4** Schematic representation of the embryologic contributions of various structures of the female urogenital system.

vesical neck as the pubovesical muscles and insert into tissues on the posterior surface of the pubic symphysis. The pubovesical muscles may facilitate bladder neck opening during voiding. Posteriorly, the longitudinal fibers fuse with the deep surface of the trigonal apex and communicate with several detrusor muscle loops at the bladder base; these loops probably aid in bladder neck closure.

## Trigone

In the bladder base is a triangular area, the trigone. The trigone has a flattened appearance with a smooth mucosal covering. The corners of the trigone are formed by three orifices: the paired ureteral orifices and the internal urethral orifice. The superior boundary of the trigone is a slightly raised area between the two ureteric orifices, called the interureteric ridge. The two ureteral openings are slitlike and, in an undistended organ, lie about 3 cm apart.

The trigone has two muscular layers: superficial and deep. The superficial layer is directly continuous with longitudinal fibers of the distal ureter, and is also continuous posteriorly with smooth muscle of the proximal urethra. The deep muscular layer of the trigone forms a dense, compact layer that fuses somewhat with detrusor muscle fibers. The deep layer is in direct communication with a fibromuscular sheath, Waldeyer's sheath, in the intravesical portion of the ureter (Fig. 1-5). The deep trigonal muscle has autonomic innervation identical to that of the detrusor, being rich in cholinergic (parasympathetic) nerves and sparse in noradrenergic (sympathetic) nerves. In contrast, the superficial

**Table 1-2**  Selected Congenital Anomalies of the Urinary Tract and Their Embryologic Causes

| Condition | Embryologic cause |
| --- | --- |
| Renal agenesis | Early degeneration of the ureteric bud |
| Pelvic kidney | Failure of kidney to ascend to the lumbar region |
| Horseshoe kidney | Fusion of lower poles of both kidneys; ascent to lumbar region prevented by root of inferior mesenteric artery |
| Urachal fistula, cyst, sinus | Variable persistence of the intraembryonic portion of allantois, from bladder to umbilicus |
| Double ureter | Early splitting of the ureteric bud |
| Ectopic ureter | Two ureteric buds develop from one mesonephric duct. One bud is in normal position; the abnormal bud moves downward with the mesonephric duct to enter into the urethra, vagina, vestibule, or uterus |
| Bladder exstrophy | Failure of the ventral wall of the urogenital sinus to increase to accommodate positional changes, followed by breakdown of the urogenital membrane |

trigonal muscle has few cholinergic nerves, but a greater number of noradrenergic nerves.

## Pelvic Ureter

As it courses retroperitoneally from the renal pelvis to the bladder, the ureter is divided anatomically into abdominal and pelvic segments, which are approximately equal in length, 12 to 15 cm each. The ureter enters the pelvis by crossing over the iliac vessels where the common iliac artery divides into the external iliac and hypogastric vessels. At this point, the ureter lies medial to the branches of the anterior division of the hypogastric artery and lateral to the peritoneum of the cul-de-sac. It is attached to the peritoneum of the lateral pelvic wall. As it proceeds more distally, the ureter courses along the lateral side of the uterosacral ligament and enters the endopelvic fascia of the parametrium (cardinal ligament). The ureter passes beneath the uterine artery approximately 1.5 cm lateral to the cervix. The distal ureter then moves medially over the lateral vaginal fornix to enter the trigone of the bladder.

The ureter has only one muscular coat that forms an irregular, helical pattern of muscle bundles with fibers oriented in almost every direction. As the ureter approaches and enters the bladder wall, its helical fibers elongate and become parallel to its lumen. The intravesical ureter is about 1.5 cm long and is divided into an intramural segment, totally surrounded by the bladder wall, and a submucosal segment directly under the bladder mucosa. The longitudinal muscle fibers of the distal ureter proceed uninterrupted into the superficial trigonal muscle.

The distal and intramural segments of the ureter are surrounded by Waldeyer's sheath. Waldeyer's sheath fuses proximally with the intrinsic musculature of the ureter and distally acts as an added fixation, linking the ureter proper to the detrusor muscle (see Fig. 1-5). Waldeyer's sheath has been described thoroughly by Tanagho (1986) and Woodburne (1968).

## Urethra

The female urethra is about 4 cm long and averages 6 mm in diameter. Its lumen is slightly curved as it passes from the retropubic space, perforates the perineal membrane, and ends with its external orifice in the vestibule directly above the vaginal opening. Throughout its length, the urethra is embedded in the adventitia of the anterior vagina.

The urethral epithelium has longitudinal folds and many small glands, which open into the urethra throughout its entire length. The epithelium is continuous externally with that of the vulva and internally with that of the bladder. It is primarily stratified squamous epithelium that becomes transitional near the bladder.

The epithelium is supported by a layer of loose fibro-elastic connective tissue, the lamina propria. The lamina propria contains many bundles of collagen fibrils and

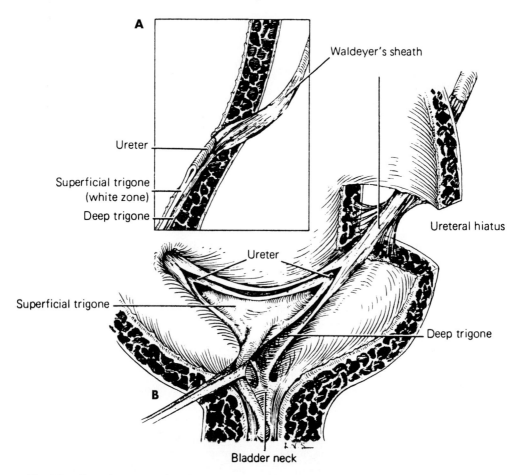

**Fig. 1-5** Normal ureterovesicotrigonal complex. **A,** Side view with Waldeyer's muscular sheath surrounding vestige of the intravesical ureter and continuing downward as the deep trigone, which extends to the bladder neck. The ureteral musculature becomes the superficial trigone, which extends to just short of the external meatus in the female. **B,** Waldeyer's sheath connected by a few fibers to the detrusor muscle in the ureteral hiatus. This muscular sheath inferior to the ureteral orifice becomes the deep trigone. The musculature of the ureters continues downward as the superficial trigone.

From Tanagho EA: Anatomy of the lower urinary tract. In Walsh PC, Gittes RF, Perlmutter AD, Stamey TA, eds: *Campbell's urology,* ed 5, Philadelphia, 1986, WB Saunders.

fibrocytes, as well as an abundance of elastic fibers oriented both longitudinally and circularly around the urethra. Numerous thin-walled veins are another characteristic feature. This rich vascular supply contributes to urethral resistance.

## Urethral Musculature

The urethral smooth muscle is composed primarily of oblique and longitudinal muscle fibers, with a few circularly oriented outer fibers. This muscle and the detrusor muscle in the bladder base form what can be called the intrinsic urethral sphincter mechanism. This smooth muscle is usually noted to be under both alpha-adrenergic and cholinergic control, although Gosling et al. (1981) found an extensive cholinergic nerve supply with few noradrenergic nerves. The longitudinally directed muscles probably shorten and widen the urethral lumen during micturition, whereas the circular smooth muscle (along with the striated urogenital sphincter muscle) contributes to urethral resistance to outflow at rest.

The striated urethral and periurethral muscles form the extrinsic urethral sphincter mechanism. It has two components: an inner portion, which lies within and adjacent to the urethral wall, and an outer portion, composed of skeletal muscle fibers of the pelvic diaphragm. The inner portion is made up of the sphincter urethrae, a striated band of muscle that surrounds the proximal two thirds of the urethra, and the compressor urethrae and urethrovaginal sphincter (known together formerly as the deep transverse perineus muscle), which consist of two straplike bands of striated muscle that arch over the ventral surface of the distal one third of the urethra (Fig. 1-6, *inset*). These three muscles, which

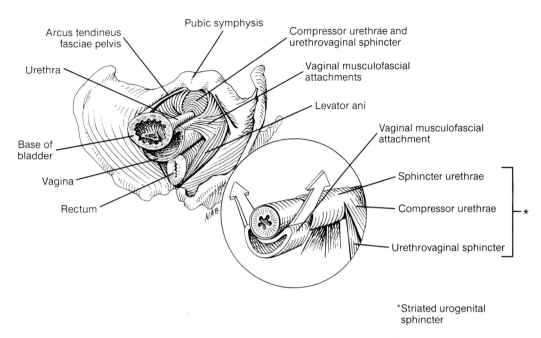

**Fig. 1-6** Diagrammatic representation showing the component parts of the urethral support and sphincteric mechanisms. Note that the proximal urethra and bladder neck are supported by the anterior vaginal wall and its musculofascial attachments to the pelvic diaphragm. *Inset,* Contraction of the levator ani muscles elevates the anterior vagina and overlying bladder neck and proximal urethra, contributing to bladder neck closure. The sphincter urethrae, urethrovaginal sphincter, and compressor urethrae are all parts of the striated urogenital sphincter.

function as a single unit, have been called by Oelrich (1983) the striated urogenital sphincter. It is composed primarily of small-diameter, slow-twitch muscle, making it ideally suited to exert tone on the urethral lumen over prolonged time periods. These muscles may also contribute (along with the levator ani) to voluntary interruption of the urine stream and to urethral closure with stress, via reflex muscle contraction.

## Urethral Support

Traditionally, support of the urethra and bladder neck was thought to be provided by the interaction of the pubourethral ligaments, the urogenital diaphragm, and the muscles of the pelvic diaphragm. Numerous investigators have described the so-called pubourethral ligaments as extending from the inferior surface of the pubic bones to the urethra. Milley and Nichols (1971) found bilaterally symmetric anterior, posterior, and intermediate pubourethral ligaments and stated that the anterior and posterior ligaments were formed, respectively, by inferior and superior fascial layers of the urogenital diaphragm. An anatomic defect of the pubourethral ligaments has been cited as a contributing factor to urinary stress incontinence in women.

Studies by DeLancey (1986, 1988, 1989, 1991) provide a more complete view of urethral support. Rather than being suspended ventrally by ligamentous structures, the proximal urethra and bladder base are supported in a slinglike fashion by the anterior vaginal wall, which is attached bilaterally to the muscles of the pelvic diaphragm (levator ani muscles) at the arcus tendineus fasciae pelvis. Similar anatomic connections between the pelvic diaphragm and vagina have been described by Olesen and Grau (1976) and others. These attachments extend caudally and blend with the superior fibers of the perineal membrane (urogenital diaphragm). The tissues, described as pubourethral ligaments, are made up of the perineal membrane and the most caudal portion of the arcus tendineus fasciae pelvis, which fix the distal urethra beneath the pubic bone. Fig. 1-6 illustrates the anatomic structures that contribute to urethral support and closure.

Anterior vaginal attachment to the pelvic diaphragm may contribute to urethral closure by providing a stable base onto which the bladder neck and proximal urethra are compressed with increases in intraabdominal pressure. These attachments also are responsible for the posterior movement of the vesical neck seen at the onset of micturition (when the pelvic floor relaxes) and for the elevation noted when a patient is instructed to arrest her urinary stream (see Fig. 1-6, *inset*). Defects in these attachments probably result in proximal urethral support defects (urethral hypermobility) and anterior vaginal prolapse (cystocele), conditions associated with stress urinary incontinence. These defects also correspond to the paravaginal fascial defects, with detachment of the vagina from its lateral connective tissue supports, described by Richardson et al. (1976).

## Vagina

The vagina is a hollow, fibromuscular tube with rugal folds that extends from the vestibule to the uterine cervix. The vagina is lined by nonkeratinizing stratified squamous epithelium that lies over a thin, loose layer of connective tissue, the lamina propria. Beneath this is the vaginal muscularis, a well-developed fibromuscular layer consisting primarily of smooth muscle with smaller amounts of collagen and elastin. Surgical terms such as *pubocervical* and *rectovaginal fascia* refer to layers that are developed as a result of separating the vaginal epithelium from the muscularis, or by splitting the vaginal muscularis layer. The muscularis is surrounded by an adventitial layer, which is a variably discrete layer of collagen, elastin, and adipose tissue containing blood vessels, lymphatics, and nerves. The adventitia represents an extension of the visceral endopelvic fascia that surrounds the vagina and adjacent pelvic organs and allows for their independent expansion and contraction.

The walls of the vagina are in contact except where its lumen is held open by the cervix. The vagina has an H-shaped lumen, with the principal dimension being transverse. As described earlier, the lateral aspects of the anterior vagina are attached on each side by fibrous connections to the levator ani muscles at the white line or arcus tendineus fasciae pelvis that extends from the pubic symphysis to each ischial spine. In addition, the upper vagina is supported by connective tissue attachments to the sacrum, coccyx, and lateral pelvic sidewalls; these are identified at surgery as the cardinal and uterosacral ligament complex. Anteriorly, the vagina lies adjacent to and supports the bladder base, from which it is separated by the vesicovaginal adventitia (endopelvic fascia). The urethra is fused with the anterior vagina, with no distinct adventitial layer separating them. The terminal portions of the ureters cross the lateral fornices of the vagina on their way to the bladder base. Posteriorly, the vagina is related to the cul-de-sac, to the rectal ampulla, and, inferiorly, to the perineal body. The rectovaginal septum is an additional layer, embryologically an extension and fusion of peritoneum from the cul-de-sac, that is attached to the posterior surface of the vaginal muscularis. A layer of adventitia separates the muscular layer of the rectum from the rectovaginal septum, except at the level of the perineal body, where there is fusion of the vaginal muscularis and connective tissue of the perineal body.

## PELVIC ORGAN SUPPORT
### Pelvic Floor

With the change from plantigrade to erect posture, the pelvis and vertebral column of humans underwent various evolutionary changes that restored balance between in-

traabdominal pressure and visceral support. The lumbosacral curve, a specific human characteristic, directs abdominal pressure forward onto the abdominal wall and nearly horizontal, flattened pubic bones. Downward pressure is directed backward onto the sacrum and the rearranged levator ani muscles, which now fill in the pelvic cavity.

The pelvic floor is made up of muscular and fascial structures that enclose the abdominal-pelvic cavity, the external vaginal opening (for intercourse and parturition), and the urethra and rectum (for elimination). The muscular components are discussed in more detail later in this chapter. The fascial components consist of two types of fascia: parietal and visceral (endopelvic). Parietal fascia covers the pelvic skeletal muscles and provides attachment of muscles to the bony pelvis; it is characterized histologically by regular arrangements of collagen. Visceral fascia is less discrete and exists throughout the pelvis as a meshwork of loosely arranged collagen, elastin, and adipose tissue through which the blood vessels, lymphatics, and nerves travel to reach the pelvic organs. By surgical convention, the visceral endopelvic fascia of the pelvis has been described as discrete "ligaments" such as the cardinal or uterosacral ligaments.

## Pelvic Diaphragm

The pelvic diaphragm collectively consists of the levator ani muscle and associated connective tissue attachments to the pelvis. The diaphragm is stretched hammocklike between the pubis in front and the coccyx behind, and is attached along the lateral pelvic walls to a thickened band in the obturator fascia, the arcus tendineus levator ani (Fig. 1-7). The levator ani functions as a unit but is described in two main parts: the diaphragmatic part (coccygeus and iliococcygeus muscles) and the pubovisceral part (pubococcygeus and puborectalis). The coccygeus muscles are paired and run from the lateral borders of the coccyx and sacrum to the ischial spines on each side, with the sacrospinous ligaments forming the tendinous components. The iliococcygeus muscle arises from the lateral pubic symphyses, travels over the pelvic sidewall (obturator internus muscle) attached to the arcus tendineus levator ani laterally, and meets in the midline at the anococcygeal raphe and the coccyx to form the levator plate. The pubovisceral portion of the levator ani arises from the inner surface of the pubic bones and passes backward to insert into the anococcygeal raphe and the superior surface of the coccyx. The levator crura are formed by the pubococcygeus and puborectalis muscles, which have attachments to the lateral aspects of the vagina and rectum. The puborectalis forms a sling behind the rectum and contributes to anal continence. The space between the levator crura through which the rectum, vagina, and urethra pass is called the genital hiatus.

The levator ani exhibits constant baseline tone and can

also be voluntarily contracted. The muscle contains both type I (slow-twitch) fibers to maintain constant tone, and type II (fast-twitch) fibers to provide reflex and voluntary contractions. Innervation is provided primarily through the anterior sacral nerve roots of S2, S3, and S4; additional innervation may be provided to the pubovisceral components through branches of the pudendal nerve, although this is controversial.

## Perineal Membrane

The perineal membrane is a triangular sheet of dense fibromuscular tissue that spans the anterior half of the pelvic outlet. It had previously been called the urogenital diaphragm and, according to DeLancey (1988), this change in name reflects the appreciation that it is not a two-layered structure with muscle in between, as had been thought. The vagina and urethra pass through the perineal membrane and are supported by it. Cephalad to the perineal membrane lies the striated urogenital sphincter muscle, which, as already mentioned, compresses the distal urethra.

## Mechanisms of Normal Support of Uterus and Vagina

Normal pelvic support is provided by interaction between the pelvic muscles (levator ani group) and connective tissue attachments. Under most conditions, the pelvic muscles are the primary support for the pelvic organs, providing a firm yet elastic base on which they rest. The connective tissue attachments stabilize the pelvic organs in the correct position to receive optimal support from the pelvic muscles. When the pelvic muscles are relaxed, as during micturition

or defecation, the connective tissue attachments temporarily hold up the pelvic organs.

When the vagina is normally supported, it provides support to the bladder and urethra, cervix, and rectum. Other than the cervix, the uterus does not have fixed supports, as indicated by its ability to enlarge without restriction during pregnancy. The upper two thirds of the vagina is in a nearly horizontal orientation in a standing woman. Connective tissue attachments stabilize the vagina at different levels, as described by DeLancey (1992) and others (Fig. 1-8). The superior and lateral connective tissue attachments (cardinal-uterosacral ligament complex, or level I) uphold the cervix and upper vagina over the levator plate and away from the genital hiatus. The mid-vagina is supported by lateral connections to the white line or arcus tendineus fasciae pelvis (level II). The lower vagina is supported predominantly by connections to the perineal membrane anteriorly and the perineal body posteriorly (level III).

## RECTUM AND ANAL SPHINCTERS

The rectum extends from its junction with the sigmoid colon to the anal orifice. The distribution of smooth muscle is typical for the intestinal tract, with inner circular and outer longitudinal layers of muscle. At the perineal flexure of the rectum, the inner circular layer increases in thickness to form the internal anal sphincter. The internal anal sphincter is under autonomic control (sympathetic and parasympathetic) and is responsible for 85% of the resting anal pressure. The outer longitudinal layer of smooth muscle becomes concentrated on the anterior and posterior walls of

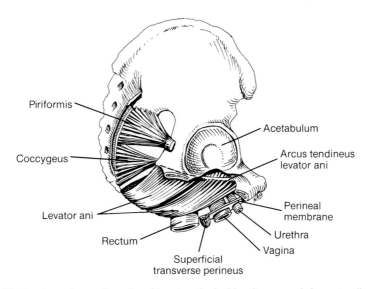

**Fig. 1-7** The levator ani, seen from the side when the ischium is removed. Arcus tendineus levator ani runs from the ischial spine to the pubic bone. Note the perineal membrane that supports distal portions of the urethra and vagina.

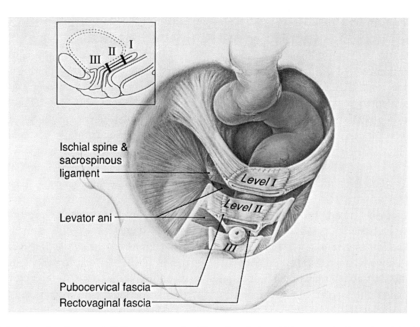

**Fig. 1-8** Levels of support of the upper and mid-vagina. In level I (suspension), endopelvic fascia suspends vagina from lateral pelvic walls. Fibers of level I extend both vertically and posteriorly toward sacrum. In level II (attachment), vagina is attached to arcus tendineus fasciae pelvis and superior fascia of levator ani muscles.

From DeLancey JOL: *Am J Obstet Gynecol* 166:1717, 1992.

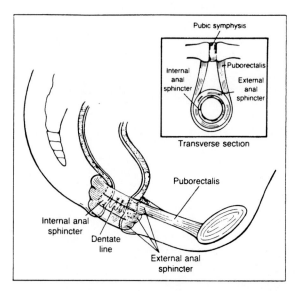

**Fig. 1-9** Diagram of the rectum, anal canal, and surrounding muscles. The puborectalis muscle forms a sling posteriorly around the anorectal junction. The external anal sphincter (skeletal muscle) surrounds the anal canal and is closely associated with the puborectalis muscle. The internal anal sphincter muscle (smooth muscle) lies within the ring of the external sphincter muscle and is a continuation of the inner circular layer of the smooth muscle of the rectal wall.

From Madoff RD, Williams JG, Caushaj PF: *N Engl J Med* 326:1003, 1992.

the rectum, with connections to the perineal body and coccyx, and then passes inferiorly on both sides of the external anal sphincter.

The external anal sphincter is composed of striated muscle that is tonically contracted most of the time and can also be voluntarily contracted. Various divisions of the external anal sphincter have been described, and although there is no consensus, recent descriptions favor superficial (combining the previous superficial and subcutaneous components) and deep compartments. The external anal sphincter functions as a unit with the puborectalis portion of the levator ani muscle group.

The anal sphincter mechanism comprises the internal anal sphincter, the external anal sphincter, and the puborectalis muscle (Fig. 1-9). As with the bladder neck and urethra, a spinal reflex causes the striated sphincter to contract during sudden increases in intraabdominal pressure, such as coughing. The anal-rectal angle is produced by the anterior pull of the puborectalis muscles. These muscles form a sling posteriorly around the anorectal junction. The anal-rectal angle was previously thought to be important in maintaining fecal continence, but its importance has been questioned. More recent studies suggest that fecal incontinence in women is often related to denervation of the muscles of the pelvic diaphragm, as well as to disruption and denervation of the external anal sphincter. This theory is discussed in Chapter 12.

# BIBLIOGRAPHY
## Embryology

Gosling JA: Anatomy. In Stanton SL, ed: *Clinical gynecologic urology,* St Louis, 1984, Mosby.

Gosling JA, Dixon J, Humpherson JR: *Functional anatomy of the urinary tract,* London, 1982, Gower.

Hilton P: The mechanism of continence. In Stanton SL, Tanagho EA, eds: *Surgery of female incontinence,* ed 2, New York, 1986, Springer-Verlag.

Langman J: *Medical embryology,* Baltimore, 1976, Williams & Wilkins.

Maizels M: Normal development of the urinary tract. In Walsh PC, Gittes RF, Perlmutter AD, Stamey TA, eds: *Campbell's urology,* ed 5, Philadelphia, 1986, WB Saunders.

Muckle CW: Developmental abnormalities of the female reproductive organs. In Sciarra JJ, ed: *Gynecology and obstetrics,* vol 1, Hagerstown, Md, 1981, Harper & Row.

Snyder HM: Anomalies of the ureter. In Gillenwater JY, Grayhack JT, Howards SS, Duckett JW, eds: *Adult and pediatric urology,* vol 2, Chicago, 1987, Mosby.

## Anatomy

Aronson MP, Lee RA, Berquist TH: Anatomy of anal sphincters and related structures in continent women studied with magnetic resonance imaging, *Obstet Gynecol* 76:846, 1990.

Curtis AH, Anson BJ, Ashley FL: Further studies in gynecological anatomy and related clinical problems, *Surg Gynecol Obstet* 74:709, 1942.

Curtis AH, Anson BJ, McVay CB: The anatomy of the pelvic and urogenital diaphragms, in relation to urethrocele and cystocele, *Surg Gynecol Obstet* 68:161, 1939.

Dalley AF: The riddle of the sphincters: the morphophysiology of the anorectal mechanism reviewed, *Am Surgeon* 53:298, 1987.

DeLancey JOL: Correlative study of paraurethral anatomy, *Obstet Gynecol* 68:91, 1986.

DeLancey JOL: Structural aspects of the extrinsic continence mechanism, *Obstet Gynecol* 72:296, 1988.

DeLancey JOL: Pubovesical ligament: a separate structure from the urethral supports ("pubo-urethral ligaments"), *Neurourol Urodyn* 8:53, 1989.

DeLancey JOL: Anatomy of the female bladder and urethra. In Ostergard DR, Bent AE, eds: *Urogynecology and urodynamics,* ed 3, Baltimore, 1991, Williams & Wilkins.

DeLancey JOL: Anatomic aspects of vaginal eversion after hysterectomy, *Am J Obstet Gynecol* 166:1717, 1992.

DeLancey JOL: Anatomy of the pelvis. In Thompson JD, Rock JA, eds: *Telinde's operative gynecology,* ed 7, Philadelphia, 1992, JB Lippincott.

DeLancey JOL, Starr RA: Histology of the connection between the vagina and levator ani muscles, *J Reprod Med* 35:765, 1990.

Dickinson RL: Studies of the levator ani muscle, *Am J Obstet Dis Women Child* 22:897, 1889.

Elbadawi A: Neuromorphologic basis of vesicourethral function: I. Histochemistry, ultrastructure and function of the intrinsic nerves of the bladder and urethra, *Neurourol Urodyn* 1:3, 1982.

Funt MI, Thompson JD, Birch H: Normal vaginal axis, *South Med J* 71:1534, 1978.

Gosling JA: The structure of the female lower urinary tract and pelvic floor, *Urol Clin North Am* 12:207, 1985.

Gosling JA, Dixon JS, Critchley HO, et al: A comparative study of the human external sphincter and periurethral levator ani muscles, *Br J Urol* 53:35, 1981.

Gosling JA, Dixon JS, Humpherson JR: *Functional anatomy of the urinary tract: an integrated text and color atlas,* Baltimore, 1982, University Park Press.

Halban J, Tandler J: Anatomie und Atiologie der Genital-prolapse (Translated by Porges RF, Porges JC: The anatomy and etiology of genital prolapse in women), *Obstet Gynecol* 15:790, 1960.

Krantz KE: The anatomy of the urethra and anterior vaginal wall, *Am J Obstet Gynecol* 62:374, 1951.

Lawson JO: Pelvic anatomy. I. Pelvic floor muscles, *Ann R Coll Surg Engl* 52:244, 1974.

Lund CJ, Fullerton RE, Tristan TA: Cinefluorographic studies of the bladder and urethra in women, *Am J Obstet Gynecol* 78:706, 1959.

Madoff RD, Williams JG, Caushaj PF: Fecal incontinence, *N Engl J Med* 326:1003, 1992.

McGuire EJ: The innervation and function of the lower urinary tract, *J Neurosurg* 65:278, 1986.

Mengert WF: Mechanics of uterine support and position, *Am J Obstet Gynecol* 31:775, 1936.

Milley PS, Nichols DH: The relationship between the pubo-urethral ligaments and the urogenital diaphragm in the human female, *Anat Rec* 170:281, 1971.

Muellner SR: The physiology of micturition, *J Urol* 65:805, 1951.

Nichols DH, Randall CL: *Vaginal surgery,* ed 3, Baltimore, 1989, Williams & Wilkins.

Oelrich TM: The striated urogenital sphincter muscle in the female, *Anat Rec* 205:223, 1983.

Olesen KP, Grau V: The suspensory apparatus of the female bladder neck, *Urol Int* 31:33, 1976.

Redman JF: Anatomy of the genitourinary system. In Gillenwater JY, Grayhack JT, Howards SS, Duckett JW, eds: *Adult and pediatric urology,* vol 1, Chicago, 1987, Mosby.

Richardson AC, Lyon JB, Williams NL: A new look at pelvic relaxation, *Am J Obstet Gynecol* 126:568, 1976.

Tanagho EA: Anatomy of the lower urinary tract. In Walsh PC, Gittes RF, Perlmutter AD, Stamey TA, eds: *Campbell's urology,* ed 5, Philadelphia, 1986, WB Saunders.

Wood BA, Kelly AJ: Anatomy of the anal sphincters and pelvic floor. In Henry MM, Swash M, eds: *Coloproctology and the pelvic floor,* ed 5, Oxford, 1992, Butterworth-Heinemann.

Woodburne RT: Anatomy of the bladder and bladder outlet, *J Urol* 100:474, 1968.

Woodburne RT: *Essentials of human anatomy,* ed 5, New York, 1976, Oxford University Press.

Zacharin RF: The suspensory mechanism of the female urethra, *J Anat* 97:423, 1963.

Zacharin RF: *Pelvic floor anatomy and the surgery of pulsion enterocoele,* New York, 1985, Springer-Verlag.

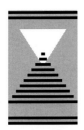

CHAPTER **2**
# Neurophysiology of the Lower Urinary Tract

J. Thomas Benson and Mark D. Walters

---

The two functions of the lower urinary tract are the storage of urine within the bladder and the timely expulsion of urine from the urethra. The precise neurologic pathways and neurophysiologic mechanisms that control micturition are complex and not completely understood. The storage and expulsion of urine are part of a complex neurophysiologic function that involves autonomic and somatic nervous systems. Function is controlled by reflex pathways, which are further modulated by central voluntary control. Precise knowledge of neuroanatomy, neurophysiology, and pharmacology is important to understand and treat many diseases of the lower urinary tract. This chapter reviews normal function and neurologic control of the lower urinary tract in women.

## GENERAL NERVOUS SYSTEM ARRANGEMENTS

The nervous system is arranged into the central and the peripheral systems. The central nervous system includes the brain and spinal cord. Twelve paired cranial and 31 paired spinal nerves with their ganglia compose the peripheral nervous system. The somatic component of the peripheral system innervates skeletal muscle, and the autonomic division innervates cardiac muscle, smooth muscle, and glands.

### Central Nervous System

Within the brain and cord, nerve cell bodies are arranged in groups of various sizes and shapes called nuclei. Fibers with a common origin and destination are called a tract; some are so anatomically distinct that they are called fasciculus, brachium, peduncle, column, or lemniscus.

Older methods of tracing the nervous system pathways consisted of inducing cell degeneration and applying appropriate stains to identify the degenerated fibers. Newer methods that do not require nerve tissue destruction and that use chemical tracers have been available since the 1970s. Such tracers as carbon-14–labeled proline move from the cell bodies to the axon terminals (orthograde) and are identified autoradiographically. Retrograde tracers, such as horseradish peroxidase, move from axon terminals to cell bodies and are identified by light and electron microscopy.

Nerve cell bodies originating high in the central nervous system send axons to the motor nuclei in the brain stem and spinal cord to exert control over the cranial and spinal nerves. The control may be positive or inhibiting, but lesions of these tracts (upper motor neuron lesions) lead to opposite-body hyperreflexia and spastic weakness caused by a net reduction of inhibiting influences.

### Peripheral Nervous System

Both somatic reflex pathways and autonomic pathways compose the peripheral nervous system, particularly as it applies to the lower urinary tract. The spinal nerve, then, has functional components dealing with somatic and visceral afferent and efferent fibers.

#### Somatic Reflex Pathway

A segmental skeletal muscle reflex consists of nerves that activate large extrafusal muscle fibers. They are affected by regulatory afferent nerves from the muscle spindles, acting through intermediate neurons. However, the urethral skeletal muscle has no spindles, so afferent regulatory activity is generated in some as yet undefined way.

Supraspinal afferent fibers similarly affect alpha-motor neurons. Alpha-motor neurons also innervate interneurons

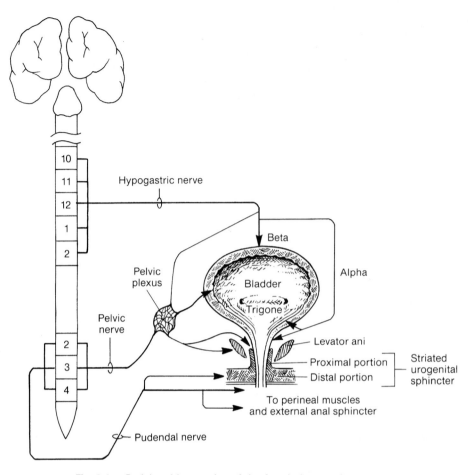

**Fig. 2-1**   Peripheral innervation of the female lower urinary tract.

in the ventral horn (Renshaw cells), which act to inhibit other alpha-motor neurons, a negative feedback response allowing more rapid firing.

Typically, motor neuron size correlates with muscle fiber type. Smaller motor neurons innervate smaller units to activate slower, less fatigable muscle fibers used for tonicity, whereas larger motor neurons activate the fast-twitch muscle fibers.

### Autonomic Pathways

The autonomic nervous system consists of general visceral efferent and general visceral afferent fibers, which ordinarily function at a subconscious level. Unlike the somatic motor system, the peripheral fibers reach the effector organ by a two-neuron chain. The preganglionic neuron arises in the intermediolateral cell column of the brain stem or spinal cord and terminates at an outlying ganglion, where the postganglionic neuron continues the impulse transmission to the end organ. Fibers arising from the intermediolateral gray column of the 12 thoracic and first two lumbar segments of the spinal cord constitute the sympathetic division of the autonomic nervous system. The parasympathetic division consists of fibers arising from the second through the fourth sacral segments and from cranial outflows.

Sympathetic nerves to the pelvic cavity originate in cord levels T5 to L2. Some preganglionic axons pass via white rami communicantes to the paravertebral sympathetic chain, synapse, and pass by gray rami communicantes to the skeletal nerves. Other preganglionic sympathetic axons pass to ganglia located at roots of arteries for which they are named (for example, lumbar splanchnic nerves terminate in inferior mesenteric and hypogastric ganglia). Postganglionic fibers from these ganglia follow the visceral arteries to the organs of the lower abdomen and pelvis. Pelvic parasympathetic system preganglionic fibers originate in spinal segments S2 through S4 and extend to ganglia located within or very near the organs they supply, thus having very short postganglionic fibers.

## NEURAL CONTROL OF THE LOWER URINARY TRACT

The urinary tract is controlled principally by local innervation acting under central nervous system modulation. Local innervation is chiefly by parasympathetic and sympathetic autonomic and peripheral somatic motor and sensory systems. A summary of the neural pathways involved in micturition is shown in Figs. 2-1 and 2-2.

FILLING/STORAGE

Inhibition of
parasympathetics

Stimulation of
sympathetics:
alpha-contraction
beta-relaxation

Stimulation of
somatic nerves to
striated urogenital
sphincter

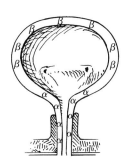

VOIDING

Stimulation of
parasympathetics

Inhibition of
sympathetics

Inhibition of
somatic nerves to
striated urogenital
sphincter

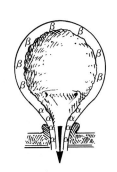

**Fig. 2-2**   Actions of the autonomic and somatic nervous systems during bladder filling/storage and voiding.

## Autonomic Nervous System

The autonomic nervous system controls the lower urinary tract by its actions on the ganglia, detrusor muscle, and smooth muscle of the trigone and urethra.

### Ganglia

Sympathetic preganglionic fibers from thoracolumbar spinal segments form white rami communicantes to corresponding chain ganglia. Postganglionic neurons reach inferior mesenteric ganglia by the lumbar splanchnic nerves and continue through the *hypogastric plexus* to the presacral fascia, across the upper posterior lateral pelvic wall, 1 to 2 cm behind and below the ureter. After these neurons join the pelvic nerves, the *pelvic plexus* is formed, running below and medial to the internal iliac vessels overlying the anterior lateral lower rectum near the anorectal junction. The plexus spreads in the lateral wall of the upper one third of the vagina beneath the uterine artery, medial to the ureter and 2 cm inferolateral to the cervix. Within the vesicovaginal space, the plexus supplies the upper vagina, bladder, proximal urethra, and lower ureter.

The parasympathetic preganglionic fibers arise from nerve roots S3 and S4 and occasionally S2. These fibers emerge from the piriformis muscle overlying the sacral foramina and enter the presacral fascia near the ischial spine at the posterior layer of the hypogastric sheath, where they contribute to the already described pelvic plexus. These parasympathetic fibers terminate in pelvic ganglia located within the wall of the bladder, a location quite vulnerable to end-organ disease such as overstretch, infection, or fibrosis.

At the ganglia, excitatory transmission occurs from activation of nicotinic acetylcholine receptors, with some ganglionic cells having secondary muscarinic receptors. Norepinephrine also acts as a neurotransmitter, and alpha-adrenergic receptors, when stimulated, depress pelvic ganglion transmission by suppression of presynaptic cholinergic neurotransmitter release. Neuropeptide agents, especially enkephalin, probably also function at ganglia; precise knowledge of transmission regulation is not available at present.

### Detrusor Innervation

Postganglionic detrusor nerve fibers diverge and store neurotransmitter agents in axonal varicosities called *synaptic vesicles*. The agent is diffused to neuromuscular bundles of 12 to 15 smooth muscle fibers enclosed in a collagen capsule that acts similarly to the tendon insertion of a muscle. Stimulating electrical pulses produce two episodes of depolarization, suggesting the release of two neurotransmitters. The first neurotransmitter is noncholinergic and nonadrenergic, and the second neurotransmitter is acetylcholine. This observation accounts for detrusor atropine resistance. Cholinergic receptors are present more in the body than in the base of the bladder, whereas adrenergic and neuropeptide receptors are more prevalent in the base. Neuropeptide receptors include vasoactive intestinal polypeptide and substance P. Histaminic and purinergic receptors may also be present in detrusor smooth muscle.

### Trigone and Urethra

The trigone is a separate anatomic and embryologic region where muscle fibers have an almost exclusively adrenergic innervation. Norepinephrine transmitter acts on alpha-receptors, which are stimulated by higher dosages and produce smooth muscle contraction, and on beta-receptors, which are stimulated by lower dosages of norepinephrine and produce smooth muscle relaxation (except in cardiac muscle). Beta-receptors are thought to be more prominent in the detrusor body, whereas alpha-receptors occur chiefly in the bladder outlet and urethra. Cholinergic development in the bladder is present at birth, whereas adrenergic development occurs later. Prostaglandins act as intracellular messengers to relax trigonal muscles.

The proximal urethra is rich in alpha-adrenergic receptors. Acetylcholine, substance P, vasoactive intestinal polypeptide, and histamine are all additional potential transmitters in the urethra.

Somatic motor control is affected by segmental innervation to the intraurethral and periurethral skeletal muscle. The exact neuropathways supplying the external urethral sphincter are controversial. The proximal intramural component of the striated urogenital sphincter muscle (sphincter urethrae, rhabdosphincter) is variably innervated by somatic efferent branches of the pelvic nerves, a component of the pelvic plexus. However, the more distal periurethral striated muscles (compressor urethrae and urethrovaginal sphincter) are innervated by the pudendal nerve, as is the skeletal muscle of the external anal sphincter and perineal muscles. The neuronal cell bodies for the sphincter urethrae and for the distal periurethral striated muscles and pelvic floor muscles are located in Onuf's somatic nucleus in the lateral aspect of the anterior horn of the gray matter of the sacral spinal cord from S2 to S4. Embryologic speculation is that pelvic caudal muscles (tail waggers), which compose the levator group in humans, are supplied from the pelvic plexus on the pelvic surface side, whereas the sphincter cloacal derivatives are supplied from the perineal aspect by the pudendal nerve.

The pudendal nerve passes between the coccygeus and piriformis muscles, leaves the pelvis through the greater sciatic foramen, crosses the ischial spine, and reenters the pelvis through the lesser sciatic foramen (see Chapter 12, Fig. 12-5). Here the nerve accompanies the pudendal vessels along the lateral wall of the ischiorectal fossa in a tunnel formed by a splitting of the obturator fascia, Alcock's canal. At the perineal membrane, the nerve divides into the inferior rectal nerve, supplying the external anal sphincter, the perineal nerve, and the dorsal nerve to the clitoris. The perineal nerve splits into a superficial branch to the labia and a deep branch to the periurethral striated muscles. There is considerable variation with the branching of the pudendal nerve.

The sphincter urethrae muscle is an integral part of the urethral wall and is made up of all slow-twitch (type 1) fibers. The periurethral muscles (compressor urethrae and urethrovaginal sphincter) are composed mostly of slow-twitch fibers (type 1) with a variable concentration of fast-twitch (type 2) fibers. These fibers combine to provide constant tonus, with emergency reflex activity mainly in the distal half of the urethra.

The response of segmental spinal reflex leading to pudendal nerve function involves several spinal cord segments. Afferent fibers involved in the reflex have both segmental and supraspinal routing. This dual routing explains the bimodal response of pudendal motor neurons when pudendal sensory nerves are stimulated, and it differs from stimulation of pelvic detrusor afferents.

The neurotransmitter at the periurethral skeletal neuromuscular junction is acetylcholine and receptors are nicotinic type. The intimate adherence of the neuromuscular junction to the striated muscle fibers conveys a resistance to blockade by neuromuscular blocking agents.

## Sensory Innervation

Detrusor proprioceptive endings exist as nerve endings in collagen bundles. They are stimulated by stretch or contraction and are responsible for the feeling of bladder fullness.

Pain and temperature nerve endings are free in bladder mucosa and submucosa. The sensory endings in the detrusor probably contain acetylcholine and substance P.

Two types of bladder sensors have been postulated, the first sensor perhaps being at the trigone, the second being stretch receptors in the bladder body. Loss of the first sensor may lead to urge incontinence because the bladder is ready to contract before sensation is noted. Sensory innervation can follow both the sympathetic and parasympathetic nerves. Urgency is transmitted along parasympathetic pathways.

Urethral sensation is carried principally by the pudendal nerve, although the pelvic nerve also contributes (Fig. 2-3). Urethral smooth muscle sensory innervation, like that of the detrusor, has both a contralateral and an ipsilateral supply.

## Central Nervous System Modulation

The detrusor and the periurethral striated muscle mechanisms have separate cortical and other higher-center regulation. The effects of such regulation are chiefly on the brain stem for the detrusor and on the sacral cord for the periurethral mechanisms.

### Cortical Pathways

Cortical-reticular axons originating from pyramidal detrusor area cells in the supramedial portion of the frontal lobes and in the genu of the corpus callosum traverse the basal ganglia and terminate in the pontomesencephalic reticular formation of the brain stem on detrusor motor nuclei in the nucleus lateralis dorsalis. These detrusor motor nuclei receive suppressive afferents from basal ganglia, coordinating afferents from the cerebellum, and sensory cord afferents

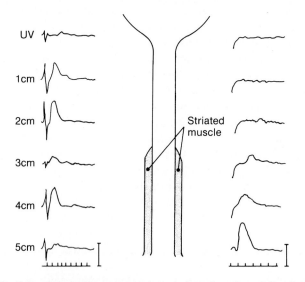

**Fig. 2-3** Longitudinal sensory innervation of urethra. Column on *left* shows responses evoked in the pelvic nerve. Column on *right* shows responses evoked in the pudendal nerve.

From Bradley WE: Physiology of urinary bladder. In Walsh PC, Perlmutter AD, Gittes RF, et al, eds: *Campbell's urology,* ed 5, Philadelphia, 1986, WB Saunders.

from tension receptors in the detrusor muscle, which synapse here to constitute the "long routing" detrusor reflex. Fibers from the raphe nuclei of the reticular formation may moderate responsiveness to different phases of the sleep-wake cycle or emotional states.

Efferents of the brain stem detrusor motor nuclei go to detrusor motor neurons in the intermediolateral cell column from the T10 to L1 and the S2 to S4 segments of the cord. It is speculated that because the detrusor reflex is a brain stem function rather than a spinal function, temporal amplification can occur, allowing for complete bladder emptying.

Pudendal cortical pathways affect periurethral striated muscle innervation by direct descending paths originating in the central vertex of the pudendal cerebral cortical area and going to pudendal nuclei in the ventromedial portion of the ventral gray matter of the S1 to S3 cord segments. At this level, the pudendal motor nuclei act as a segmental skeletal muscle reflex.

Ascending axons from periurethral striated muscle go to the pudendal cortical area, possibly synapsing in the nucleus ventralis posterolateralis of the thalamus, the brain's chief relay station.

Sensory afferents from both pudendal and detrusor pelvic nerves send input to the anterior vermis of the cerebellum, which then originates an axon relay to the cortex in the dentate nucleus. Fibers for both detrusor and pudendal proprioception and exteroception (pain, temperature, and touch) ascend in posterior columns and spinothalamic tracts, respectively.

Neurotransmitters involved in these pathways include acetylcholine and peptides, especially substance P, and enkephalin. Neurotransmitter agents are stored in astrocytes, which may also regulate extracellular concentrations.

### Other Higher Centers

The basal ganglia clearly have an effect on detrusor reflex control, which is probably suppressive. The neurotransmitter dopamine, manufactured in the substantia nigra by enzymatic conversion of catecholamines, is important for the control of somatic movements related to posture. Exhaustion of dopamine from the body is found in the 1 million patients suffering from Parkinson's disease, characterized by slowness of movement, gait disturbance, tremor, and—in 45% to 75%—hyperreflexia of the bladder.

The limbic system in the temporal lobes exerts controls affecting all autonomic functions and is a favored site for epileptiform activity. Enkephalin is a notable neurotransmitter here as well as in the reticular formation.

The hypothalamus function, although poorly delineated, is known to involve beta-endorphin neurotransmitters, the opioid peptides constituting an entire class of brain neurotransmitters.

The cerebellum, where gamma-aminobutyric acid (GABA) is prominent along with standard neurotransmitters, regulates muscle tone and coordinates movement.

Disease in this area produces spontaneous, high-amplitude bladder hyperreflexia.

The brain stem's importance in the lower urinary tract function has been known since 1921, when Barrington ablated this area in cats and produced permanent urinary retention. Brain stem neurotransmitters include substance P, GABA, and serotonin, which is produced from tryptophan.

### Spinal Cord

By adolescence, disparity in growth of the spinal cord and the vertebral column leads to the cord's terminating around the first lumbar vertebra. The adult conus medullaris is quite short and contains the entire S1 to S5 segment. Although the thoracolumbar levels are important in sympathetic autonomic influence of the lower urinary tract, the conus medullaris has greater significance because autonomic detrusor nuclei and pudendal somatic nuclei are housed in the intermediolateral and ventromedial anterior gray matter, respectively. The conus medullaris also houses neurons involved with defecation and sexual function, with relays for cortical separation of these visceral functions (encephalization) developing after birth.

Urine storage and evacuation reflexes actively involve this area of the cord and have been classified by Mahoney et al. (1977) (Table 2-1); however, the reflex pathways are mostly theoretical, few having been demonstrated in humans. In experimental animals, three pathways have been demonstrated. The first, the proximal urethra to the detrusor, facilitates detrusor reflex, which may be important when considering proximal urethral relationships to bladder instability. The second pathway, periurethral striated muscle to the detrusor for detrusor inhibition, is used for biofeedback therapy of unstable bladder conditions. The third pathway is sacral cord afferent fibers to lumbar cord efferent fibers for depression of ganglion transmission.

## MECHANISMS OF NORMAL BLADDER FILLING, STORAGE, AND VOIDING

Our understanding of the neurophysiology of micturition developed from a large body of literature based primarily on animal models. Precise neural pathways involved in voiding remain controversial. The concepts presented here are based primarily on those by Bradley et al. (1974) and DeGroat et al. (1979), as synthesized by Blaivas (1982) and McGuire (1986). Fig. 2-4 is a summary of the major neurologic pathways involved in bladder filling and voiding.

### Filling and Storage

During physiologic bladder filling, little or no increase in intravesical pressure is observed, despite large increases in urine volume. This process, called accommodation, is caused primarily by passive elastic and viscoelastic properties of the smooth muscle and connective tissue of the bladder wall. During filling, muscle bundles in the bladder wall undergo reorganization, and the muscle cells are

**Table 2-1**  Proposed Reflexes That Influence Urine Storage and Evacuation

| Pathway | Result |
| --- | --- |
| **Reflexes Involved in Bladder Storage** | |
| Sympathetic detrusor to detrusor reflex | Inhibits detrusor in response to increased detrusor tension |
| Detrusor-urethral stimulating reflex | Increased detrusor tension stimulates urethral smooth muscle |
| Perineal-detrusor inhibition | Inhibits detrusor in response to perineal sphincter muscles |
| Urethrosphincter guarding | Contracts external striated sphincter in response to trigone tension |
| **Micturition Initiation Reflexes** | |
| Perineodetrusor facilitative | Decreasing pelvic floor muscle tone stimulates detrusor |
| Detrusor-detrusor facilitative | Increased detrusor tension stimulates detrusor |
| **Reflexes to Maintain Micturition** | |
| Detrusor-urethral inhibiting | Detrusor to segmental inhibition of urethral smooth muscle |
| Detrusor-sphincter inhibiting | Detrusor to segmental inhibition of external striated sphincter |
| Urethrodetrusor facilitative | Proximal urethra segmental reflex to stimulated detrusor |
| Urethrobulbar detrusor facilitative | Proximal urethra reflex to stimulate detrusor via brain stem |
| Urethrosphincteric inhibiting | Urethra to external striated sphincter segmental reflex |
| **Micturition Cessation Reflex** | Pelvic floor afferent fibers to brain stem to inhibit detrusor |

From Benson JT: *Obstet Gynecol Clin North Am* 16:733, 1989.

elongated up to four times their length. As bladder filling progresses and at a certain bladder wall tension, a desire to void is felt, although it has not been determined where in the brain this sensation is processed. Mechanoreceptors in the bladder wall are activated, and action potentials run with afferent parasympathetic pelvic nerves to the spinal cord at the level of S2 to S4.

As filling increases to a critical intravesical pressure, or with rapid bladder filling, detrusor muscle contractility is probably inhibited by activation of a spinal sympathetic reflex. The sympathetic efferents that influence micturition arise at the T10 through L2 area and synapse in the inferior mesenteric and pelvic ganglia. This reflex, with sensory afferent activity through the pelvic nerve and efferent activity through the hypogastric nerve, results in inhibition of detrusor contractility and facilitation of bladder relaxation. As noted by McGuire (1986), three sympathetic neural responses to afferent pelvic nerve firing associated with increasing bladder volume have been demonstrated experimentally: beta-receptor-mediated relaxation of the detrusor musculature, alpha-receptor-mediated increase in urethral smooth muscle activity and urethral pressure, and inhibition of ganglionic transmission in the pelvic (vesical) ganglia, which, in effect, inhibits sacral parasympathetic outflow to the bladder. These actions are illustrated in Fig. 2-2.

During bladder filling, outlet resistance increases by reflex stimulation of alpha-adrenergic receptors within the smooth muscle of the bladder neck and proximal urethra. In addition, stimulation of the striated external sphincter occurs, resulting from increased efferent somatic (pelvic and pudendal) nerve activity. As noted earlier, innervation of the proximal intramural portion of the striated urogenital sphincter (sphincter urethrae) is from somatic components of the pelvic nerve, via the pelvic plexus. Innervation of the distal striated urogenital sphincter (compressor urethrae and urethrovaginal sphincter) is via the pudendal nerve. These responses have been shown to both increase intraurethral pressure and inhibit preganglionic detrusor motor neurons in the intermediolateral cell columns of the sacral spinal cord. The mechanisms responsible for switching reflexes from storage to voiding rely on axodendritic contacts between parasympathetic, sympathetic, and somatic pathways in the spinal cord.

## Voiding

Normal voiding is a voluntary act involving reflex-coordinated relaxation of the urethra and sustained contraction of the bladder until emptying is complete. In healthy women, the micturition reflex is probably not a simple segmental sacral reflex, but is modulated supraspinally in the pontine micturition center. Voluntary control of the micturition reflex is mediated by connections between the frontal cerebral cortex and the pons. Voluntary control of the external urethral sphincter is via the corticospinal pathway connecting the frontal cortex with the pudendal nucleus in the ventral horn of the sacral spinal cord. Bradley et al. (1974) believe that connections between the sensorimotor cortex and the pudendal nucleus control voluntary sphincter activity and that voiding is controlled voluntarily by complex interactions among cortical areas (frontal cortex), subcortical areas (thalamus, hypothalamus, basal ganglia, and limbic system), and brain stem (mesencephalic-pontine-medullary reticular formation).

With filling to bladder capacity, stimuli from the bladder cause afferent discharges in the pelvic nerve, which traverse pathways in the spinal cord to synapse in a supraspinal

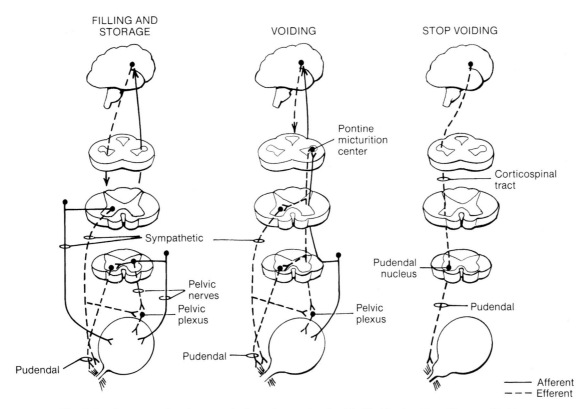

**Fig. 2-4** Summary of major neurologic pathways involved in bladder function. *Storage:* Bladder distention results in afferent pelvic nerve discharge. After synapse in pudendal nucleus, efferent pudendal nerve impulses result in contraction of external urethral sphincter. At same time, afferent sympathetic discharges traverse hypogastric nerve. After synapse in sympathetic nuclei, efferent firing causes (1) inhibition of transmission of postganglionic parasympathetic neuron, which inhibits detrusor contraction, and (2) increased tone at bladder neck. Net effect is that urethral pressure remains greater than detrusor pressure, facilitating urine storage. *Voiding:* Afferent pelvic nerve discharges ascend in spinal cord and synapse in pontine micturition center. Descending afferent pathways cause (1) inhibition of pudendal firing, which relaxes external sphincter, (2) inhibition of sympathetic firing, which opens bladder neck and permits postganglionic parasympathetic transmission, and (3) pelvic parasympathetic firing, which causes detrusor contraction. Net result is that relaxation of external sphincter causes decrease in urethral pressure, followed almost immediately by detrusor contraction, and voiding ensues. *Stop:* Voluntary interruption of urinary stream. Descending corticospinal pathways emanating from motor complex synapse in pudendal nucleus, resulting in contraction of external sphincter. Urethral pressure increases above detrusor pressure, interrupting stream.

Modified from Blaivas JG: *J Urol* 127:958, 1982.

micturition center in the pontine mesencephalic reticular formation. Voiding is initiated voluntarily or when the bladder volume is so large that it is no longer possible to suppress micturition. To initiate voiding, the external urethral sphincter relaxes voluntarily via somatic motor neurons from the ventral horn. Efferent impulses from the pontine micturition center run in the reticulospinal tracts to inhibit pudendal firing (relaxing the external sphincter) and to stimulate parasympathetic neurons situated in the intermediolateral cell column at levels S2 through S4, causing detrusor contraction. During voiding, sympathetic efferents are inhibited, which opens the bladder neck and permits postganglionic parasympathetic transmission.

Urodynamically, the micturition reflex begins with sudden and complete relaxation of the striated muscles of the urethra and pelvic floor and a decrease in urethral pressure. Several seconds later, intravesical pressure is increased by a highly controlled coordinated contraction of the bulk of the detrusor muscle. Descent and funneling of the bladder neck and proximal urethra occur and urine flow begins.

Brain stem modulation of the micturition reflex allows for a detrusor contraction long enough to evacuate intravesical contents completely. With voluntary termination of voiding or with the stop test, the striated muscles of the urethra and pelvic floor contract to elevate the bladder base, increase intraurethral pressure, and empty the urethra of urine. The detrusor muscle is reflexly inhibited and intravesical pressure returns to normal.

## CLINICAL PHARMACOLOGY OF THE LOWER URINARY TRACT

Thorough understanding of the neurologic control of the urinary bladder and its outlet allows one to intelligently use pharmacologic agents to manage many types of lower urinary tract dysfunction. Basic concepts of pharmacologic treatment are summarized within a functional scheme of therapy for micturition disorders, as developed by Wein et al. (1991). More specific guidelines for pharmacologic treatments of various lower urinary tract complaints and reviews of the clinical studies using these agents are found in the chapters describing individual urogynecologic disorders.

Most pharmacologic agents produce their effects by combining with cell receptors. The drug-receptor interaction initiates a series of biochemical and physiologic changes that characterize the effects produced by the agent. In general, drugs alter lower urinary tract function by affecting synthesis, transport, storage, and release of the neurotransmitter; the combination of the neurotransmitter with postjunctional receptors; or the inactivation, degradation, or reuptake of the neurotransmitter.

Most drugs used to treat lower urinary tract disorders were developed originally for their actions on other organ systems whose functions are also controlled by innervation or drug-receptor interaction. The pharmacologic effects on other organ systems are responsible for many of the unwanted side effects of these agents. Improving specificity and selectivity of the therapeutic agents is an important area of future development in uropharmacology.

Clinically, pharmacologic agents can be grouped into those that facilitate bladder emptying and those that facilitate urine storage (see Box 2-1). Patients with disorders of bladder emptying usually have voiding dysfunction; drugs that improve bladder emptying do so by increasing bladder contractility or by decreasing outlet resistance. Patients with disorders of urine storage often present with urinary incontinence, which is usually caused by either an overactive detrusor or an incompetent urethral sphincter mechanism. Agents that facilitate urine storage act by inhibiting bladder contractility, thereby increasing bladder capacity, or by increasing outlet resistance. The most effective and commonly used agents act on either the parasympathetic or sympathetic systems.

### Therapy to Facilitate Bladder Emptying
*Increasing Intravesical Pressure*

A major portion of the final common pathway in a physiologic bladder contraction is stimulation of the muscarinic cholinergic receptor sites at the postganglionic, parasympathetic neuromuscular junction. Parasympathetic nerve stimulation causes the release of acetylcholine (Ach) at postsynaptic, parasympathetic receptor sites. Ach release produces muscarinic and nicotinic effects; one of the muscarinic effects is contraction of the detrusor muscle and relaxation of the trigone. Muscarinic receptors have been

---

**Box 2-1**
### DRUG EFFECTS ON LOWER URINARY TRACT FUNCTION

**Therapy to Facilitate Bladder Emptying**

Increasing intravesical pressure/bladder contractility
  Parasympathomimetic agents
  Prostaglandins
  Blockers of inhibition
    Alpha-adrenergic antagonists
    Opioid antagonists
Decreasing outlet resistance
  At the level of the smooth sphincter
    Alpha-adrenergic antagonists
    Beta-adrenergic agonists
  At the level of the striated sphincter
    Skeletal muscle relaxants
      Centrally acting relaxants
      Dantrolene
      Baclofen
    Alpha-adrenergic antagonists

**Therapy to Facilitate Urine Storage**

Inhibiting bladder contractility/decreasing sensory input/increasing
  bladder capacity
    Anticholinergic agents
    Musculotropic relaxants
    Calcium antagonists
    Beta-adrenergic agonists
    Prostaglandin inhibitors
    Tricyclic antidepressants
    Dimethyl sulfoxide
    Potassium channel openers
Increasing outlet resistance
    Alpha-adrenergic agonists
    Tricyclic antidepressants
    Beta-adrenergic antagonists
    Estrogen
    Beta-adrenergic agonists

Modified from Wein AJ, Arsdalen KV, Levin RM: Pharmacologic therapy. In Krane RJ, Siroky MB, eds: *Clinical neurourology*, ed 2, Boston, 1991, Little, Brown.

categorized into $M_1$, $M_2$, and $M_3$ subtypes based on their affinity for cholinergic ligands. The human bladder is endowed with $M_2$ and $M_3$ receptors; it appears that bladder contraction is mediated by the $M_3$ type.

Ach itself cannot be used for therapeutic purposes because of actions at central and ganglionic levels and because of its rapid hydrolysis by acetylcholinesterase and nonspecific cholinesterase. Bethanechol chloride exhibits a selective Ach-like action on the urinary bladder and gut with little or no action at therapeutic dosages on ganglia or the cardiovascular system. It is cholinesterase-resistant and causes a contraction of smooth muscle from the bladder, bladder neck, and urethra, thus preventing coordinated and complete bladder emptying. Although it has been used extensively for treatment of postoperative and postpartum urinary retention, it is no longer considered to be effective to facilitate voiding.

Other pharmacologic methods of achieving a cholinergic effect include the use of cholinesterase agents, dopamine antagonists (metoclopramide), and alpha-adrenergic blocking agents (to block the inhibitory effect of sympathetics on pelvic parasympathetic ganglionic transmission). In addition, prostaglandins may facilitate bladder emptying by inducing detrusor contraction and maintaining smooth muscle tone.

### Decreasing Outlet Resistance

The lower urinary tract has alpha- and beta-adrenergic receptor sites, the functions of which have been discussed. Facilitation of bladder emptying could be achieved by the use of alpha-adrenergic antagonists, which decrease outlet resistance by smooth muscle relaxation of the bladder neck and proximal urethra. Some investigators have suggested that these agents may affect striated sphincter tone as well. Alpha-sympathetic blocking agents have thus been used to treat both smooth sphincter dyssynergia and detrusor-striated sphincter dyssynergia. Wein et al. (1991) published a review of the effectiveness of these agents.

## Therapy to Facilitate Urine Storage
### Decreasing Bladder Contractility

Hyperactivity of the bladder during filling may present as involuntary detrusor contractions, decreased bladder compliance, or sensory urgency. The pathophysiology and treatment of detrusor instability and hyperreflexia are discussed thoroughly in Chapter 24. Pharmacologic agents used to treat detrusor overactivity are directed toward inhibiting bladder contractility or decreasing sensory input during filling. Atropine and atropine-like agents depress detrusor overactivity of any cause by inhibiting muscarinic cholinergic receptor sites. Propantheline bromide is an oral agent with this mechanism of action; however, side effects limit its use. Tolterodine tartrate is a competitive muscarinic receptor antagonist that appears to have greater selectivity for the urinary bladder, a feature that may lead to fewer side

effects in clinical practice. Hyoscyamine and hyoscyamine sulfate are other anticholinergic agents used clinically, but controlled studies demonstrating their effectiveness on detrusor overactivity are lacking.

Smooth muscle relaxants are commonly used to treat detrusor overactivity. These agents reportedly act directly on smooth muscle at a site that is metabolically distal to the cholinergic receptor mechanism. In addition to being musculotropic relaxants, these agents also possess variable antimuscarinic and local anesthetic properties. The drugs most commonly used include oxybutynin chloride, dicyclomine hydrochloride, and flavoxate hydrochloride.

Tricyclic antidepressants, particularly imipramine hydrochloride, have prominent systemic anticholinergic effects, weak antimuscarinic effects on bladder smooth muscle, antihistaminic effects, and local anesthetic properties. Imipramine also appears to increase bladder outlet resistance by a peripheral blockade of noradrenaline uptake. Thus, it may be effective for the treatment of urine storage disorders by both decreasing bladder contractility and increasing outlet resistance.

Other drugs that have been used to decrease bladder contractility include calcium antagonists, beta-adrenergic agonists, prostaglandin inhibitors, and dimethyl sulfoxide.

### Increasing Outlet Resistance

Because of the preponderance of alpha-adrenergic receptor sites in the bladder neck and proximal urethra, alpha-adrenergic agonists have been used to produce urethral smooth muscle contraction, thereby increasing resting urethral pressure and resistance to outflow. The pharmacologic actions and clinical uses of these agents are discussed in Chapter 13. Beta-adrenergic blocking agents may be expected to increase urethral resistance as well potentiating an alpha-adrenergic effect. However, few studies have tested this hypothesis and clinical effects are likely to be small.

Estrogens affect adrenergic nerves by influencing excitability, neuronal influences on the muscle, receptor density and sensitivity, and transmitter metabolism. The clinical use of estrogen to augment lower urinary tract function is also discussed in Chapter 13.

## BIBLIOGRAPHY

Barrington FJ: The nervous mechanism of micturition, *Q J Exp Physiol* 8:33, 1914.

Barrington FJ: The relation of the hindbrain to micturition, *Brain* 44:23, 1921.

Beck RP: Neuropharmacology of the lower urinary tract in women, *Obstet Gynecol Clin North Am* 16:753, 1989.

Benson JT: Neurophysiologic control of lower urinary tract, *Obstet Gynecol Clin North Am* 16:733, 1989.

Blaivas JG: The neurophysiology of micturition: a clinical study of 550 patients, *J Urol* 127:958, 1982.

Blaivas JG: Pathophysiology of lower urinary tract dysfunction, *Urol Clin North Am* 12:216, 1985.

Bradley WE: Cerebro-cortical innervation of the urinary bladder, *Tohoku J Exp Med* 131:7, 1980.

Bradley WE: Physiology of urinary bladder. In Walsh PC, Perlmutter AD, Gittes RF, et al, eds: *Campbell's urology,* ed 5, Philadelphia, 1986, WB Saunders.

Bradley WE, Timm GW, Scott FB: Innervation of the detrusor muscle and urethra, *Urol Clin North Am* 1:3, 1974.

DeGroat WC: Nervous control of the urinary bladder in the cat, *Brain Res* 87:201, 1975.

DeGroat WC, Booth AM, Krier J, et al: Neural control of the urinary bladder and large intestine. In Brooks CM, Koizumi K, Sato A, eds: *Integrative functions of the autonomic nervous system,* Amsterdam, 1979, Elsevier/North Holland, Biomedical Press.

DeGroat WC, Ryall RW: Recurrent inhibition in sacral parasympathetic pathways to the bladder, *J Physiol* 196:579, 1968.

Downie JW, Armour JA: Relation of afferent nerve activity in the pelvic plexus with pressure, length, and wall strain in the urinary bladder of the cat, *Soc Neurosci Abstr* 8:858, 1982.

Edvardsen P: Changes in urinary-bladder motility following lesions in the nervous system in cats, *Acta Neurol Scand* 42:25, 1966.

Elbadawi A: Neuromorphologic basis of vesicourethral function. I. Histochemistry, ultrastructure, and function of intrinsic nerves of the bladder and urethra, *Neurourol Urodyn* 1:3, 1982.

Finkbeiner A, Welch L, Bissada N: Uropharmacology. IX. Direct acting smooth muscle stimulants and depressants, *Urology* 12:128, 1978.

Fletcher TF, Bradley WE: Neuroanatomy of the bladder-urethra, *J Urol* 119:153, 1978.

Gibson A: The influence of endocrine hormones on the autonomic nervous system, *J Auton Pharmacol* 1:331, 1981.

Gosling JA, Dixon JS: The structure and innervation of smooth muscle in the wall of the bladder neck and proximal urethra, *Br J Urol* 47:549, 1975.

Gosling JA, Dixon JS, Critchley HOD: A comparative study of the human external sphincter and periurethral levator ani muscles, *Br J Urol* 53:35, 1981.

Jünemann K, Thüroff J: Innervation. In Brubaker LT, Saclarides TJ, eds: *The female pelvic floor: disorders of function and support,* Philadelphia, 1996, FA Davis.

Kelin LA: Urge incontinence can be a disease of bladder sensors, *J Urol* 139:1010, 1988.

Kulseng-Hanssen S, Klevmark B: Continence mechanism. In Drive JO, Hilton P, Stanton SL, eds: *Micturition,* London, 1990, Springer-Verlag.

Mahoney DT, Laberte RO, Blais DJ: Integral storage and voiding reflexes: neurophysiologic concept of continence and micturition, *Urology* 10:95, 1977.

McGuire EJ: The innervation and function of the lower urinary tract, *J Neurosurg* 65:278, 1986.

Mundy AP: Clinical physiology of the bladder, urethra and pelvic floor. In Mundy AP, Stephenson TP, Wein AJ, eds: *Urodynamics: principles, practice and application,* New York, 1984, Churchill Livingstone.

Ostergard DR: Neurological control of micturition and integral voiding reflexes. In Ostergard DR, ed: *Gynecologic urology and urodynamics,* ed 2, Baltimore, 1985, Williams & Wilkins.

Pernow B: Substance P, *Pharmacol Rev* 35:85, 1983.

Raezer D, Wein AJ, Jacobowitz D, et al: Autonomic innervation of canine urinary bladder: cholinergic and adrenergic contributions and interaction of sympathetic and parasympathetic systems in bladder function, *Urology* 2:211, 1973.

Sillen U: Central neurotransmitter mechanisms involved in the control of urinary bladder function, *Scand J Urol Nephrol* 58(suppl):1, 1980.

Steers WD: Physiology and pharmacology of the bladder and urethra. In Walsh PC, Retik AB, Vaughan ED, et al, eds: *Campbell's urology,* ed 7, Philadelphia, 1998, WB Saunders.

Swash M: Innervation of the bladder, urethra and pelvic floor. In Drive JO, Hilton P, Stanton SL, eds: *Micturition,* London, 1990, Springer-Verlag.

Tanagho EA, Miller ER: Initiation of voiding, *Br J Urol* 42:175, 1970.

Taylor P: Cholinergic agonists. In Gilman AG et al, eds: *Goodman and Gilman's the pharmacological basis of therapeutics,* ed 7, New York, 1985, Macmillan.

Torrens M: Human physiology. In Torrens M, Morrison JFB, eds: *The physiology of the lower urinary tract,* London, 1987, Springer-Verlag.

Tulloch AG: Sympathetic activity of internal urethral sphincter in empty and partially filled bladder, *Urology* 5:353, 1975.

Uvelius B, Gabella G: Relation between cell length and force production in urinary bladder smooth muscle, *Acta Physiol Scand* 110:357, 1980.

Walters MD: Mechanisms of continence and voiding, with International Continence Society classification of dysfunction, *Obstet Gynecol Clin North Am* 16:773, 1989.

Wang P, Luthin GR, Ruggieri MR: Muscarinic acetylcholine receptor sub-types mediating urinary bladder contractility and coupling to GTP binding proteins, *J Pharmacol Exp Ther* 273:959, 1995.

Wein AJ: Pharmacology of incontinence, *Urol Clin North Am* 22:557, 1995.

Wein AJ, Arsdalen KV, Levin RM: Pharmacologic therapy. In Krane RJ, Siroky MB, eds: *Clinical neurourology,* ed 2, Boston, 1991, Little, Brown.

Wein AJ, Barrett DM: *Voiding function and dysfunction,* Chicago, 1988, Mosby.

Winter DL: Receptor characteristics and conduction velocities in bladder efferents, *J Psychiatr Res* 8:225, 1971.

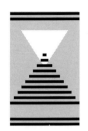

CHAPTER **3**

# Epidemiology and Social Impact of Urinary and Fecal Incontinence

Anne M. Weber and Mark D. Walters

Urinary and fecal incontinence are common diseases that in the past were considered to be a natural result of aging and an inevitable problem with which women must contend. However, many studies show that both types of incontinence have multiple and broad-reaching effects that influence daily activities, social interactions, and self-perceptions of health. This chapter reviews epidemiologic issues related to urinary and fecal incontinence, including prevalence, risk factors, and the social, psychologic, sexual, and economic effects of urinary and fecal incontinence in women who live in the community and in nursing homes.

## PREVALENCE AND INCIDENCE

Because the prevalence of urinary and fecal incontinence increases with age, the changing demographics of the U.S. population will result in even more affected women. Based on projections from the Bureau of the Census, the proportion of postmenopausal women will increase from 23% of the population in 1995 to 33% in 2050. The proportion of women aged 85 and older will triple, from about 2% of the population in 1995 to about 6% in 2050.

## Urinary Incontinence

The estimated prevalence of urinary incontinence in women varies widely because of differences in populations studied, the methods used to collect data, and definitions of disease. Incorrect estimates may result from biases in sample surveys and underreporting due to embarrassment. Herzog and Fultz (1990) found an 83% agreement between self-reported data and clinicians' assessments of incontinence. For these reasons, estimates from the literature should be considered only as close approximations.

There is considerable variation in the estimated prevalence of any urinary incontinence, that is, any urine loss during a 12-month period in women in the community. There is a significant prevalence even in women not traditionally thought to be at risk for urinary incontinence. In a study of nulliparous college athletes, 28% reported ever experiencing urine loss during athletic activity, and in two thirds it occurred more than rarely. Studies have reported the prevalence of any urinary incontinence among older people as ranging from 8% to 41%.

When the severity of urine loss is defined as "daily," "weekly," or "most of the time," the reported prevalence ranges from 3% to 14% for women in the community. This estimate corresponds more closely to the clinical estimate of disease because it probably identifies women who consider the involuntary urine loss to be a social or hygienic problem. The prevalence of urinary incontinence in women in nursing homes is much higher than in women in the community, ranging from 40% to 70%, especially in facilities where residents have more severe functional impairments.

The incidence of incontinence is defined as the probability of becoming incontinent during a defined period of time, given continence at the onset of the time period. Because few long-term longitudinal studies have been performed, little information about the incidence of urinary incontinence is available. One study showed a 1-year incidence rate of about 20% for women, with most of those cases being mild incontinence. Those who changed their severity level of incontinence were most likely to progress from mild to moderate symptoms, and in type of incontinence, from single symptoms (stress or urge) to mixed.

These estimates include both chronic and acute causes of urinary incontinence. Acute, transient causes such as infection, drug use, and delirium often regress after treatment. Thus, there is a yearly fluctuation of development and regression of incontinence among individuals. About 12% of incontinent women per year have regression of urinary incontinence.

## Fecal Incontinence

As with urinary incontinence, the prevalence of fecal incontinence varies by the definition used and the population surveyed. There is no consensus on what constitutes severe or clinically important fecal incontinence, but many studies use a frequency of incontinent episodes of once a week or more, or requiring sanitary protection. The prevalence of anal incontinence (loss of gas or stool) in the general population was reported in one study to be 2.2%, with 10% of those experiencing incontinent episodes more than once a week. The prevalence of fecal incontinence in elderly people in the community is higher, ranging from 3.7% to 18.4%. Fecal incontinence occurs commonly in women with urinary incontinence ("double incontinence") and pelvic organ prolapse, with a prevalence of fecal incontinence of 21% in one study of women with urinary incontinence and prolapse. Women in nursing homes experience fecal incontinence at an even higher rate of up to 50%. Information on the incidence of fecal incontinence is unavailable, as is information on progression from mild or infrequent fecal incontinence to more severe forms.

## RISK FACTORS FOR URINARY AND FECAL INCONTINENCE
### Sex

Urinary incontinence is two to three times more common in women than in men. The gender difference is most pronounced among adults under 60 years of age because of the very low prevalence of urinary incontinence in younger men. These sex differences are consistent whether the measure is any incontinence, severe incontinence, or irritative bladder symptoms. The symptom of stress incontinence is uncommon in men, but voiding problems are more common, especially in elderly men, in part caused by prostate conditions.

Some studies show a higher prevalence of fecal incontinence in women than in men, although a study by Johanson and Lafferty (1996) reported that fecal incontinence was 1.3 times more common in men than in women. Obviously, women are uniquely susceptible to damage to fecal continence mechanisms at vaginal childbirth, but how this influences the prevalence and causes of fecal incontinence in women compared to men is unknown. Studies of anorectal function show that, compared to men, women have lower anal squeeze pressures, greater perineal descent, and more evidence of nerve damage to the pelvic muscles and anal sphincters.

## Age

Many studies have confirmed that the prevalence of urinary incontinence increases with age. Brown et al. (1996) reported daily incontinence in 12.5% of women less than 80 years old, 19% between 80 and 89, and 31.1% in women aged 90 years and older. Multivariate analysis established age as a risk factor for incontinence, with a 30% greater prevalence for each 5-year increase in age.

Reasons for increased prevalence of urinary incontinence with age are not completely understood. Normal aging is characterized by decline in the reserve capacity of all organ systems. As in other muscles, the volume and number of muscle cells in the urethral sphincter decrease with age. Bladder capacity, ability to postpone voiding, bladder compliance, and urinary flow rate decrease with age in both sexes. Uninhibited bladder contractions and elevated postvoid residual urine volume increase with age. Maximal urethral closure pressure and functional urethral length decrease with age in women. These changes in bladder and urethral function may be related directly to aging and indirectly to the development of various medical conditions that affect bladder function. Another important age-related change is an alteration in the pattern of fluid excretion. Whereas younger people excrete the bulk of their daily ingested fluid before bedtime, the pattern reverses with age so that one or two episodes of nocturia per night may be normal.

Urinary symptoms are found in over half of institutionalized elderly people. In addition to the various urologic diagnoses of incontinence, nonurologic causes of incontinence such as behavioral problems, immobility, medication use, and diabetes often are present. Jirovec and Wells (1990) observed that when multiple variables were examined together, mobility emerged as the best predictor of urinary control, followed by cognitive impairment. Therapy should always include a combination of urologic treatments with nonurologic, behavioral treatments in dealing with urinary incontinence in nursing home residents.

Some but not all studies of fecal incontinence show increased prevalence with age. Kok et al. (1992) reported fecal incontinence in 4.2% of women aged 60 to 84 years and 16.9% in women aged 85 and over. Increasing prevalence of fecal incontinence with age was shown by Talley et al. (1992) in women but not in men. Johanson and Lafferty (1996) did not observe a progressive increase in prevalence with age in women, but found a higher rate in women less than 30 years old and in women over age 50.

As with urinary function, the effect of age on anorectal function is multifactorial. Increasing age may lead to increased perineal descent, nerve dysfunction measured by slowed pudendal nerve conduction, and decreased anorectal sensation. One study showed a decrease in resting anal pressure with age, and another study showed a decrease in anal pressure at voluntary contraction ("squeeze") with age. These changes interact with other aspects of patients' functional status and may result in symptoms, particularly in association with cognitive impairments or physical limitations.

Women in nursing homes are especially vulnerable to fecal incontinence caused by fecal impaction. Many factors may contribute to impaction, such as decreased fluid and dietary fiber intake, limited physical activity, medication effects, and lack of attention to regular bowel habits. Despite the availability of simple, effective preventive techniques and treatment, fecal impaction is responsible for at least half of all cases of fecal incontinence in women in nursing homes.

## Race

Little information is available on racial differences in the occurrence of urinary incontinence, and no reports are available for fecal incontinence. Traditionally, white women have been thought to be at higher risk for incontinence and other disorders of pelvic support than nonwhite women. This may reflect different levels of risk based on genetic or anatomic attributes, lifestyle factors such as diet, exercise, and work habits, or cultural expectations and tolerance of symptoms. A study of 30 Chinese female cadavers revealed that the general anatomic relationship of the levator ani muscles and urethra was similar to that found in Western women. However, the levator ani muscle bundles in the Chinese cadavers were judged to be thicker and to extend more laterally on the arcus tendineus than in white cadavers. Furthermore, the fascia of the pelvic diaphragm was particularly dense. Although this work was uncontrolled and subjective, it provides one explanation for a possible racial difference in the prevalence of pelvic support defects and incontinence.

Recent reports describe a significant prevalence of urinary incontinence and other urinary symptoms in women of nonwhite races, including black, Hispanic, and Japanese women. There may be differences in the distribution of presenting symptoms or confirmed diagnoses, with two reports showing a higher prevalence of detrusor instability in black or Hispanic women than in white women.

## Childbirth

Many studies have shown a higher rate of urinary incontinence in parous women than in nulliparous women. Most of the increase occurs in women with one vaginal birth compared to women with none, although the prevalence increases in smaller increments for each subsequent birth after the first. Among types of incontinence, stress incontinence consistently shows the strongest associations with parity. Little or no association is found between urge incontinence and parity.

Damage to pelvic tissues at vaginal birth has been implicated as a major factor leading to stress urinary incontinence and other pelvic support abnormalities. Vaginal birth may directly damage pelvic muscles and connective tissue attachments. Vaginal delivery leads to loss of pelvic muscle strength in the immediate postpartum period,

although most or all of this strength may be recovered with aggressive pelvic muscle exercises. Women who have had cesarean births demonstrate greater pelvic muscle strength during and after the postpartum period than women delivered vaginally.

In addition to direct muscle damage, pelvic muscle dysfunction may be caused by nerve damage as a result of trauma or stretch injury to the pelvic nerves during vaginal birth. In a study of 128 women during pregnancy and after delivery, 16% had abnormal nerve function measured by prolonged pudendal nerve latency after delivery, but it remained prolonged after 6 months in only a third of these. Women with incontinence or pelvic organ prolapse or both have significantly higher rate of denervation of the pelvic muscles than asymptomatic women. In a study of urinary incontinence at 3 months postpartum, vaginal birth was an adverse risk factor (incontinence in 36.2% of women after spontaneous deliveries and 35.3% after forceps) and cesarean delivery was a protective factor, although not completely so (incontinence in 23.6%). The prevalence of incontinence in women having three or more cesarean deliveries was similar to women who delivered vaginally.

Childbirth has been linked to damage that may result in fecal incontinence. Pregnancy itself does not have a significant effect on anal sphincter morphology or function, so changes in sphincter function are more likely caused by mechanical trauma at vaginal birth rather than hormonal changes of pregnancy. In addition to potential damage to pelvic muscles, connective tissue, and nerves, both the internal and external anal sphincters are at risk for damage during vaginal birth, even without a recognized sphincter separation (third- or fourth-degree perineal laceration or episiotomy). By using anal sonography in women before and after delivery, Sultan et al. (1993a) found that 35% of primiparous women sustained external or internal anal sphincter damage, although only 3% were recognized at the time of delivery. Forty percent of multiparous women had preexisting sphincter defects, increasing only slightly to 44% after the index delivery. None of the women delivered by cesarean birth sustained anal sphincter damage. Only a third of women with sphincter defects had anal incontinence or fecal urgency, suggesting redundancy of function that maintains continence despite some damage.

Traditional obstetric teaching has recommended performance of episiotomies to protect pelvic tissue integrity, but recent evidence has shown that not only does median episiotomy fail to prevent damage, but its use actually increases overt sphincter damage. Despite primary repair after third- or fourth-degree perineal lacerations, 85% of women have persistent structural sphincter defects and 50% remain symptomatic.

These data suggest that childbirth adversely affects lower urinary tract and anorectal function. However, childbirth per se does not explain all cases of urinary and fecal incontinence. Further research is needed to define the roles of pregnancy and childbirth in the causes of urinary and fecal incontinence and other pelvic support defects and, in particular, to identify changes in obstetric practice that would reduce the risk of developing these conditions.

## Menopause

The vagina and urethra have similar epithelial linings because of their common embryologic origin. Urinary cytologic changes are similar to those of vaginal cytology during the menstrual cycle, during pregnancy, and after menopause. In women, several studies have identified high-affinity estrogen receptors in the pubococcygeal muscle, urethra, and bladder trigone, but receptors are found infrequently in the rest of the bladder. Estrogen deficiency urogenital atrophy is at least partly responsible for sensory symptoms and decreased resistance to infection often found after menopause. Estrogen therapy reduces the incidence of bladder infections in postmenopausal women with recurrent infections.

Normal urethral function in women is affected by age and estrogen status. Maximum urethral pressure and urethral length increase from infancy to about 25 years of age and then decrease with advancing age. A further decrease in functional urethral length occurs after menopause, possibly because of estrogen deprivation. Decreased urethral vascularity and abnormal smooth and skeletal muscle efficiency may contribute to low resting urethral pressure and an abnormal stress response. Finally, age- and estrogen-induced changes in collagen of the pelvic connective tissue may allow for the development and progression of urethral detachment, urinary incontinence, and pelvic organ prolapse.

Despite good evidence that estrogen plays a role in maintaining normal urinary function, it is less certain whether it has pharmacologic use in the prevention or treatment of incontinence. Estrogen replacement therapy in young continent nulliparous women who are hypoestrogenic because of premature ovarian failure results in little change in urethral function. Although a meta-analysis suggested that estrogen may subjectively improve urinary incontinence in postmenopausal women, a subsequent randomized, placebo-controlled trial did not demonstrate any improvement in subjective or objective outcomes related to urinary incontinence or quality of life.

The effect of age on fecal incontinence has been discussed, but little is known about the potential independent effects of menopause or estrogen status on fecal incontinence. Estrogen receptors have been demonstrated in the external anal sphincter, but the influence of estrogen on anorectal function is not yet known.

## Smoking

In a large case control study of continent and incontinent women, Bump and McClish (1992) noted a significant association between cigarette smoking and the development of all forms of urinary incontinence. Women who smoked (including former and current smokers) were two to three times more likely to have incontinence than nonsmokers. Smokers generated greater increases in bladder pressure with coughing, thus overcoming the sphincteric continence mechanism.

No information is available on the effect of smoking or obesity on fecal incontinence.

## Obesity

Obesity is more common in women with urinary incontinence than in continent women. In a study of 2589 women, Mommsen and Foldspang (1994) found that, irrespective of other risk factors, body mass index was positively associated with urinary incontinence, especially stress incontinence. It may be that obese women generate higher intraabdominal pressures that overwhelm the continence mechanism. Weight loss may result in resolution of incontinence without further specific therapy. In a study of 12 incontinent women who had surgically induced weight loss, 75% had resolution of incontinence, both subjectively and objectively, after 1 year. Significant changes were seen on urodynamic testing, including decreases in the magnitude of bladder pressure increases with coughing, bladder to urethra pressure transmission with cough, and urethral mobility.

Surgical treatment of incontinence is technically more difficult, and postoperative complications are more common in obese patients, especially with retropubic procedures. Obesity may also decrease the long-term effectiveness of incontinence surgery, although this has not been consistently reported.

## PSYCHOSOCIAL IMPACT OF URINARY AND FECAL INCONTINENCE

Loss of control of urine, gas, and stool can have a significant impact on the social well-being of affected people. Indeed, the International Continence Society's definition of urinary incontinence, "a condition in which involuntary loss of urine is a social or hygienic problem," requires that all women with clinically significant urinary incontinence have some degree of social distress. Although there is no consensus about the definition of fecal incontinence, it seems appropriate to include social and hygienic concerns in determining the impact of the problem for each woman. Urinary and fecal incontinence and related psychosocial distress constitute a spectrum related to the actual severity of the loss of control and to the woman's perception of her disability. A summary of potential psychosocial consequences of urinary and fecal incontinence is shown in Table 3-1. In contrast to urinary incontinence, there is little specific information available on social, psychologic, and sexual changes caused by fecal incontinence. It is likely that many of the changes are similar, if not more pronounced, because of the greater stigma and shame associated with fecal incontinence.

**Table 3-1**   Summary of Consequences of Urinary and Fecal Incontinence

| Individual | Family | Health care professional |
|---|---|---|
| Psychologic symptoms | Caregiver burden and emotional stress | Negative feelings and behaviors toward |
|   Insecurity | Impaired interpersonal relationships |   patients with urinary incontinence |
|   Anger | Economic worries | Reaction formation |
|   Apathy | Health deterioration of primary caregiver |   Overindulgence |
|   Dependence | Potential for abuse or neglect |   Excessive permissiveness |
|   Guilt | Decision to institutionalize |   Excessive caring |
|   Indignity | Delayed discharge from institutional care | Extra care responsibilities |
|   Feeling of abandonment | | Staff frustration, depression, and guilt |
|   Shame | | Reduction in staff morale |
|   Embarrassment | | "Burn-out" syndrome |
|   Depression | | |
|   Denial | | |
| Sense of self | | |
|   Loss of self-confidence/self-esteem | | |
|   Sexual difficulties | | |
|   Lack of attention to personal hygiene | | |
| Social interaction | | |
|   Reduction in social activities | | |
|   Socially disengaged | | |
|   Socially isolated | | |
|   Psychologic and functional decline | | |
|   Potential for institutionalization | | |

Modified from Ory MG, Wyman JF, Yu L: *Clin Geriatr Med* 2:657, 1986.

## Social Changes

Many techniques have been used to measure psychosocial impact of urinary incontinence, and condition-specific quality of life instruments have been developed and validated for use in research and clinical settings. In an excellent review, Wyman et al. (1990) examined epidemiologic and clinical studies addressing the psychosocial impact of urinary incontinence on community-dwelling women. They noted wide variations among studies regarding patient populations surveyed, methods of evaluation, and definitions used. Reports of interference with social activities ranged from 8% to 52%. Areas affected included social, domestic, physical, occupational, and leisure activities. Sufferers may give up or restrict certain household chores, church attendance, shopping, traveling, vacations, physical recreation, entertainment events outside the home, and hobbies. They may avoid activities outside the home if they are unsure of restroom locations. Some incontinent people become increasingly isolated as they limit social activities and social contacts. Even incontinent homebound women, when compared with continent homebound women, have significantly fewer social interactions, particularly with family members. Spousal relationships appear to be most impaired, perhaps because of an additional adverse effect on sexual relationships.

Urinary incontinence among very old people can lead to such disability and dependency that family or home caregivers have difficulty coping and responding to increased demands. Incontinence may be the last straw in a family's attempts to care for an elderly person at home. Incontinence is a major factor leading to institutionalization of the elderly, especially in patients with dementia. In one study, 5% of incontinent nursing home residents indicated that incontinence was the main reason for nursing home admission, and it was a secondary reason for many more.

Studies relating measures of perceived social impact with objective measures of incontinence have yielded inconsistent results. Norton (1982) noted that the degree of disability as reported on questionnaire does not correlate with the amount of incontinence. In contrast, Wyman et al. (1990) found significant but modest positive relationships between psychosocial impact scores and the number of incontinent episodes reported in a diary, as well as the amount of fluid lost with a perineal pad test. Some studies noted more social restriction with stress incontinence than with urge incontinence, whereas others reported more abnormal psychosocial impact with detrusor instability. These inconsistencies in the literature indicate that the patient's threshold for tolerance of urinary incontinence and perceived disability or distress may be wide and is probably influenced by other, still undefined factors.

It is widely accepted that urinary incontinence is underrecognized and undertreated. Fewer than half of people with urinary incontinence in the community consult their health care providers about the problem. The reasons for this include embarrassment, easy availability of absorbent products, low expectations of benefit from treatment, and lack of information regarding options for treatment. In a recent questionnaire study of 1140 men and women aged 65 and older, 58% indicated that urinary incontinence was one of the results of normal aging, and 62% did not know of treatments for incontinence other than absorbent underpants and catheters.

The few studies on the prevalence of fecal incontinence have also documented underreporting by patients, with fewer than one third reporting the symptom to their doctor. The same factors could apply as for urinary incontinence, probably with an even greater degree of shame and reluctance to admit to such a problem.

## Psychologic Changes

Urinary incontinence is a complex phenomenon with multiple causative factors, including psychogenic causes. Early studies, perhaps because of insufficient understanding of the pathophysiology, stressed the psychosomatic aspects of urinary complaints. Psychiatric analyses of women with lower urinary tract symptoms described somatization, hysteria, depression, anxiety, and abnormal levels of situational life stresses. Such disorders have been considered to be etiologic of lower urinary tract dysfunction, specifically urethral syndrome, unstable bladder, and urinary retention. Urinary incontinence has been implicated as one expression of "masked depression" often seen in gynecologic patients. Most of these studies were methodologically flawed by biases in patient selection and interview techniques, lack of appropriate control groups, and little application of statistical analyses.

More recent studies have used personality testing in patients with urinary incontinence. Using the Eysenck Personality Inventory questionnaire, Berglund et al. (1994) recorded significantly higher scores for somatic and psychic anxiety in incontinent patients than in controls. Chiverton et al. (1996) found a strong correlation between low self-esteem, depression, and urinary incontinence. Walters et al. (1990) found that compared to matched continent controls, many incontinent women had Minnesota Multiphasic Personality Inventory profiles that were clinically significant, reflecting moodiness, feelings of helplessness and sadness, pessimism, and general hypochondriasis and somatization. No differences in profile scores were found between women with detrusor instability and those with genuine stress incontinence. Taken together, these studies suggest that anxiety, depression, and other psychologic abnormalities may be related to urinary incontinence. Because most objective studies report similar test results with the various diagnoses of incontinence, it is more likely that psychologic changes are related to the symptom and related disability and distress than to specific urogynecologic conditions. This possibility is consistent with literature that correlates significant declines in the frequency of once-pleasurable activities with depression. Because most studies are retrospective, however, the direction of any cause-and-effect relationship remains to be determined.

It is unknown whether the psychologic changes described in incontinent patients are amenable to treatment. In patients with sensory urgency and detrusor instability, bladder-retraining drills and pharmacotherapy with propantheline bromide result in significant reductions in state anxiety on follow-up testing. Psychotherapy in patients with detrusor instability results in fewer somatic symptoms but no reduction in state anxiety. In a study of bladder retraining for the treatment of detrusor instability, Oldenburg and Millard (1986) reported improvement in psychologic symptoms regardless of urologic response. Although preliminary and somewhat conflicting, these studies suggest that psychologic factors associated with urinary incontinence can be modified with therapy.

## Sexual Changes

The close anatomic proximity of the bladder, urethra, and rectum with the vagina allows for an association between lower urinary tract or anorectal dysfunction and sexual difficulties. The effects can be bidirectional; sexual activity can cause or aggravate bladder or anorectal problems, and bladder or anorectal problems can lead to sexual dysfunction. Examples of conditions in which vaginal intercourse affects the lower urinary tract are the increase in urinary tract infections with intercourse, especially in vaginal diaphragm users, and dyspareunia experienced by women with urethral diverticula. Women may experience urgency to void during or immediately after sexual intercourse. Intercourse may also produce rectal urgency and the fear or occurrence of fecal incontinence in affected women.

Urine loss occurs during vaginal intercourse in 24% to 56% of incontinent women. This complaint is rarely volunteered, probably because of embarrassment. Urine loss may occur with penetration, during clitoral stimulation, or with orgasm. Hilton (1988) demonstrated that 70% of those who became incontinent on penetration had genuine stress incontinence and 4% had detrusor instability, whereas of those who complained of incontinence at orgasm, 42% had genuine stress incontinence and 35% had detrusor instability.

The association between urologic symptoms and sexual problems may occur in several ways. Urinary symptoms may be a direct cause of sexual difficulties, where none previously existed. Alternatively, urinary symptoms may be used (consciously or unconsciously) as an excuse to avoid sexual contact in the presence of a preexisting but unacknowledged sexual problem. Conditions common in incontinent women, such as advanced age and estrogen deficiency related to menopause, may adversely affect sexual activity due to vaginal atrophy, decreased lubrication and vaginal secretions, and fewer orgasmic contractions. Declining general health of the woman and her partner with advancing age also may affect sexual activity. In a study of women with and without urinary incontinence and pelvic organ prolapse, age was the most important predictor of sexual function, rather than the presence or absence of incontinence or prolapse. Thus, many complex factors affect the quality of sexual function.

Sexual function may be positively or negatively affected by the surgical treatment of urinary incontinence. Haase and Skibsted (1988) studied 55 sexually active women who underwent a variety of operations for stress incontinence or pelvic organ prolapse. Postoperatively, 24% of the patients experienced improvement in their sexual satisfaction, 67% experienced no change, and 9% experienced deterioration. Improvement often resulted from cessation of urinary incontinence. Deterioration was always caused by dyspareunia after posterior colporrhaphy. These authors concluded that the prognosis for an improved sexual life is good after surgery for stress incontinence but that posterior colpoperineorrhaphy causes dyspareunia in some patients.

## ECONOMIC ISSUES

Despite the prevalence of urinary incontinence, studies of its economic impact are scarce, primarily because of the absence of reliable prevalence, risk factor, and cost data and because of wide diversity of treatment methods. Most available economic studies have focused on the cost of caring for elderly incontinent people in nursing homes because the data are easier to obtain there than in a community setting.

Estimated costs of urinary incontinence should include direct and indirect costs, as well as costs of treating complications related to incontinence. Direct costs are the resources from the economy used to diagnose, treat, care for, and rehabilitate incontinent patients. Indirect costs of incontinence include lost productivity, consequences of incontinence ranging from skin ulcers to mortality, and the cost of time spent by unpaid caregivers. Box 3-1 lists the direct and indirect costs of urinary incontinence. The sum of direct and indirect costs of urinary incontinence reflects the total economic burden on the entire economy. Not every incontinent patient incurs all of these costs, but data describing precise resource use as a result of urinary incontinence are not available.

Based on multiple assumptions regarding prevalence and cost information, Hu (1994) estimated that the total direct and indirect economic cost of urinary incontinence for the entire economy in 1994 dollars was $16.4 billion. This included $11.2 billion for people in the community and $5.2 billion in nursing homes. The single largest cost item, either in the community (60%) or in nursing homes (62%), was for routine care and supplies (laundry, pads, absorbent underpants). Costs related to evaluation and treatment amounted to only 0.5% of all costs in the community and only 0.26% of total costs in nursing homes. In another study, elderly

**Box 3-1**
## COSTS OF URINARY INCONTINENCE

**Direct Costs**

Diagnostic and
  evaluation costs
  Physician consultation
    and examination
  Laboratory
  Diagnostic procedures
Treatment costs
  Surgery
  Drugs
Routine care costs
  Nursing labor
  Supplies
  Laundry
Rehabilitation costs
  Nursing labor
  Supplies

Incontinence consequence costs
  Skin breakdowns
  Urinary tract infections
  Falls
  Additional nursing home
    admissions
  Longer hospital stays

**Indirect Costs**

Time costs of unpaid caregivers
  for treating and caring for incontinent elderly people
Loss of productivity because of
  morbidity
Loss of productivity because of
  mortality

From Hu TW: *J Am Geriatr Soc* 38:292, 1990.

incontinent people incurred greater costs for home care services, and the effective use of resources was questioned because patterns of care suggested palliative rather than rehabilitative services.

Despite the large economic burden of urinary incontinence in nursing homes, whether interventions decrease or increase overall costs remains unknown. Borrie and Davidson (1992) demonstrated that more active evaluation and treatment of incontinence in nursing homes could result in considerable cost savings. However, in studies of behavioral therapy (prompted voiding) for incontinent nursing home residents, although residents receive the benefits of reduced incontinence and nursing homes realize some cost savings in laundry and supplies, the increased work load for personnel may increase the cost of treatment over the level of cost savings. At least for the short term, behavioral therapy to improve incontinence in institutionalized elderly may cost more than the direct cost normally incurred by the nursing home. Quality of life and other second-order benefits must be considered if continence rehabilitation is to be cost-effective. In the community, behavioral therapy would not incur labor costs and so may be more cost-effective, although this has not been studied. Medical and surgical treatments for incontinence have not been evaluated for cost-effectiveness in nursing home settings. Studies reflecting cost of incontinence treatment in the community have typically compared the cost of one treatment to another, rather than to the cost of no treatment.

# BIBLIOGRAPHY

## Prevalence and Incidence

Brown JS, Seeley DG, Fong J, et al: Urinary incontinence in older women: who is at risk? *Obstet Gynecol* 87:715, 1996.

Herzog AR, Diokno AC, Brown MB, et al: Two-year incidence, remission, and change patterns of urinary incontinence in noninstitutionalized older adults, *J Gerontol* 45:M67, 1990.

Herzog AR, Fultz NH: Prevalence and incidence of urinary incontinence in community-dwelling populations, *J Am Geriatr Soc* 38:273, 1990.

Jameson JS, Chia YW, Kamm MA, et al: Effect of age, sex and parity on anorectal function, *Br J Surg* 81:1689, 1994.

Johanson JF, Lafferty J: Epidemiology of fecal incontinence: the silent affliction, *Am J Gastroenterol* 91:33, 1996.

Kok ALM, Voorhorst FJ, Burger CW, et al: Urinary and faecal incontinence in community-residing elderly women, *Age Ageing* 21:211, 1992.

Laurberg S, Swash M: Effects of aging on the anorectal sphincters and their innervation, *Dis Colon Rectum* 32:737, 1989.

Nelson R, Norton N, Cautley E, et al: Community-based prevalence of anal incontinence, *JAMA* 274:559, 1995.

Nygaard IE, Thompson FL, Svengalis SL, et al: Urinary incontinence in elite nulliparous athletes, *Obstet Gynecol* 84:183, 1994.

Ouslander JG, Schnelle JF: Incontinence in the nursing home, *Ann Intern Med* 122:438, 1995.

Talley NJ, O'Keefe EA, Zinsmeister AR, et al: Prevalence of gastrointestinal symptoms in the elderly: a population-based study, *Gastroenterology* 102:895, 1992.

Tobin GW, Brocklehurst JC: Faecal incontinence in residential homes for the elderly: prevalence, aetiology and management, *Age Ageing* 15:41, 1986.

## Risk Factors

Bump RC: Racial comparisons and contrasts in urinary incontinence and pelvic organ prolapse, *Obstet Gynecol* 81:421, 1993.

Bump RC, McClish DK: Cigarette smoking and urinary incontinence in women, *Am J Obstet Gynecol* 167:1213, 1992.

Bump RC, McClish DK: Cigarette smoking and pure genuine stress incontinence of urine: a comparison of risk factors and determinants between smokers and nonsmokers, *Am J Obstet Gynecol* 170:579, 1994.

Bump RC, Sugerman HJ, Fantl JA, et al: Obesity and lower urinary tract function in women: effect of surgically induced weight loss, *Am J Obstet Gynecol* 167:392, 1992.

Carlile A, Davies I, Rigby A, et al: Age changes in the human female urethra: a morphometric study, *J Urol* 139:532, 1988.

Cosner KR, Dougherty MC, Bishop KR: Dynamic characteristics of the circumvaginal muscles during pregnancy and postpartum, *J Nurse Midwifery* 36:221, 1991.

Fantl JA, Bump RC, Robinson D, et al: Efficacy of estrogen supplementation in the treatment of urinary incontinence. The Continence Program for Women Research Group, *Obstet Gynecol* 88:745, 1996.

Fantl JA, Cardozo L, McClish DK: Estrogen therapy in the management of urinary incontinence in postmenopausal women: a meta-analysis. First report of the Hormones and Urogenital Therapy Committee, *Obstet Gynecol* 83:12, 1994.

Fantl JA, Newman DK, Colling J, et al: Managing acute and chronic urinary incontinence, Clinical Practice Guideline No 2, 1996 update, Rockville, MD, 1996, U.S. Department of Health and Human Services, Public Health Service, Agency for Health Care Policy and Research, AHCPR Pub No 96-0686.

Foldspang A, Mommsen S, Lam GW, Elving L: Parity as a correlate of adult female urinary incontinence prevalence, *J Epidemiol Community Health* 46:595, 1992.

Haadem K, Ling L, Ferno M, et al: Estrogen receptors in the external anal sphincter, *Am J Obstet Gynecol* 164:609, 1991.

Iosif CS, Batra S, Ek A: Estrogen receptors in the human female lower urinary tract, *Am J Obstet Gynecol* 141:817, 1981.

Jackson SL, Weber AM, Hull TL, et al: Fecal incontinence in women with urinary incontinence and pelvic organ prolapse, *Obstet Gynecol* 89:423, 1997.

Jirovec MM, Wells TJ: Urinary incontinence in nursing home residents with dementia: the mobility-cognition paradigm, *Appl Nurs Res* 3:112, 1990.

Kamm MA: Obstetric damage and faecal incontinence, *Lancet* 334:730, 1994.

Karram MM, Yeko TR, Sauer MV, et al: Urodynamic changes following hormonal replacement therapy in women with premature ovarian failure, *Obstet Gynecol* 74:208, 1989.

Klein MC, Gauthier RJ, Robbins JM, et al: Relationship of episiotomy to perineal trauma and morbidity, sexual dysfunction, and pelvic floor relaxation, *Am J Obstet Gynecol* 171:591, 1994.

Mattox TF, Bhatia NN: The prevalence of urinary incontinence or prolapse among white and Hispanic women, *Am J Obstet Gynecol* 174:646, 1996.

McCallin PF, Taylor ES, Whitehead RW: A study of the changes in the cytology of the urinary sediment during the menstrual cycle and pregnancy, *Am J Obstet Gynecol* 60:64, 1950.

Mommsen S, Foldspang A: Body mass index and adult female urinary incontinence, *World J Urol* 12:319, 1994.

Nakanishi N, Tatara K, Naramura H, et al: Urinary and fecal incontinence in a community-residing older population in Japan, *J Am Geriatr Soc* 45:215, 1997.

O'Donnell BF, Drachman DA, Barnes HJ, et al: Incontinence and troublesome behaviors predict institutionalization in dementia, *J Geriatr Psychiatry Neurol* 5:45, 1992.

Raz R, Stamm WE: A controlled trial of intravaginal estriol in postmenopausal women with recurrent urinary tract infections, *N Engl J Med* 329:753, 1993.

Rother P, Loffler S, Dorschner W, et al: Anatomic basis of micturition and urinary continence. Muscle systems in urinary bladder neck during ageing, *Surg Radiol Anat* 18:173, 1996.

Rud T: Urethral pressure profile in continent women from childhood to old age, *Acta Obstet Gynecol Scand* 59:335, 1980.

Ryhammer AM, Laurberg S, Bek KM: Age and anorectal sensibility in normal women, *Scand J Gastroenterol* 32:278, 1997.

Sampselle CM: Changes in pelvic muscle strength and stress urinary incontinence associated with childbirth, *J Obstet Gynecol Neonatal Nurs* 19:371, 1990.

Semmelink HJF, de Wilde PCM, van Houwelingen JC, et al: Histomorphometric study of the lower urogenital tract in pre- and postmenopausal women, *Cytometry* 11:700, 1990.

Smith ARB, Hosker GL, Warrell DW: The role of partial denervation of the pelvic floor in the aetiology of genitourinary prolapse and stress incontinence of urine. A neurophysiological study, *Br J Obstet Gynaecol* 96:24, 1989.

Sorensen M, Tetzschner T, Rasmussen OO, et al: Sphincter rupture in childbirth, *Br J Surg* 80:392, 1993.

Sultan AH, Kamm MA, Hudson CN: Pudendal nerve damage during labor: prospective study before and after childbirth, *Br J Obstet Gynaecol* 101:22, 1994.

Sultan AH, Kamm MA, Hudson CN, et al: Anal-sphincter disruption during vaginal delivery, *N Engl J Med* 329:1905, 1993a.

Sultan AH, Kamm MA, Hudson CN, et al: Effect of pregnancy on anal sphincter morphology and function, *Int J Colorect Dis* 8:206, 1993b.

Wilson PD, Herbison RM, Herbison GP: Obstetric practice and the prevalence of urinary incontinence three months after delivery, *Br J Obstet Gynaecol* 103:154, 1996.

Zacharin RF: "A Chinese anatomy": the pelvic supporting tissues of the Chinese and Occidental female compared and contrasted, *Aust NZ J Obstet Gynaecol* 17:1, 1977.

## Psychosocial Changes

Abrams P, Blaivas JG, Stanton SL, et al: The standardization of terminology of lower urinary tract function, *Scand J Urol Nephrol* 114(suppl):5, 1988.

Barnick C, Cardozo L: Sexual and bladder dysfunction: how are they related? *Female Patient* 14:63, 1989.

Berglund AL, Eisemann M, Lalos O: Personality characteristics of stress incontinent women: a pilot study, *J Psychosom Obstet Gynaecol* 15:165, 1994.

Berglund AL, Eisemann M, Lalos A, et al: Social adjustment and spouse relationships among women with stress incontinence before and after surgical treatment, *Soc Sci Med* 42:1537, 1996.

Branch LG, Walker LA, Wetle TT, et al: Urinary incontinence knowledge among community-dwelling people 65 years of age and older, *J Am Geriatr Soc* 42:1257, 1994.

Burgio KL, Ives DG, Locher JL, et al: Treatment seeking for urinary incontinence in older adults, *J Am Geriatr Soc* 42:208, 1994.

Chiverton PA, Wells TJ, Brink CA, et al: Psychological factors associated with urinary incontinence, *Clin Nurse Spec* 10:229, 1996.

Clark A, Romm J: Effect of urinary incontinence on sexual activity in women, *J Reprod Med* 38:679, 1993.

Epstein S, Jenike MA: Disabling urinary obsessions: an uncommon variant of obsessive-compulsive disorder, *Psychosomatics* 31:450, 1990.

Grimby A, Milsom I, Molander U, et al: The influence of urinary incontinence on the quality of life of elderly women, *Age Ageing* 22:82, 1993.

Haase P, Skibsted L: Influence of operations for stress incontinence and/or genital descensus on sexual life, *Acta Obstet Gynecol Scand* 67:659, 1988.

Hilton P: Urinary incontinence during sexual intercourse: a common, but rarely volunteered, symptom, *Br J Obstet Gynaecol* 95:377, 1988.

McDowell BJ, Engberg SJ, Rodriguez E, et al: Characteristics of urinary incontinence in homebound older adults, *J Am Geriatr Soc* 44:963, 1996.

Norton C: The effects of urinary incontinence in women, *Int Rehabil Med* 4:9, 1982.

Oldenburg B, Millard RJ: Predictors of long term outcome following a bladder re-training programme, *J Psychosom Res* 30:691, 1986.

Ory MG, Wyman JF, Yu L: Psychosocial factors in urinary incontinence, *Clin Geriatr Med* 2:657, 1986.

Shumaker SA, Wyman JF, Uebersax JS, et al: Health-related quality of life measures for women with urinary incontinence: the Incontinence Impact Questionnaire and the Urogenital Distress Inventory, *Qual Life Res* 3:291, 1994.

Uebersax JS, Wyman JF, Shumaker SA, et al: Short forms to assess life quality and symptom distress for urinary incontinence in women: the Incontinence Impact Questionnaire and the Urogenital Distress Inventory, *Neurourol Urodyn* 14:131, 1995.

Vierhout ME, Gianotten WL: Mechanisms of urine loss during sexual activity, *Eur J Obstet Gynecol Reprod Biol* 52:45, 1993.

Walters MD, Taylor S, Schoenfeld LS: Psychosexual study of women with detrusor instability, *Obstet Gynecol* 75:22, 1990.

Wyman JF, Harkins SW, Fantl JA: Psychosocial impact of urinary incontinence in the community-dwelling population, *J Am Geriatr Soc* 38:282, 1990.

### Economic Issues

Baker DI, Bice TW: The influence of urinary incontinence on publicly financed home care services to low-income elderly people, *Gerontologist* 35:360, 1995.

Borrie MJ, Davidson HA: Incontinence in institutions: costs and contributing factors, *Can Med Assoc J* 147:332, 1992.

Cummings V, Holt R, van der Sloot C, et al: Costs and management of urinary incontinence in long-term care, *J Wound Ostomy Continence Nurs* 22:193, 1995.

Hu T: Impact of urinary incontinence on health-care costs, *J Am Geriatr Soc* 38:292, 1990.

Hu T: The cost impact of urinary incontinence on health care services. Paper presented at National Multi-Specialty Nursing Conference on Urinary Continence, Phoenix, AZ, 1994.

Schnelle JF, Keeler E, Hays RD, et al: A cost and value analysis of two interventions with incontinent nursing home residents, *J Am Geriatr Soc* 43:1112, 1995.

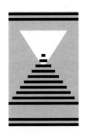

CHAPTER 4

# Description and Classification of Lower Urinary Tract Dysfunction and Pelvic Organ Prolapse

Mark D. Walters

## CLASSIFICATION SYSTEMS OF LOWER URINARY TRACT DYSFUNCTION

The purpose of any classification system is to facilitate understanding of the etiology and pathophysiology of disease, to help establish and standardize treatment and research guidelines, and to avoid confusion among those who are concerned with the problem. A number of classification systems for voiding disorders and stress urinary incontinence have been developed. These classifications have been based on various anatomic, radiographic, and urodynamic findings. The advantages, disadvantages, and applicability of the various classification systems of voiding dysfunction have been described by Wein and Barrett (1988). This chapter reviews two practical systems for the classification of voiding dysfunction in women. In addition, the differential diagnosis of urinary incontinence in women is discussed. It is hoped that the nomenclature used in these classification systems will become more widely understood and used and that further research will be aimed at defining their clinical applicability.

### International Continence Society Classification

In 1973 the International Continence Society (ICS) established a committee for the standardization of terminology of lower urinary tract function. Five of the first six reports from this committee were published. These reports were revised, extended, and collated in a monograph (see Appendix A). Following is a summary of their findings.

The lower urinary tract is composed of the bladder and urethra, which work together as a functional unit to promote storage and emptying of urine. Although a complete urodynamic investigation is not necessary for all symptomatic patients, some clinical or urodynamic assessment of the filling and voiding phases is essential for each patient. It is useful to examine bladder and urethral activity separately in each phase. If urodynamic studies are performed, results should clearly reflect the patient's symptoms and signs.

### Filling and Storage Phase

The ICS classification of abnormalities of the storage and voiding phases is outlined in Box 4-1. Cystometry is used to examine the bladder during filling and storage. Function should be described in terms of bladder (detrusor) activity, sensation, capacity, and compliance.

Detrusor activity may be normal or overactive. Overactive detrusor function is characterized by involuntary detrusor contractions during filling. They may be spontaneous or provoked and cannot be suppressed completely. Overactive detrusor function in the absence of a known neurologic abnormality is called *unstable detrusor;* overactivity caused by disturbance of the nervous control mechanisms is called *detrusor hyperreflexia.* These conditions are often associated with the symptom of urinary urgency. Urgency associated with overactive detrusor function is called motor urgency; urgency associated with bladder hypersensitivity is called sensory urgency.

Urethral function during storage can be assessed clinically (direct observation of urine loss with cough or Valsalva maneuver), urodynamically (urethral closure pressure profilometry and leak point pressure measurements), or radiographically (cystourethrography with or without video). The urethral closure mechanism may be normal or incompetent. An incompetent urethral closure mechanism is one that allows leakage of urine in the absence of a detrusor contraction. Leakage may occur whenever intravesical pressure exceeds intraurethral pressure (genuine stress incontinence) or when there is an involuntary fall in urethral pressure (unstable urethra). The definition and significance of the latter condition await additional data.

Urinary incontinence is an involuntary (urethral or extraurethral) loss of urine that can be demonstrated objectively and is a social or hygienic problem for the patient. Urinary incontinence is a symptom, a sign, and a condition. Urinary incontinence as a symptom means that the patient states she has involuntary urine loss. Types of incontinence symptoms include stress incontinence, urge incontinence, enuresis, postmicturition dribble, and continuous incontinence. The sign of stress incontinence denotes the observation of urine loss from the external urethral meatus synchronously with physical exertion such as a cough or Valsalva maneuver. Postmicturition dribble and continuous leakage are other signs of incontinence. Because symptoms and signs of urinary incontinence are sometimes misleading, accurate diagnosis often requires urodynamic investigation in addition to careful history and physical examination.

The ICS defines the following conditions of urinary incontinence:

*Genuine stress incontinence* is the involuntary loss of urine that occurs when, in the absence of a detrusor contraction, the intravesical pressure exceeds the maximum urethral pressure.

*Reflex incontinence* is the loss of urine caused by detrusor hyperreflexia or involuntary urethral relaxation in the absence of the sensation usually associated with the desire to void. This condition is seen only in patients with neuropathic bladder or urethral disorders.

*Overflow incontinence* is any involuntary loss of urine associated with overdistention of the bladder.

---

**Box 4-1**

**THE INTERNATIONAL CONTINENCE SOCIETY CLASSIFICATION OF LOWER URINARY TRACT DYSFUNCTION**

I. Storage phase
  A. Bladder function during storage
    1. Detrusor activity
      a. Normal
      b. Overactive
    2. Bladder sensation
      a. Normal
      b. Increased (hypersensitivity)
      c. Reduced (hyposensitivity)
      d. Absent
    3. Bladder capacity
    4. Bladder compliance
  B. Urethral function during storage
    1. Normal
    2. Incompetent
II. Voiding phase
  A. Detrusor function during voiding
    1. Normal
    2. Underactive
    3. Acontractile
  B. Urethral function during voiding
    1. Normal
    2. Obstructive
      a. Overactive
      b. Mechanical

---

## Voiding Phase

During the voiding phase, the detrusor muscle may be normal, underactive, or acontractile. Normal voiding usually is achieved by a voluntarily initiated detrusor contraction that is sustained and can be suppressed. An underactive detrusor during micturition implies that the detrusor contraction is of inadequate magnitude or duration to effect bladder emptying within a normal time span. Detrusor areflexia is defined as acontractility caused by an abnormality of nervous control and denotes the complete absence of centrally coordinated contraction.

During voiding, urethral function may be normal or obstructed. Obstruction may be caused by urethral overactivity, as in detrusor-external sphincter dyssynergia, or by mechanical obstruction, as with a urethral stricture or tumor.

Simultaneous measurement of intravesical or detrusor pressure and urine flow is necessary to determine whether the patient's voiding is obstructive. In general, high detrusor pressures with low flow rates suggest an obstructive problem, whereas low detrusor pressures with low flow rates imply that the problem is one of detrusor underactivity or acontractility. Simultaneous external urethral sphincter electromyography is necessary to determine whether an obstructive voiding pattern is secondary to urethral overactivity or mechanical obstruction.

## Functional Classification

Wein (1981) classified voiding dysfunction on a functional basis, describing the dysfunction simply in terms of whether the deficit is primarily one of the filling/storage phase or the voiding phase. Each section is subcategorized into whether the deficit is one of the bladder or the outlet. The expanded functional classification, as suggested by Wein (1998), is shown in Box 4-2.

A reasonably accurate urodynamic description is required for proper use of this system for a given voiding problem, but an exact diagnosis is not required for treatment. Several deficits can be present in the same patient, and all of them must be recognized to properly use this classification system.

## DIFFERENTIAL DIAGNOSIS OF URINARY INCONTINENCE

Among women complaining of urinary incontinence, the differential diagnosis includes genitourinary and nongenitourinary conditions (Box 4-3). As previously mentioned, genitourinary disorders include problems of bladder filling and storage, as well as extraurethral disorders such as fistula and congenital abnormalities. Nongenitourinary conditions that cause urinary incontinence generally are functional conditions that occur simultaneously with normal or abnormal urethral and bladder function. These conditions are most common in elderly women.

The most common urine storage disorder in women is genuine stress incontinence. Bladder filling disorders caused by overactive detrusor function are the second most common cause of urinary incontinence. Underactive or acontractile detrusor function may result in voiding dysfunction or urinary incontinence. As previously mentioned, involuntary loss of urine associated with overdistention of the bladder is called overflow incontinence. This condition is less prevalent in women and is usually associated with diabetes, neurologic diseases, severe genital prolapse, or postsurgical obstruction.

Functional incontinence is associated with cognitive, psychologic, or physical impairments that make it difficult to reach the toilet or interfere with appropriate toileting. With these conditions, continent women may not have enough time to avoid an accident. Functional causes also may act synergistically with other urinary problems. For example, women with manageable detrusor instability may become incontinent if another disease or physical problem keeps them from reaching the toilet. Physical conditions that may cause functional incontinence include joint abnormalities, arthritic pain, or muscular weakness. An unfamiliar setting, lack of convenient toilet facilities, or other environmental factors can aggravate this condition. Psychologic difficulties and repressed or hostile behavior may be related to incontinence, especially in the institutionalized elderly. Finally, iatrogenic factors, such as drugs, can cause or aggravate incontinence (see Chapter 5).

The relative likelihood of each condition causing incontinence varies with the age and health of the individual (Fig. 4-1). Among ambulatory incontinent women, the most common condition is genuine stress incontinence, which represents 50% to 70% of cases. Detrusor abnormalities

---

### Box 4-2
## EXPANDED FUNCTIONAL CLASSIFICATION

**Failure to Store**

*Because of the bladder*
Detrusor hyperactivity
    Involuntary contractions
        Neurologic disease, injury, or degeneration
        Bladder outlet obstruction
        Inflammation
        Idiopathic cause
    Decreased compliance
        Neurologic disease
        Fibrosis
        Idiopathic cause
Detrusor hypersensitivity
    Inflammation
    Infection
    Neurologic disease
    Psychologic cause
    Idiopathic cause

*Because of the outlet*
Stress incontinence (hypermobility related)
Nonfunctional bladder neck–proximal urethra (intrinsic sphincter dysfunction)

**Failure to Empty**

*Because of the bladder*
Neurologic disease
Myogenic cause
Psychologic cause
Idiopathic cause

*Because of the outlet*
Anatomic abnormality
Urethral compression: extramural (e.g., vaginal mass, prolapse, hematocolpos)
    Urethral mass (intramural or intraluminal)
    Urethral stricture
    Bladder neck contracture
Functional cause
    Smooth sphincter dyssynergia
    Striated sphincter dyssynergia

---

Modified from Wein AJ: Pathophysiology and categorization of voiding dysfunction. In Walsh PC, Retik AB, Vaughan ED, et al, eds: *Campbell's urology*, ed 7, Philadelphia, 1998, WB Saunders.

---

### Box 4-3
## DIFFERENTIAL DIAGNOSIS OF URINARY INCONTINENCE IN WOMEN

**Genitourinary Etiology**

*Filling/storage disorders*
Genuine stress incontinence
Detrusor instability (idiopathic)
Detrusor hyperreflexia (neurogenic)
Mixed types
Overflow incontinence

*Fistula*
Vesical
Ureteral
Urethral

*Congenital*
Ectopic ureter
Epispadias

**Nongenitourinary Etiology**

Functional
Neurologic
Cognitive
Environmental
Pharmacologic
Metabolic

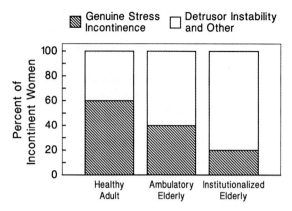

**Fig. 4-1** Estimated likelihood of conditions causing incontinence in women in various age categories.

and mixed forms (usually genuine stress incontinence and detrusor instability) account for 20% to 40% of incontinence cases. Among elderly, noninstitutionalized incontinent women evaluated in referral centers, genuine stress incontinence is found less often (30% to 46%), and detrusor abnormalities and mixed disorders are more common than in younger ambulatory women, occurring in 29% to 61% of cases. However, in a urodynamic study of elderly community-dwelling women with incontinence, Diokno et al. (1988) reported a prevalence of detrusor abnormalities of only 12%, probably reflecting a healthier group of women. Institutionalized elderly women who are incontinent have detrusor overactivity (with or without impaired bladder contractility) in 38% to 61% of cases and genuine stress incontinence in only 16% to 21% of cases.

## DESCRIPTION AND STAGING OF PELVIC ORGAN PROLAPSE

As with voiding dysfunction, a systematic description and classification of pelvic organ prolapse are useful to help document and communicate the severity of the problem, establish treatment guidelines, and improve the quality of research by standardizing definitions. Two general classification systems are in use, although it is likely that the ICS terminology will eventually be used by clinicians and researchers in the future.

For many years, the severity of pelvic organ prolapse has been described using criteria modified from Beecham (1980) and Baden et al. (1968). This system is simple to use; it is widely understood among gynecologic surgeons and has been found to have reasonable interobserver variability for all segments of the vagina and for uterine support. This system is described in Box 4-4. The most dependent position of the pelvic organs during maximum straining or standing is used. Classification of rectoceles can be aided by performing a rectovaginal examination.

In 1996, Bump et al. described the ICS standardization of terminology of female pelvic organ prolapse. In this system, the pelvic organ anatomy is described during physical examination of the external genitalia and vaginal canal. Segments of the lower reproductive tract replace the terms *cystocele, enterocele, rectocele,* and *urethrovesical junction* because these terms imply an unrealistic certainty as to the structures on the other side of the vaginal bulge, particularly in women who have had previous prolapse surgery. The examiner sees and describes the maximum protrusion noted by the patient during her daily activities. The details of the examination, including criteria for the endpoint of the examination and full development of the prolapse, should be specified. Suggested criteria for demonstration of maximum prolapse include one or all of the following: any protrusion of the vaginal wall has become tight during straining by the patient; traction on the prolapse causes no further descent; the subject confirms that the size of the prolapse and the extent of the protrusion seen by the examiner are as extensive as the most severe protrusion she has had (a small hand-held mirror to visualize the protrusion may be helpful); and a standing/straining examination confirms that the full extent of the prolapse was observed in the other positions used. Details about the patient position, types of vaginal specula or retractors, the type and intensity of straining used to develop the prolapse maximally, and the fullness of the bladder should be stated.

This descriptive system contains a series of site-specific measurements of the woman's pelvic organ support. Prolapse in each segment is evaluated and measured relative to the hymen (not introitus), which is a fixed anatomic landmark that can be identified consistently and precisely. The anatomic position of the six defined points for measurement should be centimeters above or proximal to the hymen (negative number) or centimeters below or distal to the hymen (positive number), with the plane of the hymen being defined as zero. For example, a cervix that protrudes 3 cm distal to the hymen should be described as +3 cm.

Six points (two on the anterior vaginal wall, two in the superior vagina, and two on the posterior vaginal wall) are located with reference to the plane of the hymen (Fig. 4-2). In describing the anterior vaginal wall, the term *anterior vaginal wall prolapse* is preferable to *cystocele* or *anterior enterocele* unless the organs involved are identified by ancillary tests. There are two anterior sites:

Point Aa: A point located in the midline of the anterior vaginal wall 3 cm proximal to the external urethral meatus, corresponding to the proximal location of the urethrovesical crease. By definition, the range of position of point Aa relative to the hymen is −3 to +3 cm.

Point Ba: A point that represents the most distal (i.e., most dependent) position of any part of the upper anterior vaginal wall from the vaginal cuff or anterior vaginal fornix to point Aa. By definition, point Ba is at −3 cm in the absence of prolapse and would have a positive value equal to the position of the cuff in women with total posthysterectomy vaginal eversion.

Two points are on the superior vagina. These points represent the most proximal locations of the normally positioned lower reproductive tract.

Point C: A point that represents either the most distal (i.e., most dependent) edge of the cervix or the leading edge of the vaginal cuff (hysterectomy scar) after total hysterectomy.

Point D: A point that represents a location of the posterior fornix in a woman who still has a cervix. It represents a level of uterosacral ligament attachment to the proximal posterior cervix. It is included as a point of measurement to differentiate suspensory failure of the uterosacral cardinal ligament complex from cervical elongation. Point D is omitted in the absence of the cervix.

Two points are located on the posterior vaginal wall. Analogous to anterior prolapse, posterior prolapse should be

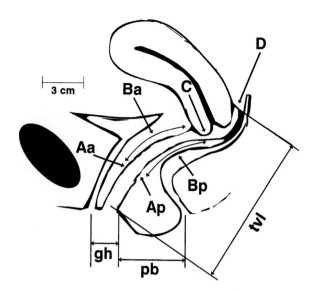

**Fig. 4-2**  Six sites (points *Aa, Ba, C, D, Bp,* and *Ap*), genital hiatus *(gh)*, perineal body *(pb)*, and total vaginal length *(tvl)* used for pelvic organ support quantitation.

From Bump RC, Mattiasson A, Bo K, et al: The standardization of terminology of female pelvic organ prolapse and pelvic floor dysfunction, *Am J Obstet Gynecol* 175:10, 1996.

discussed in terms of segments of the vaginal wall rather than the organs that lie behind it. Thus, the term *posterior vaginal wall prolapse* is preferable to *rectocele* or *enterocele* unless the organs involved are identified by ancillary tests. If small bowel appears to be present in the rectovaginal space, the examiner should comment on this fact and clearly describe the basis for this clinical impression (e.g., by observation of peristaltic activity in the distended posterior vagina or palpation of loops of small bowel between an examining finger in the rectum and one in the vagina). In such cases, a "pulsion" addendum to the point Bp position may be noted (e.g., Bp equals +5 [pulsion]; see following text for further discussion).

Point Bp: A point that represents the most distal (i.e., most dependent) position of any part of the upper posterior vaginal wall from the vaginal cuff of posterior vaginal fornix to point Ap. By definition, point Bp is at −3 cm in the absence of prolapse and would have a positive value equal to the position of the cuff in a woman with total posthysterectomy vaginal eversion.

Point Ap: A point located in the midline of the posterior vaginal wall 3 cm proximal to the hymen. By definition, the range of position point Ap relative to the hymen is −3 to +3 cm.

Other landmarks include the genital hiatus, which is measured from the middle of the external urethral meatus to the posterior midline hymen. The perineal body is measured from the posterior margin of the genital hiatus to the midanal opening. The total vaginal length is the greatest depth of the vagina in centimeters when point C or D is

| anterior wall **Aa** | anterior wall **Ba** | cervix or cuff **C** |
|---|---|---|
| genital hiatus **gh** | perineal body **pb** | total vaginal length **tvl** |
| posterior wall **Ap** | posterior wall **Bp** | posterior fornix **D** |

**Fig. 4-3**   Three-by-three grid for recording quantitative description of pelvic organ support.

From Bump RC, Mattiasson A, Bo K, et al: The standardization of terminology of female pelvic organ prolapse and pelvic floor dysfunction, *Am J Obstet Gynecol* 175:10, 1996.

reduced to its full normal position. The points and measurements are presented in Fig. 4-2.

The positions of points Aa, Ba, Ap, Bp, C, and (if applicable) D with reference to the hymen are measured and recorded. Positions are expressed as centimeters above or proximal to the hymen (negative number) or centimeters below or distal to the hymen (positive number), with the plane of the hymen defined as zero. Measurements may be recorded as a simple line of numbers (e.g., –3, –3, –7, –9, –3, –3, 9, 2, 2 for points Aa, Ba, C, D, Bp, Ap, total vaginal length, genital hiatus, and perineal body, respectively). Alternatively, a 3 × 3 grid can be used to concisely organize the measurements, as shown in Fig. 4-3, or a line diagram of a configuration can be drawn, as shown in Figs. 4-4 and 4-5. Fig. 4-4 is a grid and line diagram contrasting measurements indicating normal support to those of posthysterectomy vaginal eversion. Fig. 4-5 is a grid and line diagram representing predominant anterior and posterior vaginal wall prolapse with partial vault descent.

The profile for quantifying prolapse provides a precise description of anatomy for individual patients. An ordinal staging system of pelvic organ prolapse is suggested using these measurements and can be useful for the description of populations and for research comparisons. Stages are

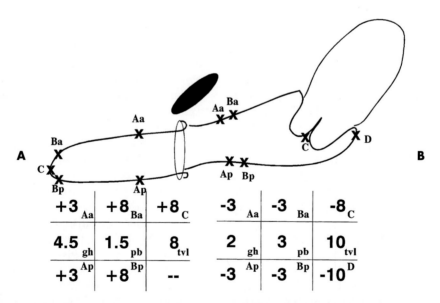

| +3 Aa | +8 Ba | +8 C |
|---|---|---|
| 4.5 gh | 1.5 pb | 8 tvl |
| +3 Ap | +8 Bp | -- |

| -3 Aa | -3 Ba | -8 C |
|---|---|---|
| 2 gh | 3 pb | 10 tvl |
| -3 Ap | -3 Bp | -10 D |

**Fig. 4-4**   **A**, Grid and line diagram of complete eversion of vagina. Most distal point of anterior wall (point *Ba*), vaginal cuff scar (point *C*), and most distal point of the posterior wall (point *Bp*) are all at same position (+8) and points *Aa* and *Ap* are maximally distal (both at +3). Because total vaginal length equals maximum protrusion, this is stage IV prolapse. **B**, Normal support. Points *Aa* and *Ba* and points *Ap* and *Bp* are all –3 because there is no anterior or posterior wall descent. Lowest point of the cervix is 8 cm above hymen (–8) and posterior fornix is 2 cm above this (–10). Vaginal length is 10 cm, and genital hiatus and perineal body measure 2 and 3 cm, respectively. This represents stage 0 support.

From Bump RC, Mattiasson A, Bo K, et al: The standardization of terminology of female pelvic organ prolapse and pelvic floor dysfunction, *Am J Obstet Gynecol* 175:10, 1996.

assigned according to the most severe portion of the prolapse when the full extent of the protrusion has been demonstrated. For a stage to be assigned to an individual subject, it is essential that her quantitative description be completed first. The five stages of pelvic organ support (0-IV) are described in Box 4-5.

Ancillary techniques for describing pelvic organ prolapse include performance of a digital rectal examination while the patient is straining; digital assessment of the contents of the rectovaginal septum during examination to differentiate between a "traction" enterocele (the posterior cul-de-sac is pulled down by the prolapsing cervix or

---

**Box 4-5**
## STAGES OF PELVIC ORGAN PROLAPSE

Stage 0    No prolapse is demonstrated. Points Aa, Ap, Ba, and Bp are all at −3 cm and either point C or D is between −TVL (total vaginal length) cm and −(TVL-2) cm (i.e., the quantitation value for point C or D is ≤−[TVL-2] cm). Fig. 4-4, *B*, represents stage 0.

Stage I    The criteria for stage 0 are not met, but the most distal portion of the prolapse is >1 cm above the level of the hymen (i.e., its quantitation value is <−1 cm).

Stage II    The most distal portion of the prolapse is ≤1 cm proximal to or distal to the plane of the hymen (i.e., its quantitation value is ≥−1 cm but ≤+1 cm).

Stage III    The most distal portion of the prolapse is >1 cm below the plane of the hymen but protrudes no further than 2 cm less than the total vaginal length in centimeters (i.e., its quantitation value is >+1 cm but <+[TVL-2] cm). Fig. 4-5 *A*, represents stage III Ba and Fig. 4-5, *B*, represents stage III Bp prolapse.

Stage IV    Essentially, complete eversion of the total length of the lower genital tract is demonstrated. The distal portion of the prolapse protrudes to at least (TVL-2) cm (i.e., its quantitation value is ≥+[TVL-2] cm). In most instances, the leading edge of stage IV prolapse is the cervix or vaginal cuff scar. Fig. 4-4, *A*, represents stage IV C prolapse.

From Bump RC, Mattiasson A, Bo K, et al: The standardization of terminology of female pelvic organ prolapse and pelvic floor dysfunction, *Am J Obstet Gynecol* 175:10, 1996.

---

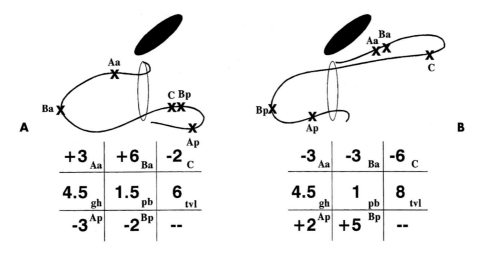

**Fig. 4-5** **A,** Grid and line diagram of predominant anterior support defect. Leading point of prolapse is upper anterior vaginal wall, point *Ba* (+6). There is significant elongation of bulging anterior wall. Point *Aa* is maximally distal (+3) and vaginal cuff scar is 2 cm above hymen (C = −2). Cuff scar has undergone 4 cm of descent because it would be at −6 (total vaginal length) if it were perfectly supported. In this example total vaginal length is not maximum depth of vagina with elongated anterior vaginal wall maximally reduced but rather depth of vagina at cuff with point *C* reduced to its normal full extent, as specified in text. This represents stage III Ba prolapse. **B,** Predominant posterior support defect. Leading point of prolapse is upper posterior vaginal wall, point *Bp* (+5). Point *Ap* is 2 cm distal to hymen (+2) and vaginal cuff scar is 6 cm above hymen (−6). Cuff has undergone only 2 cm of descent because it would be at −8 (total vaginal length) if it were perfectly supported. This represents stage III Bp prolapse.

From Bump RC, Mattiasson A, Bo K, et al: The standardization of terminology of female pelvic organ prolapse and pelvic floor dysfunction, *Am J Obstet Gynecol* 175:10, 1996.

vaginal cuff but is not distended by intestines) and a "pulsion" enterocele (the intestinal contents of the enterocele distend the rectal-vaginal septum and produce a protruding mass); cotton swab testing for the measurement of urethral axis mobility (Q-tip test); measurement of perineal descent; measurement of the transverse diameter of the genital hiatus or of the protruding prolapse; measurement of vaginal volume; description and measurement of rectal prolapse; and examination techniques differentiating between various types of defects (e.g., central versus paravaginal defects of the anterior vaginal wall). Cystoscopy and photography can be useful in describing pelvic organ prolapse. Imaging procedures include ultrasonography, contrast radiography, computed tomography, and magnetic resonance imaging. Intraoperative evaluation of pelvic support defects is intuitively attractive but of unproven value. The effect of anesthesia, diminished muscle tone, and loss of consciousness are of unknown magnitude and direction. Limitations because of the position of the patient must be evaluated.

Precise characterization of pelvic floor muscle strength and the description of functional symptoms are important. The reader is referred to the ICS committee document for further details (Bump et al., 1996).

## BIBLIOGRAPHY
### Classification of Urinary Incontinence

Abrams P, Blaivas JG, Stanton SL, et al: Sixth report on the standardization of terminology of lower urinary tract function. Procedures related to neurophysiological investigations: electromyography, nerve conduction studies, reflex latencies, evoked potentials and sensory testing, *World J Urol* 4:2, 1986; *Scand J Urol Nephrol* 20:161, 1986.

Abrams P, Blaivas JG, Stanton SL, et al: The standardization of terminology of lower tract function, *Scand J Urol Nephrol* 114(suppl):5, 1988.

Bates P, Bradley WE, Glen E, et al: First report on the standardization of terminology of lower urinary tract function. Urinary incontinence. Procedures related to the evaluation of urine storage: cystometry, urethral closure pressure profile, units of measurement, *Br J Urol* 48:39, 1976; *Eur Urol* 2:274, 1976; *Scand J Urol Nephrol* 11:193, 1976; *Urol Int* 32:81, 1976.

Bates P, Bradley WE, Glen E, et al: Second report on the standardization of terminology of lower urinary tract function. Procedures related to the evaluation of micturition: flow rate, pressure measurement, symbols, *Acta Urol Jpn* 27:1563, 1977; *Br J Urol* 49:207, 1977; *Scand J Urol Nephrol* 11:197, 1977.

Bates P, Bradley WE, Glen E, et al: Third report on the standardization of terminology of lower urinary tract function. Procedures related to the evaluation of micturition: pressure flow relationships, residual urine, *Br J Urol* 52:348, 1980; *Eur Urol* 6:170, 1980; *Acta Urol Jpn* 27:1566, 1980; *Scand J Urol Nephrol* 12:191, 1980.

Bates P, Bradley WE, Glen E, et al: Fourth report on the standardization of terminology of lower urinary tract function. Terminology related to neuromuscular dysfunction of lower urinary tract, *Br J Urol* 52:333, 1981; *Urology* 17:618, 1981; *Scand J Urol Nephrol* 15:169, 1981; *Acta Urol Jpn* 27:1568, 1981.

Bent AE, Richardson DA, Ostergard DR: Diagnosis of lower urinary tract disorders in postmenopausal patients, *Am J Obstet Gynecol* 145:218, 1983.

Blaivas JG: Classification of stress urinary incontinence, *Neurourol Urodyn* 2:103, 1983.

Blaivas JG, Olsson CA: Stress incontinence: classification and surgical approach, *J Urol* 139:727, 1988.

Castleton CM, Duffin HM, Asher MJ: Clinical and urodynamic studies in 100 elderly incontinent patients, *BMJ* 282:1103, 1981.

Diokno AC, Brown MB, Brock BM, et al: Clinical and cystometric characteristics of continent and incontinent non-institutionalized elderly, *J Urol* 140:567, 1988.

Enhorning G: Simultaneous recording of intravesical and intraurethral pressure, *Acta Chir Scand* 276(suppl):1, 1961.

McGuire EJ, Lytton B, Pepe V, et al: Stress urinary incontinence, *Am J Obstet Gynecol* 47:255, 1976.

Ouslander J, Staskin D, Raz S, et al: Clinical versus urodynamic diagnosis in an incontinent female geriatric population, *J Urol* 37:68, 1987.

Quigley GJ, Harper AC: The epidemiology of urethral-vesical dysfunction in the female patient, *Am J Obstet Gynecol* 151:220, 1985.

Resnick NM, Yalla SV, Laurino E: The pathophysiology of urinary incontinence among institutionalized elderly persons, *N Engl J Med* 320:1, 1989.

Wein AJ: Classification of neurogenic voiding dysfunction, *J Urol* 125:605, 1981.

Wein AJ: Pathophysiology and categorization of voiding dysfunction. In Walsh PC, Retik AB, Vaughan ED, et al, eds: *Campbell's urology,* ed 7, Philadelphia, 1998, WB Saunders.

Wein AJ, Barrett DM: *Voiding function and dysfunction,* Chicago, 1988, Mosby.

Williams ME, Pannill FC: Urinary incontinence in the elderly, *Ann Intern Med* 97:895, 1982.

### Classification of Pelvic Organ Prolapse

Baden WF, Walker T: Fundamental, symptoms, and classification. In Baden WF, Walker T, eds: *Surgical repair of vaginal defects,* Philadelphia, 1992, JB Lippincott.

Baden WF, Walker T, Lindsey JH: The vaginal profile, *Tex Med* 64:56, 1968.

Beecham CT: Classification of vaginal relaxation, *Am J Obstet Gynecol* 136:957, 1980.

Bump RC, Mattiasson A, Bo K, et al: The standardization of terminology of female pelvic organ prolapse and pelvic floor dysfunction, *Am J Obstet Gynecol* 175:10, 1996.

Hall AF, Theofrastous JP, Cundiff GW, et al: Interobserver and intraobserver reliability of the proposed International Continence Society, Society of Gynecologic Surgeons, and American Urogynecology Society pelvic organ prolapse classification system, *Am J Obstet Gynecol* 175:467, 1996.

Kobak WH, Rosenberger K, Walters MD: Interobserver variation in the assessment of pelvic organ prolapse, *Int Urogynecol J* 7:121, 1996.

Porges RF: A practical system of diagnosis and classification of pelvic relaxations, *Surg Gynecol Obstet* 117:769, 1963.

PART II
*Evaluation*

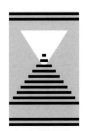

CHAPTER **5**

# Evaluation of Urinary Incontinence
## History, Physical Examination, and Office Tests

Mark D. Walters

Urinary incontinence can be a symptom of which patients complain, a sign demonstrated on examination, or a condition (i.e., diagnosis) that can be confirmed by definitive studies. When a woman complains of urinary incontinence, appropriate evaluation includes exploring the nature of her symptoms and looking for physical findings. The history and physical examination are the first and most important steps in the evaluation. A preliminary diagnosis can be made with simple office and laboratory tests, with initial therapy based on these findings. If complex conditions are present, if the patient does not improve after initial therapy, or if surgery is being considered, definitive, specialized studies are necessary.

## HISTORY AND PHYSICAL EXAMINATION
### History

Early in the interview, one should elicit a description of the patient's main complaint, including duration and frequency. A clear understanding of the severity of the problem or disability and its effect on quality of life should be sought. Assessment of mobility and living environment is especially important in certain patients. Questions should be asked about access to toilets or toilet substitutes and about social factors such as living arrangements, social contacts, and caregiver involvement.

Box 5-1 lists questions that are helpful in evaluating incontinence in women. The first question is designed to elicit the symptom of stress incontinence (i.e., urine loss with events that increase intraabdominal pressure). The symptom of stress incontinence is usually (but not always) associated with the diagnosis of genuine stress incontinence. Questions 2 through 9 help elicit the symptoms associated with detrusor instability. The symptom of urge incontinence is present if the patient answers question 3 affirmatively. Frequency (questions 4 and 5), bedwetting (question 6), leaking with intercourse (question 8), and a sense of urgency (questions 2 and 7) are all associated with detrusor instability. Questions 9 and 10 help to define the severity of the problem. Questions 11 through 13 screen for urinary tract infection and neoplasia, and questions 14 through 16 are designed to elicit symptoms of voiding dysfunction.

After the urologic history, thorough medical, surgical, gynecologic, neurologic, and obstetric histories should be obtained. Certain medical and neurologic conditions, such as diabetes, stroke, and lumbar disk disease, may cause urinary incontinence. Furthermore, strong coughing associated with chronic pulmonary disease can markedly worsen symptoms of stress incontinence. A bowel history should be noted because chronic severe constipation has been associated with voiding difficulties, urgency, stress incontinence, and increased bladder capacity. A history of hysterectomy, vaginal repair, pelvic radiotherapy, or retropubic surgery should alert the physician to the possibility of prior surgical trauma to the lower urinary tract.

A complete list of the patient's medications (including nonprescription medications) should be sought to determine whether individual drugs might influence the function of the bladder or urethra, leading to urinary incontinence or voiding difficulties. A list of drugs that commonly affect lower urinary tract function is shown in Table 5-1. In these cases, altering drug dosage or changing to a drug with similar therapeutic effectiveness, but with fewer lower urinary tract side effects, will often improve or "cure" the offending urinary tract symptom.

## Box 5-1

### HELPFUL QUESTIONS IN THE EVALUATION OF FEMALE URINARY INCONTINENCE

1. Do you leak urine when you cough, sneeze, or laugh?
2. Do you ever have such an uncomfortable strong need to urinate that if you don't reach the toilet you will leak?
3. If "yes" to question 2, do you ever leak before you reach the toilet?
4. How many times during the day do you urinate?
5. How many times do you void during the night after going to bed?
6. Have you wet the bed in the past year?
7. Do you develop an urgent need to urinate when you are nervous, under stress, or in a hurry?
8. Do you ever leak during or after sexual intercourse?
9. How often do you leak?
10. Do you find it necessary to wear a pad because of your leaking?
11. Have you had bladder, urine, or kidney infections?
12. Are you troubled by pain or discomfort when you urinate?
13. Have you had blood in your urine?
14. Do you find it hard to begin urinating?
15. Do you have a slow urinary stream or have to strain to pass your urine?
16. After you urinate, do you have dribbling or a feeling that your bladder is still full?

## Urinary Diary

Patient histories regarding frequency and severity of urinary symptoms are often inaccurate and misleading. Urinary diaries are more reliable and require the patient to record volume and frequency of fluid intake and of voiding, usually for a 1- to 7-day period. Episodes of urinary incontinence and associated events or symptoms such as coughing or urgency are noted. The number of times voided each night and any episodes of bedwetting are recorded the next morning. The maximum voided volume also provides a relatively accurate estimate of bladder capacity. The physician should review the frequency/volume charts with the patient and corroborate or modify the initial diagnostic impression. If excessive frequency and volume of fluid intake are noted, restriction of excessive oral fluid intake (combined with scheduled voiding) may improve symptoms of stress and urge incontinence by keeping the bladder volume below the threshold at which urinary leaking results.

## Gynecologic Examination

General, gynecologic, and lower neurologic examinations should be performed on every incontinent woman. The pelvic examination is of primary importance. Vaginal discharge can mimic incontinence, so evidence of this problem should be sought and, if present, treated. Vulvar

**Table 5-1** Medications That Can Affect Lower Urinary Tract Function

| Type of medication | Lower urinary tract effects |
| --- | --- |
| Diuretics | Polyuria, frequency, urgency |
| Caffeine | Frequency, urgency |
| Anticholinergic agents | Urinary retention, overflow incontinence |
| Alcohol | Sedation, impaired mobility, diuresis |
| Narcotic analgesics | Urinary retention, fecal impaction, sedation, delirium |
| Psychotropic agents | |
|    Antidepressants | Anticholinergic actions, sedation |
|    Antipsychotics | Anticholinergic actions, sedation |
|    Sedatives/hypnotics | Sedation, muscle relaxation, confusion |
| Alpha-adrenergic blockers | Stress incontinence |
| Alpha-adrenergic agonists | Urinary retention |
| Beta-adrenergic agonists | Urinary retention |
| Calcium-channel blockers | Urinary retention, overflow incontinence |

and vaginal atrophy consistent with hypoestrogenemia suggests that the urethra and periurethral tissues are also atrophic. Palpation of the anterior vaginal wall and urethra may elicit urethral discharge or tenderness that suggests a urethral diverticulum, carcinoma, or inflammatory condition of the urethra.

The presence and severity of anterior vaginal relaxation, including cystocele and proximal urethral detachment and mobility, or anterior vaginal scarring, are estimated. Associated pelvic support abnormalities, such as rectocele, enterocele, and uterovaginal prolapse, are noted. The amount or severity of prolapse in each vaginal segment should be measured and recorded according to guidelines noted in Chapter 4. A bimanual examination is performed to rule out coexistent gynecologic pathology, which can occur in up to two thirds of patients. The rectal examination further evaluates for pelvic pathology and fecal impaction, the latter of which may be associated with voiding difficulties and incontinence in elderly women. Urinary incontinence has been shown to improve or resolve after the removal of fecal impactions in institutionalized geriatric patients.

## Neurologic Examination

Urinary incontinence may be the presenting symptom of neurologic disease. The screening neurologic examination should evaluate mental status as well as sensory and motor function of both lower extremities. Mental status is determined by noting the patient's level of consciousness, orientation, memory, speech, and comprehension. Disorders associated with mental status aberrations that may produce neurourologic abnormalities include senile and presenile dementia, brain tumors, and normal pressure hydrocephalus.

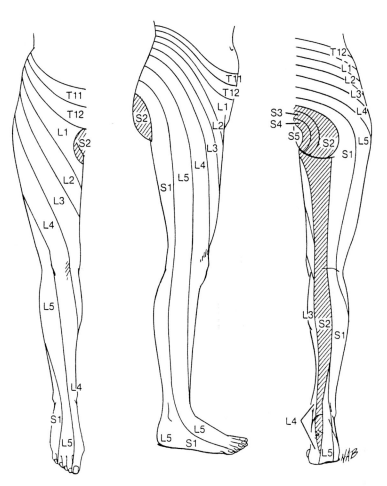

**Fig. 5-1**    Sensory dermatomes of the lower extremities and perineum. Shaded area represents sacral segments 2, 3, and 4.

Modified from Boileau Grant JC: *Grant's atlas of anatomy,* ed 6, Baltimore, 1972, Williams & Wilkins.

Evaluation of the motor and sensory systems may identify an occult neurologic lesion or can help determine the level of a known lesion. Common diseases associated with motor abnormalities that can produce urologic disturbances include Parkinson's disease, multiple sclerosis, cerebrovascular disease, infections, and tumors. Sacral segments 2 through 4, which contain the important neurons controlling micturition, are particularly important (Fig. 5-1). To test motor function, the patient extends and flexes the hip, knee, and ankle and inverts and everts the foot. The strength and tone of the bulbocavernosus muscle and external anal sphincter are estimated digitally. The patellar, ankle, and plantar reflex responses are tested. Sensory function along the sacral dermatomes is tested by using light touch and pinprick on the perineum and around the thigh and foot.

Two reflexes may help in the examination of sacral reflex activity. In the anal reflex, stroking the skin adjacent to the anus causes reflex contraction of the external anal sphincter muscle. The bulbocavernosus reflex involves contraction of the bulbocavernosus and ischiocavernosus muscles in re-

sponse to tapping or squeezing of the clitoris. Unfortunately, these reflexes can be difficult to evaluate clinically and are not always present, even in neurologically intact women.

## TECHNIQUES FOR MEASURING URETHRAL MOBILITY

Examination of the anterior vaginal wall is inaccurate in predicting the amount of urethral mobility. It is difficult with physical examination to differentiate between cystocele and rotational descent of the urethra and the two often coexist. Measuring urethral mobility aids in the diagnosis of genuine stress incontinence and in planning treatment for this condition (bladder neck suspension versus periurethral injection of bulking agents). Several tests are available for estimating the amount of urethral mobility in women.

### Radiologic Assessment

Lateral cystourethrography in the resting and straining view can identify mobility or fixation of the bladder neck, funneling of the bladder neck and proximal urethra, and degree of cystocele. The voiding component can identify a urethral diverticulum, fistula, obstruction, or vesicoureteral reflux. Videocystourethrography allows a dynamic assessment of the anatomy and function of the bladder base and urethra during retrograde filling with contrast material and during voiding. It is most helpful in sorting out causes of complex incontinence problems. However, it is invasive, expensive, and not widely available. For these reasons, other methods are usually used to measure urethral mobility in incontinent women.

## Ultrasonography

Ultrasonography is an alternative method of evaluating the urethrovesical anatomy. When compared to bead-chain cystourethrography, fluoroscopy, and the Q-tip test, perineal and vaginal ultrasonography accurately displays descent of the urethrovesical junction, opening of the bladder neck, and detrusor contractions. This technique appears to hold promise as a noninvasive and accurate method of evaluating the position and mobility of the urethrovesical junction and proximal urethra in incontinent women.

## Q-Tip Test

Placement of a cotton swab in the urethra to the level of the vesical neck and measurement of the axis change with straining can be used to demonstrate urethral mobility. To perform the Q-tip test, a sterile, lubricated cotton-tipped applicator is inserted transurethrally into the bladder, then withdrawn slowly until definite resistance is felt, indicating that the cotton tip is at the bladder neck. This is best accomplished with the patient in the supine lithotomy position during a pelvic examination. The resting angle of the applicator stick in relation to the horizontal is measured with a goniometer or protractor. The patient is then asked to cough and perform a Valsalva maneuver, and the maximum straining angle from the horizontal is measured. Results are not affected by the amount of urine in the bladder. Care should be taken to ensure that the cotton tip is not in the bladder or at the mid-urethra because this results in a falsely low measurement of urethral mobility.

Although maximum straining angle measurements greater than 30 degrees are generally considered to be abnormal, few data are available to differentiate normal from abnormal measurements. Urethral mobility in continent women is probably related to age, parity, and support defects of the anterior vaginal wall. Walters and Diaz (1987) noted that asymptomatic women with a mean parity of two and a mean age of 32 years had an average resting Q-tip angle of 18 degrees and an average maximum straining angle of 54 degrees. Women with genuine stress incontinence had a significantly higher maximum straining angle of 73 degrees, although there was wide overlap in measurements between the continent and incontinent women. These data indicate that arbitrary cutoff values around 30 degrees are too low to define "normal" urethral mobility for parous women.

## PERINEAL PAD TESTS

Perineal pad weighing may be used when one wants to document objectively the presence and amount of urine loss. The test should approximate activities in daily life and should evaluate as long a period as possible, yet be practical. A 1-hour period of testing is recommended and can be extended for additional 1-hour periods if the result of the first test is not considered representative of the symptoms by either the patient or the physician. Alternatively, the test can be performed after filling the bladder to a defined volume or at home over a 24-hour period.

The total amount of urine lost during the test period is determined by weighing a collecting device such as an absorbent pad. The pad should be worn inside waterproof underpants or should have a waterproof backing. Care should be taken to use a collecting device of adequate capacity. Immediately before the test begins the collecting device is weighed to the nearest gram. A typical test schedule is started without the patient voiding and with drinking approximately 500 ml of fluid. A period of walking, coughing, exercise, and hand-washing is done. At the end of the 1-hour test the collecting device is removed and weighed. If the test is regarded as representative, the patient voids and the volume is recorded; if not, the test is repeated for an additional hour.

If the collecting device becomes saturated or filled during the test, it should be removed, weighed, and replaced. The total weight of urine lost during the test period is taken to be equal to the gain in weight of the collecting device(s). In interpreting the results of the test, it should be remembered that a weight gain of up to 1 g may be due to weighing errors, sweating, or vaginal discharge.

Two critical variables determine the sensitivity of pad weighing: the amount of fluid in the bladder during exercise and the type of activity used to generate increased intraabdominal pressure. Lose et al. (1986) found that pad weight correlated significantly with the fluid load on the bladder (i.e., the initial volume plus diuresis). Pad weighing has acceptable test-retest reliability and is easy to perform in a clinical setting. However, it has low sensitivity and poor correlation between pad gain and videographic assessment of incontinence severity. These shortcomings have limited acceptance of pad weighing as a routine part of the evaluation of incontinence.

Phenazopyridine hydrochloride (Pyridium) is sometimes used to aid clinicians in differentiating urinary continence from incontinence in women with disturbing vaginal wetness. Patients are given Pyridium tablets and instructed to wear a sanitary pad for a given time. The pad is then removed and examined. Red-orange staining is taken as evidence that urine loss has occurred. Although this test may occasionally be useful, Wall et al. (1990) demonstrated that although all incontinent women had pad staining, 52% of healthy continent women also had staining, reflecting a high rate of false-positive tests.

## OFFICE DIAGNOSTIC TESTS
### Laboratory

Few laboratory tests are necessary for the evaluation of incontinence. A clean midstream or catheterized urine sample should be obtained for dipstick urinalysis. Urine culture and sensitivity should be obtained when the dipstick test indicates infection. Acute cystitis can present with multiple irritative symptoms, such as dysuria, frequency, urgency, incontinence, and voiding difficulty. In these cases, treatment of the infection usually eradicates the symptoms. However, bacteriuria is often asymptomatic, especially in the elderly. Boscia et al. (1986) demonstrated that no differences in urinary symptoms were found when elderly bacteriuric subjects were compared with themselves when they were nonbacteriuric. In view of these conflicting data, it seems reasonable to examine the urine for infection in all incontinent patients and, if bacteriuria is found, to prescribe appropriate antibiotics and reevaluate the patient in several weeks.

Blood testing (BUN, creatinine, glucose, and calcium) is recommended if compromised renal function is suspected or if polyuria (in the absence of diuretics) is present. Urine cytology is not recommended in the routine evaluation of the incontinent patient. However, patients with hematuria (2 to 5 RBC/hpf) or acute onset of irritative voiding symptoms in the absence of urinary tract infection require cystoscopy and cytology to exclude bladder neoplasm.

### Evaluation of Bladder Filling and Voiding

The office evaluation of incontinence should involve some assessment of voiding, detrusor function during filling, and competency of the urethral sphincteric mechanism. During the assessment, one should try to determine the specific circumstances leading to the involuntary loss of urine. If possible, such circumstances should be reproduced and directly observed during clinical evaluation. The examination is most easily initiated with the patient's bladder comfortably full. The patient is allowed to void as normally as possible in private. The time to void and the amount of urine voided are recorded. The patient then returns to the examination room and the volume of residual urine is noted by transurethral catheterization. If a sterile urine sample has not yet been obtained for analysis, it can be obtained at this time. A 50-ml syringe without its piston or bulb is attached to the catheter and held above the bladder. The patient is then asked to sit or stand and the bladder is filled by gravity by pouring 50-ml aliquots of sterile water into the syringe (Fig. 5-2). The patient's first bladder sensation and maximum bladder capacity are noted. The water level in the syringe should be closely observed during filling, as any rise in the column of water can be secondary to a detrusor contraction. Unintended increases in intraabdominal pressure by the patient should be avoided.

The catheter is then removed and the patient is asked to cough in a standing position. Loss of small amounts of urine

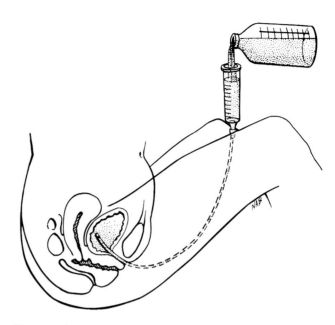

**Fig. 5-2** Office evaluation of bladder filling function. In sitting or standing position with a catheter in the bladder, the bladder is filled by gravity by pouring sterile water into the syringe.

in spurts simultaneous with the coughs strongly suggests a diagnosis of genuine stress incontinence. Prolonged loss of urine, leaking 5 to 10 seconds after coughing, or no urine loss with provocation indicates that other causes of incontinence, especially detrusor instability, may be present. Interpretation of these office tests can be difficult because of artifact introduced by rises in intraabdominal pressure caused by straining or patient movement. Borderline or negative tests should be repeated to maximize their diagnostic accuracy.

## MAKING THE DIAGNOSIS

Based on the clinical evaluation, the physician can formulate a presumptive diagnosis and initiate treatment, using the algorithm in Fig. 5-3 as a guide. Similar guidelines for evaluation of incontinence were proposed by Fantl et al. (1996) and have been used with success in elderly patients. The initial goal should be to diligently seek out and treat all reversible causes of urinary incontinence and voiding difficulty (see Box 5-2). Complex causes of incontinence are triaged for urodynamic testing or for consultation (see Box 5-3).

After the evaluation, patients can be categorized as having probable genuine stress incontinence or probable detrusor instability (with or without coexistent stress incontinence). For either diagnosis, appropriate behavioral or medical therapy can be given and a substantial percentage of patients expected to respond. Even patients with mixed disorders (coexistent genuine stress incontinence and detrusor instability) respond to various forms of conservative therapy in about 60% of cases.

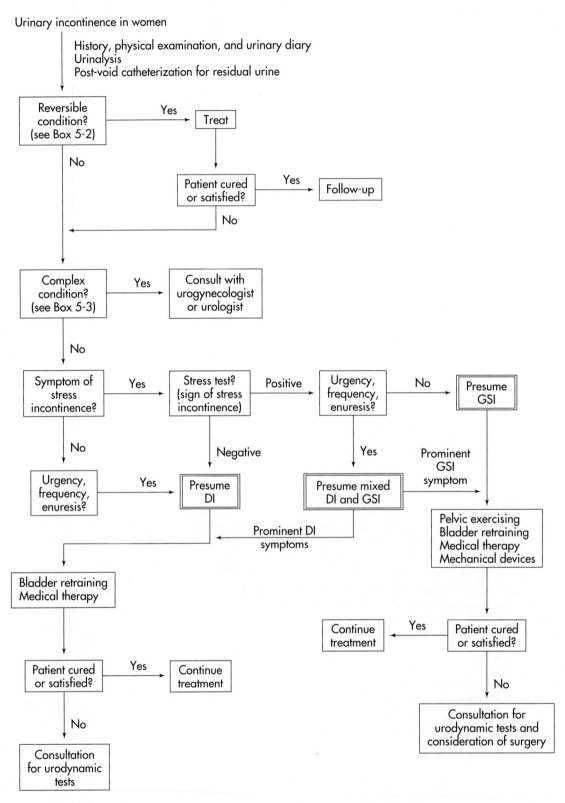

**Fig. 5-3**   Algorithm for clinical assessment of urinary incontinence in women. *GSI,* Genuine stress incontinence; *DI,* detrusor instability.

**Box 5-2**

**REVERSIBLE CONDITIONS THAT CAUSE OR CONTRIBUTE TO URINARY INCONTINENCE**

Conditions affecting the lower urinary tract
  Urinary tract infection
  Urethritis
  Atrophic vaginitis/urethritis
  Pregnancy/vaginal delivery
  Stool impaction
Drug side effects (see Table 5-1)
Increased urine production
  Metabolic (hyperglycemia, hypercalcemia)
  Excess fluid intake
  Volume overload
Impaired ability or willingness to reach toilet
  Delirium
  Chronic illness, injury, or restraint that interferes with
    mobility
  Psychologic

**Box 5-3**

**SITUATIONS THAT WARRANT CONSULTATION FOR THE EVALUATION AND TREATMENT OF LOWER URINARY TRACT DYSFUNCTION**

Uncertain diagnosis and inability to develop a reasonable treatment plan based on the basic diagnostic evaluation. Uncertainty in diagnosis may occur when there is lack of correlation between symptoms and clinical findings.
Failure to respond to the patient's satisfaction to an adequate therapeutic trial, and the patient is interested in pursuing further therapy.
Consideration of surgical intervention, particularly if previous surgery failed or the patient has a high surgical risk.
The presence of other comorbid conditions:
  • Incontinence associated with recurrent symptomatic urinary tract infection
  • Persistent symptoms of difficult bladder emptying
  • History of previous antiincontinence surgery, radical pelvic surgery, or pelvic radiation therapy
  • Symptomatic pelvic prolapse, especially if beyond hymen
  • Abnormal postvoid residual urine
  • Neurologic condition such as multiple sclerosis or spinal cord lesions or injury
Fistula or suburethral diverticulum.
Hematuria without infection.

## DIAGNOSTIC ACCURACY OF OFFICE EVALUATIONS

The findings of a careful history and physical examination predict the actual incontinence diagnosis with reasonable accuracy. Women who have the symptom of stress incontinence as their only complaint have a 64% to 90% chance of having genuine stress incontinence confirmed on diagnostic urodynamic testing. Of these patients, 10% to 30% are found to have detrusor instability (alone or coexistent with genuine stress incontinence). Other rare conditions that can cause the symptom of stress incontinence are urethral diverticulum, genitourinary fistula, ectopic ureter, and urethral instability. Physical findings associated with genuine stress incontinence are anterior vaginal relaxation, urethral hypermobility, and observed transurethral loss of urine with coughing.

Sensory urgency, urge incontinence, diurnal and nocturnal frequency, and bedwetting all have been associated with unstable bladder. The more of these abnormal urinary symptoms the patient has, the greater the chance that she has an unstable bladder. Cantor and Bates (1980) observed that 81% of patients with three or more of these symptoms had detrusor instability on cystometry. The physical findings of abnormal neurologic examination and absent urethral hypermobility in a woman with incontinence have been associated with overactive detrusor function.

Is the determination of urethral mobility useful in diagnosing the cause of urinary incontinence? Urethrocystographic findings, such as the posterior urethrovesical angle, funneling of the proximal urethra on straining, and angle of urethral inclination, do not differ between continent

and incontinent women with pelvic relaxation. Numerous authors have shown that although the bead-chain cystourethrogram and Q-tip test accurately reflect the amount of urethral mobility with stress, they are of little value in differentiating genuine stress incontinence from detrusor instability. Furthermore, serial addition of the measurement of urethral inclination with a Q-tip to the history and pelvic examination does not appreciably change the sensitivity or specificity for diagnosing genuine stress incontinence. However, because most women with primary genuine stress incontinence have urethral hypermobility, a negative test should cause one to question that diagnosis, perhaps indicating the need to perform urodynamic testing. Clearly, the measurement of urethral mobility should not be used to differentiate urethral sphincter incompetence from abnormalities of voiding or detrusor function because these diagnoses require the measurement of detrusor pressure during filling and emptying.

Although the determination of urethral mobility is not useful in the diagnosis of urinary incontinence, it may provide some information about which surgical therapy is most appropriate. In patients with genuine stress incontinence, anterior colporrhaphy, needle urethropexy, or a retropubic suspension procedure is used when urethral hypermobility is found to coexist with relatively normal intrinsic urethral sphincteric function. When urethral hypermobility is found in a patient with findings of intrinsic sphincter deficiency, a sling procedure is usually recommended. When the urethra is nonmobile or intrinsically functionless, periurethral injection of bulking agents or artificial urinary sphincter is likely to provide better results. Thus, measurement of urethral mobility can aid the surgeon in choosing one group of surgical procedures over another, but cannot determine which procedures yield the best results in each clinical situation.

Retrograde bladder filling provides an assessment of bladder sensation and an estimate of bladder capacity. Patients without urgency and frequency who note a sensation of bladder fullness and have an estimated bladder capacity that is within normal range probably have normal bladder filling function. There seems to be no clear consensus about the definition of normal bladder capacity. Values range from 300 to 750 ml. However, large bladder capacities are not always pathologic. Weir and Jaques (1974) showed that 33% of women with bladder capacities greater than 800 ml were urodynamically normal and only 13% had true bladder atony.

In the absence of symptoms of voiding difficulty, patients usually have normal voiding function. The incidence of asymptomatic voiding dysfunction among women with other urologic complaints is only about 3%. Normal values for postvoid residual urine measurements have not been established. Volumes less than 50 ml indicate adequate bladder emptying and volumes greater than 200 ml can be considered inadequate emptying. Clinical judgment must be exercised in interpreting the significance of postvoid residual urine volumes, especially in the intermediate range of 50 to 200 ml. Because isolated instances of elevated residual urine volume may not be significant, the test should be repeated when abnormally high values are obtained. Among women with symptoms of voiding difficulty and those who appear to void abnormally or have retention, more sophisticated testing is required to determine the causes and the mechanism of the voiding dysfunction.

## INDICATIONS FOR URODYNAMIC TESTS

The physician must recognize that even under the most typical clinical situations, the diagnosis of incontinence based only on clinical evaluation may be uncertain. This diagnostic uncertainty may be acceptable if medical or behavioral treatment (as opposed to surgery) is planned because of the low morbidity and cost of these treatments and because the ramifications of noncure (continued incontinence) are not severe. When surgical treatment of stress incontinence is planned, urodynamic testing is recommended to confirm the diagnosis.

As noted, consultation should be considered for complex cases that may require urodynamic testing or surgical treatment. Whenever objective clinical findings do not correlate with or reproduce the patient's symptoms, urodynamic testing is indicated for diagnosis. Finally, when trials of therapy are used, patients must be followed up periodically to evaluate response. If the patient fails to improve to her satisfaction, appropriate further testing is indicated.

## BIBLIOGRAPHY
### History and Physical Examination

Bannister JJ, Laurence WT, Smith A, et al: Urological abnormalities in young women with severe constipation, *Gut* 29:17, 1988.

Benson JT: Gynecologic and urodynamic evaluation of women with urinary incontinence, *Obstet Gynecol* 66:691, 1985.

Blaivas JG, Zayed AAH, Kamal BL: The bulbocavernosus reflex in urology: a prospective study of 299 patients, *J Urol* 126:197, 1981.

Diokno AC, Wells TJ, Brink CA: Comparison of self-reported voided volume with cystometric bladder capacity, *J Urol* 137:698, 1987.

Fantl JA, Wyman JF, Wilson MS, et al: Diuretics and urinary incontinence in community-dwelling women, *Neurourol Urodyn* 9:25, 1990.

Gormley EA, Griffiths DJ, McCracken PN, et al: Polypharmacy and its effect on urinary incontinence in a geriatric population, *Br J Urol* 71:265, 1993.

Hilton P, Stanton SL: Algorithmic method for assessing urinary incontinence in elderly women, *BMJ* 282:940, 1981.

Julian TM: Pseudoincontinence secondary to unopposed estrogen replacement in the surgically castrate premenopausal female, *Obstet Gynecol* 70:382, 1987.

Larson G, Victor A: The frequency-volume chart in genuine stress incontinent women, *Neurourol Urodyn* 1:23, 1992.

Walters MD, Realini JP: The evaluation and treatment of urinary incontinence in women: a primary care approach, *J Am Board Fam Pract* 5:289, 1992.

Williams ME, Gaylord SA: Role of functional assessment in the evaluation of urinary incontinence, National Institutes of Health Consensus Development Conference on Urinary Incontinence in Adults, Bethesda, MD, October 3-5, 1988, *J Am Geriatr Soc* 38:296, 1990.

Wyman JF, Choi SC, Harkins SW, et al: The urinary diary in evaluation of incontinent women: a test-retest analysis, *Obstet Gynecol* 71:812, 1988.

### Techniques for Measuring Urethral Mobility

Bergman A, McCarthy TA, Ballard CA, et al: Role of the Q-tip test in evaluating stress urinary incontinence, *J Reprod Med* 32:273, 1987.

Bhatia NN, Ostergard DR, McQuown D: Ultrasonography in urinary incontinence, *Urology* 29:90, 1987.

Crystle CD, Charme LS, Copeland WE: Q-tip test in stress urinary incontinence, *Obstet Gynecol* 38:313, 1971.

Fantl JA, Hurt WG, Bump RC, et al: Urethral axis and sphincteric function, *Am J Obstet Gynecol* 155:554, 1986.

Gordon D, Pearce M, Norton P: Comparison of ultrasound and lateral chain urethrocystography in the determination of bladder neck position and descent, *Neurourol Urodyn* 5:181, 1987.

Karram MM, Narender N, Bhatia MD: The Q-tip test: standardization of the technique and its interpretation in women with urinary incontinence, *Obstet Gynecol* 71:807, 1988.

Koelbl H, Hanzal E, Bernaschek G: Sonographic urethrocystography: methods and applications in patients with genuine stress incontinence, *Int Urogynecol J* 2:25, 1991.

Kohorn EI, Scioscia AL, Jeanty P, et al: Ultrasound cystourethrography by perineal scanning for the assessment of female stress urinary incontinence, *Obstet Gynecol* 68:269, 1986.

Montella JM, Ewing S, Cater J: Visual assessment of urethrovesical junction mobility, *Int Urogynecol J* 8:13, 1997.

Mouritsen L, Strandberg C, Jensen AR, et al: Inter- and intra-observer variation of colpo-cysto-urethrography diagnoses, *Acta Obstet Gynecol Scand* 72:2000, 1993.

Schaer GN, Koechli OR, Schuessler B, et al: Perineal ultrasound for evaluating the bladder neck in urinary stress incontinence, *Obstet Gynecol* 85:220, 1995.

Walters MD, Diaz K: Q-tip test: a study of continent and incontinent women, *Obstet Gynecol* 70:208, 1987.

## Perineal Pad Tests

Abrams P, Blaivas JG, Stanton SL, et al: The standardization of terminology of lower urinary tract function recommended by the International Continence Society, *Int Urogynecol J* 1:45, 1990.

Fantl JA, Harkins SW, Wyman JF, et al: Fluid loss quantitation test in women with urinary incontinence: a test-retest analysis, *Obstet Gynecol* 70:739, 1987.

Haylen BT, Frazer MI, Sutherst JR: Diuretic response to fluid load in women with urinary incontinence: optimum duration of pad test, *Br J Urol* 62:331, 1988.

Jakobsen H, Vedel P, Andersen JT: Which pad-weighing test to choose: ICS one hour test, the 48 hour home test or a 40 min test with known bladder volume? *Neurourol Urodyn* 4:23, 1987.

Jorgensen L, Lose G, Anderson JT: One hour pad-weighing test for objective assessment of female urinary incontinence, *Obstet Gynecol* 69:39, 1987.

Kinn A-C, Larsson B: Pad test with fixed bladder volume in urinary stress incontinence, *Acta Obstet Gynecol Scand* 55:369, 1987.

Klarskov P, Hald T: Reproducibility and reliability of urinary incontinence assessment with a 60 min test, *Scand J Urol Nephrol* 18:293, 1984.

Lose G, Gammelgaard J, Jorgenson TJ: The one-hour pad-weighing test: reproducibility and the correlation between the test result, the start volume in the bladder, and the diuresis, *Neurourol Urodyn* 5:17, 1986.

Richmond DH, Sutherst JR, Brown MC: Quantification of urine loss by weighing perineal pads. Observation on the exercise regimen, *Br J Urol* 59:224, 1987.

Sutherst JR, Brown MC, Richmond D: Analysis of the pattern of urine loss in women with incontinence as measured by weighing perineal pads, *Br J Urol* 58:273, 1986.

Versi E, Cardozo L: Perineal pad weighing versus videographic analysis in genuine stress incontinence, *Br J Obstet Gynaecol* 93:364, 1986.

Versi E, Orrego G, Hardy E, et al: Evaluation of the home pad test in the investigation of female urinary incontinence, *Br J Obstet Gynaecol* 103:162, 1996.

Wall LL, Want K, Robson I, et al: The pyridium pad test for diagnosing urinary incontinence, *J Reprod Med* 35:682, 1990.

Walters MD, Dombroski RA, Prihoda TJ: Perineal pad testing in the quantitation of urinary incontinence, *Int Urogynecol J* 1:3, 1990.

## Office Diagnostic Tests

Abrams P: The practice of urodynamics. In Mundy AR, Stephenson TP, Wein AJ, eds: *Urodynamics,* Edinburgh, 1984, Churchill Livingstone.

Abrams P, Feneley R, Torrens M: The clinical contribution of urodynamics. In Chism DG, ed: *Urodynamics,* New York, 1983, Springer-Verlag.

Boscia JA, Kobasa WD, Abrutyn E, et al: Lack of association between bacteriuria and symptoms in the elderly, *Am J Med* 81:979, 1986.

Brocklehurst JC, Dillane JB, Griffiths L, et al: The prevalence and symptomatology of urinary infection in an aged population, *Gerontol Clin* 10:242, 1968.

Eastwood HDH, Warrell R: Urinary incontinence in the elderly female: prediction in diagnosis and outcome of management, *Age Ageing* 13:230, 1984.

Fantl JA, Newman DK, Colling J, et al: *Urinary incontinence in adults: acute and chronic management.* Clinical Practice Guideline No 2, 1996 Update, Rockville MD, March 1996, U.S. Department of Health and Human Services, Public Health Service, Agency for Health Care Policy and Research, AHCPR Pub No 96-0682.

Marshall VF, Marchetti A, Krantz K: The correction of stress incontinence by simple vesicourethral suspension, *Surg Gynecol Obstet* 88:509, 1949.

Migliorini GD, Glenning PP: Bonney's test: fact or fiction? *Br J Obstet Gynaecol* 94:157, 1987.

Poston G, Joseph A, Riddle P: The accuracy of ultrasound and the measurement of changes in bladder volume, *Br J Urol* 55:361, 1983.

Sourander LB: Urinary tract infection in the aged. An epidemiological study, *Ann Med Intern Fenn* 55(suppl 45):1, 1966.

Stanton SL: Voiding difficulties and retention. In Stanton SL (ed): *Clinical gynecologic urology,* St Louis, 1984, Mosby.

Stanton SL, Ozsoy C, Hilton P: Voiding difficulties in the female: prevalence, clinical and urodynamic review, *Obstet Gynecol* 61:144, 1983.

Utz DC, Zincke H: The masquerade of bladder cancer in situ as interstitial cystitis, *J Urol* 111:160, 1974.

Wein AJ, Barrett DM: *Voiding function and dysfunction,* Chicago, 1988, Mosby.

Weir J, Jaques PF: Large capacity bladder, *Urology* 4:544, 1974.

## Diagnostic Accuracy of Office Evaluation and Indications for Urodynamic Testing

Arnold EP, Webster JR, Loose H, et al: Urodynamics of female incontinence: factors influencing the results of surgery, *Am J Obstet Gynecol* 117:805, 1973.

Byrne DJ, Hamilton Stewart PA, Gray BK: The role of urodynamics in female urinary stress incontinence, *Br J Urol* 59:228, 1987.

Cantor TJ, Bates CP: Comparative study of symptoms and objective urodynamic findings in 214 incontinent women, *Br J Obstet Gynaecol* 87:889, 1980.

Drutz HP, Mandel F: Urodynamic analysis of urinary incontinence symptoms in women, *Am J Obstet Gynecol* 134:789, 1979.

Farrar DJ, Whiteside CG, Osborne JL, et al: A urodynamic analysis of micturition symptoms in the female, *Surg Gynecol Obstet* 144:875, 1975.

Fischer-Rasmussen W, Hansen RI, Stage P: Predictive values of diagnostic tests in the evaluation of female urinary stress incontinence, *Acta Obstet Gynecol Scand* 65:291, 1986.

Jensen JK, Nielsen FR, Ostergard DR: The role of patient history in the diagnosis of urinary incontinence, *Obstet Gynecol* 83:904, 1994.

Kadar N: The value of bladder filling in the clinical detection of urine loss and selection of patients for urodynamic testing, *Br J Obstet Gynaecol* 95:698, 1988.

Karram MM, Bhatia NN: Management of coexistent stress and urge urinary incontinence, *Obstet Gynecol* 73:4, 1989.

Korda A, Krieger M, Hunter P, et al: The value of clinical symptoms in the diagnosis of urinary incontinence in the female, *Aust NZ J Obstet Gynecol* 27:149, 1987.

Moolgaoker AS, Ardran GM, Smith JC, et al: The diagnosis and management of urinary incontinence in the female, *J Obstet Gynaecol Br Commonw* 79:481, 1972.

Ouslander JG: Diagnostic evaluation of geriatric urinary incontinence, *Clin Geriatr Med* 2:715, 1986.

Ouslander J, Staskin D, Raz S, et al: Clinical versus urodynamic diagnosis in an incontinent female geriatric population, *J Urol* 37:68, 1987.

Quigley GJ, Harper AC: The epidemiology of urethral-vesical dysfunction in the female patient, *Am J Obstet Gynecol* 151:220, 1985.

Sand PK, Hill RC, Ostergard DR: Incontinence history as a predictor of detrusor stability, *Obstet Gynecol* 71:257, 1988.

Swift SE, Ostergard DR: Evaluation of current urodynamic testing methods in the diagnosis of genuine stress incontinence, *Obstet Gynecol* 86:85, 1995.

Walters MD, Shields LE: The diagnostic value of history, physical examination, and the Q-tip cotton swab test in women with urinary incontinence, *Am J Obstet Gynecol* 159:145, 1988.

Webster GD, Sihelnik SA, Stone AR: Female urinary incontinence: the incidence, identification, and characteristics of detrusor instability, *Neurourol Urodyn* 3:235, 1984.

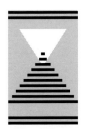

CHAPTER **6**

# Urodynamics: Cystometry

Mickey M. Karram

---

---

The term *urodynamics* means observation of the changing function of the lower urinary tract over time. Urodynamic tests have been slow to achieve acceptance and are by no means universally used; however, in recent years there has been a resurgence of interest in the hydrodynamic and neurophysiologic aspects of the storage and evacuation of urine. An abundance of new diagnostic procedures, methodologies, and testing equipment have made it exceedingly difficult for the clinician to decide what tests are necessary to adequately evaluate lower urinary tract dysfunction in women.

To understand the fundamental value of urodynamics, one should realize that the female bladder responds similarly to a variety of pathologies. Symptoms do not always reflect accurately the physiologic state of the bladder. For example, a patient may feel that her bladder is full when it is nearly empty, or that her bladder is contracting when it is not. Nevertheless, the evaluation of a woman with lower urinary tract complaints should not exclude the basic history and physical examination. The validity of any urodynamic diagnosis is linked to the patient's symptoms and the reproduction of these symptoms during the testing session. To obtain the most accurate, clinically relevant interpretation of urodynamic studies, the urodynamicist should clearly understand lower urinary tract function and correlate

urodynamic data with other clinical information. Ideally, the urodynamicist should be the physician who takes the history, performs the physical examination, interprets other tests, explains the diagnosis, and develops a reasonable management plan.

Results of urodynamic investigations should be recorded in a way that can be communicated among physicians and other health care personnel. For this reason, the recommendations detailed in the standardization reports of the International Continence Society (ICS) should be followed (see Appendix A).

Chapters 6 through 8 discuss urodynamic modalities used in the evaluation of filing, storage, and evacuation of urine. The intent is to give the reader a clear understanding of the rationale, technique, utility, and limitations of each test.

## PRINCIPLES OF CYSTOMETRY

The first cystometer dates back to 1872 when Schatz accidentally discovered a crude technique for measuring bladder pressure while trying to record intraabdominal pressure. Shortly thereafter, DuBois studied the effects of changes in body position on intravesical and intrarectal pressures and observed that the desire to void was associated with contraction of the detrusor muscle. The currently popular water cystometer was designed by Lewis in 1939. The later use of air and carbon dioxide as filling media further simplified the procedure.

Cystometry is a urodynamic test that measures the pressure and volume relationship of the bladder. It is used to assess detrusor activity, sensation, capacity, and compliance. Every factor has unique implications, and before any definitive conclusions can be reached, each parameter must be examined in association with symptoms and clinical findings.

A normal bladder has the power of accommodation; it can maintain an almost constant low intravesical pressure throughout filling, regardless of volume. A normal woman should be able to suppress voiding even at maximum capacity. Then, in an acceptable environment, she should be able to initiate a voiding reflex of sufficient magnitude to empty her bladder.

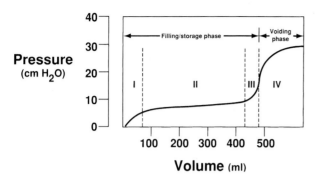

**Fig. 6-1** Normal cystometrogram. Note filling phase is divided into an initial slight rise in bladder pressure (phase I), followed by a tonus limb reflecting bladder accommodation (phase II). At maximum capacity, the detrusor muscle and elastic bladder wall tissue are stretched to their limits, causing a rise in bladder pressure (phase III). A detrusor contraction then is initiated voluntarily and the patient voids (phase IV).

Modified from Wein AJ, Barrett DM: *Voiding function and dysfunction,* Chicago, 1988, Mosby.

The basic principle of cystometry is the coupling of a manometer to the bladder lumen. A filling medium is instilled into the bladder and, as it fills, intravesical pressure is measured against volume. Testing apparatuses range from simple single-channel methods, which are performed manually or electronically, to complex methods combining electronic measurements of bladder, abdominal, and urethral pressure, together with electromyography and fluoroscopy.

A cystometrogram has two phases: a filling/storage phase and an emptying (voiding) phase (Fig. 6-1). The filling phase is subdivided into a brief initial rise in pressure to achieve resting bladder pressure, followed by a tonus limb that reflects vesicoelastic properties of accommodation of the smooth muscle and collagen of the bladder wall. There may be a third increase in the pressure, which is attributed to stretching of detrusor muscle and collagenous elements of the bladder wall beyond their limits at bladder capacity. During this third stage, the patient is still able to suppress voiding. A detrusor contraction then is initiated voluntarily and the patient voids.

## DEFINITIONS AND NORMAL CYSTOMETRIC PARAMETERS

The International Continence Society has defined certain terms that are used in the reporting of cystometric results.

Intravesicle pressure is the pressure within the bladder. Abdominal pressure is taken to be the pressure surrounding the bladder. It is generally estimated from rectal, vaginal, or, less commonly, extraperitoneal pressure.

Detrusor pressure is the component of intravesical pressure that is created by both active and passive forces in the bladder wall. It is estimated by subtracting abdominal pressure from intravesical pressure.

Bladder sensation is difficult to evaluate because of its subjective nature. During the testing session, it is assessed by questioning the patient about her feeling of bladder fullness. Commonly used descriptive terms include the following:

First desire to void (the woman is aware that the bladder is filling and feels that she could void)

Normal desire to void (the feeling that leads the patient to pass urine at the next convenient moment, but voiding can be delayed if necessary)

Strong desire to void (persistent desire to void without the fear of leakage)

Urgency (strong desire to void accompanied by fear of leakage or fear of pain)

Maximum cystometric capacity in patients with normal sensation is the volume at which the patient feels she can no longer delay micturition. In the absence of sensation it is the volume at which the clinician decides to terminate filling.

Functional bladder capacity, or voided volume is assessed from a frequency/volume chart (urinary diary).

Maximum (anesthetic) bladder capacity is the volume measured after filling during a deep general or regional anesthetic. The fluid temperature, filling pressure, and filling time should be specified.

Compliance (C) is the change in volume for a change in pressure. It is calculated by dividing the volume change ($\Delta V$) by the change in detrusor pressure ($\Delta P_{det}$) during that change in bladder volume ($C = \Delta V / \Delta P_{det}$). Compliance is expressed in milliliters per centimeter $H_2O$.

A female bladder normally experiences a first desire to void at a volume of approximately 150 to 250 ml, a normal desire to void at 300 to 400 ml, and a strong desire to void at 400 to 600 ml. During filling, an initial rise in true detrusor pressure between 2 and 8 cm $H_2O$ usually occurs. The average pressure rise is approximately 6 cm $H_2O$ and never exceeds 15 cm $H_2O$. Provocation of a normal bladder by rapid filling, change of posture, coughing, or catheter movement should not normally incite any abnormal rises in detrusor pressure.

## EQUIPMENT

It is beyond the scope of this chapter to discuss all commercially available cystometers, but reviews by Blaivas (1990) and Rowan et al. (1987) give the most current information. The simplest cystometer is a water manometer connected by a Y tube to both a reservoir and a catheter. A variation of this technique is discussed in Chapter 5.

Commercially available cystometers can be broadly classified into single-channel and multichannel machines (subtracted cystometry). Single-channel cystometry involves the placement into the bladder of a pressure-measuring catheter that produces an electronic signal, creating a graph on a recording device (Fig. 6-2). Multichannel cystometry relies on the measurement of both abdominal ($P_{abd}$) and intravesical pressures ($P_{ves}$), thereby enabling one to distinguish changes in intraabdominal pressure from changes in intra-

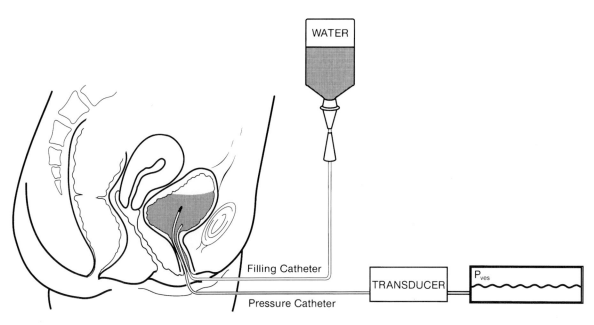

**Fig. 6-2**  Single-channel cystometry. *P~ves~*, Bladder pressure.

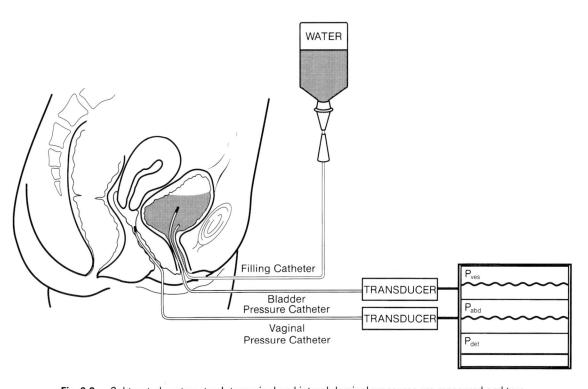

**Fig. 6-3**  Subtracted cystometry. Intravesical and intraabdominal pressures are measured and true detrusor pressure is electronically derived ($P_{ves} - P_{abd}$). $P_{ves}$, Bladder pressure; $P_{abd}$, abdominal pressure; $P_{det}$, detrusor pressure.

vesical pressure (Fig. 6-3). Abdominal pressure can be measured via either transrectal or transvaginal catheters. We prefer vaginally placed catheters because they are more comfortable and easier to clean and maintain, and measurements are not cluttered by rectal peristalsis. Electronic subtraction of intraabdominal from intravesical pressure allows for the calculation of true detrusor pressure ($P_{det}$).

Subtracted cystometry may be enhanced further by additional measurement of urethral pressure ($P_{ure}$). This measurement allows for the calculation of urethral closure pressure ($P_{ucp}$), which is the difference between urethral and bladder pressures. Certain machines also allow for the simultaneous measurement of electromyographic (EMG) activity and the performance of flow studies (Fig. 6-4).

## METHODOLOGY

Despite the widespread use of cystometry, the optimal technique for performing the test is unknown. The following section addresses the various technical aspects, controversies, and techniques for performing cystometry.

### Filling Media

The commonly used infusants for cystometry include water, carbon dioxide, and radiographic contrast material. In 1971, Merrill et al. introduced the use of carbon dioxide, which has become popular in North America. It is particularly suitable for office studies because it is clean and quick, and can be instilled at rates of up to 300 ml/min. Nevertheless, the following reservations about the use of gas during cystometry exist. First, it further decreases the physiologic nature of the test. Second, if gas is used, the bladder volume cannot be assessed because $CO_2$ is compressible. Third, $CO_2$ dissolves in urine to form carbonic acid, which irritates and reduces functional bladder capacity. Fourth, abdominal pressure is not usually measured during $CO_2$ cystometry, making interpretation more difficult. Finally, when $CO_2$ is used for filling cystometry, it is impossible to perform a stress test or voiding studies.

Water or physiologic saline is the most commonly used filling medium unless radiologic screening is also being performed, in which case contrast medium is used. The cystometric findings are not affected by the choice of liquid medium.

### Position of Patient and Provoking Maneuvers

Cystometry should mimic everyday stresses on the bladder as much as possible. Thus, it is preferable to perform the test with the patient in the sitting or standing position. During cystometry, the bladder should be provoked by a series of tests that usually include coughing, heel bouncing, walking in place, and listening to running water. These maneuvers may provoke uninhibited detrusor contractions or induce stress incontinence.

Physical factors may influence the positioning of patients during urodynamic tests; for example, in elderly patients or those with neurologic disease, it may be difficult to undertake cystometry in any position other than supine.

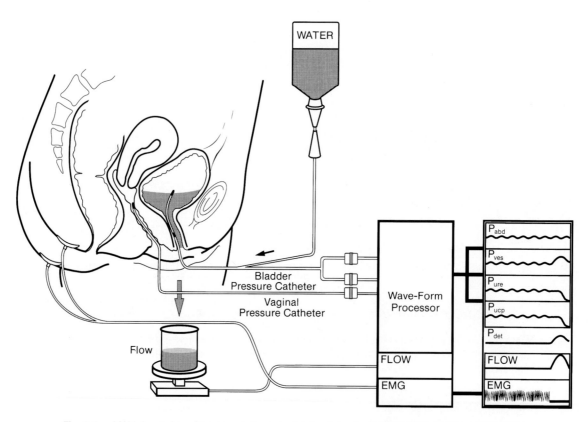

**Fig. 6-4** Multichannel urodynamics. Intravesical, intraabdominal, and intraurethral pressures are measured. True detrusor pressure ($P_{det}$) and urethral closure pressure ($P_{ucp}$) are electronically derived. EMG and flow studies are also performed. $P_{ves}$, Bladder pressure; $P_{abd}$, abdominal pressure; $P_{det}$, detrusor pressure; $P_{ure}$, urethral pressure; $P_{ucp}$, urethral closure pressure; *EMG*, electromyography.

## Temperature of Fluid

Most laboratories use fluid at room temperature, although some investigators believe that the instillation of warm or cold fluid may provoke abnormal bladder activity. The instillation of ice water (Bor's test) is occasionally used as a test for neurologic disorders.

## Technique of Bladder Filling

Theoretically, the most physiologic method of filling is by diuresis, combined with a suprapubically placed pressure line. The long time needed to investigate the patient prohibits natural filling as a practical method of performing cystometry in most centers. Therefore, cystometry is usually performed through a transurethrally placed catheter. Filling is accomplished using either simple gravity or a water pump. The bladder is filled through either a small catheter or, preferably, a separate channel on the pressure-measuring catheter.

## Rate of Bladder Filling

The ICS attempted to standardize filling rates by describing three ranges: slow fill is less than 10 ml/min, medium fill is 10 to 100 ml/min, and rapid or fast fill is greater than 100 ml/min. Patients with normal lower urinary tract function can tolerate most fast-fill rates. The effect of the filling rate on an unstable bladder is still poorly understood, but fast-fill methods may be more effective in provoking detrusor overactivity. For this reason, medium- or fast-fill techniques are more widely used. In patients with neurologic abnormalities, slow fill is essential to reduce artifactual bladder activity.

## Types of Catheters

A variety of catheters have been used for cystometry. Simple or manual cystometry can be performed with a transurethral Foley catheter. Electronically monitored studies require more sophisticated balloon or microtransducer catheters. Water-filled balloon catheters or water perfusion catheters have been used with moderate success. These catheters are inexpensive, disposable, and easy to use. However, more sophisticated laboratories usually use sensitive microtransducer catheters (Fig. 6-5). These catheters are available with one to six microtransducers on the catheter. They have small diameters, are flexible, and can measure rapid changes in pressure accurately during repetitive coughing or other provoking maneuvers. Disadvantages include their expense, their need to be replaced after approximately 100 studies, and their tendency to produce rotational artifacts; pressure readings may vary depending on the orientation of the transducer to the bladder or urethral wall.

## Technique of Cystometry

The technique of multichannel subtracted urethrocystometry used in our laboratory is as follows:

1. The patient presents with a symptomatically full bladder. She voids spontaneously in a uroflow chair. A postvoid residual urine volume is obtained via a transurethral catheter. With the catheter in place, approximately 50 ml of sterile, room-temperature saline or water is placed into the bladder to facilitate placement of the microtransducer catheters and to decrease the amount of initial artifact secondary to the bladder wall collapsing around the microtip.

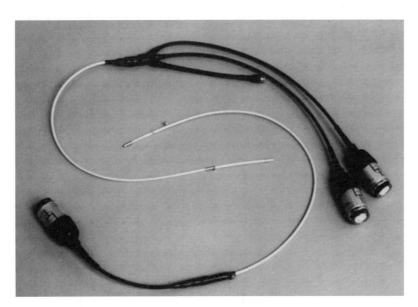

**Fig. 6-5**  Two microtransducer catheters. One catheter has a single microtransducer and is used for estimating abdominal pressure. The other catheter has two microtransducers approximately 6 cm apart used to measure intravesical and intraurethral pressure. This catheter also contains a fluid filling port.

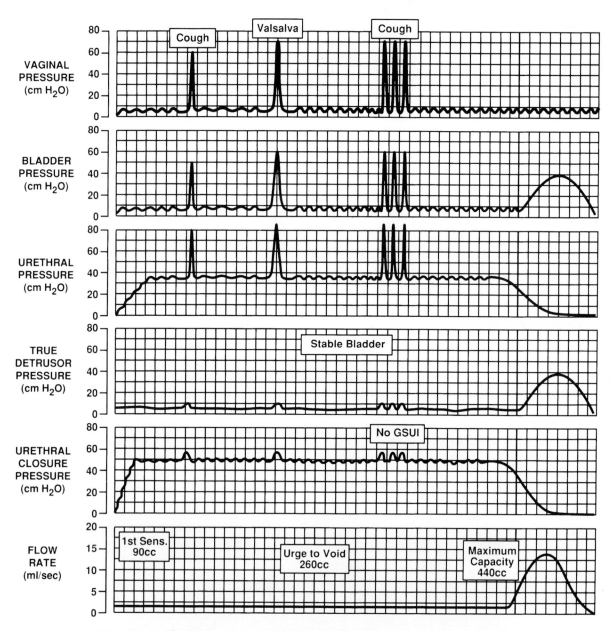

**Fig. 6-6**  Normal filling and voiding subtracted cystometry. Note that provocation in the form of coughing and straining does not provoke any abnormal rise in true detrusor pressure. At maximum capacity on command, a detrusor contraction is generated and voiding is initiated. *GSUI,* Genuine stress urinary incontinence.

2. The microtransducer catheters are connected to the appropriate cables and to the tubing from the water pump. The machine is calibrated with the catheters in water and all channels are set at zero. A small amount of water is flushed through the tubing to remove any air.
3. With the patient in the supine position on a birthing or urodynamic chair, the abdominal catheter is placed into the vagina and taped to the inside of the leg. If the patient has severe vaginal prolapse or has undergone previous vaginal surgery resulting in a narrowed vagina, the catheter is placed into the rectum. A dual microtrans-

ducer catheter with a filling port is then placed into the bladder. The patient is moved to a sitting position and the catheter secured to a mechanical puller (if urethral pressure studies are anticipated) or to the inside of the leg, so that the proximal transducer is near the mid-urethra (area of maximum urethral closure pressure).
4. After the catheters are appropriately placed, the subtraction is checked by asking the patient to cough. Cough-induced pressure spikes should be seen on the $P_{ves}$, $P_{abd}$, and $P_{ure}$ channels, but not on the true detrusor pressure channel. If there is an inappropriate deflection on $P_{det}$, it

is usually secondary to inaccurate placement of the vaginal (or rectal) catheter. If repositioning the catheter does not correct the problem, all connections and calibration techniques should be rechecked.

5. Bladder filling is begun. First sensation, initial urge to void, and maximum capacity are recorded. Throughout the filling portion of the examination, the patient is asked to perform provocative activities, such as coughing and straining. The external urethral meatus is constantly observed for any involuntary urine loss. Leak point pressures can be obtained at various bladder volumes. Any abnormal rise in true detrusor pressure is noted. If the patient's symptoms are reproduced during filling, then the test can be completed in the sitting position. If they are not, the patient should be asked to stand and perform provocative maneuvers in an attempt to reproduce her symptoms.

6. At the completion of filling, urethral pressure and flow studies can be performed, if indicated. These tests are discussed in Chapters 7 and 8. Fig. 6-6 illustrates an example of filling and voiding urethrocystometry. No urodynamic abnormalities are noted in this study.

## INDICATIONS FOR CYSTOMETRY

The indications for cystometry are somewhat controversial. Each patient must be evaluated individually. Based on clinical findings and planned treatments, the physician must decide whether cystometry is indicated and, if it is, whether it should be performed via a simple office test or with more sophisticated electronic testing. In our opinion, an electronic single-channel study does not offer any more information than does a carefully performed nonelectronic test. We believe the only reason to perform electronic urodynamic testing is to measure pressures from several anatomic sites, thus obtaining subtracted pressures of importance.

Indications for single-channel cystometry versus subtracted or multichannel cystometry have been debated extensively; however, few comparisons exist in the literature. One study by Ouslander et al. (1987) reported a sensitivity of 75% in geriatric patients undergoing simple supine cystometry when compared to multichannel testing. Sutherst and Brown (1984) compared single-channel and multichannel urodynamics in a blinded crossover study of 100 incontinent women. They noted single-channel studies to be 100% sensitive and 89% specific compared to multichannel studies. Multichannel cystometry may have a higher sensitivity for recognizing low-pressure detrusor contractions, which have sometimes been called "subthreshold detrusor instability." Multichannel techniques also improve the specificity of cystometry by avoiding false positive test results created by increases in abdominal pressure. Whether the cost of multichannel testing is justified for most patients remains to be proved. Box 6-1 lists suggested indications for subtracted cystometry.

**Box 6-1**

### INDICATIONS FOR MULTICHANNEL SUBTRACTED CYSTOMETRY

Complicated history
Inconclusive single-channel studies
Stress incontinence before surgical correction
Urge incontinence not responsive to therapy
Recurrent urinary loss after previous surgery for stress incontinence
Frequency, urgency, and pain syndromes not responsive to therapy
Nocturnal enuresis not responsive to therapy
Lower urinary tract dysfunction after pelvic radiation or radical pelvic surgery
Neurologic disorders
Continuous leakage
Suspected voiding difficulties

## VIDEO-URODYNAMIC TESTING

Video-urodynamic studies of the lower urinary tract represent a combination of video-cystourethrography and standard urodynamic techniques. Video-urodynamics requires equipment for cystometry, plus an image intensifier and a videotape recorder. In addition, various interface modules are necessary, depending on the exact design of the system. A television camera positioned above the recorder with a mixing device projects the recording channels on a television monitor alongside the radiographic image of the bladder (Fig. 6-7). Radio-opaque filling medium is used for video-urodynamic studies. As with all other urodynamic studies, every effort must be made to limit the inhibitory effect of the additional machinery and personnel imposed on the patient.

Potential advantages of video-urodynamic studies include the consolidation of multiple evaluation modalities into one examination, thereby providing information about lower urinary tract anatomy and function under various provocative environments. Descent of the bladder neck, milk-back of urine from the urethra to the bladder, and bladder neck funneling all may be visualized during simultaneous recording and imaging of bladder, urethral, and abdominal pressures. Asymptomatic abnormalities such as urethral or bladder diverticula also may be noted. The major disadvantages of video-urodynamic testing are the radiation exposure, cost, and technical expertise and support necessary for its use.

The indications for video-urodynamic studies are controversial. Some authorities believe that no additional information is obtained when these studies are compared to more conventional nonimaged multichannel studies; however, others believe that valuable additional information can be obtained from simultaneous imaging, especially in recurrent

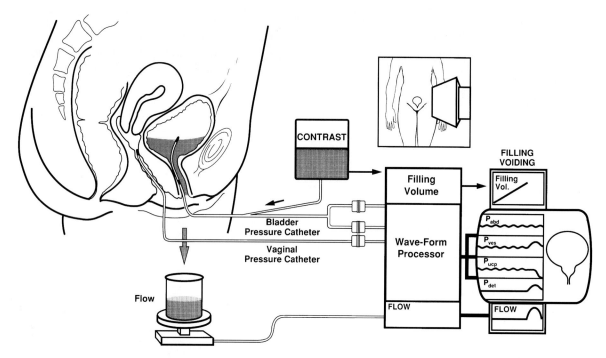

**Fig. 6-7** Video-urodynamic testing. Multichannel urodynamic tests are performed under fluoroscopy, thus allowing simultaneous visualization of the lower urinary tract during recording of pressures. $P_{ves}$, Bladder pressure; $P_{abd}$, abdominal pressure; $P_{det}$, detrusor pressure; $P_{ucp}$, urethral closure pressure.

cases of incontinence or complicated neurologic conditions. Visualizing bladder neck opening at rest and during straining may help differentiate stress incontinence secondary to bladder neck hypermobility from intrinsic sphincter deficiency.

## AMBULATORY URODYNAMICS (AUDS)

The largest deficiency of currently available urodynamic techniques is that laboratory observations may not always represent accurately physiologic behavior of the bladder and urethra. At times, the urodynamicist cannot reproduce the patient's symptoms in the laboratory setting. Several companies have recently developed commercially available AUDS systems. This equipment uses indwelling catheter-mounted transducers that are connected to a microcomputer worn over the patient's shoulder. This allows freedom of movement to the extent that the patient can reproduce the activities that incite lower urinary tract dysfunction. In principle these systems are the same as those used for conventional urodynamics, and the same basic methodology applies. AUDS should be considered when conventional urodynamics fail to provide a pathophysiologic explanation for the patient's symptoms. The most common example of this is in a patient who complains of incontinence that cannot be objectively demonstrated and has failed nonsurgical modes of therapy. Before more invasive therapy such as surgery is considered, AUDS could be used to objectively

demonstrate the incontinence. AUDS systems are also helpful in determining whether detrusor instability or urethral incompetence is the main cause of incontinence in women for whom surgery is being contemplated.

The technique for performing AUDS as described by Abrams (1997) involves the recording of three micturition cycles: a resting cycle when the patient sits in a chair, an ambulant cycle when the patient moves around the hospital, and an exercising cycle, which should include any specific incontinence-provoking measures. Once the three cycles are recorded the information is downloaded to a computer for analysis. This analysis is time consuming and requires considerable expertise.

Ideally the data acquired should include information on voiding and urine leakage. The recent development of an electronic urine-loss detector has markedly improved AUDS. This device fits into a commercially available female pad. The advantage of electronic urine loss detection is that it is noted instantaneously and therefore does not depend on the patient filling in her diary. It is also very useful in patients who cannot sense urine loss. The AUDS unit should allow the connection of a flowmeter so that the urine flow rate can be recorded synchronously with intravesicle and intraabdominal pressure. This is particularly important if bladder outlet obstruction is suspected. The equipment should have an event marker, which the patient uses in conjunction with a diary to signal sensations such as first desire to void, urgency, or leakage.

Besides providing objective evidence and the cause of the patient's lower urinary tract symptoms, additional interesting information is being generated by AUDS. Present ideas on bladder compliance, detrusor instability, and voiding function are being questioned. AUDS studies performed on asymptomatic, neurologically intact volunteers have shown a 30% incidence of detrusor instability. It has been previously suspected that bladder compliance is related to the speed of bladder filling, and AUDS has confirmed this fact (Kulseng-Hanson, 1996). Finally, voiding pressures during AUDS in females have been shown to be significantly higher than those obtained during conventional urodynamics.

AUDS testing has some drawbacks. During the investigation there is no control on the validity of the measured signals. For this reason it is important that before the patient is sent away with the monitor, the catheter position must be checked and the patient must be adequately instructed.

Ambulatory monitoring of the upper and lower urinary tract is still developing and is currently performed only in specialized urodynamic centers. A real breakthrough in the technique will be the development of automated analysis and quantitative interpretation.

## CYSTOMETRY: ABNORMAL STUDIES

Abnormalities of bladder filling are categorized into abnormal detrusor activity, compliance, sensation, and capacity. If urethral pressure is being measured simultaneously, the urethral response to filling and provocation can be elicited. For descriptive purposes, these abnormalities tend to be compartmentalized; however, no single urodynamic finding should be taken in isolation. Many patients have more than one cystometric abnormality (Fig. 6-8).

Any significant rise in true detrusor pressure during filling or provocation should be interpreted as abnormal detrusor activity or compliance. A pressure increase of 15 cm $H_2O$ has been used by the ICS to differentiate between normal and abnormal. It has recently become apparent that this cutoff is too arbitrary, and any pressure rise must be assessed in terms of the patient's symptoms. The most recent ICS recommendations have redefined detrusor overactivity to be any rise in true detrusor pressure that is felt not to be caused by normal bladder compliance.

Although it is useful to categorize pressure changes during cystometry, the different patterns that occur are not mutually exclusive. Examples of the various cystometric findings in detrusor overactivity are shown in Fig. 6-9. Detrusor overactivity may present as phasic contractions that return to baseline after each contraction or as phasic contractions in which there is a gradual rise in pressure. A steady rise in true detrusor pressure indicates a low-compliance bladder. When this type of pattern is noted, an organic reason for the poor bladder compliance, such as interstitial cystitis, should be ruled out. The clinical relevance of these various patterns is not fully understood. The management of detrusor overactivity is discussed in Chapter 24.

Sensory abnormalities are classified as either hypersensitive or hyposensitive. Hypersensitive bladder behavior is similar whether there is a definable cause, such as interstitial cystitis, or whether the cause is unknown. In these patients, catheterization is often painful. Volumes at first sensation of bladder filling, first desire to void, and maximum capacity are reduced. Sensory urgency is present when the patient experiences a strong desire to void at abnormally low bladder volumes in the absence of any rise in true detrusor pressure (Fig. 6-10, *A*). Bladder overactivity may be associated with hypersensitivity from causes such as radiation therapy and interstitial cystitis. Therapy may result in bladder stability; however, the symptoms of frequency and urgency may persist if the bladder remains hypersensitive.

Urodynamically, the hyposensitive bladder behaves similarly, whatever the cause. The bladder has a large capacity and a flat cystometrogram (Fig. 6-10, *B*). At maximum capacity, there may rarely be a rise in pressure as the limits of compliance are reached. This rise does not represent a detrusor contraction and there may be little or no sensation to filling up to this point. Weir and Jaques (1974) noted that 30% of patients with bladder capacities over 800 ml were able to generate a normal detrusor contraction and void to completion on command. A hyposensitive, overdistended bladder, in itself, is not necessarily an indication of pathology.

During cystometry, functional and cystometric bladder capacity should be differentiated. Maximum cystometric capacity is a somewhat subjective measure of the total volume of fluid the patient can tolerate comfortably during bladder filling. Functional bladder capacity is the amount of urine the bladder can hold under natural conditions. This amount can be checked easily by asking the patient to drink a large amount of water and hold it until she feels a maximum sensation to void. She then urinates, and a postvoid residual urine volume is measured. The sum of the volumes of urine voided plus the residual urine provides the maximal functional bladder capacity. The artifacts of catheter insertion, the environment of cystometric examination, and the presence of medical personnel may change the patient's bladder capacity. Thus, it is important to interpret bladder capacity data as derived from cystometry on a comparative basis with the patient's functional capacity as determined on frequency volume charts.

Both local and systemic conditions can result in abnormal bladder capacity. Box 6-2 reviews the differential diagnosis of low-volume and high-volume bladder capacity.

When urethral pressure is measured simultaneously during filling cystometry, several abnormal urethral responses may be seen. The most common is an incompetent urethral sphincter (Fig. 6-11). This finding usually results from genuine stress incontinence; rarely it is caused by uninhibited urethral relaxation. The term *urethral instability*

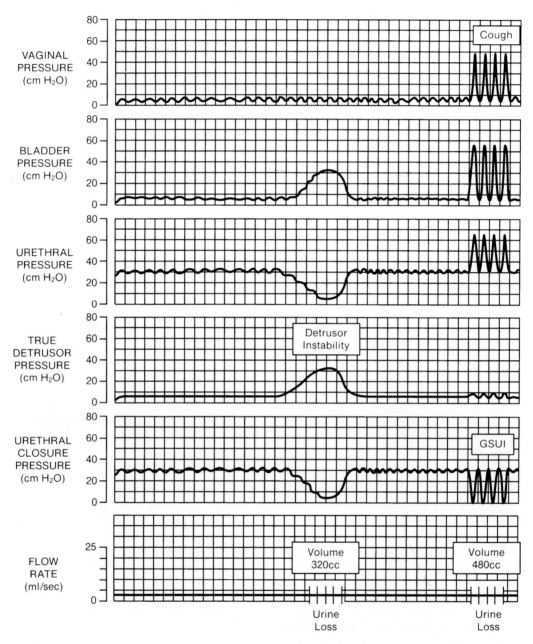

**Fig. 6-8** Multichannel urethrocystometry in a patient with combined detrusor instability and genuine stress incontinence. *GSUI,* Genuine stress urinary incontinence.

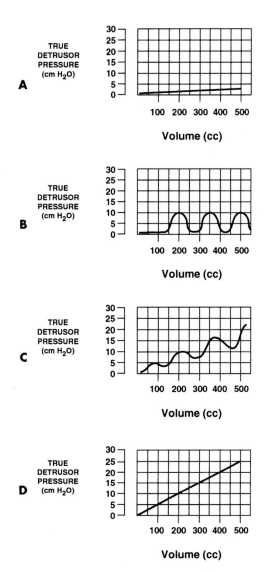

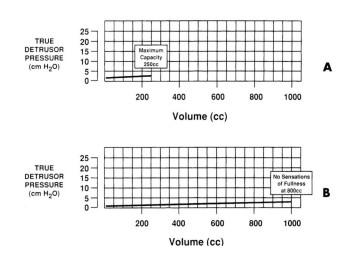

**Fig. 6-10**   **A,** Urodynamic diagnosis of sensory urgency. Patient experiences severe urgency at abnormally low bladder capacity in the absence of any significant rise in true detrusor pressure. **B,** Urodynamic diagnosis of hyposensitive bladder. Patient experiences no sensation of fullness at abnormally high bladder volume.

**Fig. 6-9**   Various detrusor responses to filling: **A,** Normal filling cystometry; **B,** Phasic contractions that return to baseline; **C,** Phasic contractions with gradual rise in true detrusor pressure; **D,** Steady rise in true detrusor pressure (low-compliance bladder).

has been used by some investigators to describe abnormal fluctuations in urethral pressure during filling. The clinical significance of this finding is controversial and is discussed in more detail in Chapter 8.

## SUMMARY

Cystometry is the most important and most commonly performed urodynamic test. It assesses bladder filling and storage and is also important in evaluating bladder emptying, when used in conjunction with the other urodynamic and radiologic tests. Although it is clinically useful, its limitations should be recognized. Gynecologists should become familiar with cystometry so that they can perform and interpret basic office tests and work with urogynecologic or urologic consultants when more sophisticated tests are indicated.

---

**Box 6-2**
### DIFFERENTIAL DIAGNOSIS OF LOW-VOLUME AND HIGH-VOLUME BLADDER

**Low Volume**

Detrusor instability (idiopathic)
Detrusor hyperreflexia (neurogenic)
Genuine stress incontinence
Hypersensitive bladder (sensory urgency)
Interstitial cystitis
Radiation cystitis or fibrosis
Bladder tumor
Urinary tract infection
Emotional factors

**High Volume**

Chronic outlet obstruction
Uterovaginal prolapse
Urethral stricture
Urethral tumor
Neuropathy
Diabetes mellitus
Hypothyroidism
Tabes dorsalis
Pernicious anemia
Lumbospinal disk disease
Previous radical pelvic surgery
Multiple sclerosis
Habitual infrequent voiding

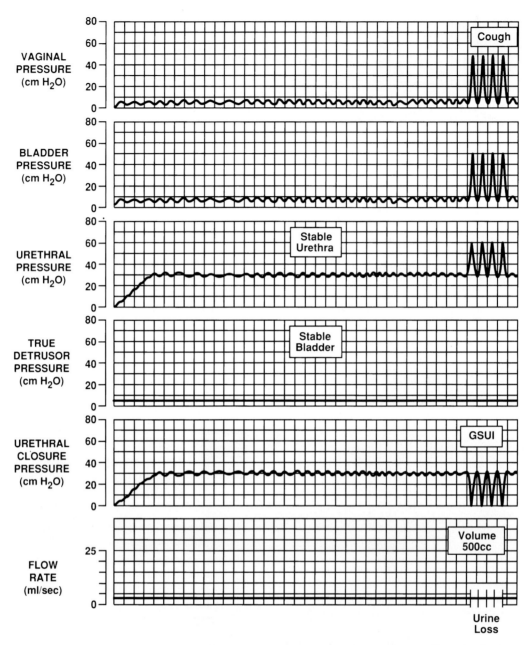

**Fig. 6-11** Urodynamic diagnosis of the condition of genuine stress incontinence. There is visual loss of urine in the absence of any rise in true detrusor pressure with complete pressure equalization. *GSUI,* Genuine stress urinary incontinence.

## BIBLIOGRAPHY

Abrams P: *Urodynamics,* ed 2, London, 1997, Springer.

Abrams P, Blaivas JG, Stanton SL, et al: The standardization of terminology of lower urinary tract function, *Scand J Urol Nephrol* 114(suppl):5, 1988.

Arnold EP: Cystometry: postural effects in incontinent women, *Urol Int* 29:185, 1974.

Arnold EP, Webster JR, Loose H, et al: Urodynamics of female incontinence: factors influencing the results of surgery, *Am J Obstet Gynecol* 117:805, 1973.

Barnick CG, Cardozo LD, Benness C: Use of routine videocystourethrography in the evaluation of female lower urinary tract dysfunction, *Neurourol Urodyn* 8:447, 1989.

Bates CP, Whiteside CG, Turner-Warwick R: Synchronous cine/pressure/flow cystourethrography with special reference to stress and urge incontinence, *Br J Urol* 42:714, 1970.

Bates P, Bradley WE, Glen E, et al: First report on the standardization of terminology of the lower urinary tract function. Urinary incontinence. Procedures related to the evaluation of urine storage: cystometry, urethral closure pressure profile, units of measurement, *Br J Urol* 48:39, 1976; *Eur Urol* 2:274, 1976; *Scand J Urol Nephrol* 11:193, 1976; *Urol Int* 32:81, 1976.

Bhatia NN, Bradley WE, Haldeman S: Urodynamics: continuous monitoring, *J Urol* 128:963, 1982.

Bhatia NN, Bradley WE, Haldeman S, et al: Continuous ambulatory urodynamic monitoring, *Br J Urol* 54:357, 1982.

Blaivas JG: Multichannel urodynamic studies, *Urology* 23:421, 1984.

Blaivas JG: Machines for measuring urodynamics, *Contemp Obstet Gynecol* 35:99, 1990.

Bradley WE, Timm GW, Scott FB: Cystometry: III. Cystometers, *Urology* 5:843, 1975.

Bradley WE, Timm GW, Scott FB: Cystometry: V. Bladder sensation, *Urology* 6:654, 1975.

Bump RC: The urodynamic laboratory, *Obstet Gynecol Clin North Am* 16:795, 1989.

Cardozo L: *Urogynecology,* New York, 1997, Churchill Livingstone.

Cass AS, Ward BD, Markland C: Comparison of slow and rapid fill cystometry using liquid and air, *J Urol* 104:104, 1970.

Colstrup H, Andersen JT, Walter S: Detrusor reflex instability in male intravesical obstruction. Fact or artefact? *Neurourol Urodyn* 1:183, 1982.

Coolsaet BL, Blok C, Van Venrooij GE, et al: Subthreshold detrusor instability, *Neurourol Urodyn* 4:309, 1985.

DuBois P: Über den Druck in der Harnblase, *Arch Klin Med* 17:248, 1876.

Enhorning G: Simultaneous recording of intravesical and intraurethral pressure, *Acta Chir Scand* 276(suppl):1, 1961.

Fossberg E, Beisland HO, Sauder S: Sensory urgency in females. Treatment with phenylpropanolamine, *Eur Urol* 7:157, 1981.

Gleason DM, Bottaccini MR, Reilly RJ: Comparison of cystometrograms and urethral profiles with gas and water media, *Urology* 9:155, 1977.

Jorgensen L, Lose G, Andersen JT: Cystometry: $H_2O$ or $CO_2$ as filling medium? A literature survey of the influence of the filling medium on the qualitative and the quantitative cystometric parameters, *Neurourol Urodyn* 7:343, 1988.

Kulseng-Hanson S, Klevmark B: Ambulatory urethro-cysto-rectometry: a new technique, *Neurourol Urodyn* 7:119, 1988.

Kulseng-Hanson S, Klevmark B: Ambulatory urodynamic monitoring of women, *Scand J Urol Nephrol* 179(suppl 30):27, 1996.

Lapides J, Friend CR, Ajemian EP: Denervation supersensitivity as a test for neurogenic bladder, *Surg Gynecol Obstet* 114:141, 1962.

Lewis LG: A new clinical recording cystometer, *J Urol* 41:638, 1939.

Massey A, Abrams P: Urodynamics of the female lower urinary tract, *Urol Clin North Am* 12:231, 1985.

McCarthy TA: Validity of rectal pressure measurements as indication of intraabdominal pressure changes during urodynamic evaluation, *Urology* 20:657, 1982.

McGuire EJ, Savastano JA: Stress incontinence and detrusor instability/urge incontinence, *Neurourol Urodyn* 4:313, 1985.

Melzer M: The urecholine test, *J Urol* 108:729, 1972.

Merrill DC, Bradley WE, Markland C: Air cystometry. I. Technique and definition of terms, *J Urol* 106:678, 1971.

Merrill DC, Bradley WE, Markland C: Air cystometry. II. A clinical evaluation of normal adults, *J Urol* 108:85, 1972.

Merrill DC, Rotta JA: A clinical evaluation of detrusor denervation supersensitivity using air cystometry, *J Urol* 111:27, 1974.

O'Donnell PD: *Urinary incontinence,* St Louis, 1997, Mosby.

Ouslander JG, Staskin D, Raz S, et al: Clinical versus urodynamic diagnosis in an incontinent geriatric female population, *J Urol* 137:68, 1987.

Penders L, De Leval J: Simultaneous urethrocystometry and hyperactive bladders: a manometric differential diagnosis, *Neurourol Urodyn* 4:89, 1985.

Rowan D, James ED, Kramer AE, et al: Urodynamic equipment: technical aspects. Produced by the International Continence Society Working Party on Urodynamic Equipment, *J Med Eng Technol* 1:57, 1987.

Sand PK, Bowen LW, Ostergard DR: Uninhibited urethral relaxation: an unusual cause of incontinence, *Obstet Gynecol* 68:645, 1986.

Sand PK, Hill RC, Ostergard DR: Supine urethroscopic and standing cystometry as screening methods for the detection of detrusor instability, *Obstet Gynecol* 70:57, 1987.

Sutherst JR, Brown MC: Comparison of single and multichannel cystometry in diagnosing bladder instability, *BMJ* 288:1720, 1984.

Torrens M, Abrams P: Cystometry: symposium on clinical urodynamics, *Urol Clin North Am* 6:71, 1979.

Van Waalwijk van Doorn ESC, Gommer E: Ambulatory urodynamics, *Curr Opin Obstet Gynecol* 7:378, 1995.

Van Waalwijk van Doorn ESC, Remmers A, Janknegt RA: Conventional and extramural ambulatory urodynamic testing of the lower urinary tract in female volunteers, *J Urol* 147:1319, 1992.

Wein AJ, Barrett DM: *Voiding function and dysfunction,* Chicago, 1988, Mosby.

Weir J, Jacques PF: Large-capacity bladder: a urodynamic survey, *Urology* 4:544, 1974.

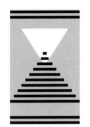

CHAPTER *7*

# *Urodynamics: Voiding Studies*

Mickey M. Karram

Normal micturition depends on a multitude of complex factors that must be coordinated to facilitate bladder emptying. Voiding consists of a combination of bladder contraction and outlet relaxation so that emptying is rapid and complete. The neurophysiologic mechanisms involved in micturition are complex and have been discussed elsewhere. Disturbances in any of the connections in the voiding mechanism can produce abnormal micturition.

Various urodynamic techniques have been devised to study voiding. Uroflowmetry is the simplest and most commonly used of these investigations. Drake described one of the first clinically useful urinary flowmeters in 1948. A kymograph was attached to a receptacle for the voided urine and rotated at a known speed, and a tracing of voided urine volume against time was obtained. Drake was the first to record average flow rates in men and noted that flow rates increased significantly with increasing volumes. In 1956 von Garrelts described the first electronic urine flowmeters, which consisted of a tall urine-collecting cylinder with a pressure transducer in the base. The pressure transducer measured the pressure exerted by an increase in the column of urine as the patient voided. Because of the direct relationship between the volume voided and the pressure recorded, von Garrelts was able to produce electronically a direct recording of urine flow rate.

## UROFLOWMETRY

Uroflowmetry, or the measure of urine volume voided over time, is a simple and noninvasive test. It is performed by asking the patient to void in a special commode. Urine is funnelled into a flowmeter that records volume versus time (Fig. 7-1). It is important to get a representative flow pattern; this pattern depends on a number of factors. First, the patient should understand the simple nature of the test and be as relaxed as possible to have a normal desire to void at the time of the study. Second, the patient should be allowed to void in private because tension and embarrassment can artificially reduce the maximum flow achieved. Third, if there is doubt about the accuracy of the test, it is important to ask the patient whether he or she felt it was representative. If the patient believes that the test was not typical, it should be repeated.

## Definitions and Normal Parameters

Urine flow may be described in terms of flow rate and flow pattern and may be continuous or intermittent. Flow rate $(Q)$ is defined as the volume of fluid expelled via the urethra per unit time and is expressed in milliliters per second (ml/sec). Certain information is necessary in interpreting the tracing, including the volume voided, the environment and position in which the patient passed urine, whether the bladder filled naturally or by a catheter, and whether diuresis was stimulated by fluid or diuretics. If filling was by catheter, then the type of fluid used should be stated; it should also be stated whether the flow study was part of another investigation. Maximum flow rate ($Q_{max}$) is the maximum measured value of the flow rate. Voided volume is the total volume expelled via the urethra. Flow time ($Q_{time}$) is the time over which measurable flow occurs. Average flow rate ($Q_{ave}$) is voided volume divided by flow time. Time to maximum flow is the elapsed time from onset of flow to maximum flow. Drach et al. (1979) observed that the mean maximum flow rate in asymptomatic women was $26 \pm 14$ ml/sec, with an average voided volume of 224 ml. Flow time, maximum flow rate, and average flow rate all increase with corresponding increases in volume voided. Flow rates are higher in women than in men and in pregnant versus nonpregnant women. Little variation in flow rates with menstrual cycles, menopause, or increasing age has been reported.

Most experts agree that one can consider a study normal if the patient voids at least 200 ml over 15 to 20 seconds and it is recorded as a smooth single curve with a maximum flow rate greater than 20 ml/sec (Fig. 7-2). Maximum flow rates of less than 15 ml/sec with a voided volume greater than 200 ml are generally considered abnormal. However, because flow rate is determined by the relationship between detrusor force and urethral resistance and because these factors may vary considerably and still produce adequate bladder emptying, a precise definition of a normal or a low flow rate cannot be made. In general, depending on the clinical situation, borderline low flow rates require further urodynamic testing.

Residual urine is the volume of urine remaining in the bladder immediately after the completion of micturition. It is most accurately measured via a transurethral catheter, but also can be estimated by radiographic studies or ultrasound examination. A consistently high residual urine volume generally indicates increased outlet resistance, decreased bladder contractility, or both. Absent postvoid residual urine is compatible with normal urinary tract function, but also can exist in the presence of significant filling and storage disorders (incontinence) or with disorders of emptying in which the intravesical pressure is sufficient to overcome increased outlet resistance. What constitutes an abnormally high residual urine volume is not universally established. Previous investigators empirically have chosen volumes of 50 or 100 ml to indicate normal residual urine volumes. However, it is best to state the residual urine volume only in the context of the total voided volume. Normality should be described as a percentage of the total voided volume. We believe that most asymptomatic women should void spontaneously at least 80% of their total intravesical volume.

## Interpretation

Curve patterns refer to the configuration of the uroflowmetric curve. Continuous flow showing a rapidly increasing flow rate reaching the maximum within one third of the total voiding time is usually considered normal (Fig. 7-2).

Flow is considered intermittent when the flow rate drops and subsequently increases (Fig. 7-3, *B* and *C*). Intermittent flow rates are described as multiple-peak patterns when there is a downward deflection of the flow rate that does not

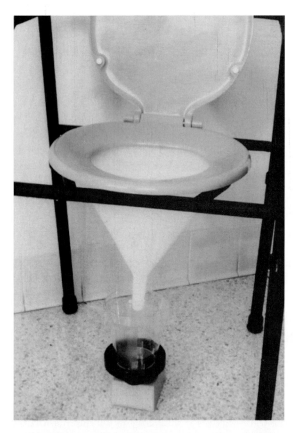

**Fig. 7-1**  Special commode and flowmeter used for spontaneous uroflowmetry.

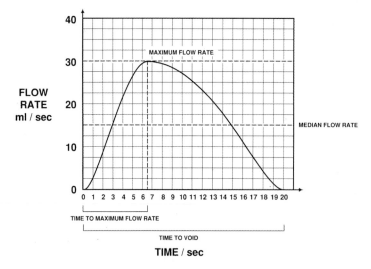

**Fig. 7-2**  Graphic representation of normal uroflow curve.

reach 2 ml/sec (Fig. 7-3, *B*). If the downward deflection of the flow rate reaches 2 ml/sec or less, it is called interrupted pattern (Fig. 7-3, *C*). Uroflowmetric parameters can be obtained from multiple peak patterns by reconstructing the curve, as shown in Fig. 7-4. The peak flow rate is determined by the highest horizontal segment that has a duration of at least 1 second. The peak flow rate then is connected to an ascending and descending limb. Deflections from the reconstructed curve are analyzed individually. Uroflowmetric parameters on curves with interrupted flow patterns are usually not estimated.

Obstructed voiding patterns are much less common in women than in men and usually produce a low, flat tracing (Fig. 7-3, *D*). Abnormal flow tracings caused by detrusor underactivity with abdominal straining or by intermittent urethral sphincter activity are characterized by slow changes in flow rate, producing a wavelike tracing. Each rise or fall in flow rate represents either a contraction of the abdominal and diaphragmatic muscles or a contraction of the external striated sphincter (Fig. 7-3, *B* and *C*).

A patient who voids very quickly can produce what has been called a *superflow* pattern in which there is very little outlet resistance. This pattern can be seen in patients with severe stress incontinence (Fig. 7-3, *A*).

Abnormal uroflowmetric parameters can occur secondary to factors that affect detrusor contractility, urethral resistance, or both.

Detrusor contractility can be affected by neuropathic lesions, pharmacologic manipulation, intrinsic detrusor muscle or bladder wall dysfunction, or psychogenic inhibition.

Urethral resistance can be altered by tissue trophic changes producing atrophy or fibrosis, drug effects such as alpha-adrenergic stimulators, neuropathic striated muscle contraction, pain or fear, and urethral axis distortion secondary to severe pelvic relaxation. Outlet obstruction secondary to an intraurethral lesion or stricture is exceedingly rare in women. Extraurethral lesions, such as vaginal masses or cysts, and large enterocele or rectocele may compress the urethra, resulting in obstructed voiding.

Detrusor–external sphincter dyssynergia is a condition in which there is lack of coordination between the detrusor muscle and the external striated sphincter. This leads to obstructed voiding and is always secondary to a neurologic lesion, most classically high spinal cord trauma.

## Clinical Applicability

Flow studies are much less useful in women than in men. Over half of cases of lower urinary tract dysfunction in men

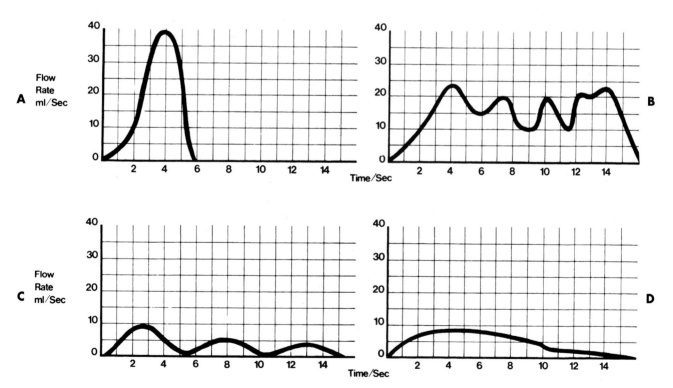

**Fig. 7-3** Graphic representation of various uroflow patterns. **A,** Superflow commonly seen with poor urethral resistance. **B,** Intermittent multiple-peak pattern. **C,** Intermittent interrupted pattern. **D,** Abnormal flow rate characteristic of detrusor outlet obstruction.

From Karram MM: Urodynamics. In Benson JT, ed: *Female pelvic floor disorders: investigation and management,* New York, 1992, Norton Medical Books.

are related to outflow obstruction, whereas only about 4% of cases of lower urinary tract dysfunction in women are related to voiding problems. Nevertheless, uroflowmetry is a simple urodynamic investigation that is useful as a preliminary screening test to distinguish patients who need more extensive studies from those who do not. It is also an integral part of the full urodynamic studies performed for more complex problems. Some clinical situations in which spontaneous uroflowmetry may be useful are briefly discussed here.

1. Symptoms suggestive of voiding dysfunction: If uroflow measures are normal in patients complaining of symptoms consistent with voiding difficulty, further investigation is unnecessary. Abnormal flow rates would require further urodynamic testing.
2. Frequency and urgency syndromes: It is often necessary to find the urodynamic abnormality responsible for the symptom complex of frequency, nocturia, urgency, and urge incontinence. Flow studies are only preliminary to cystometry in this situation. Flow studies also can be used to evaluate treatment response. One study by Bergman et al. (1989) on patients with urethral syndrome noted a significant improvement in uroflow parameters after urethral dilation in patients who were subjectively improved, whereas no significant change was observed in patients who remained symptomatic.
3. Before pelvic surgery: Stanton et al. (1983) showed that symptoms are an unreliable guide to the presence of voiding difficulty. They recommended that women undergoing pelvic surgery, particularly suprapubic procedures for incontinence and radical pelvic surgery, and those who are elderly, have neurologic disease, or have had past pelvic surgery should have uroflowmetry performed. On the other hand, Bhatia and Bergman (1986) noted that neither abnormal peak flow rates (defined as less than 20 ml/sec during uroflowmetry with voided volumes greater than 200 ml) nor high postvoid residual urine volumes were

predictive of prolonged postoperative voiding difficulties in patients undergoing surgery for stress incontinence.

4. Neurologic disease: When neurologic disease affects the lower urinary tract, various degrees of voiding dysfunction can result. Uroflowmetry is preliminary to more detailed urodynamic tests and at times can be helpful in the diagnosis, management, and prognosis of these patients.

## PRESSURE-FLOW STUDIES

Because urine flow studies can provide only limited information, pressure-flow studies represent a natural progression. Flow rate depends on both the outlet resistance and the contractile properties of the detrusor. A low flow rate may be associated with a high voiding pressure or a below-normal voiding pressure. Similarly, the finding of a normal flow rate does not exclude bladder outlet obstruction because normal flow may be maintained by a high voiding pressure.

Some women have normal flow rates in the absence of a detrusor contraction. This may be because sphincteric relaxation, either alone or assisted by increased intraabdominal pressure from straining, is sufficient to produce a normal flow rate. Pressure-flow studies are essential for a complete functional classification of lower urinary tract disorders and an objective assessment of the basis of a patient's voiding dysfunction.

### Definitions

The following are definitions of standardized terminology proposed by the International Continence Society (Fig. 7-5).

- Premicturition pressure is the intravesical pressure recorded immediately before the initial isovolumetric contraction. It should be the same as the resting pressure at maximum cystometric capacity.
- Opening pressure is the pressure recorded at the onset of measured flow. There is a delay of approximately 0.5 to 1 second in the recording of flow because of the time taken for urine to reach the flowmeter.
- Opening time is the time elapsed from the initial rise in detrusor pressure to the onset of flow. This is the initial isovolumetric contraction period of micturition.
- Maximum voiding pressure is the maximum value of the measured pressure during voiding.
- Pressure at maximum flow is the pressure recorded at the time of maximum flow. Any delay in the recording of flow rate must be allowed for.
- Contraction pressure at maximum flow is the difference between the pressure at maximum flow and the premicturition pressure.
- After-contraction describes the common findings of a pressure increase after flow ceases. The etiology and significance of this event are unknown.

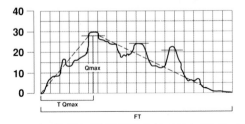

**Fig. 7-4** Uroflowmetric curve with multiple-peak pattern. $Q_{max}$, Maximum flow rate; $TQ_{max}$, time to maximum flow rate; *FT*, flow time.

Adapted from Fantl AJ, Smith PJ, Schneider V, et al: *Am J Obstet Gynecol* 145:1017, 1983.

- To formalize the relationship of pressure and flow, various urethral resistance factors have been proposed. Initially, urethral resistance (UR) was defined as $UR = Pressure/Q_{max}^2$. However, this calculation of resistance fell into dispute largely because it was based on the hydrodynamics of laminar flow through rigid straight tubes. In reality the urethra is neither rigid nor straight, and flow is often turbulent, not laminar. In 1987 the ICS recommended that pressure-flow data be presented graphically, plotting one quantity against the other (Rowan et al., 1987).

## Methodology

These studies are usually performed after a cystometric evaluation. In most patients it is clear when bladder filling should be stopped. However, if the patient has little sensation, it is important to use the functional bladder capacity from the frequency-volume chart as a guide to cystometric capacity. At this point, if a separate filling catheter is being used it is removed; the intravesical catheter is left in place. An intravaginal or intrarectal catheter records intraabdominal pressure to assess whether the patient uses a Valsalva maneuver to void and to electronically derive true detrusor pressure. Thus these studies involve the monitoring of abdominal, intravesical, and true detrusor pressure synchronously with flow. External sphincter electromyographic (EMG) activity, as well as urethral pressure, also may be measured. To ensure that proper pressure transmission is occurring, the patient should be asked to cough before being allowed to void. With the patient in a sitting position, she is then instructed to void to completion if possible (Fig. 7-6). It is very important during the voiding phase to respect the patient's privacy. Few women are able to void in the presence of others, so it may be necessary for the practitioner to leave the room for her to initiate voiding. Once flow is initiated, the patient can be asked to interrupt the stream suddenly (stop test). This test attempts to establish voluntary control of micturition and also obtains isometric detrusor pressure.

## Interpretation

Pressure-flow studies are invasive because the patient is asked to void around catheters, sometimes with EMG needles in place. It is important to appreciate the limitations

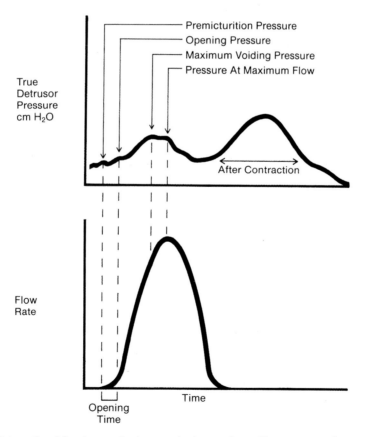

**Fig. 7-5** International Continence Society terminology and specific parameters for pressure-flow studies.

From Karram MM: Urodynamics. In Benson JT, ed: *Female pelvic floor disorders: investigation and management,* New York, 1992, Norton Medical Books.

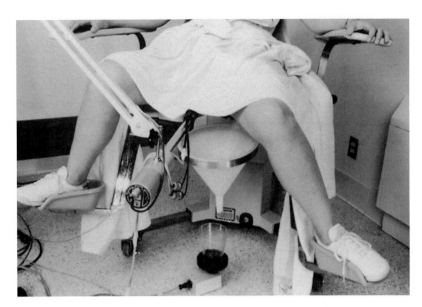

**Fig. 7-6** Technique for performing pressure-flow studies. The patient must be able to void around the catheters.

of pressure-flow studies, as well as the differences between the patient's performance during urodynamic testing and her normal voiding. This is best judged by asking the patient and by comparing the noninstrumented urine flow rate with the flow rate obtained from the pressure-flow study.

Voiding in a urodynamic laboratory can be affected by a variety of factors. It is estimated that approximately 30% of women who void without problems at home are unable to void on command in the urodynamic laboratory. This is hardly surprising because they are surrounded by complex equipment, have catheters in their bladder and vagina or rectum, and are usually being observed by strangers.

Fast filling or overfilling of the bladder may make normal voiding difficult. Studies that compared ambulatory urodynamics (natural bladder filling) with conventional urodynamics show that voiding pressures are higher with natural filling. This implies that the detrusor may be incompletely stimulated, partially inhibited, or mechanically less efficient if it is overfilled or filled too fast.

During the voiding phase, the detrusor muscle may be normal, acontractile, or underactive. Normal voiding is usually achieved by a voluntarily initiated detrusor contraction that is sustained and can be suppressed. An underactive detrusor during micturition implies that the detrusor contraction is of inadequate magnitude or duration (or both) to effect bladder emptying within a normal time span. Detrusor areflexia is defined as acontractility caused by an abnormality of nervous control and denotes the complete absence of a centrally coordinated contraction.

During voiding, urethral function may be normal or obstructed. A normal urethra is relaxed throughout voiding. Obstruction may be secondary to urethral overactivity or a mechanical obstruction, such as a urethral stricture or tumor.

Urethral obstruction for whatever reason leads to increased voiding pressures. In mechanical obstruction, which is rare in females, the voiding pressures are constantly elevated. If the obstruction is caused by urethral overactivity, the voiding pressures may fluctuate. Urethral overactivity is characterized by the urethra contracting during voiding or the urethra failing to relax. In detrusor-sphincter dyssynergia, the patient's phasic contractions of the intrinsic urethral striated muscle are simultaneous with the detrusor contraction. This produces a very high voiding pressure and an interrupted flow. The urodynamic characteristic of this type of urethral overactivity is a fall in flow rate accompanied by a rising detrusor pressure that then falls when the urethra relaxes, leading to a resumption of urine flow. Another form of urethral overactivity is called dysfunctional voiding. This is most commonly seen in children who are neurologically normal but complain of urinary incontinence or recurrent infections. The interrupted flow in these children is caused by pelvic floor overactivity rather than contractions of the intrinsic striated muscle.

Depending on age, menopausal status, total voided volume, and the presence or absence of lower urinary tract dysfunction, women void by any combination of a detrusor contraction, abdominal straining, and urethral relaxation (Table 7-1 and Figs. 7-7 and 7-8).

It is difficult to ascertain whether abdominal straining that occurs during a pressure-flow study is real or artifactually induced by the surroundings and presence of indwelling catheters. The patient should always be asked to void normally and in as relaxed a way as possible. If the patient has an acontractile detrusor, voiding can be achieved only by straining (Fig. 7-8). If the detrusor contracts during voiding but the patient also strains, then the tracing is more

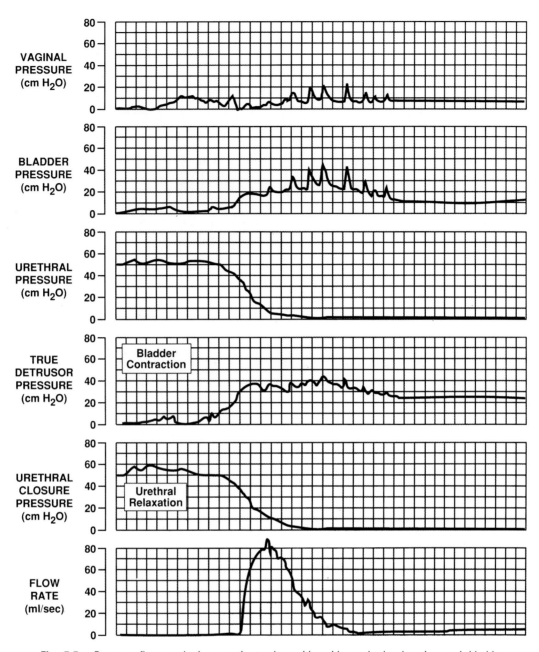

**Fig. 7-7**   Pressure-flow study in a patient who voids with urethral relaxation and bladder contraction. Note minimal Valsalva effort.

difficult to interpret. It is also difficult to understand precisely what effect straining has on urine flow. In patients without obstruction, straining increases flow, but it does not produce the same increase in flow as that achieved by a detrusor pressure rise of the same magnitude. However, in obstructed patients, straining does not increase flow.

Although pressure-flow studies are an established and accepted urodynamic modality, what constitutes a normal voiding mechanism is incompletely understood, as is the normal range for detrusor pressure during voiding in women. Most of the previously published literature has been

**Table 7-1**   Potential Voiding Mechanisms on Pressure-Flow Studies in Neurologically Intact Women

| Urethral relaxation | Bladder contraction | Abdominal straining |
|---|---|---|
| Present | Absent | Absent |
| Present | Present | Absent |
| Present | Absent | Present |
| Present | Present | Present |

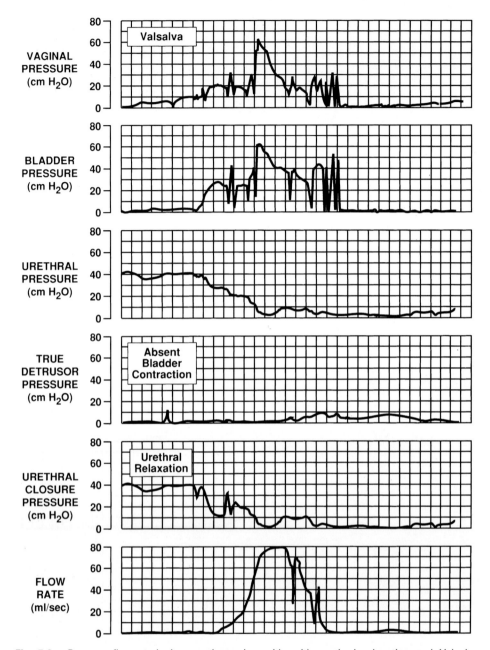

**Fig. 7-8** Pressure-flow study in a patient who voids with urethral relaxation and Valsalva maneuver. Note that bladder contraction is absent.

derived from male subjects in which pressures are abnormally high secondary to more frequent outflow obstruction.

As previously mentioned, to better evaluate the detrusor during voiding, one may perform a stop-flow test (Fig. 7-9). In many patients, if voiding is suddenly interrupted by sphincter action, the detrusor pressure rises rapidly. This behavior reflects a fundamental myogenic property of the contracting detrusor: a trade-off between the pressure generated and the flow delivered. The detrusor pressure attained on stopping (isometric detrusor pressure) should be a more reliable measure of detrusor contractions than the

detrusor pressure during voiding, which also depends on flow rate and urethral resistance.

The routine clinical use of the stop test has some disadvantages. A high isometric detrusor pressure implies a good detrusor contraction, but a low or absent rise in pressure does not necessarily imply lack of a detrusor contraction. The detrusor contraction may be reflexly inhibited when the urethra is closed, or flow may be interrupted by inhibiting the detrusor instead of increasing outlet resistance. In addition, the patient may be unable to interrupt her stream completely on command. These situations can lead

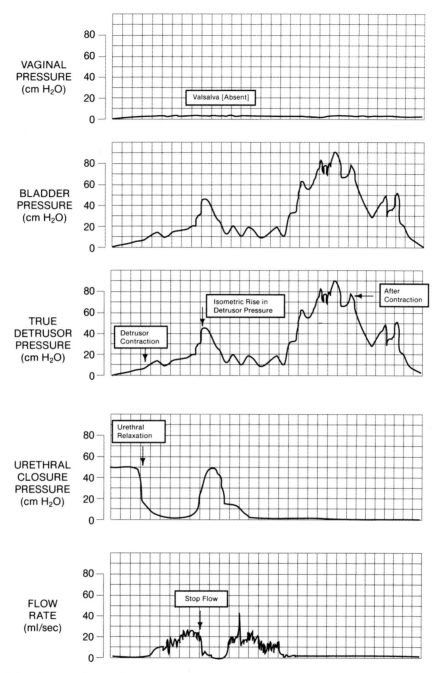

**Fig. 7-9**   Pressure-flow study with stop test. Note isometric rise in detrusor pressure simultaneous with stoppage of flow.

to a falsely low isometric detrusor pressure. For these reasons, the test is probably more accurate when the urethra is physically occluded with a catheter or by elevation of the anterior vaginal wall.

## Clinical Applicability

The main clinical use of pressure-flow studies is to document the mechanism of abnormal voiding. If a patient has symptoms and signs of abnormal voiding, has low flow rates, and voids with a high detrusor pressure, she is

probably voiding against an obstruction. On the other hand, if a patient has low flow rates and voids with minimal or no rise in detrusor pressure, then her voiding dysfunction is probably secondary to an acontractile or underactive detrusor (Fig. 7-10). The limiting factor is that there is no clear cutoff between normal and abnormally high detrusor pressure during voiding.

The clinical setting in which pressure-flow studies are most useful in women is in the patient who has undergone pelvic surgery and has developed postoperative voiding

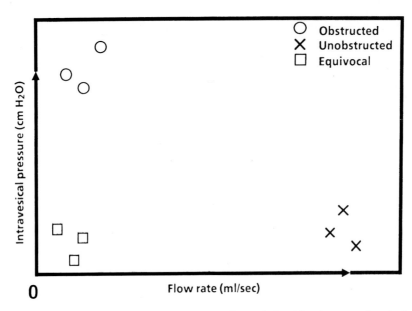

**Fig. 7-10** Recommended presentation of pressure-flow relationships for normal and abnormal voiding.
From Walters MD: *Obstet Gynecol Clin North Am* 16:773, 1989.

dysfunction. The dysfunction may be secondary to denervation, resulting in an underactive or acontractile detrusor, or the dysfunction may be secondary to increased outlet resistance produced from the surgery. Voiding dysfunction or retention occurs in 5% to 20% of patients after various operations to correct stress incontinence. It is always a clinical dilemma whether urethrolysis or a takedown of the repair will restore normal voiding. Filling cystometry and pressure-flow studies are helpful in this setting. If the patient is able to void around a catheter and is noted to have a high detrusor pressure with a low flow rate, then the patient is obstructed and relieving the obstruction should improve voiding (Nitti, 1994).

Bhatia and Bergman (1984) performed pressure-flow studies on 30 patients with stress incontinence before retropubic urethropexy. They noted that no patient who voided with a detrusor contraction greater than 15 cm $H_2O$ preoperatively required prolonged bladder drainage (more than 7 days). Eighty-four percent of patients who used significant abdominal straining in addition to urethral relaxation during voiding required prolonged postoperative catheterization. Thus these studies may be useful prognostically to predict postoperative voiding difficulty in patients undergoing antiincontinence surgery.

## COMBINED STUDIES

Pressure-flow studies performed under fluoroscopy can be a useful diagnostic urodynamic procedure. The size of the bladder and the presence of trabeculations, bladder diverticula, and vesicoureteral reflux can be visualized. Competence of the sphincter can be assessed and the patient's ability to initiate and stop micturition can be observed. The site of significant outflow obstruction usually can also be detected. The technique of these studies is discussed in Chapter 6.

When neurogenic voiding dysfunction is present or suspected, EMG activity of the external striated sphincter should be recorded. These studies are discussed in Chapter 9.

## SUMMARY

Any condition that affects detrusor contractility or urethral resistance can impair micturition. Uroflowmetry is a simple noninvasive test that can be used to document voiding dysfunction objectively. Because it does not provide direct information on expulsive forces or outlet resistance, it is probably best considered a screening test.

Pressure-flow studies provide information on detrusor and abdominal pressure. They are helpful in differentiating voiding dysfunction secondary to obstruction from that secondary to an underactive detrusor. They also may give useful information to predict postoperative voiding dysfunction after urethropexy. However, these tests are invasive and unpredictable; 20% to 30% of patients are not able to void around the catheters and artifacts are difficult to assess. More research is needed to define normal voiding parameters in women and to determine the value of these tests in clinical practice.

# BIBLIOGRAPHY

Abrams P: Uroflowmetry. In Stanton SL, ed: *Clinical gynecologic urology,* St Louis, 1984, Mosby.

Abrams P, Blavas JG, Stanton SL, et al: Sixth report on the standardization of terminology of lower urinary tract function. Procedures related to neurophysiological investigations: electromyography, nerve conduction studies, reflex latencies, evoked potentials and sensory testing, *World J Urol* 4:2, 1986; *Scand J Urol Nephrol* 20:161, 1986.

Abrams P, Torrens M: Urine flow studies, *Urol Clin North Am* 6:71, 1979.

Backman KA: Urinary flow during micturition in normal women, *Acta Chir Scand* 130:357, 1965.

Barnick CG, Cardozo LD, Benness C: Use of routine videocystourethrography in the evaluation of female lower urinary tract dysfunction, *Neurourol Urodyn* 8:447, 1989.

Bergman A, Bhatia NN: Uroflowmetry: spontaneous versus instrumented, *Am J Obstet Gynecol* 150:788, 1984.

Bergman A, Bhatia NN: Uroflowmetry for predicting postoperative voiding difficulties in women with stress urinary incontinence, *Br J Obstet Gynaecol* 92:835, 1985.

Bergman A, Karram M, Bhatia N: Urethral syndrome: a comparison of different treatment modalities, *J Reprod Med* 34:157, 1989.

Bhatia NN, Bergman A: Urodynamic predictiablity of voiding following incontinence surgery, *Obstet Gynecol* 63:85, 1984.

Bhatia NN, Bergman A: Use of preoperative uroflowmetry and simultaneous urethrocystometry for predicting risk of prolonged postoperative bladder drainage, *Urology* 28:440, 1986.

Bhatia NN, Bergman A, Karram MM: Changes in urethral resistance following incontinence surgery, *Urology* 34:200, 1989.

Bradley WE: Urologically oriented neurological examination. In Ostergard DR, ed: *Gynecologic urology and urodynamics,* ed 2, Baltimore, 1985, Williams & Wilkins.

Chancellor MB, Killholma P: Urodynamic evaluation of patients following spinal cord injury, *Semin Urol* 10:83, 1992.

Cucchi A: Acceleration of flow rate as a screening test for detrusor instability in women with stress incontinence, *Br J Urol* 65:17, 1990.

Diokno AC, Normolle DP, Brown MB, et al: Urodynamic tests for female geriatric urinary incontinence., *Urology* 36:431, 1990.

Drach GW, Ignatoff J, Layton T: Peak urinary flow rate: observations in female subjects and comparison to male subjects, *J Urol* 122:215, 1979.

Drake WM: The uroflowmeter: an aid to the study of lower urinary tract, *J Urol* 59:650, 1948.

Enhorning G: Simultaneous recording of intravesical and intraurethral pressure, *Acta Chir Scand* 276 (suppl):4, 1961.

Fantl AJ: Clinical uroflowmetry. In Ostergard DR, ed: *Gynecologic urology and urodynamics,* ed 2, Baltimore, 1985, Williams & Wilkins.

Fantl AJ, Smith PJ, Schneider V, et al: Fluid weight uroflowmetry in women, *Am J Obstet Gynecol* 145:1017, 1983.

Griffiths DJ: Uses and limitations of mechanical analogies in urodynamics, *Urol Clin North Am* 6:143, 1979.

Griffiths DJ: Basics of pressure-flow studies, *World J Urol* 13:30, 1995.

Haylen BT, Ashby D, Sutherst JR, et al: Maximum and average flow rates in normal male and female populations: the Liverpool nomograms, *Br J Urol* 64:30, 1989.

Haylen BT, Parys BT, Anyaegbunam WI, et al: Urine flow rates in male and female urodynamic patients compared with Liverpool nomograms, *Br J Urol* 65:483, 1990.

Karl C, Gerlach R, Hannappel J, et al: Uroflow measurements: their information yield in a long-term investigation of pre- and postoperative measurements, *Urol Int* 41:270, 1986.

Massey A, Abrams P: Urodynamics of the female lower urinary tract, *Urol Clin North Am* 12:231, 1985.

Meunier P: Study of micturition parameters in healthy young adults using a uroflowmetric method, *Eur J Clin Inv* 13:25, 1983.

Mundy AP: Clinical physiology of the bladder, urethra and pelvic floor. In Mundy AP, Stephenson TP, Wein AJ, eds: *Urodynamics: principles, practice and applications,* New York, 1984, Churchill Livingstone.

Nitti VW, Raz S: Obstruction following anticontinence procedures: diagnosis and treatment with transvaginal urethrolysis, *J Urol* 152:93, 1994.

Rowan D, James ED, Kramer AEJL, et al: Urodynamic equipment technical aspects, *J Med Eng Technol* 11:57, 1987.

Saxton HM: Urodynamics: the appropriate modality for the investigation of frequency, urgency, incontinence, and voiding difficulties, *Radiology* 175:307, 1990.

Stanton SL, Ozsoy C, Hilton P: Voiding difficulties in the female: prevalence, clinical and urodynamic review, *Obstet Gynecol* 61:144, 1983.

Susset JG, Brissot RB, Regnier CH: The stop-flow technique: a way to measure detrusor strength, *J Urol* 127:489, 1982.

Susset JG, Picker P, Kretz M, et al: Critical evaluation of uroflometers and analysis of normal curves, *J Urol* 109:874, 1983.

Tanagho EA: Urodynamics: uroflowmetry and female voiding patterns. In Ostergard DR, ed: *Gynecologic urology and urodynamics,* ed 2, Baltimore, 1985, Williams & Wilkins.

Tanagho EA, McCurrey E: Pressure and flow rate as related to lumen caliber and entrance configuration, *J Urol* 105:583, 1971.

Tanagho EA, Miller ER: Initiation of voiding, *Br J Urol* 42:175, 1970.

van Garrelts B: Analysis of micturition: a new method of recording the voiding of the bladder, *Acta Chir Scand* 112:326, 1956.

van Garrelts B, Strandell P: Continuous recording of urinary flow-rate, *Scand J Urol Nephrol* 6:224, 1972.

Walter S, Olesen KP, Nordling J, et al: Bladder function in urologically normal middle aged females, *Scand J Urol Nephrol* 13:249, 1979.

Walters MD: Mechanism of continence and voiding, with International Continence Society classification of dysfunction, *Obstet Gynecol Clin North Am* 16:773,1989.

Yalla SV, Blunt KJ, Fam BA, et al: Detrusor–urethral sphincter dyssynergia, *J Urol* 118:1026, 1977.

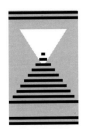

CHAPTER **8**

# Urodynamics: Urethral Pressure Profilometry and Leak Point Pressures

Mickey M. Karram and John R. Miklos

There is no general consensus on how best to evaluate urethral function in women with lower urinary tract dysfunction. Ideally, urethral function is assessed quantitatively in the hope of providing objective parameters that can be used to make important clinical decisions. Urinary continence depends on the pressure in the urethra exceeding the pressure in the bladder at all times, even with increases in abdominal pressure. Contributing to normal urethral compliance and pressure are smooth and striated urethral muscles; fibroelastic tissue of the urethral wall; vascular tension caused by the rich, spongy network around the urethra; and extrinsic compression from surrounding pelvic floor musculature. The urethra lies on the supportive layer composed of the endopelvic fascia and the anterior vaginal wall. This layer is structurally stable because of its bilateral attachment (as a hammock) to the arcus tendineus fasciae pelvis and the levator ani. Intraabdominal pressures compress the urethra to close its lumen; that is, urethral closure pressure during stress rises because the urethra is compressed.

Attempts to evaluate and quantify the urethra's role in storage and voiding disorders have led to the development and use of urethral pressure profilometry and leak point pressure studies. Urethral pressure profilometry is a graphic representation of pressure within the urethra at successive points along its length. Leak point pressure is a measurement of the amount of abdominal pressure or detrusor pressure required to overcome outlet resistance and produce incontinence. This chapter reviews the methodology, interpretation variables, and clinical applications of these tests.

## URETHRAL PRESSURE PROFILOMETRY

The first attempt to measure urethral pressure was published in 1923 by Victor Bonney, who used the technique of retrograde sphincterometry. This method was replaced by a balloon catheter in 1936. Karlson (1953) introduced the technique of simultaneous measurement of intraurethral and intravesical pressure (urethrocystometry), and in 1969 the fluid profusion method was described by Brown and Wickham. More recent technology has introduced the use of microtransducer catheters.

### Definitions

The International Continence Society has standardized terminology relating to urethral pressure profilometry.

A urethral pressure profile (UPP) indicates the intraluminal pressure along the length of the urethra with the bladder at rest. When describing this method, one should specify the catheter type and size, the measurement technique, the rate of infusion (if the Brown and Wickham technique is used), the rate of catheter withdrawal, the bladder volume, and the position of the patient.

The maximum urethral pressure is the maximum pressure of the measured profile.

The maximum urethral closure pressure is the difference between the maximum urethral pressure and the intravesical pressure.

The functional urethral length is the length of the urethra along which the urethral pressure exceeds the intravesical pressure and the anatomic urethral length is the total length of the urethra (Fig. 8-1).

The pressure transmission ratio (PTR) is the increment in urethral pressure on stress as a percentage of the simultaneously reported increment in vesical pressure. For stress profiles obtained during coughing, PTRs can be obtained at any point along the urethra. If single values are given, the position of the urethra should be stated. If several PTRs are defined at different points along the urethra, a pressure transmission profile is obtained. The term *transmission* is

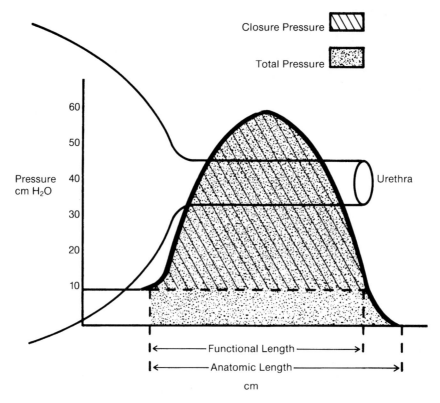

**Fig. 8-1** Urethral pressure profile demonstrating total urethral pressure, urethral closure pressure, and anatomic and functional urethral length.

From Karram MM: Urodynamics. In Benson JT, ed: *Female pelvic floor disorders: investigation and management,* New York, 1992, Norton Medical Books.

commonly used, but *transmission* implies a completely passive process. Such an assumption is not yet justified by scientific evidence because a role for muscular activity cannot be excluded.

## Methodology

Urethral pressure can be measured with balloon catheters, membrane catheters, perfusion techniques, or microtransducers. With balloon catheters, the frequency of the response is determined by the catheter-manometer system. It integrates the pressure over the length and circumference of the whole balloon. This reduces the disturbances caused by local variations and averages are obtained rather than a point of measurement. The system has a rise time of 40 ms, so it probably cannot give an accurate indication of urethral response to physiologic stresses. In addition, the balloon is deformed by pressure variations that affect the cross-sectional area of the balloon, so the measurements are distorted.

Perfusion techniques involve the use of one- or two-channel catheters with side holes through which saline or gas is perfused with a motorized syringe pump. The advantage of this system is that the infused fluid prevents blockage. However, any sudden rise in pressure results in tissue contact initially blocking the side hole, resulting in a raised pressure until the infusing fluid clears the blockage. Not all fluid systems have an adequate frequency response time to measure stress profiles.

Microtransducers are currently the most widely used catheters for urethral pressure studies in the United States. These catheters have two microtransducers mounted 6 cm apart. The distal transducer in the bladder measures bladder pressure, whereas the more proximal catheter is manually or mechanically withdrawn through the urethra. Microtransducers have an adequate response time for all aspects of urethral pressure profilometry. The sidewall mounting of the transducer provides a more reproducible recording of both mechanical and fluid pressures in a collapsible tube. Some investigators have used multiple transducers along the urethra to assess stationary recordings of UPPs.

Hilton and Stanton (1983) suggested a standard technique for performing UPPs using microtransducer catheters. We use a similar technique (Fig. 8-2).

1. With the patient in the sitting position at maximum cystometric capacity (usually after filling cystourethrometry), the catheter is secured to a mechanical puller. The orientation of the transducer on the catheter is directed laterally to the 9 o'clock position.

2. As the proximal transducer is pulled through the urethra, the resting or static urethral pressure is recorded on graph

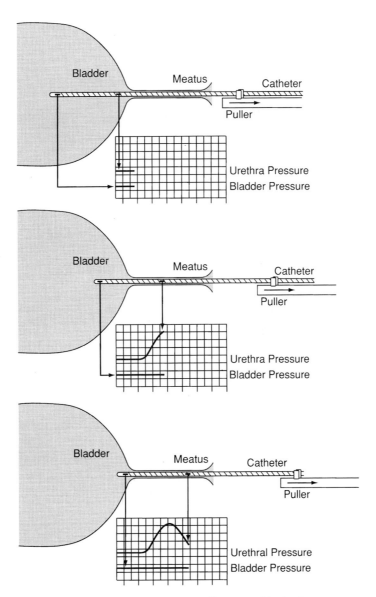

**Fig. 8-2**    Technique of static urethral pressure profilometry with simultaneous measurement of bladder pressure. Study begins with both microtransducers in the bladder *(top)*. As the catheter is mechanically withdrawn through the urethra *(middle and bottom)*, urethral and bladder pressures are recorded.

paper that is moving at the same speed as the catheter. The urethral closure pressure ($P_{ure} - P_{ves}$) is recorded on a separate channel. The proximal sensor is then mechanically reinserted into the bladder, and a second profile is obtained to ensure consistency and reproducibility of results. A minimum of two profiles are averaged to obtain final results.

3. To perform a cough or stress pressure profile, the same procedure is repeated with the patient coughing repetitively while the catheter is withdrawn through the urethra. The patient should cough at a consistent intensity, every 2 to 3 seconds, which corresponds approximately to every 2 to 3 mm of functional urethral length. It is important that the recorder be set so that the entire ampli-

tude of each cough spike in the bladder and urethra remains on the chart paper (Fig. 8-3). The external urethral meatus is visualized for involuntary loss of urine.

## Interpretation Variables

Urethral pressure is measured by inserting a transducer, mounted on a catheter into a normally coapted lumen. In reality, what is being measured is the force exerted by the walls of the urethra on the transducer. If the urethra were a tube with a circular lumen, the occlusive forces would be equal around its circumference; however, because the urethra is a collapsed tube with the anterior and posterior walls in apposition, the occlusive forces are unequally distributed around the urethra. Thus, certain factors must be

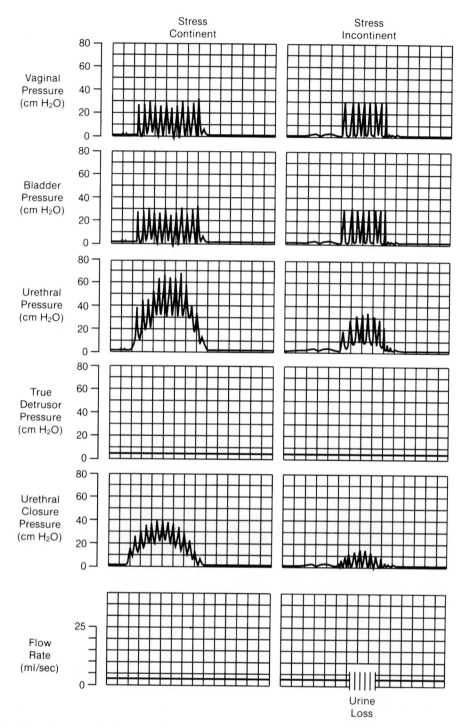

**Fig. 8-3** Dynamic (cough) pressure profile in continent patient *(left)* (note good pressure transmission) and in incontinent patient *(right)* (note poor pressure transmission).

taken into consideration to ensure the reproducibility of urethral pressure studies.

Studies on orientation of the microtransducer within the urethral lumen have noted that the pressure is highest when the transducer is placed anteriorly and lowest when it is placed posteriorly. For this reason, most studies are per-

formed with the transducer in the lateral positions, providing more standardized measurement. In addition, the pressure measurement depends on the size and stiffness of the catheter as well as the form of the pressure sensor. Catheter sizes ranging from 8 to 12 French and withdrawal speeds of 1 to 40 cm per minute do not significantly affect urethral pressure results. The position of the patient and bladder volume should also be standardized. It has been noted that urethral pressure increases with increasing bladder volumes in continent, neurologically intact females. Most tests are performed in the supine or sitting position. The normal response to the assumption of a more upright posture is an increase in the maximum urethral closure pressure of about 23%. In some abnormal patients this increase may not occur, and in women with neurogenic bladders, the increase in pressure may be excessive (greater than 100%). When performing stress pressure profiles, Schick (1985) noted that PTRs decrease as the strength of cough increases. Therefore, reproducibility requires comparable strengths of coughs during these tests.

A normal female UPP is symmetric in shape, and asymmetry is generally caused by a faulty measurement technique. The values for normal urethral pressures in the literature are all taken from very small series. Recently, Abrams (1997) published values for maximum urethral pressure in patients who have no lower urinary tract abnormality noted on clinical or urodynamic assessment. He noticed a significant deterioration in closure pressure with an increase in age, noting a mean maximum urethral pressure of 90 cm $H_2O$ in patients less than 25 years old, with a significant decrease over time to a mean of 65 cm $H_2O$ in patients older than 64 years. This is similar to previous data published by Rud (1980), who noted that maximum urethral pressure decreases with changes in vascularization that are inevitable with increasing age. Also, previous studies indicate that there is a trend toward lower urethral closure pressures and shorter functional length in stress incontinent patients than in patients who are stress continent.

## Clinical Applications

The clinical applications of urethral pressure studies are very controversial. Some investigators believe that urethral pressure studies are clinically useful in certain conditions, while others believe that they have no clinical utility.

### Diagnosis of Genuine Stress Incontinence

Over the years many investigators have attempted to use urethral pressure studies to explain the pathogenesis of urinary incontinence and to diagnose genuine stress incontinence. However, the lack of consistent associations of UPP variables with diagnoses confirmed by video-urodynamic testing has limited its acceptance. Versi et al. (1990) examined 24 urethral pressure variables and used kappa statistical analysis to determine which variables were the most discriminatory. Although there was a significant difference in maximum urethral closure pressure between patients with genuine stress incontinence and continent women, there was a large overlap between the two groups. They concluded that no single parameter of a urethral pressure study could be used to diagnose genuine stress incontinence.

PTR is a test of the dynamic response of the urethra to increases in intraabdominal pressure. It requires simultaneous measurement of urethral and vesical pressures during coughing, allowing the calculation of the relative amounts of abdominal pressure transmitted to each structure. The PTR can be used to quantitate urethral closure during stress. It is calculated by dividing a cough-induced urethral pressure increase by the bladder pressure increase and multiplying by 100 (Fig. 8-4). Bump et al. (1988) performed PTRs on 110 subjects and noted that women with genuine stress incontinence had significantly lower mean PTRs than continent women. Rosenzweig et al. (1991) performed PTRs on 63 patients with stress incontinence before and after Burch colposuspension. They observed no difference in preoperative PTRs between UPPs with and without leakage of urine. They could not determine a threshold PTR that was associated with urine loss. However, they did note that the higher the postoperative pressure ratio, the more likely the surgical success. Consequently, PTRs should not be considered diagnostic tests to help determine the type of incontinence, but tests more aimed at assessing urethral function and position.

### Diagnosis of Intrinsic Sphincter Deficiency

Urethral pressure profilometry can be used in the planning of the type of surgery indicated to correct genuine stress incontinence. Numerous retrospective studies have noted that a low maximum urethral closure pressure is a predictor of poor outcome for conventional antiincontinence surgery that suspends or stabilizes the bladder neck. It has been suggested that in patients with lower maximum urethral closure pressures, intrinsic sphincter deficiency (ISD) is the cause of their incontinence. Thus, an operation more aimed at obstructing the urethra, such as a suburethral sling, injection of a bulk-enhancing agent, or possibly an artificial urinary sphincter, should be used. Others, though identifying the potential of a low urethral pressure as a risk factor for failure of suspension surgeries, do not consider that the increased complication rate of sling procedures is justified because a reasonable cure rate can still be obtained with a colposuspension. The concept of a static low urethral closure pressure being a risk factor for failure of suspension procedures was initially reported by McGuire (1981), and later by Sand et al. (1987), both in a retrospective fashion. Sand et al. (1987) reported on 86 women undergoing Burch colposuspension. They noted that the failure rate was three times higher in patients with preoperative closure pressures less than 20 cm $H_2O$ than in those who had urethral closure pressures greater than 20 cm $H_2O$. Other studies have also noted the failure rate with various stress incontinence procedure surgeries to be higher in patients with low urethral closure pressures. Some of these studies have used a cutoff of 20 cm $H_2O$, but in other studies no cutoff point was stated.

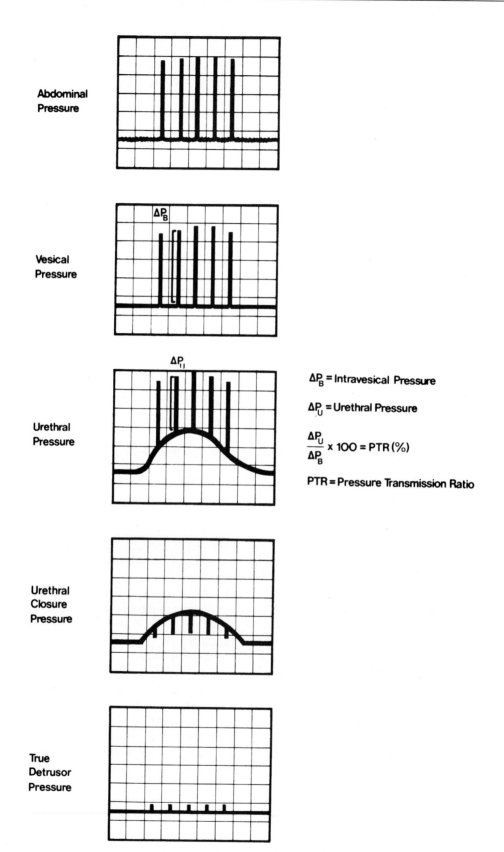

**Fig. 8-4**   Method of calculation of pressure transmission ratio during cough pressure profile.

From Karram MM: Urodynamics. In Benson JT, ed: *Female pelvic floor disorders: investigation and management,*
New York, 1992, Norton Medical Books.

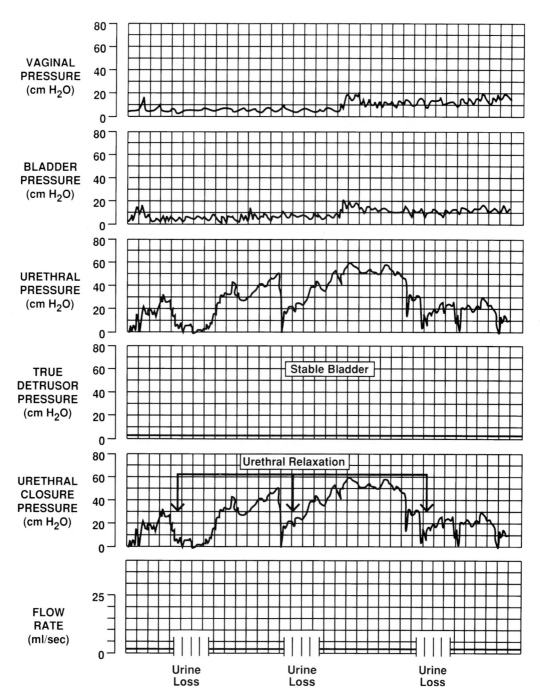

**Fig. 8-5**   Multichannel urodynamic tracing of a patient with urethral instability (uninhibited urethral relaxation). Note bladder pressure remains stable and there is visual loss of urine, simultaneous with drop in urethral pressure.

## Diagnosis of Urethral Instability

When measurements of urethral pressure are performed during filling cystometry, it is not uncommon to note fluctuations in urethral pressure. Normally these fluctuations are synchronous with the heartbeat because of normal urethral vascular pulsation. Artifactual pressure fluctuations caused by urethral catheter movement are common and should not be confused with the following conditions. The association between variations in urethral pressure (at the point of maximum urethral closure pressure at rest) and abnormal detrusor function has been examined. This phenomenon is known as urethral instability, which has been defined by the International Continence Society as an involuntary fall in intraurethral pressure in the absence of any rise in true detrusor pressure, resulting in the leakage of urine (Fig. 8-5). Others have defined urethral instability as simply unstable urethral pressures in which large fluctuations of urethral pressure, not necessarily associated with incontinence, occur (Fig. 8-6).

Although uninhibited urethral relaxation is a well-documented cause of incontinence, it is very rare and its management is currently controversial. This form of urethral instability may actually be a form of detrusor instability in which urethral pressure loss occurs, but the detrusor contraction is not perceived because the urethra is open and a urethral-vesical equilibrium exists.

Tapp et al. (1988b) investigated the correlation between unstable urethral pressure and clinical symptoms by comparing women with significant versus nonsignificant variations in mean urethral closure pressure. His analysis was carried out for absolute cutoff points and also for the ratio change in mean urethral closure pressure to resting mean urethral closure pressure. He concluded that there was no significant difference in clinical symptoms between these two groups. It is apparent that the actual significant level of fluctuation in mean urethral pressure and the overall clinical relevance of this entity is subject to debate.

## Diagnosis of Urethral Diverticulum

Although suburethral diverticulas are best diagnosed by radiologic studies or endoscopic studies, it has been reported that the presence of a biphasic curve on a UPP indicates the possibility of a diverticulum. However, this configuration may also occur in some cases of genuine stress incontinence, especially in women who have previously undergone incontinence surgery. The typical UPP in patients with suburethral diverticulum shows a loss of urethral pressure at the level of the diverticular ostium. If the diverticulum is proximal to the maximum urethral pressure, the operation of choice should be diverticulectomy; however, if it is distal to this point, marsupialization (Spence procedure) can be considered.

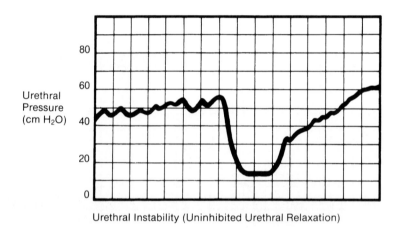

Urethral Instability (Uninhibited Urethral Relaxation)

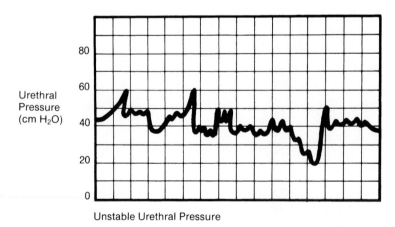

Unstable Urethral Pressure

**Fig. 8-6** Graphic representation to show difference between urethral instability (uninhibited urethral relaxation) and unstable urethral pressure.

From Karram MM: Urodynamics. In Benson JT, ed: *Female pelvic floor disorders: investigation and management,* New York, 1992, Norton Medical Books.

## LEAK POINT PRESSURES

An alternative method to evaluate or objectively assess urethral resistance and function is the leak point pressure. Abdominal and detrusor leak point pressures determine urethral resistance to two different expulsive forces. As far as the urethra is concerned, these two forces (abdominal and detrusor pressure) are the sum total of the forces acting on the urethra to cause leakage.

### Definitions

An abdominal or stress (cough or Valsalva maneuver) leak point pressure is a measure of the stress competence of the urethra or a measure of the ability of the urethra to resist the expulsive forces of abdominal pressure. It is the amount of abdominal pressure (in cm $H_2O$) required to overcome urethral resistance and produce urine leakage.

A detrusor or bladder leak point pressure is a measurement of the resistance of the urethra to detrusor pressure as an expulsive force. A detrusor leak point pressure is related to upper tract function in that a high detrusor leak point pressure is associated with the propensity for upper tract deterioration.

Leak point pressures, abdominal and bladder, actually reflect outlet resistance at the time these forces individually induce leakage. Neither leak point pressure reflects the strength or character of the detrusor contraction.

### Methodology

Ideally, the technique of performing an abdominal leak point pressure should be standardized and performed exactly the same way each time to allow comparison between patients and to make posttreatment studies meaningful. Many controversies exist regarding the technique of this test. These include catheter size, bladder volume, type of provocation, patient positioning, how the actual rise in pressure is determined, and how best to perform the test in the presence of genital prolapse. In abdominal leak point pressure measurements it is essential that the cystometrogram is stable (i.e., there is no significant increase in detrusor pressure during filling). If abnormal bladder compliance does exist, leak point pressure testing will underestimate urethral sphincter resistance.

The technique we use for measuring abdominal leak point pressures is as follows. With a 6-French dual-sensor microtip transducer in the bladder, subtracted filling cystometry is performed to a bladder volume of 150 to 200 ml. Assuming no abnormalities in bladder compliance are present, leak point pressure measurements are performed at this volume. In the sitting position, the patient performs a gradually more vigorous Valsalva maneuver until leakage occurs. The lowest bladder pressure at which leaking occurs is considered the abdominal leak point pressure (Fig. 8-7, *A*). If a Valsalva maneuver cannot produce enough abdominal pressure to produce leakage or the patient is unable to strain on command, then coughing is used as the provoca-

tive maneuver. Because coughing is a more "rapid" process than straining, attainment of accurate and reproducible values is more difficult. The patient is asked to cough repetitively, and the external urethral meatus is visualized for leakage. Once leakage has occurred, the strength of the cough is reduced until the cough that generates the minimal amount of abdominal pressure required to produce leakage is isolated (Fig. 8-7, *B*). These maneuvers are then performed several times in the hope of documenting reproducible values. If patients do not leak with either a Valsalva maneuver or repetitive coughing, the catheter is removed from the bladder and the provocative maneuvers are repeated with the abdominal pressure being measured via an intravaginal or intrarectal catheter. Filling cystometry is then continued to maximum cystometric capacity, and the leak point pressure measurements are repeated. Although these numbers are usually significantly lower than those noted at 150 to 200 ml, they can be useful in objectively documenting and following the severity of the disease after various modes of nonsurgical or surgical therapy.

To perform a bladder leak point pressure, the filling cystometrogram is performed at a slower filling rate, usually 25 ml/min. The patient is typically supine for this study. Filling continues to the point at which leakage occurs and is identified by either direct observation or fluoroscopy. The total bladder pressure (i.e., detrusor and abdominal pressures) is measured and recorded as the bladder leak point pressure. In some patients the pressure may occur at very large volumes and high pressures. Once a bladder pressure of 40 cm $H_2O$ is reached, the study can be terminated as ongoing filling above this pressure can be dangerous.

### Interpretation Variables

Variables in performing this study revolve around the lack of standardization. Multiple parameters have been shown to affect the abdominal leak point pressure measurements. These include catheter caliber, catheter location (vaginal versus intravesical), bladder volume, the use of coughing versus Valsalva maneuver as the provocation, patient position, and the use of an absolute or change in measured pressure.

More subjects demonstrate urine loss during Valsalva maneuvers with a 3-French rather than 8-French transurethral catheter, and the abdominal leak point pressures obtained with the 3-French catheter are consistently lower. At least two investigators have shown that removal of the transurethral catheter and measurement of the intraabdominal pressure rise with an intravaginal or intrarectal catheter consistently lowered abdominal leak point pressure by up to 20 cm $H_2O$, suggesting that the transurethral catheters are obstructive.

An inverse relationship exists between bladder volume and abdominal leak point pressures. Miklos et al. (1995) performed Valsalva leak point determination at various bladder volumes and found a 19-cm $H_2O$ fall in the leak

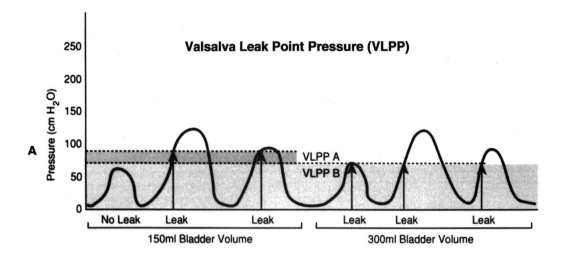

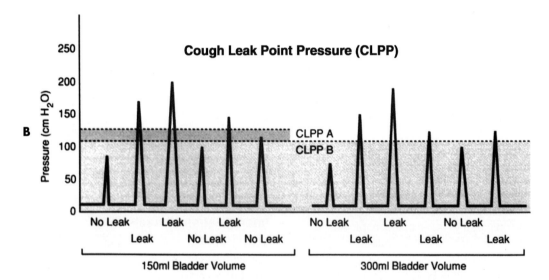

**Fig. 8-7** **A,** Graphic representation of Valsalva leak point pressure measurement at bladder volumes of 150 ml and 300 ml. Leak point pressures tend to decrease with increased bladder volume. **B,** Graphic representation of cough leak point pressure at bladder volumes of 150 ml and 300 ml. Note the difficulty involved in isolating the cough that generates the minimal amount of abdominal pressure required to produce leakage.

point pressure as the volume increased from 150 ml to more than 400 ml.

Although the effect of patient positioning on leak point pressure measurements has not yet been studied, one could postulate that if the patient moves from a supine to an upright position, the value of the leak point pressure diminishes, provided a mechanical obstruction such as a large prolapse is not accentuated in the erect position.

Another area of controversy concerns the use of coughing versus a Valsalva maneuver as the technique for provoking urine loss. Cough-induced leak point pressures are consistently higher than Valsalva-induced leak point pressures. A major concern with coughing is that it is

technically more difficult to control the intensity of a cough and to pinpoint the absolute lowest value associated with urine loss. Unfortunately, some patients demonstrate incontinence only with coughing because Valsalva-induced incontinence has only a 70% to 80% sensitivity in detecting stress incontinence. Valsalva leak point pressures have been shown to have excellent reproducibility, with test-retest correlation coefficients of more than 0.9. The test-retest reliability of a cough-induced leak point pressure has not been studied.

Finally, how should the actual number be determined? Some investigators have used a subtracted value or an increase in intravesical pressure over the baseline resting intravesical pressure, whereas others used the absolute increase in intravesical pressure, which reflects the increase plus the resting baseline pressure.

## Clinical Applications

The abdominal leak point pressure is being used as a severity measure for dysfunction of the urethral sphincteric mechanism with implications regarding surgical management. Many urologists and urogynecologists use abdominal leak point pressures below 60 cm $H_2O$ to define ISD or type III stress incontinence. Operations that reposition the urethra (colposuspension) may result in a higher failure rate in patients with ISD; thus, operations that at least partially obstruct the urethra such as the suburethral sling may be used. These concepts are not universally accepted and to date no surgical outcome data are available. These recommendations are based mostly on data published by McGuire et al. (1993), who performed leak point pressures on 125 women with genuine stress incontinence. They noted that 76% of patients who had a leak point pressure less than 60 cm $H_2O$ were noted to have type III incontinence on video-urodynamic testing. They defined type III incontinence as proximal urethral pressures less than 10 cm $H_2O$ or a nonfunctioning open internal sphincter. Two studies have correlated leak point pressures with subjective degrees of stress incontinence in women. Both studies defined grade 3 incontinence as loss of urine with minimal activity or gravitational incontinence. McGuire et al. (1993) noted that 81% of patients with leak point pressures less than 60 cm $H_2O$ had grade 3 incontinence, whereas Nitti and Combs (1996) noted that 75% and 50% of patients with grade 3 incontinence had leak point pressure less than 90 cm $H_2O$ and 60 cm $H_2O$, respectively.

In summary, we feel that the measurement of abdominal leak point pressure is a simple urodynamic study that can objectively quantitate the severity of genuine stress incontinence. This may be clinically useful in selecting surgical procedures for women with genuine stress incontinence and in the follow-up of patients who have received various modes of therapy but are not completely cured. In the future, it may also help investigators communicate with each other and standardize subjective terms such as *improvement*.

## CONTROVERSIES AND CORRELATIONS

Urethral pressure and leak point pressure studies are two different urodynamic tests aimed at objectively quantifying urethral function. Until recently, intrinsic urethral sphincter deficiency was believed to be a condition that occurred only after injury to the urethra. ISD was felt to commonly occur secondary to anterior vaginal wall surgery, previous bladder neck surgery, pelvic radiation, or thoracolumbar neurologic lesions. The diagnosis has recently become much more commonly used, based mostly on the more liberal use of these tests.

Numerous investigators have attempted to correlate urethral pressures and leak point pressures. Two studies (Sultana, 1995; Swift and Ostergard, 1995) noted a statistically significant but clinically weak correlation between maximum urethral closure pressure and Valsalva leak point pressure, measured as the absolute increase in intravesical pressure. These studies noted correlation coefficients around 0.5 to 0.6. However, studies by Bump et al. (1995) and McGuire et al. (1993) noted no correlation between maximum urethral closure pressure and Valsalva leak point pressures. The inconsistencies in these findings are due at least in part to differences in the technique of performing Valsalva leak point pressure measurements. More recently, McLennan and Bent (1998) studied the relationship between a positive supine empty stress test, Valsalva leak point pressure, and maximum urethral closure pressure. They concluded that a positive supine empty stress test is a useful screening test for a low leak point pressure but not a low urethral closure pressure.

## SUMMARY

The clinical applications of urethral pressure profilometry and abdominal leak point pressures are controversial. Until the techniques for performing these tests are standardized, clinical applicability will remain controversial. Although these tests show promise in the various clinical situations discussed, they should not be the sole determinant for important management issues, most notably, choice of surgical intervention. These decisions should be based on the patients' subjective complaints, important physical findings, these and other urodynamic test results, and the patients' desires and expectations. Further research into the function of the urethra, as well as randomized surgical trials of common operations, will help to clarify the clinical role of these tests.

## BIBLIOGRAPHY
### Urethral Pressure Profilometry

Abrams P: *Urodynamics,* ed 2, London, 1997, Springer.

Abrams P, Blaivas JG, Stanton SL, et al: The standardization of terminology of lower tract function, *Scand J Urol Nephrol* 114(suppl):5, 1988.

Asmussen M, Ulmsten U: Simultaneous urethrocystometry and urethral pressure profile measurement with a new technique, *Acta Obstet Gynecol Scand* 54:385, 1975.

Asmussen M, Ulmsten U: The role of urethral pressure profile measurement in female patients with urethral carcinoma, *Ann Chir Gynecol* 71:122, 1982.

Baker KR, Drutz HP: Retropubic colpourethropexy: clinical and urodynamic evaluation in 289 cases, *Int Urogynecol J* 2:196, 1991.

Bhatia NN, McCarthy TA, Ostergard DR: Urethral pressure profiles of women with diverticula, *Obstet Gynecol* 58:375, 1981.

Blaivas JG, Olsson CA: Stress incontinence: classification and surgical approach, *J Urol* 139:727, 1988.

Bonney V: On diurnal incontinence of urine in women, *J Obstet Gynaecol Br Emp* 30:358, 1923.

Bowen LW, Sand PK, Ostergard DR: Unsuccessful Burch retropubic urethropexy: a case controlled urodynamic study, *Am J Obstet Gynecol* 160:452, 1989.

Brown M, Wickham JEA: The urethral pressure profile, *Br J Urol* 41:211, 1969.

Bump RC, Copeland WE, Hurt WG, et al: Dynamic urethral pressure profilometry pressure transmission ratio determinations in stress-incontinent and stress-continent subjects, *Am J Obstet Gynecol* 159:749, 1988.

Bump RC, Fantl JA, Hurt WG: Dynamic urethral pressure profilometry pressure transmission ratio determinations after continence surgery: understanding the mechanism of success, failure, and complications, *Obstet Gynecol* 72:870, 1988.

Cardozo L: *Urogynecology,* New York, 1997, Churchill Livingstone.

Edwards L, Malvern J: The urethral pressure profile: theoretical considerations and clinical applications, *Br J Urol* 46:325, 1974.

Enhorning G, Miller ER, Hinman F: Urethral closure studies with cine roentgenography and bladder urethral recording, *Surg Gynecol Obstet* 118:507, 1964.

Fantl AJ, Hurt WG, Bump RC, et al: Urethral axis and sphincteric function, *Am J Obstet Gynecol* 155:554, 1986.

Farghaly SA, Shah J, Worth P: The value of transmission–pressure ratio in the assessment of female stress incontinence, *Arch Gynecol* 237(suppl): 366 (abst 14.42.01), 1985.

Ghoneim MA, Gottembourg JL, Freton J, et al: Urethral pressure profile. Standardization of technique and study of reproducibility, *Urology* 5:632, 1975.

Hilton P: Unstable urethral pressure: toward a more relevant definition, *Neurourol Urodyn* 6:411, 1988.

Hilton P, Stanton SL: A clinical and urodynamic evaluation of the Burch colposuspension for genuine stress incontinence, *Br J Obstet Gynaecol* 90:934, 1983.

Horbach NS, Blanco JS, Ostergard DR, et al: A suburethral sling procedure with polytetrafluoroethylene for the treatment of genuine stress incontinence in patients with low urethral closure pressure, *Obstet Gynecol* 71:648, 1988.

Karlson S: Experimental studies in functioning of the female urinary bladder and urethra, *Acta Obstet Gynecol Scand* 32:285, 1953.

Kauppila A, Penttinen J, Häggman V: Six-microtransducer catheter connected to computer in evaluation of urethral closure function of women, *Urology* 33:159, 1989.

Koonings PP, Bergman A, Ballard CA: Low urethral pressure and stress urinary incontinence in women: risk factor for failed retropubic surgical procedure, *Urology* 36:245, 1990.

Kujansuu E: The effect of pelvic floor exercises on urethral function in female stress urinary incontinence: a urodynamic study, *Ann Chir Gynecol* 72:28, 1982.

Kulseng-Hanssen S: Prevalence and pattern of unstable urethral pressure in one hundred seventy-four gynecologic patients referred for urodynamic investigation, *Am J Obstet Gynecol* 146:895, 1983.

McGuire EJ: Urodynamics findings in patients after failure of stress incontinence operations, *Prog Clin Biol Res* 78:351, 1981.

McGuire EJ, Lytton B, Pepe V, et al: Stress urinary incontinence, *Obstet Gynecol* 47:255, 1976.

Millar HD, Baker LE: Stable ultraminiature catheter-tip pressure transducer, *Med Biol Eng* 11:86, 1973.

O'Donnell PD: *Urinary incontinence,* St Louis, 1997, Mosby.

Plevnik S: Model of the proximal urethra: measurement of the urethral stress profile, *Urol Int* 31:23, 1976.

Richardson DA: Value of the cough pressure profile in the evaluation of patients with stress incontinence, *Am J Obstet Gynecol* 155:808, 1986.

Rosenzweig BA, Bhatia NN, Nelson AL: Dynamic urethral pressure profilometry pressure transmission ratio: what do the numbers really mean? *Obstet Gynecol* 77:586, 1991.

Rud T: Urethral pressure profile in continent women from childhood to old age, *Acta Obstet Gynecol Scand* 59:331, 1980.

Sand PK, Bowen LW, Ostergard DR: Uninhibited urethral relaxation: an unusual cause of incontinence, *Obstet Gynecol* 68:645, 1986.

Sand PK, Bowen LW, Panganiban R, et al: The low pressure urethra as a factor in failed retropubic urethropexy, *Obstet Gynecol* 69:399, 1987.

Schick E: Objective assessment of resistance of female urethra to stress, *Urology* 26:518, 1985.

Tanagho EA, Meyers FH, Smith DR: Urethral resistance: its components and implications, *Invest Urol* 7:135, 1969.

Tapp AJS, Cardozo L, Hills B, et al: Who benefits from physiotherapy? *Neurourol Urodyn* 7:259, 1988a.

Tapp AJS, Cardozo L, Versi E, et al: The prevalence of variation of resting urethral pressure in women and its association with lower urinary tract function, *Br J Urol* 61:314, 1988b.

Tapp AJS, Hills B, Cardozo L: Randomized study comparing pelvic floor physiotherapy with the Burch colposuspension, *Neurourol Urodyn* 8:356, 1989.

Ulmsten U, Hendriksson L, Iosif S: The unstable female urethra, *Am J Obstet Gynecol* 144:93, 1982.

Versi E: Discriminant analysis of urethral pressure profilometry data for the diagnosis of genuine stress incontinence, *Br J Obstet Gynaecol* 97:251, 1990.

Versi E, Cardozo L: Urethral instability: diagnosis based on variations of the maximum urethral pressure in normal climacteric women, *Neurourol Urodyn* 5:535, 1986.

Versi E, Cardozo L, Brincat M, et al: Correlation of urethral physiology and skin collagen in postmenopausal women, *Br J Obstet Gynaecol* 95:147, 1988.

Versi E, Cardozo L, Studd J: Distal urethral compensatory mechanisms in women with an incompetent bladder neck who remain continent, and the effect of the menopause, *Neurourol Urodyn* 9:579, 1990.

Ward GH, Hosker GL: The anisotropic nature of urethral occlusive forces, *Br J Obstet Gynaecol* 92:1279, 1985.

Weil A, Reyes H, Bischoff P, et al: Modification of urethral rest and stress profiles after different types of surgery for urinary stress incontinence, *Br J Obstet Gynaecol* 91:46, 1984.

### Leak Point Pressures

Bump RC, Elser DM, Theofrastous JP, et al: Valsalva leak point pressures in women with genuine stress incontinence: reproducibility, effect of catheter caliber, and correlations with other measures of urethral resistance, *Am J Obstet Gynecol* 173:551, 1995.

Decter RM, Harpster L: Pitfalls in determination of leak point pressure, *J Urol* 148:588, 1992.

Gray M, King CJ: Urodynamic evaluation of the intrinsically incompetent sphincter, *J Urol Nurs* 13:67, 1993.

McCormack M, Pike J, Kiruluta G: Leak point of incontinence: a measure of the interaction between outlet resistance and bladder capacity, *J Urol* 150:1452, 1993.

McGuire EJ, Fitzpatrick CC, Wan J, et al: Clinical assessment of urethral sphincter function, *J Urol* 150:1452, 1993.

McGuire EJ, Woodside JR, Bordern TA, et al: Prognostic value of urodynamic testing in myelodysplastic patients, *J Urol* 126:205, 1981.

McLennan MT, Bent AE: Supine empty stress test as a predictor of low Valsalva leak point pressure, *Neurourol Urodyn* 7(17):121, 1998.

Miklos Jr, Sze EHM, Karram MM: A critical appraisal of methods of measuring leak point pressures in women with stress incontinence, *Obstet Gynecol* 86:86, 1995.

Nitti VW, Combs AJ: Correlation of Valsalva leak point pressure with subjective degree of stress urinary incontinence in women, *J Urol* 155:281, 1996.

O'Connel HE, McGuire EJ: Leak point pressure. In O'Donnell PD: *Urinary incontinence,* St Louis, 1997, Mosby.

Sultana CJ: Urethral closure pressure and leak-point pressure in incontinent women, *Obstet Gynecol* 86:839, 1995.

Swift SE, Ostergard DR: A comparison of stress-leak-point pressure in incontinent women, *Obstet Gynecol* 85:704, 1995.

Swift SE, Ostergard DR: Evaluation of current urodynamic test methods in the diagnosis of genuine stress urine incontinence, *Obstet Gynecol* 86:85, 1995.

Swift SE, Utrie JW: The need for standardization of the Valsalva leak point pressure, *Int Urogyn J* 7:227, 1996.

Theofrastous JP, Bump RC, Elser DM, et al: Correlation of urodynamic measure of urethral resistance with clinical measures of incontinence severity in women with pure genuine stress incontinence, *Am J Obstet Gynecol* 173:407, 1995.

Wan J, McGuire EJ, Bloom DA, et al: Stress leak point pressure: a diagnostic took for incontinent children, *J Urol* 150:700, 1993.

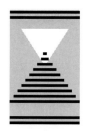

CHAPTER **9**

# Electrophysiologic Testing

J. Thomas Benson

In the patient presenting with urinary incontinence or a voiding disturbance, it is important to consider the possible neurologic causes that may be associated with the symptoms. When the history, physical examination, and urodynamic findings suggest the possibility of nervous system impairment, the adjunctive use of electrophysiologic testing is useful to determine whether neuropathy is a significant component of the patient's problem and, if it is, to localize the area of the central, peripheral, or autonomic nervous system chiefly affected. Thus, the older patient with urge incontinence and headaches, the younger patient with incontinence and difficulty voiding, the patient with low back pain and overflow incontinence, and the patient with stress urinary and anal incontinence may have the respective underlying disorders of brain tumor, multiple sclerosis, intervertebral disk disease, and pudendal neuropathy diagnosed and treated appropriately.

This chapter describes pelvic floor electrodiagnostic techniques including surface and needle electromyography (EMG), nerve conduction and terminal latency studies, evoked potentials, and reflex response studies. The clinical, urodynamic, and electrophysiologic findings to be expected with neuropathy in various areas, from the cerebral cortex to the peripheral pelvic floor nerves, are also described.

Because of the widespread technical advances and great increase in the amount of information about human neurourology, concepts are continually undergoing modification and change. This presentation concentrates on the present aspects of clinically useful knowledge, although modification of many concepts will soon be needed.

## ELECTROPHYSIOLOGIC STUDIES

Electrical activity is produced by intracellular and intercellular neuronal activity. Within the nerve cell and its processes are semipermeable, lipoprotein, bilayered membranes with irregular distributions of ions on either side. This ionic distribution leads to a difference in resting electrical potential across the membrane (inside negative, outside positive). An impulse can be transmitted (action potential), causing change in these potentials with a resultant ionic current flow that can be recorded electrically.

Many nerve cell axons have a myelin sheath, capacitating this current flow, which is interrupted at intervals called nodes of Ranvier (Fig. 9-1). The amount of myelinization determines the diameter of the nerve, and the larger nerves with more myelinization have greater conduction speeds (Table 9-1). The conduction velocity along the axon is proportional to the internodal distance. The internodal distance is decreased in neuropathy of axonal degeneration or demyelination origin. The velocity of the current flow is recorded in nerve conduction studies.

Interneuronal conduction occurs at nerve synapses and at neuroeffector junctions such as muscle fibers. Interneuronal communication is performed chemically by neurotransmitters, which either excite (depolarize) or inhibit (hyperpolarize) the postsynaptic membrane. Specific receptor proteins for each neurotransmitter are in the membranes on both sides of the synapse, and binding opens channels for the current flow.

### Electromyography

In a muscle, the fibers innervated by branches emanating from the motor neuron of a single anterior horn cell are called a *motor unit*. The electrical activity of motor units in a muscle is recordable as motor unit action potentials (MUAPs) (Fig. 9-2). The study of electrical potentials generated by the depolarization of muscle is electromyography (EMG).

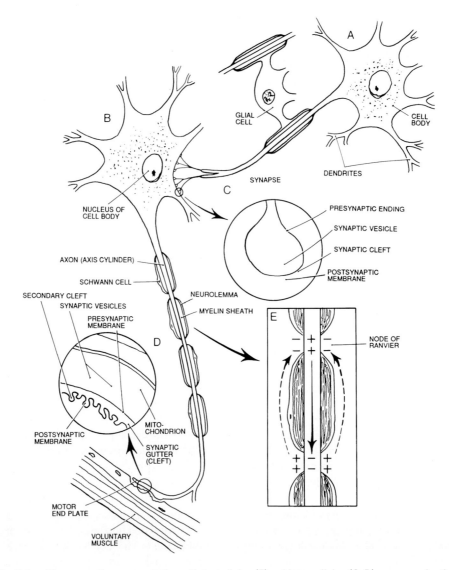

**Fig. 9-1** Diagrammatic representation of intracellular *(E)* and intercellular *(C, D)* nerve conduction.

From Manter JT: *Essentials of clinical neuroanatomy and neurophysiology,* ed 7, Philadelphia, 1987, FA Davis.

EMG is used primarily to study striated muscle, which is easy because of sodium-mediated high-current flow. Smooth muscles, being phylogenetically earlier, depend on calcium ion exchange with low current generation. This smaller current density is more difficult to study, requiring micro-electrode intracellular recording devices.

Motor unit territories within skeletal muscles are variable in size, ranging from 2 to 10 mm. Their electrical activity may be recorded by surface electrodes, which cover large areas and show aggregate effects of many MUAPs, or by various types of needle electrodes, which record smaller areas of activity. The EMG potentials must be amplified and filtered and may be visualized on an oscilloscope screen or heard through audio amplifiers, which is more sensitive than visualization. These potentials are of small amplitude (20 to 2000 µV) and are very brief (3 to 15 ms). To be recorded, therefore, the amplifiers and recording device must have wide-frequency response capabilities, from 30 to 10,000 Hz.

## Surface Electrodes

Surface electrodes are commonly used in conjunction with urodynamic studies. Two electrodes are placed: the active placed close to the muscle under study and a remote electrode placed at a more distant site. If necessary, both recording electrodes can be placed over the active muscle. The EMG recording apparatus amplifies, filters, and displays the voltage changes. To record simultaneously low-frequency urodynamic data (e.g., cystometrics, uroflow) and high-frequency EMG data requires an analog converter, which records the EMG activity in a semiquantitative estimation of the EMG potentials per second.

Skin surface electrodes are often used to record perineal EMG (Fig. 9-3). Monopolar electrodes are placed on either side of the anal orifice. A disposable surface recording electrode, such as a silver chloride disk, can be mounted on a self-adhesive sticker. It is important to reduce the electrical resistance of the skin by washing and drying the

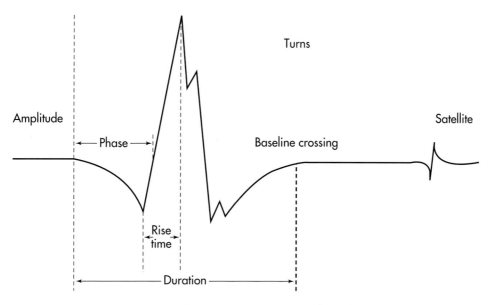

**Fig. 9-2**  Motor unit action potential (MUAP).

**Table 9-1**  Classification of Nerve Fibers

| Sensory and motor fibers | Sensory fibers | Largest fiber diameter | Fastest conduction velocity (M/sec) | General comments |
|---|---|---|---|---|
| A-alpha | Ia | 22 | 120 | Motor: The large alpha motor neurons of lamina IX, innervating extrafusal muscle fibers<br>Sensory: The primary afferent fibers of muscle spindles |
| A-alpha | Ib | 22 | 120 | Sensory: Golgi tendon organs, touch and pressure receptors |
| A-beta | II | 13 | 70 | Motor: The motor neurons innervating both extrafusal and intrafusal (muscle spindle) fibers<br>Sensory: The secondary afferent fibers of muscle spindles, touch and pressure receptors, and pacinian corpuscles (vibratory sensors) |
| A-gamma | | 8 | 40 | Motor: The small gamma motor neurons of lamina IX, innervating intrafusal fibers (muscle spindles) |
| A-delta | III | 5 | 15 | Sensory: Small, lightly myelinated fibers; touch pressure, pain, and temperature |
| B | | 3 | 14 | Motor: Small, lightly myelinated preganglionic autonomic fibers |
| C | IV | 1 | 2 | Motor: All postganglionic autonomic fibers (all are unmyelinated)<br>Sensory: Unmyelinated pain and temperature fibers |

From Manter JT: *Essentials of clinical neuroanatomy and neurophysiology*, ed 7, Philadelphia, 1987, FA Davis.

area and applying electrode paste to ensure firm adherence between electrode and skin. Other surface electrodes useful in pelvic floor studies are depicted in Figs. 9-4 to 9-7.

With surface electrodes, electromyographic pattern recordings depict the net electrical activity occurring in the muscle. Surface electrodes therefore demonstrate an electronically generated summation of muscular electrical activity but are incapable of distinguishing abnormal from normal individual motor unit potentials.

When surface electrodes are used in conjunction with the cystometrogram, a gradual increase in EMG activity is usually seen as the bladder is filled. Normally, when a detrusor contraction occurs, the EMG activity of the pelvic floor ceases. Two subgroups of abnormal coordination between electrical activity in the perineal musculature and

bladder pressure recordings are uninhibited involuntary sphincter relaxation and detrusor-sphincter dyssynergia, where the sphincter and detrusor contract *involuntarily* at the same time.

There are problems with the diagnosis of detrusor-sphincter dyssynergia and with terminology. True detrusor-sphincter dyssynergia occurs with a neurologic lesion, generally located between the pons and the sacral outflow to the lower urinary tract. Many times examiners find increased EMG activity during detrusor contractions, which is behaviorally caused and not attributable to neurologic lesions (e.g., Valsalva action causes increase in perineal EMG activity and must be monitored). Activity of other surrounding musculature (such as gluteal) can contribute to the overall electrical activity measured when using surface electrodes.

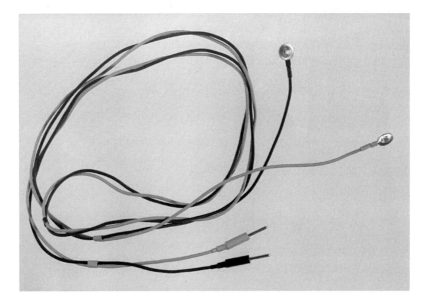

**Fig. 9-3** Surface electrodes.

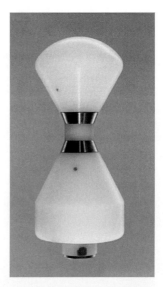

**Fig. 9-4** Anal plug electrode with bipolar concentric recording surfaces mounted on a Teflon, hourglass-shaped plug.

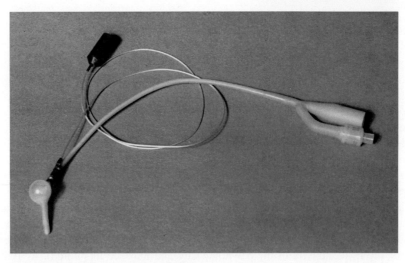

**Fig. 9-5** Foley catheter ring electrode: two lengths of platinum wire protected by a plastic coating and positioned 1 cm distal to the Foley balloon.

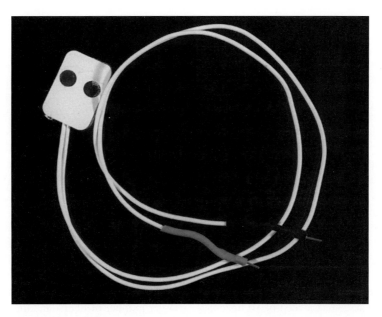

**Fig. 9-6** Vaginal silver chloride electrodes attached to a disposable, flexible vinyl foam tampon.

Simultaneous detrusor-perineal activity without cord defects has been designated as nonneurogenic neurogenic bladder. Precise recordings can distinguish features present in nonneurogenic neurogenic bladder and patients with true detrusor-sphincter dyssynergia. In the latter, dyssynergic EMG activity augments before and concomitant with the detrusor contraction, diminishing before the contraction subsides, whereas the nonneurogenic discrepancy tends to have quiet EMG activity before the beginning of the detrusor contraction, which augments as the contraction subsides.

### Needle EMG

Inserting a needle electrode into skeletal musculature allows analysis of individual motor units and is the superior technique used by the electromyographer for studying peripheral skeletal neuromuscular disease. The needle electrodes by design may be monopolar, concentric, or single-fiber in type, varying in dimensions and in the metal used.

### Monopolar Needle EMG

The monopolar needle electrode is made of solid stainless steel wire, 0.3 to 0.5 mm in diameter, which is insulated with Teflon except at its sharp tip. A second electrode used as a remote reference may be a surface disk or a subcutaneous needle. The monopolar electrode is less painful for the subject and less expensive. Compared with concentric needles, the recorded MUAPs have higher amplitudes, although durations are similar. The monopolar electrode is less selective, however, which may be a disadvantage when trying to isolate single recruited MUAPs, and they have more recording artifact.

Artifacts create considerable difficulty for the novice electromyographer. Sixty-cycle voltage patterns may arise from appliances (even when turned off) or fluorescent lights. Improper grounding or defective needle insulation may

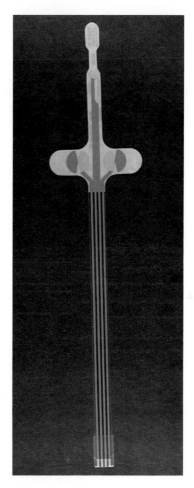

**Fig. 9-7** St. Mark's disposable pudendal electrodes to be placed over index finger of a disposable glove. Stimulating anode and cathode are located at fingertip, recording electrodes at base of finger.

cause markedly distorted tracings. The ground plate should be clean and applied over bone (e.g., the iliac crest) using conductive paste. Needle insulation may be examined under a microscope.

### Concentric Needle EMG

Concentric electrodes have a hollow cannula, which serves as the reference electrode; extending down the shaft to the tip is an insulated fine wire with a beveled tip, which is the active electrode. The advantage of the concentric electrode is its more predictable surface area, which produces more reliable measurements of MUAP variables.

Amplifier settings influence recorded electrical activity. Gain settings determine the size of the electrical activity, which is observable, and by convention the MUAP is recorded at a standard 100 µV per division. Filters are set at a low and high end, usually 2 to 3 Hz and 8 kHz or higher, respectively. The sweep speed determines the spread of the potential on the oscilloscope screen. A sweep of 10 ms/cm is used for most displays, although it is often easier to observe the characteristics of a MUAP when it is recorded at 5 ms/cm.

Concentric needle study of sphincter musculature begins as soon as the needle is inserted into the muscle. Characteristic noise occurs when a muscle is penetrated (insertional activity), normally quieting soon after insertion. In the early period after denervation of skeletal muscle, increased membrane electrical sensitivity is typically seen as fibrillation potentials (small and short single-fiber action potentials) or positive waves (Fig. 9-8). However, sphincter EMG is problematic because small MUAPs are normally present and, unlike other skeletal muscle in the body, complete electrical silence is present only during elimination. Recognizing fibrillation activity in the sphincters requires electromyographic skill. In addition to fibrillations, spontaneous, abrupt onset and cessation potentials (called complex repetitive discharges) and random fasciculation potentials are found in denervated muscle.

As a person increases voluntary effort, the firing rate of activated motor units increases and, finally, more motor units are recruited. This recruitment pattern describes the relationship of the rate of firing of individual motor units to the number of active motor units recorded with the EMG electrode. In denervating states with loss of some motor units, the recruitment pattern is reduced; with increasing effort there is a reduction in the number of newly recruited motor units, and those already activated discharge at a greater frequency than expected. Normally, at full contraction, there is so much recruitment that individual MUAPs can no longer be identified; this phenomenon is called *interference pattern*. Coughing typically produces a dramatic interference pattern in pelvic floor musculature. With dropout of motor units, a full interference pattern is not found. Care must be taken to ensure that the patient is expending maximal voluntary effort.

Observation of tonic firing of motor units in the sphincter is ideal for individual motor unit analyses. A trigger delay on the electrodiagnostic equipment is helpful because it allows a motor unit to appear repeatedly at the same point on the oscilloscope screen. The duration, amplitude, and number of turns can then be assessed (see Fig. 9-2).

Analyses of motor units from the normal urethral sphincter reveal durations less than 6 ms, amplitudes between 0.15 and 0.5 mV, and no more than 5 turns of 100 µV or more amplitude. More turns represent polyphasia. The number of phases in a MUAP is equal to the number of baseline zero crossings plus 1, and MUAPs having greater than four phases are considered *polyphasic*.

After nerve damage, muscle becomes reinnervated by regrowth of the axon from the site of the lesion or by collateral axonic regrowth. With the latter, the surviving motor axons sprout within the muscle, sending out branches to denervated muscle fibers. Hence, a single axon supplies a larger number of fibers, and the motor unit develops a more complex wave form with each new muscle fiber, giving rise to a new phase in the MUAP.

The immature axon conducts impulses slowly, which increases the duration of the motor unit potential. Thus, the EMG pattern seen in established reinnervation is characterized by a lower number of high-amplitude, longer-duration, polyphasic motor units firing at a rapid rate. The amplitude of a MUAP depends on the size of the muscle fiber, which is proportional to the square of the diameter. Hence, a 100-µm-diameter muscle fiber produces an action potential roughly four times larger than that of a 50-µm fiber. The amplitude also relates to the distance from the electrode to the muscle fiber, decreasing exponentially as the distance increases. The rise time, which determines the steepness of the potential (see Fig. 9-2), also decreases with distance.

### Single-Fiber EMG

Single-fiber EMG (SFEMG) is a selective recording technique that uses a concentric needle electrode to identify and record action potentials from individual muscle fibers. The technique is selective because of the small recording surface (25 µm in diameter) exposed at a port at the side of the electrode 3 mm from the tip. This distance allows examination of an area approximately 350 µm diameter. In our laboratory, the high filter setting is 10,000 Hz and the low setting is 350 Hz. The images are triggered and delayed using a gain setting of 100 µV to trigger. In other skeletal muscle work, 200 µV is used as the triggering potential, but in sphincter work measuring smaller muscle fibers, 100 µV as a trigger is now standard. The number of fibers supplied by a branch axon (hence, firing essentially simultaneously) is observed, as each fiber creates an action potential (Fig. 9-9).

Measurements are made visually from the oscilloscope screen. At least 20 sites within the muscle are studied, usually requiring four needle insertions, which analyze five

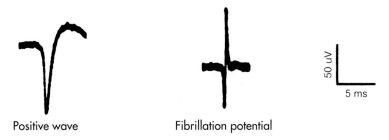

Positive wave          Fibrillation potential

**Fig. 9-8** Positive wave (by convention, downward is positive) and fibrillation potential. Signs of abnormal increased insertional activity.

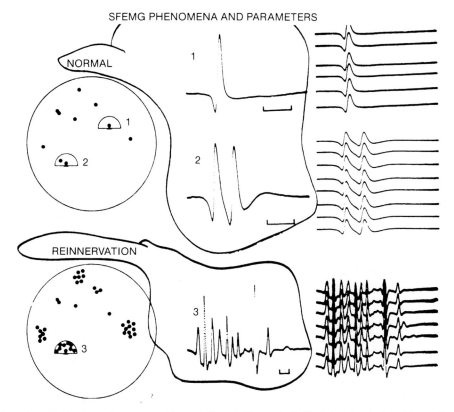

**Fig. 9-9** Single-fiber phenomena: Normal *(1* and *2)* muscle field pickup in circle with resultant MUAPs. Reinnervation *(3)* muscle field pickup of "bunched" muscle fibers supplied by single axon with resultant MUAPs.

different action potentials with each insertion. The time base of the amplifier is set at 2 to 5 ms per division. All potentials with a component greater than 100 μV must be included in the calculation of the mean derived from the 20 recordings. The fiber density in SFEMG recordings increases after the age of about 60 years, so that average fiber density in a normal 30-year-old is approximately 1.4, at age 65 about 1.5, and at age 75, 1.75.

## Conduction Studies

Electrical activity traveling through a nerve process can be measured by stimulating the nerve to depolarize it, thereby achieving a propagated action potential traveling away from the site of the stimulus. One may record the traveling potential directly from the nerve or when the impulse reaches a muscle, at which point the compound muscle action potential (CMAP) may be recorded. Propagation of the impulse along a nerve fiber in the same direction as occurs physiologically is called *orthodromic conduction;* propagation in the opposite direction is called *antidromic conduction.* Nerve conduction rates vary directly with the size of the nerve. Conduction velocities are also affected by temperature, with cooling slowing superficial nerve velocity by 0.7 to 2.4 m/sec for each degree centigrade. Generally, age has little significance or effect on conduction velocities until after age 60. One may not conclude that there is no peripheral neuropathy merely because nerve conduction velocities are normal.

The stimulation is accomplished by using two electrodes, a cathode and an anode. The cathode depolarizes the nerve and the anode hyperpolarizes it. The cathode should be located closer to the recording electrode along the pathway of the propagated action potential so that the action potential does not have to cross a hyperpolarized portion, thus avoiding the possibility of anodal block. The electrodes can be surface electrodes or monopolar needles.

The CMAP generated is called the M wave. The stimulus must be supramaximal; that is, all nerve fibers to the muscle must be depolarized simultaneously. Supramaximal stimulation is achieved when increasing the stimulus no longer increases the resulting amplitude of the M wave. The recording parameters are the latency in milliseconds from the nerve stimulation until the initial deflection, the amplitude of the CMAP in millivolts, the duration in milliseconds, and the configuration, which is normally a smooth curve with an initial negative component (upward deflection) followed by a terminal positive component.

Recording is accomplished with both active and reference electrodes. When studying the CMAP generated after stimulation of a nerve, the resultant latency includes the time for the nerve conduction plus the time for neuromuscular junction transmission and muscle fiber depolarization, so it is not nerve conduction alone, but rather a terminal latency. Only a small stimulus intensity is required to achieve supramaximal stimulation of a nerve, and it is generally below the threshold regarded as painful. The stimulus pulse width must be standardized because it affects the latency, and the sweep speed must be adjusted to visualize the resulting potentials.

Stimulus artifact is a reaction from the stimulus that may interfere with the recorded response, especially when studying latencies of short distance. The stimulus artifact can be minimized by keeping the stimulus intensity and duration as low as possible. Other techniques to minimize stimulus artifact include reducing current leakage across the skin surface by proper preparation, keeping the receptive electrodes in proximity to each other, separating the stimulator wires from the recording system to avoid induction currents, and rotating the stimulating anode to either side of the cathode.

Placement of the ground electrode on the patient is necessary, but position is not extremely critical. If convenient, the electrode is positioned between the stimulating and recording electrodes. Amplifier settings must be constant because increasing the sensitivity of the amplifier may shorten the latency value. Motor responses (CMAPs) are usually of greater amplitude and of longer duration than sensory responses recorded from the nerve itself.

### Pudendal Nerve Terminal Motor Latency (PNTML)

Kiff and Swash (1984) devised a method for stimulating the pudendal nerve transrectally using electrodes mounted on a disposable glove (see Fig. 9-7). The stimulating electrodes are located on the fingertip, and the recording electrodes are found at the base of the finger. The pudendal nerve is stimulated transrectally near its passage in Alcock's canal by the ischial spine, and the response is obtained from the inferior hemorrhoidal division of the pudendal nerve supplying the anal sphincter (Fig. 9-10). Both right and left nerves may be tested. Our laboratory PNTML mean is $2.2 \pm 0.4$ ms, comparable to results of other laboratories. The amplitudes of the CMAP obtained by the St. Mark's technique has been found to have variability secondary to the location of the recording electrodes (base of the examining finger). Such variability is due to the size of the examiner's finger and the variable intraanal location in respect to the external anal sphincter. Therefore, standard positioning of the recording electrodes on paraanal skin (3 or 9 o'clock position for active electrodes and 6 o'clock for reference electrodes with patient in the lithotomy position)

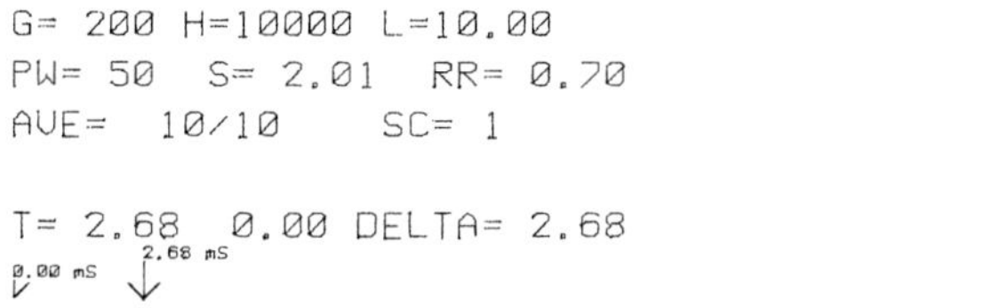

```
G= 200  H=10000 L=10.00
PW= 50  S= 2.01  RR= 0.70
AVE=  10/10    SC= 1

T= 2.68  0.00 DELTA= 2.68
0.00 mS   2.68 mS
```

**Fig. 9-10** Pudendal nerve terminal motor latency (PNTML). *G*, Gain in microvolts per (vertical) division; *H*, high-frequency filter setting in hertz; *L*, low-frequency filter setting in hertz; *PW*, pulse width of stimulus in microseconds; *S*, sweep speed of display in milliseconds per (horizontal) division; *RR*, repetition rate of stimulus (per second); *Ave*, number of responses averaged; *SC*, scale; *T*, time in milliseconds (determined by vertical marker placement); *Delta*, time from stimulus to vertical marker. Top two responses are with pudendal nerve stimulated (replicated response); bottom line, a "control" with stimulation not applied to pudendal nerve.

results in more consistency in amplitude, allowing this valuable parameter to be useful clinically. Our laboratory amplitude mean is $99 \pm 44$ μV with a range of 34 to 182 and interrater variability of 1%. Another advantage of this modification is that the stimulation (still performed with the St. Mark's cathode and anode) can be performed vaginally, a much more comfortable procedure for most women than intraanal stimulation.

### *Perineal Nerve Terminal Motor Latency (PeNTML)*

Stimulating the pudendal nerve as previously described for PNTML and recording with the Foley catheter ring electrode (see Fig. 9-5) enable one to obtain the right and left PeNTML to the urethral sphincter. This nerve branch of the pudendal nerve supplies the area of anatomic distribution, which is even more affected by vaginal delivery than is the PNTML. Our laboratory reports a mean PeNTML of $2.29 \pm 0.3$ ms. There is anatomic variability of the perineal branch of the pudendal nerve, even from side to side in the same patient. If the perineal nerve branches from the pudendal trunk distal to the point of stimulation at the ischial spine, the Foley mounted ring electrodes will record a negative-positive waveform similar to other CMAPs. However, if the urethral rhabdosphincter is supplied by a nerve supply separate from one arising from a pudendal trunk (e.g., an intrapelvic pathway from direct sacral branches), such a waveform may not be produced.

Evidence of more proximal peripheral neuropathy in pelvic floor disorders has been obtained with direct spinal cord stimulation using surface electrodes and recording the latency of response in the anal and urethral sphincters. However, the large voltage stimulus required for this procedure precludes its approval for use by the Food and Drug Administration. Selective sacral nerve needle stimulation can be used. Magnetic stimulators are now being developed that may provide direct stimulation tests to evaluate more effectively the proximal pelvic floor nerves.

## Evoked Response

An evoked response is the summation of potentials recorded from central nervous tissue (spinal cord or cortex) that have been stimulated from a peripheral site. Because electrical activity is occurring throughout the body tissues and can be detected by the recording electrodes, it is necessary to obtain multiple responses so that the evoked potential, which is usually only a few microvolts in amplitude, can be identified against the background activity. Computer averaging within the recording system allows the individual responses, which occur in a time-locked relationship to the stimulus, to be increased in clarity against the background; the randomly occurring background activity progressively lessens in prominence.

Pudendal cortical evoked responses, obtained by stimulation of the dorsal nerve of the penis in men, can be obtained by lateral paraclitoral stimulation in women. The two cortical recording electrodes are placed as follows: the active electrode is placed midline, 2 cm posterior to the halfway mark between the inion and the nasion, and the reference electrode is placed in the upper mid-forehead. Recording electrodes may also be placed over the vertebral column at levels L1 (active electrode) and L5 (reference electrode), which correspond to the cord levels of the cauda equina (Fig. 9-11). Then, using two channels, the evoked responses can be simultaneously recorded from the cortex and the lumbar spine. Such lumbar spine recording of pudendal stimuli is technically difficult in women, however.

Similar recordings may be obtained by stimulating posterior to the medial malleolus at the posterior tibial nerve (Fig. 9-12). These evoked responses are often called *somatosensory,* but it must be emphasized that these responses have nothing to do with examining sensory functioning. Thus, sensory evoked responses do not offer objective means of assessing bladder sensory function and are useful only for indicating indirectly that tracts are intact from the point of stimulation to the point of response. This same information can be obtained for the area of the cauda equina and spinal cord by the more commonly used posterior tibial nerve. These studies determine conduction times as peripheral (from stimulus to L1), central (L1 to cortex), or total (stimulus to cortex). Localization of lesions is suggested as peripheral (delayed peripheral and total) or cord (normal peripheral, delayed central, and total). Cortical lesions may have absent response.

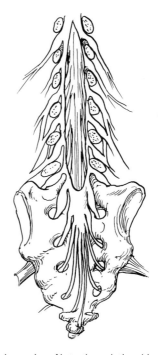

**Fig. 9-11**  Cauda equina: Note the relationship to first and fifth lumbar vertebra where electrodes may be placed.

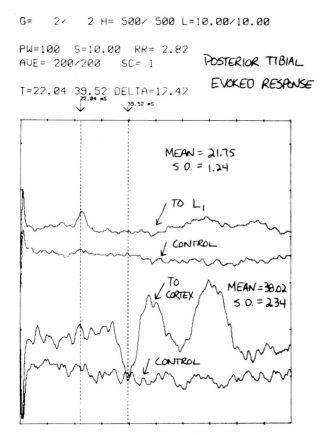

G=    2/    2 H= 500/ 500 L=10.00/10.00

PW=100   S=10.00   RR= 2.82
AVE= 200/200     SC= 1

POSTERIOR TIBIAL
EVOKED RESPONSE

T=22.04  39.52  DELTA=17.47
22.04 mS      39.52 mS

MEAN = 21.75
S.O. = 1.24

TO L₁

CONTROL

TO CORTEX

MEAN = 38.02
S.O. = 2.34

CONTROL

**Fig. 9-12**   Evoked response from stimulation of posterior tibial nerve. Top two lines represent response at L1 vertebra (and control) and bottom two lines, the response at cerebral cortex (and control). *G*, Gain; *H*, high-frequency filter; *L*, low-frequency filter settings for lumbar and cortical responses, respectively. Parameter definitions as in Fig. 9-10.

## Reflex Response and Sensory Study

Stimulation delivered by the Foley catheter ring electrode produces a reflex response at the external anal sphincter, which Bradley has called *electromyelography* (*myelo* referring to the spinal cord) (Fig. 9-13). This reflex stimulus may be in the urethra or may be moved into the bladder to stimulate the bladder. It therefore incorporates detrusor and urethral sensory afferents, conus medullaris synapses, and pudendal motor neurons. The stimulus has a pulse duration of 50 μs, is paired with interspike interval of 5 ms, and can be increased by increments using a constant current stimulator to determine the sensory threshold. Normal urethral perception ranges from 3 to 10 mA, with a mean of 5, whereas bladder perception normally ranges 20 to 25 mA. The stimulus level is three to four times sensory threshold. Separate responses are obtained and are accepted when similar latencies are seen. The responses are not averaged because there is enough variability to make averaging unproductive. The response is easily obtained, and the latency is measured at the onset. Our laboratory mean is 59.0 ± 9.0 ms.

Cauda equina or pelvic plexus injury is characterized by diminished amplitude or absence of this response. If reflex response is present but the patient has lost sensation, the lesion is in the sensory cortex or ascending spinal cord tracts. The patient can suppress or eliminate the response during voiding; failure to do so indicates a suprasacral tract disorder. Finding normal electromyelography and normal sphincter EMG effectively excludes a lower motor neuron lesion of S2 through S4.

Reflex response may also be obtained when stimulating at the clitoris and picking up with electrodes at the anal sphincter. The stimulus at the clitoris may be either right- or left-sided, and the pickup at the anal sphincter can be performed with surface electrodes or with concentric needles that are placed into the right and left external anal sphincter musculature. In placing the needles, EMG is used to make certain that the needles are placed within the muscle. Stimulating at the clitoris creates pudendal nerve afferent stimulus, which reflexly goes to the cord and results in response contraction in the external anal sphincter that can be lateralized, either right or left. Using auditory response in conjunction is helpful. This allows lateralization of both afferent and efferent response to test dorsal and ventral roots in the sacral portion of the cord. These roots are often affected in cauda equina disease. This reflex is not affected in pelvic plexus disorder. In our laboratory this reflex has a latency of 33 ± 4 ms. Sensory values can be obtained as well because most patients perceive sensation between 3 and 9 mA. The response usually requires a stimulus that is approximately three times the threshold of perception.

## "Supersensitivity" Testing

Cannon's law of denervation states that once an organ is deprived of its efferent nerve supply, it develops supersensitivity to its neuromuscular transmitter. This is particularly true of smooth muscle. In cases of detrusor hypoactivity, a neurogenic etiology (detrusor areflexia) may be documented by injection of bethanechol chloride (Urecholine, 5 mg subcutaneously) after baseline cystometry, followed by rapid fill cystometric studies at 5-minute intervals. A positive test is indicated by a rise in intravesical pressure more than 15 cm $H_2O$. Bladders that demonstrate such denervation have damage to the postganglionic parasympathetic nerve fibers.

## CLINICAL CONDITIONS

The nervous system relationship to the lower urinary tract is extremely complex, and simplification, although clinically useful, will never be totally accurate. Every nervous system physiologic control over the urinary tract has positive and negative aspects, and either can dominate in a given clinical situation. Although the following suggestions can be useful in clinical evaluation, they do not describe situations that are

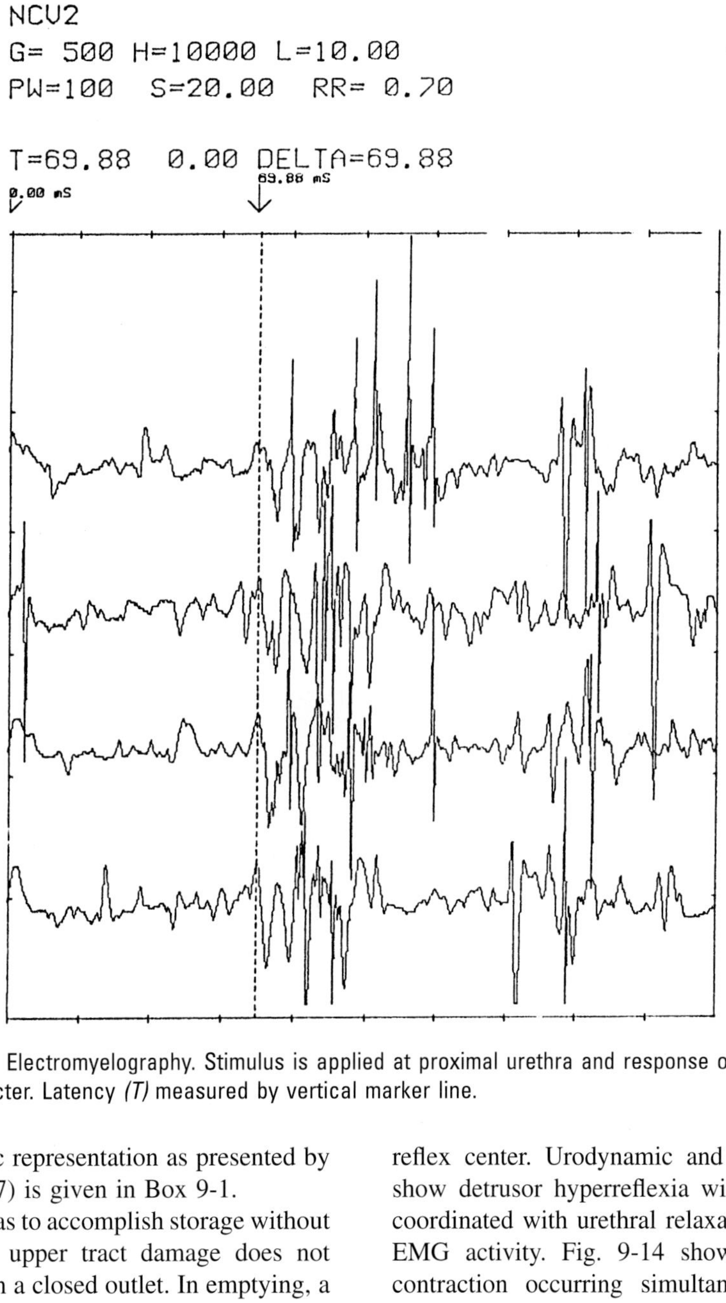

NCV2
G= 500 H=10000 L=10.00
PW=100  S=20.00  RR= 0.70

T=69.88  0.00 DELTA=69.88
                69.88 mS
0.00 mS
↓                ↓

**Fig. 9-13**  Electromyelography. Stimulus is applied at proximal urethra and response obtained at anal sphincter. Latency (T) measured by vertical marker line.

always present. A schematic representation as presented by Torrens and Morrison (1987) is given in Box 9-1.

The lower urinary tract has to accomplish storage without increased pressure so that upper tract damage does not occur. Storage must occur in a closed outlet. In emptying, a complex reflex mechanism must be mediated under autonomic, central, and peripheral nervous system control. The Barrington's center in the anterior pontine region of the brain stem acts as the detrusor reflex coordinating and augmenting center. This reflex of bladder emptying can be thought of as being facilitated or inhibited by various components of the nervous system. That concept is applied in the following clinical descriptions.

## Cortical Lesions

The only region of the cerebral cortex consistently associated with detrusor dysfunction when damaged is the superior frontal gyrus-septal area. Lesions in this area interfere with voluntary inhibition of the pontine detrusor

reflex center. Urodynamic and electrophysiologic testing show detrusor hyperreflexia with contractions, which are coordinated with urethral relaxation and decreased surface EMG activity. Fig. 9-14 shows a coordinated detrusor contraction occurring simultaneously with a petit mal seizure. The contraction is of large magnitude, with the pons augmentation intact.

Such cortical lesions prevent voluntary postponement of voiding. Urge incontinence results when sensation is intact. If sensation is not intact, involuntary voiding (enuresis) occurs. With larger lesions, social concern about incontinence is lost.

A separate cortical area regulates upper motor neuron control of the pudendal nerve. This pudendal nucleus is located in paracentral lobule cortical areas. Lesions here may be involved with hemiparesis and may produce upper motor neuron findings with contralateral extensor plantar reflexes and increased deep tendon reflexes. These lesions can be characterized electrophysiologically by inability to

**Box 9-1**

**SIMPLIFIED SCHEME OF INTERACTION OF VARIOUS LEVELS OF THE NERVOUS SYSTEM IN MICTURITION**

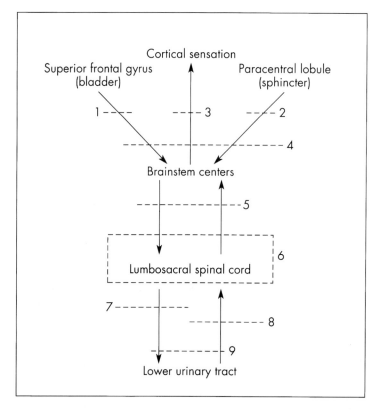

The locations of certain possible nervous lesions are denoted by numbers and explained as follows:

*1,* Lesions isolating the superior frontal gyrus prevent voluntary postponement of voiding. If sensation is intact, this produces urge incontinence. If the lesion is larger, there is additional loss of social concern about incontinence.

*2,* Lesions isolating the paracentral lobule, sometimes associated with a hemiparesis, cause spasticity of the urethral sphincter and retention. This is painless if sensation is abolished. Minor degrees of this syndrome may cause difficulty in the initiation of micturition.

*3,* Pathways of sensation are not known accurately. In theory, an isolated lesion of sensation above the brain stem would lead to unconscious incontinence. Defective central conduction of sensory information would explain nocturnal enuresis.

*4,* Lesions above the brain stem centers lead to involuntary voiding that is coordinated with sphincter relaxation.

*5,* Lesions below brain stem centers but above the lumbosacral spinal cord lead, after a period of bladder paralysis associated with spinal shock, to involuntary reflex voiding that is not coordinated with sphincter relaxation (detrusor/sphincter dyssynergia).

*6,* Lesions destroying the lumbosacral cord or the complete nervous connections between the central and peripheral nervous system result in a paralyzed bladder that contracts only weakly in an autonomous fashion because of its remaining ganglionic innervation. However, if the lumbar sympathetic outflow is preserved in the presence of conus or cauda equina destruction, then there may be some residual sympathetic tone in the bladder neck and urethra that may be sufficient to be obstructive.

*7,* A lesion of the efferent fibers alone leads to a bladder of decreased capacity and decreased compliance associated experimentally with an increased number of adrenergic nerves.

*8,* A lesion confined to the afferent fibers produces a bladder that is areflexic with increased compliance and capacity.

*9,* Because there are ganglion cells in the bladder wall, it is technically impossible to decentralize the bladder completely, but congenital absence of bladder ganglia may exist, producing megacystis.

From Torrens M, Morrison JFB, eds: *The physiology of the lower urinary tract,* London, 1987, Springer-Verlag.

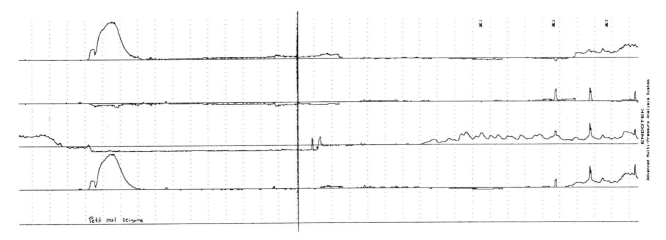

**Fig. 9-14** Multichannel cystometric study. Lines *(top to bottom):* vesical pressure, abdominal pressure, urethral pressure, detrusor pressure.

quiet electrical activity in the pelvic floor, as measured by loss of voluntary influence on electromyelography amplitude reflex, failure to suppress sphincter EMG activity during voiding, or more simply by exaggerated surface EMG perineal musculature activity. This exaggeration and spasticity may be associated with difficulty in initiating micturition. This paracentral lobule syndrome is uncommon.

The sphincter is an example of a muscle that does not have a fully crossed relationship with the motor cortex because stimulation of the motor cortex on either side can cause contractions on both sides of the sphincter musculature. Cortical inhibition of sphincteric activity is aided partly by inhibition of spinal origin.

## Suprasacral Cord Areas

The nature of a voiding or urinary storage disturbance that occurs with spinal cord disease depends on the site and extent of the injury, type of recovery, and presence or absence of other neurologic or urogynecologic disorders.

Lower urinary tract neurons with long ascending axons reach the pons micturition area to mediate chiefly facilitative effects. These axons enter sacral posterior roots and pass in the spinothalamic and posterior spinal tracts. Lesions affecting these compartments can lead to detrusor areflexia and increased compliance. Correspondingly, intentional sectioning (sacral dorsal rhizotomy) prevents bladder contractions and increases capacity. Effector pathways from the pons to the lower cord are chiefly inhibitory, and lesions affecting these cord areas lead to small nonamplified, poorly coordinated detrusor contractions of short duration, with resultant increased residual urine. Hence, higher cord lesions vary in clinical manifestation.

The usual response to spinal cord injury is complete bladder paralysis followed by return of some lower urinary tract function within months. This return of reflexes may be in response to demand, a demonstration of the body's neuroplasticity. Many patients develop automatic bladder in

which the bladder contracts in response to distention. This intrinsic power is less than normal, so residual volumes generally increase.

Lesions below the pons, with resultant loss of bladder and sphincter activity coordination, generally lead to detrusor-sphincter dyssynergia, further complicating residual urine problems. These problems can be severe enough to affect the upper urinary system. Generally, this complication occurs when the bladder pressure exceeds 40 cm $H_2O$. Almost all suprasacral cord injuries produce dysfunction of both the bladder and the outlet, the detrusor becoming hyperreflexic and the outlet demonstrating varying degrees of dyssynergia. When the bladder becomes trabeculated and fibrotic, the small detrusor contractions may empty the bladder (hence no residual urine), but upper tract deterioration may continue to progress secondary to high intravesical pressure.

Neurophysiologic studies in patients with suprasacral spinal cord disease may demonstrate normal peripheral and prolonged total and central conduction times. Urodynamic studies document detrusor hyperreflexia, with or without detrusor-sphincter dyssynergia, depending on the lesion. Electromyelography and sphincter EMG studies often do not show abnormalities, although facilitation of the electromyelographic reflex response and lack of volitional control over it could be expected. Deep tendon hyperreflexia and impaired lower extremity sensation may be found on physical examination.

## Sacral Cord Area

Lesions involving the sacral cord lead to lower motor neuron disorders with possible absence of both detrusor and urethral sphincteric activity. Causes include tumor, arachnoiditis, and trauma. Symmetric saddle distribution of sensory loss, sensory disassociation, and mild lower limb motor loss without atrophy are found. The detrusor activity may be further reduced by a block of long routing detrusor afferent nerves, compounding the areflexia. This type of bladder decentralization may result in loss of subjective sensation to large volumes, but poor compliance and increased pressure are more common. When the bladder pressure exceeds urethral closing pressure, incontinence occurs. This incontinence usually is due to poor bladder volume tolerance, coupled with abnormal urethral function. Obstruction to the incontinence (as by antiincontinence surgery) may place the upper tracts in jeopardy.

Findings in these patients include trabeculation on cystoscopy, positive bethanechol supersensitivity test, abnormal sphincter EMG (lower motor neuron disease), usually abnormal electromyelography, decreased sensation, and prolonged peripheral and total conduction times.

## Cauda Equina

Because the cauda equina conveys the afferent and efferent nerves from the sacral cord, the findings with injury here are similar to those found with sacral cord injury. Clinically, however, they differ because in most patients cauda equina injury is a result of vertebral injury below T12 or intervertebral disk protrusion usually in the L4-L5 or L5-S1 spaces. The saddle distribution of sensory loss is less symmetric than with sacral cord lesions, and sensory dissociation is absent. Pain is more severe and motor deficits are asymmetric but more profound with atrophy present. Many of these patients have autonomic parasympathetic interruption with decreased urinary flow, as measured by uroflowmetry. Elevated postvoid residual urine volumes and occasional urinary retention are common. Urinary incontinence may be caused by urine overflow, which is often accentuated by maintained alpha-adrenergic activity or loss of urethral competency secondary to lower motor neuron disease of the striated external urethral sphincter.

Urodynamic studies show abdominal-type voiding, absent detrusor activity, abnormal sphincter EMG, and abnormal electromyelography with prolonged peripheral conduction times. Bethanechol supersensitivity test is usually positive.

Electrophysiologic testing of the lower limbs as well as of the nerves to the pelvis is necessary to assist in the diagnosis of cauda equina and sacral cord syndromes.

## Pelvic Plexus Injury

The pelvic plexus may be affected by surgical procedures involving the lower colorectal or gynecologic systems. Patients may present with micturition disturbances after pelvic surgery, and distinction between damage in the pelvic plexus and damage in the cauda equina may be aided by electrophysiologic techniques.

The pelvic plexus contains sympathetic postganglionic, parasympathetic preganglionic, visceral afferent, and some sacral somatic nerves. Patients with pelvic plexus injury do not have noticeable perineal sensory loss. Sensory disturbances may be seen in the bladder when damage occurs to the afferent innervation through autonomic nerves in the pelvic plexus, thus increasing the micturition threshold. Pelvic plexus injury may lead to parasympathetic denervation and detrusor areflexia, occasionally with markedly decreased compliance. Complicating this situation, alpha-adrenergic denervation leads to incompetency at the bladder neck so that incontinence may be associated with the frustrating difficulty in initiating urination. Thus, there is decreased bladder compliance, detrusor hypoactivity, incompetence of the bladder neck, and diminished urethral closure pressures.

Electromyelography generally is abnormal. Clitoral anal reflex and perineal and pudendal terminal motor latencies generally are unaffected, being beyond the area of injury. Evoked responses from bladder base may be affected, but pudendal or posterior tibial evoked responses are often unaffected, a finding helpful in differentiating pelvic plexus from cauda equina injury. Pelvic plexus injury may be associated with hyposensitivity in the bladder and urethra. Sphincter EMG is variable depending on whether the nerve supply is through direct pelvic plexus somatic nerve or pudendal pathways.

## Distal Pudendal Neuropathy

With the advent of pudendal and perineal nerve terminal motor latency studies, single-fiber density studies, and other sphincter EMG studies, there is increased appreciation of the significance of distal pudendal nerve injury. It is strongly related both to urinary and fecal incontinence and to pelvic organ prolapse. The association of changes in latency with EMG changes in the sphincters can demonstrate neuropathy. Twenty percent of women show such changes after vaginal delivery. The strong relationship between pudendal neuropathy and genuine stress urinary incontinence and anal incontinence suggests possible methods for prevention of these disorders. In patients demonstrating persistence of this neurophysiologic abnormality after vaginal delivery, change in management of subsequent deliveries may be considered to prevent the profound sequelae of pelvic floor neuropathy in later years.

## BIBLIOGRAPHY
### Electrophysiologic Studies

Benson JT: Neurophysiologic control of lower urinary tract, *Obstet Gynecol Clin North Am* 16:733, 1989.

Benson JT: Electrodiagnosis. In Benson JT, ed: *Female pelvic floor disorders*, New York, 1992, WW Norton.

Benson JT: Clinical neurophysiological techniques in urinary and fecal incontinence. In Ostergard DR, Bent AE, eds: *Urogynecology and urodynamics*, Baltimore, 1996, Williams & Wilkins.

Blaivas JG, Singha HP, Zayed AA, et al: Detrusor-external sphincter dyssynergia, *J Urol* 125:542, 1981.

Borirakchanyavat S, Aboseif SR, Carroll PR, et al: Continence mechanism of the isolated female urethra: an anatomical study of the intrapelvic somatic nerves, *J Urol* 158:822, 1997.

Bradley WE, Timm GW, Rockswold GL, et al: Detrusor and urethral electromyelography, *J Urol* 114:69, 1975.

Cannon WB: A law of denervation, *Am J Med Sci* 198:737, 1959.

Haldeman S, Bradley WE, Bhatia N: Evoked responses from the pudendal nerve, *J Urol* 12:974, 1982.

Haldeman S, Bradley WE, Bhatia NN, et al: Pudendal evoked responses, *Arch Neurol* 39:280, 1982.

Hinman F: Non-neurogenic neurogenic bladder (the Hinman syndrome): 15 years later, *J Urol* 136:769, 1986.

Lapides J, Friend CR, Ajemian EP, et al: A new test for neurogenic bladder, *J Urol* 88:245, 1962.

Manter JT: *Essentials of clinical neuroanatomy and neurophysiology,* ed 7, Philadelphia, 1987, FA Davis.

Powell PH, Feneley RCL: The role of urethral sensation in clinical urology, *Br J Urol* 52:539, 1980.

Rudy DC, Woodside JR: Non-neurogenic neurogenic bladder: the relationship between intravesical pressure and the external sphincter myogram, *Neurourol Urodyn* 10:169, 1991.

Snooks SJ, Swash M: Perineal nerve and transcutaneous spinal stimulation: new methods for investigation of the urethral striated sphincter musculature, *Br J Urol* 56:406, 1984.

Snooks SJ, Swash M: Pudendal nerve terminal motor latency and spinal stimulation. In Henry MM, Swash M, eds: *Coloproctology and the pelvic floor,* London, 1985, Butterworth.

## Clinical Conditions

Benson JT: Clinical application of electrodiagnostic studies of female pelvic floor neuropathy, *Int Urogynecol J* 1:3, 1990.

Kiff ES, Swash M: Normal proximal and delayed distal conduction in the pudendal nerves of patients with idiopathic (neurogenic) faecal incontinence, *J Neurol Neurosurg Psychiatry* 47:820, 1984.

Percy JP: A neurogenic factor in faecal incontinence in the elderly, *Age Ageing* 11:175, 1982.

Smith ARB, Hosker GL, Warrell DW: The role of partial denervation of the pelvic floor in the aetiology of genitourinary prolapse and stress incontinence of urine. A neurophysiological study, *Br J Obstet Gynaecol* 96:24, 1989.

Snooks SJ, Barnes PRH, Swash M: Damage to the innervation of the voluntary anal and periurethral musculature in incontinence, *J Neurol Neurosurg Psychiatry* 47:406, 1984.

Snooks SJ, Henry MM, Swash M: Anorectal incontinence and rectal prolapse: differential assessment of the innervation to puborectalis and external anal sphincter muscles, *Gut* 26:470, 1984.

Torrens M, Morrison JFB, eds: *The physiology of the lower urinary tract,* London, 1987, Springer-Verlag.

CHAPTER **10**

# Endoscopic Evaluation of the Lower Urinary Tract

Geoffrey W. Cundiff and Alfred E. Bent

## HISTORICAL PERSPECTIVE

Bozzini, in 1805, was the first to describe an endoscopic technique for evaluating the female urethra and bladder. His invention was a cumbersome cystoscope consisting of a stand that supported different-sized hollow funnels, a candle for illumination, and a reflector to direct the light into the funnel when it was placed into the urethra. Visibility with this device was limited both by poor illumination and the tendency of the operator to burn himself if the stand was tilted for a better view.

Nineteenth-century refinements to this crude instrument included the addition of a surrounding cannula and, later, a lens system to provide magnification of the field of view. The greatest drawback of the early cystoscopes was poor illumination, and innovators tried multiple techniques to overcome the problem, including reflective mirrors, an alcohol lamp, a platinum wire loop, and finally, an incandescent light source. Even with these improvements in the cystoscope and illumination, visualization was still poor without bladder distention. By the end of the nineteenth century, cystoscopy was considered to be nothing more than an ad-

junct to the established method of urethral dilation and bimanual palpation of the bladder.

Kelly's (1894) contribution to cystoscopy was a technique that provided adequate bladder distention. The Kelly cystoscope, a hollow tube without a lens, was not innovative, but his technique was. The cystoscope was introduced using an obturator, with the patient in knee-chest position. The negative intraabdominal pressure created by this position allowed air to distend the bladder when the cystoscope was introduced. A head mirror was used to reflect an electric light into the bladder for illumination. The technique was simple but provided an excellent view. Its simplicity made cystoscopy available to all physicians for the first time. Kelly's fame as a genitourinary surgeon, and as the founder of the Johns Hopkins Hospital residency training program in gynecology, the first in the nation, established cystoscopy as a gynecologic technique.

The twentieth century provided many innovations in the cystoscope. Hopkins and Kopany (1954) introduced both a fiberoptic telescope and a rod lens system, which dramatically improved light transmission and resolution. This rod lens design is the system used in today's rigid cystoscopes. Replacement of the air chamber with a series of glass rods with optically finished ends, separated by intervening air spaces, provides a wider viewing field and permits a change in the viewing angle. The innovation of angled telescopes improved the extent of visualization and facilitated more invasive procedures. Increasingly complex instruments were developed to perform operative procedures through a cystoscope, and gradually, general surgeons developed the subspecialty of urology around this new technology. The development of the subspecialty of urology coincident with the combination of gynecology and obstetrics into a single training program deemphasized cystoscopy in gynecologic training, and gynecologists gradually became less skilled in the technique.

The most recent development in cystoscopy is the flexible cystoscope. A flexible cystoscope takes advantage of the flexibility of the fiberoptic lens system to create a cystoscope that bends, thereby increasing the range of the field of view. Some authors report an improved view of the bladder neck using a flexible fiber cystoscope, whereas others advocate flexible cystoscopy to limit the necessary instrumentation and improve patient tolerance.

Robertson (1973), the father of urogynecology, reintroduced cystoscopy to gynecology with the development of the Robertson urethroscope. He addressed the deficiencies of the cystoscope for viewing the urethra by applying the rods lens technology of the Hopkins cystoscope to a shorter straight-on telescope with a nonfenestrated sheath designed specifically for viewing the urethra. He subsequently outlined a technique, dynamic urethroscopy, for evaluating incontinent women using the Robertson urethroscope. Dynamic urethroscopy offered a simple office procedure that considerably improved the diagnostic evaluation of the lower urinary tract.

## INDICATIONS

Cystourethroscopy, an invaluable procedure for today's urogynecologist, has both diagnostic and operative indications. Diagnostic indications include hematuria, irritative voiding symptoms, urinary incontinence, urethral diverticula, and urogenital fistulas.

The differential diagnosis of hematuria is extensive but falls into conditions that are primarily renal or postrenal in origin. Endoscopy is useful in the diagnosis of the postrenal conditions, including neoplasms of the bladder and urethra, urethral polyps, chronic cystitis, recurrent cystitis, interstitial cystitis, urolithiasis, and foreign bodies.

The differential diagnosis for irritative voiding symptoms is extensive, including many nebulous conditions. Possible causes include acute cystitis, chronic cystitis, trigonitis, radiation cystitis, urethral syndrome, urethral diverticula, urethritis, and interstitial cystitis. Other conditions that may cause similar symptoms include detrusor instability, sensory urgency, urolithiasis, partial urinary retention, and moderate to severe pelvic organ prolapse. Cystourethroscopy is indicated when the presenting symptoms strongly suggest a diagnosis of urethral diverticulum, interstitial cystitis, urolithiasis, or tumor, and for patients who do not respond to initial therapy. Endoscopy should be avoided in the presence of an active urinary tract infection.

There is general agreement that cystoscopy is indicated for patients complaining of persistent incontinence or voiding dysfunction following incontinence surgery, but there is less agreement about the role of cystoscopy in the baseline evaluation of patients with urinary incontinence. The refinement of urodynamic evaluation over the last three decades has demonstrated the superiority of this modality for diagnosing the common causes of urinary incontinence such as genuine stress incontinence and detrusor instability. However, although urodynamic testing excels at providing an objective assessment of lower urinary tract function, it provides little information about lower urinary tract anatomy. Urethrocystoscopy contributes an anatomic assessment of the urethra and bladder that is not achieved by

urodynamic tests alone. Anatomic abnormalities, such as urethral diverticula, urinary-vaginal fistulas, and intravesical foreign bodies causing detrusor instability, might be suspected based on history or urodynamic tests but require an anatomic assessment for confirmation. Cystourethroscopy can also reveal unsuspected neoplasia in the incontinent patient.

For many urogynecologists, cystourethroscopy also has a role in the diagnosis of intrinsic sphincteric deficiency, a condition that does not have standardized diagnostic criteria. Some advocate a single urodynamic parameter to make the diagnosis. However, in the absence of validated standard criteria for diagnosing intrinsic sphincteric deficiency, an approach that combines clinical measures of severity, urodynamic evidence of poor urethral resistance, and an anatomic evaluation of urethral coaptation seems to be warranted. Cystourethroscopy is perhaps the simplest way to achieve such an anatomic evaluation of the urethrovesical junction (UVJ).

Operative indications of cystourethroscopy in the female lower urinary tract include minor operative procedures performed through an operative cystoscope and intraoperative uses. Cystoscopy is an important adjuvant to surgery of the female genitourinary system. It is commonly used to perform and judge coaptation during periurethral injections, assess the elevation of the UVJ during needle urethropexies and suburethral sling procedures, facilitate surgical repair of urinary tract fistula and urethral diverticula, ensure the safe placement of suprapubic catheters, and evaluate the ureters and bladder mucosa for inadvertent damage at the time of surgery.

## INSTRUMENTATION
### Rigid Cystoscopy

There are three components to the rigid cystoscope: the telescope, the bridge, and the sheath (Fig. 10-1). Each component serves a different function and is available with various options to facilitate its role under different circumstances.

The telescope transmits light to the bladder cavity as well as an image to the viewer. Telescopes designed for cystoscopy are available with several viewing angles including zero degree (straight), 30 degree (forward-oblique), 70 degree (lateral), and 120 degree (retroview). The different angles facilitate the inspection of the entire bladder wall. Although the zero-degree lens is essential for adequate urethroscopy, it is insufficient for cystoscopy. The 30-degree lens provides the best view of the bladder base and posterior wall and the 70-degree lens permits inspection of the anterior and lateral walls. The retroview of the 120-degree lens is not usually necessary for cystoscopy of the female bladder but can be useful for evaluating the urethral opening into the bladder. For many applications, a single telescope is preferable. In diagnostic cystoscopy, the 30-degree telescope usu-

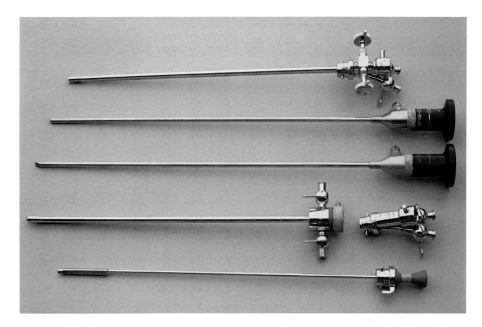

**Fig. 10-1**   Rigid endoscopes in urology and urogynecology. *Top to bottom,* Catheter-deflecting bridge; 30-degree telescope; 70-degree telescope; cystoscope sheath with bridge; obturator.

ally is sufficient, although a 70-degree telescope may be required in the presence of elevation of the UVJ. For operative cystoscopy, the 70-degree telescope is preferable. The angled telescopes have a field marker, visible as a blackened notch at the outside of the visual field opposite the angle of deflection, that helps facilitate orientation.

The cystoscope sheath provides a vehicle for introducing the telescope and distending medium into the vesical cavity. Sheaths are available in various calibers, ranging from 17 to 28 French for use in adults and smaller calibers for use in pediatrics. When placed within the sheath, the telescope, which is 15 French, only partially fills the lumen, leaving an irrigation-working channel. The smallest sheath is better tolerated for diagnostic procedures whereas the larger calibers provide space for the placement of instruments into the irrigation-working channel. The proximal end of the sheath has two irrigating ports, one for introduction of the distending medium and another for removal. The distal end of the cystoscope sheath is fenestrated to permit use of instrumentation in the angled field of view. It is also beveled, opposite the fenestrae, to increase the comfort of introduction of the cystoscope into the urethra. Bevels increase with the diameter of the cystoscope and larger sheaths may require an obturator for atraumatic placement.

The bridge serves as a connector between the telescope and sheath and forms a watertight seal with both. It may also have one or two ports for introduction of instruments into the irrigation-working channel. The Albarran bridge is a variation that has a deflector mechanism at the end of an inner sheath (Fig. 10-2). When placed in the cystoscope sheath, the deflector mechanism is located at the distal end of the inner sheath within the fenestra of the outer sheath. In

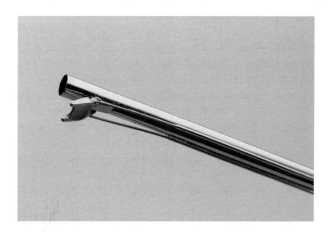

**Fig. 10-2**   Deflector at the tip of an Albarran bridge.

this location, elevation of the deflector mechanism assists the manipulation of instruments within the field of view.

## Rigid Urethroscopy

The rigid urethroscope is a modification of the cystoscope designed exclusively for evaluation of the urethra (Fig. 10-3). Because it is primarily a diagnostic instrument, it does not have a bridge. The telescope is shorter and has a zero-degree viewing angle, which provides a circumferential view of the urethral lumen as the mucosa in front of the urethroscope is distended by the distention medium. The zero-degree lens is essential for adequate urethroscopy.

The urethroscope sheath is designed to maximize distention of the urethral lumen. The proximal end of the sheath has a single irrigating port, and the telescope only partially

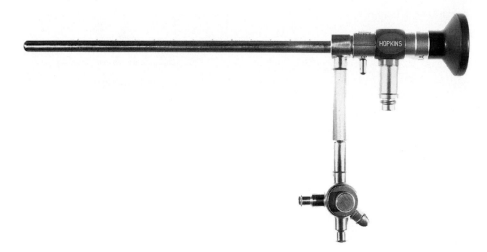

**Fig. 10-3**   Rigid urethroscope.

fills the sheath, leaving space for the irrigant to flow around it. Sheaths are available in 15-French and 24-French calibers. If tolerated, the larger sheath is useful because it provides the best view of the urethral lumen by providing more rapid fluid flow for maximal distention.

## Flexible Cystoscopy

Unlike the rigid cystoscope, the flexible cystoscope combines the optical systems and irrigation-working channel in a single unit. The coated tip is 15 to 18 French in diameter and 6 to 7 cm in length; the working unit makes up half the length. The optical system consists of a single image-bearing fiberoptic bundle and two light-bearing fiberoptic bundles. The fibers of these bundles are coated parallel coherent optical fibers that transmit light even when bent. The coating of the fibers results in a somewhat granular image and the delicate 5- to 10-μm diameter makes them susceptible to damage. Gentle handling is essential to good visualization and instrument longevity. The flexibility of the fibers permits incorporation of a distal tip-deflecting mechanism, controlled by a lever at the eyepiece, that will deflect the tip 290 degrees in a single plane. The optical fibers are fitted to a lens system that magnifies and focuses the image. A focusing knob is located just distal to the eyepiece. The irrigation-working port enters the instrument at the eyepiece opposite the deflecting mechanism.

Many urologists prefer the flexible cystoscope because of improved patient comfort, but this applies primarily to male patients. The absence of a prostate and the short length of the female urethra make rigid cystoscopy well tolerated by women. This may offset any perceived advantage of flexible cystoscopy in female patients. Moreover, there are several disadvantages to the flexible cystoscope. The flow rate of the irrigation-working channel is approximately one fourth that of a similar-size rigid cystoscope and is further curtailed by passage of instruments down this channel. Some tip

deflection is also lost with use of the instrument channel. In addition, because the view afforded by the flexible cystoscope is not as clear as that of a rigid cystoscope, greater operator skill is required to completely visualize the vesical cavity. There is no difference in the postprocedural morbidity as compared to rigid cystourethroscopy.

## Light Sources and Video Monitors

Any light source that provides adequate illumination via a fiberoptic cable is sufficient. A high-intensity (Xenon) light source is often recommended for the use of video monitoring or photography, but with recent innovations, the newest cameras require less light.

The cable attaches to the telescope at the eyepiece. Light cables are either fiberoptic or fluid-filled. The fluid-filled cables tend to be more expensive and more durable, although they add a slight tint to the light. Fiberoptic cables use flexible optic fibers that are comparable to those of the flexible cystoscope and are similarly prone to damage.

Although all cystoscopic procedures can be performed with direct visualization through the eyepiece, video monitoring eliminates awkward positioning required for direct visualization. It permits video documentation, which facilitates teaching, and often improves patient tolerance by providing distraction during the procedure. The video camera attaches directly to the eyepiece and should be maintained in an upright orientation. Changing the direction of view is accomplished by rotating the cystoscope without moving the camera itself.

## Distending Media

There are three types of distention media: nonconductive fluids, conductive fluids, and gases. Cystourethroscopy is feasible with carbon dioxide, but most practitioners prefer to use water or saline to distend the bladder and urethra. A liquid medium prevents the carbon dioxide bubbling and washes away blood or debris that can limit visualization. Moreover, the bladder volumes achieved using a liquid medium more accurately approximate physiologic volumes.

The choice of liquid medium depends on the procedure for which it is to be used. For diagnostic cystourethroscopy, sterile water is an ideal medium that is readily available and inexpensive. If absorption of a large volume of fluid into the vascular space is anticipated, an osmotic solution such as normal saline should be used. Similarly, if electrocautery is to be used, a nonconducting solution such as glycine should be used.

If a liquid medium is used, the water is instilled by gravity through a standard intravenous infusion set. The bag should be at a height of 100 cm above the patient's pubic symphysis to provide adequate flow.

## Operative Instrumentation

A wide range of instrumentation is available for use through a cystoscope. Those most pertinent to urogynecology are grasping forceps with either a rat tooth or alligator jaws, biopsy forceps, and scissors. These instruments can be obtained in semirigid or flexible varieties and come in various diameters. A flexible monopolar ball electrode is useful for electrocautery during operative cystoscopy.

## Instrument Care

Blood and debris should be removed from the equipment promptly to avoid accumulation in crevices and pitting of metal surfaces. The most common method of sterilization is immersion in a 2% activated glutaraldehyde solution (Cidex; Surgikos, Inc., Arlington, TX). Cystourethroscopic equipment should be soaked for 20 minutes and then transferred to a basin of sterile water until ready for use. Longer soaks shorten the life of the telescope by deteriorating the lens system and seals. If more permanent storage is desired, the scopes are cleaned with detergent and water, rinsed, and stored. Once a week the scopes are cleaned inside and out with alcohol and super oil used for lubrication. The irrigating ports and locking mechanisms should also be lubricated regularly.

## CYSTOURETHROSCOPIC TECHNIQUE

A complete evaluation of the lower urinary tract includes both urethroscopy and cystoscopy. A convenient approach begins with urethroscopy followed by cystoscopy. Diagnostic urethroscopy provides an evaluation of the urethral mucosa and UVJ. Diagnostic cystoscopy permits evaluation of the vesical cavity and ureteral function.

## Diagnostic Urethroscopy

The urethral meatus is cleansed with a disinfectant, and with the distention medium flowing, the urethroscope is advanced into the urethral meatus. The center of the urethral lumen is maintained in the center of the operator's visual field, and the urethral lumen, distended by the infusing medium, is followed to the UVJ. The urethral mucosa is examined for redness, pallor, exudate, and polyps as the urethroscope is advanced. The mucosa is normally pink and smooth, and a posterior longitudinal ridge, the urethral crest, may be seen. When the UVJ, typically round or horseshoe-shaped, is reached, flow is stopped and the area is observed for fronds (feathery structures with a central capillary) and polyps (bulbous structures).

Dynamic urethroscopy is performed after the bladder has a volume of 300 ml. The urethroscope is withdrawn until the UVJ closes one third of the way and the response of the UVJ to "hold your urine" and "squeeze your rectum" commands is evaluated. The urethroscope is then withdrawn until the UVJ is two-thirds closed and its response to Valsalva maneuver and cough is observed (Fig. 10-4). The normal response is UVJ closure with all of these commands.

The urethroscope is then positioned so that the UVJ is one-third closed and its response to bladder filling is observed. The bladder volumes at first sensation of filling, fullness, and maximum capacity are noted. The maneuvers at the UVJ are repeated, and the patient attempts to void. If voiding occurs, the urethra opens to the meatus and water escapes around the sheath. The normal UVJ should close over the urethroscope in response to a "hold your urine" command. The urethroscope is next withdrawn while a vaginal finger massages the urethra against the scope. Exudate or diverticular openings may be seen.

## Diagnostic Cystoscopy

Cystoscopy is performed using a 30- or 70-degree rigid telescope with a 17-French sheath. Topical anesthetics are typically avoided during urethroscopy because they can affect the color of the urethral mucosa. Following urethroscopy, however, 2% Lidocaine jelly may be used on the cystoscope sheath as a lubricant and topical anesthetic.

The cystoscope is placed into the urethral meatus with the bevel directed posteriorly and advanced to the bladder under direct vision. An obturator is not necessary when using a diagnostic 17-French sheath because downward pressure on the posterior lumen of the urethra with the blunt bevel is well tolerated by the majority of patients. The infusion of water is maintained at a slow rate until the patient reports fullness or a volume of approximately 400 ml is reached. Further infusion is not necessary unless it is required to improve the endoscopic view, in which case a small volume can be removed for patient comfort.

Orientation is easily established by identifying an air bubble anteriorly at the dome of the bladder. This serves as a landmark during the remainder of the examination. Beginning at the superior dome to the UVJ, the survey progresses in 12 sweeps, corresponding to the points of a clock (Fig. 10-5). Orientation is maintained by placing the field marker directly opposite the portion of the bladder to be inspected. The trigone and ureteral orifices are viewed by

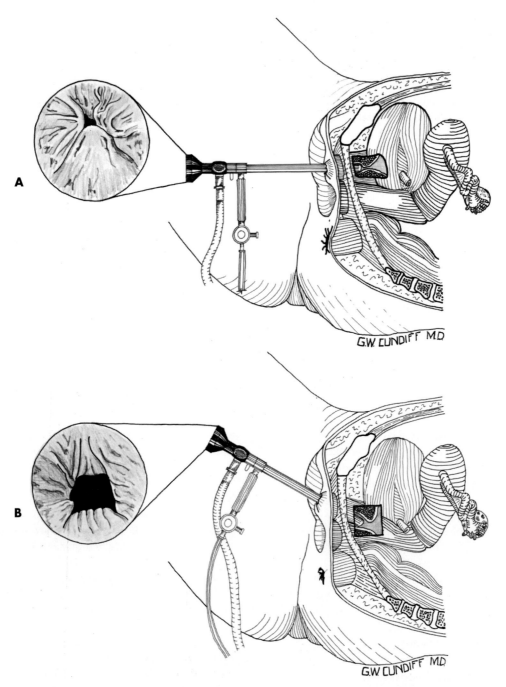

**Fig. 10-4** Evaluating urethral hypermobility using dynamic urethroscopy. **A,** Urethroscope is positioned to view the urethrovesical junction (window cut away to visualize the urethrovesical junction). **B,** As the patient coughs, the urethrovesical junction descends and opens (the urethroscope is elevated to follow the urethrovesical junction visualized through cutaway).

angling the scope downward at a 30-degree angle and laterally. Visualization of the bladder base can be difficult in patients with a large cystocele unless the prolapse is reduced with a vaginal finger. The mucosa is examined for color, vascularity, trabeculation, and abnormal lesions such as plaques or masses. Once the survey is complete, the telescope is removed while the sheath is left in place. This allows the bladder to drain and permits measurement of the volume of drained fluid. The approach to diagnostic

cystoscopy using a flexible cystoscope follows an approach similar to that described for rigid cystoscopy.

Infection is one of the leading causes of morbidity associated with cystourethroscopy, yet the actual rate of procedure-related bacteruria is not well defined. In the literature, the rate of bacteruria following cystoscopy ranges from 2.8% to 16.6%. The upper limit of the range represents significant factors of potential morbidity that have prompted many clinicians to use prophylactic antibiotics. Approaches

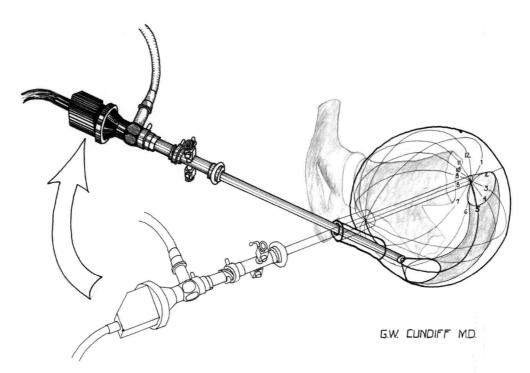

G.W. CUNDIFF M.D.

**Fig. 10-5** Diagnostic cystoscopy. A survey of vesical cavity is made by making 12 sweeps from the superior bladder to the urethrovesical junction. The 5 o'clock sweep is demonstrated.

vary considerably in terms of choice of antimicrobial agents and route of administration. Some practitioners use antibiotic bladder irrigation in lieu of oral antibiotics. The most common prophylactic regimen used for cystoscopy is probably oral nitrofurantoin. A recent double-blind randomized trial of nitrofurantoin prophylaxis for combined urodynamics and cystourethroscopy showed no difference between those receiving nitrofurantoin and placebo.

## Intraoperative Assessment of Lower Urinary Tract Integrity

The majority of ureteral injuries today occur during gynecologic operations, and lower urinary tract injury is one of the most common reasons for medical litigation against gynecologists. Estimates of the incidence of injury to the ureters during major gynecologic surgery range from 0.4% to 2.5%. The incidence of lower urinary tract injury is higher for urogynecologic surgery.

The approach to assessment of the integrity of the bladder mucosa following pelvic surgery is similar to the approach described for diagnostic cystoscopy. A thorough survey of the bladder is made with special attention to the portions of the bladder potentially jeopardized by the procedure. Inspection of the anterior and lateral aspects of the mucosa is important after a retropubic urethropexy, whereas inspection of the trigone is warranted following a difficult vaginal hysterectomy or dissection of an anterior enterocele from the bladder. Assessment of ureteral integrity should be considered after any retropubic suspension or culdeplasty and is warranted whenever there is a suspicion

of ureteral injury. Intravenous administration of indigo carmine approximately 5 minutes before initiating cystoscopy facilitates visualization of the ureteral orifices during efflux by staining the urine blue.

### Suprapubic Teloscopy

Suprapubic teloscopy is an alternative to transurethral cystoscopy for evaluating the lower urinary tract during pelvic surgery. Transurethral cystoscopy is well suited to pelvic surgery performed by a vaginal approach but is inconvenient in conjunction with an abdominal procedure. Valuable operative time is lost by closing the abdominal wound to permit repositioning and prepping for transurethral cystoscopy. Moreover, any significant cystoscopic findings mandate reopening the abdomen for surgical correction. Suprapubic teloscopy addresses this dilemma by providing a way to perform endoscopy from an abdominal approach. Because of the simplicity of the technique, suprapubic teloscopy compares favorably to the alternatives of open cystotomy or dissection of ureters in terms of required operating time and morbidity. It is an easy transition for an endoscopist experienced in cystoscopy.

Suprapubic teloscopy is an extraperitoneal technique that begins with closure of the anterior peritoneum to prevent contamination of the peritoneal cavity with spilled urine. If indigo carmine is to be used to help identify the ureteral orifices, it should be given at this juncture to permit time for renal excretion. The bladder cavity is filled through a triple-lumen transurethral Foley catheter to at least 400 ml. A 1- to 2-cm pursestring suture is placed into the muscularis layer of the dome of the bladder, using a 2-0 absorbable suture. Two absorbable stay sutures can be placed within the pursestring, but with a full-thickness purchase to facilitate introduction of the telescope. A stab incision made between the stay sutures provides an opening for insertion of the telescope. Because distention of the bladder is achieved through the transurethral catheter, the sheath and bridge are unnecessary and the telescope is inserted alone. The pursestring is tightened sufficiently to prevent leakage without limiting the movement of the telescope. A 30-degree telescope provides the best view of the trigone and ureteral orifices while also permitting a thorough bladder survey. Orientation can be achieved by identifying the transurethral Foley catheter bulb and locating the trigone beneath the bulb. If suprapubic catheterization is planned, the catheter can be placed through the same stab incision when teloscopy is completed.

### Cystoscopic Passage of Ureteral Catheters

The absence of efflux of urine from the ureteral orifices during pelvic surgery is an indication for the passage of ureteral catheters to evaluate for potential obstruction. Ureteral catheters are available in various sizes and with a number of specialized tips. The most useful catheters for assessing ureteral patency are the general purpose catheter and the whistle tip catheter. Although available from 3 to 12 French, the most useful catheter calibers are in the 4- to 7-French range. They have graduated centimeter markings for judging the length of insertion.

Once the ureteral orifice is located, the ureteral catheter is advanced into the field of view. Although the deflecting mechanism of the Albarran bridge facilitates ureteral catheterization, it is usually not essential to its completion. The catheter is placed just outside the fenestrated end of the cystoscope, with the catheter tip oriented in the axis of the ureteral lumen. The tip is threaded into the ureteral orifice by advancing the entire cystoscope. Once the tip enters the ureteral orifice, the catheter is gently advanced until it meets resistance as it passes into the renal pelvis, which is generally 25 to 30 cm. If the catheter is to be left in place, it should be secured to a transurethral catheter and connected to a drainage device. Gentle technique is essential to preventing hematuria and resulting colic. Other potential complications include perforation and ureteral spasm, but with proper methods the risk of complication is small.

### Operative Cystoscopy

Operative cystoscopy is generally done by urologists. However, several minor procedures are easily performed in the office by urogynecologists during diagnostic cystoscopy. These include biopsy of mucosal lesions and removal of small foreign bodies or intravesical sutures.

Because of the focal length of the optics, the best view is immediately in front of the telescope; this is where operative procedures should take place. Following introduction of the cystoscope into the bladder and instillation of a sufficient volume of fluid to view the entire vesical wall, the instrument is introduced into the operative port and advanced until it is visible just at the end of the cystoscope. Gross movements are made by moving the cystoscope, and minor adjustments are made by moving the instrument itself. This approach keeps the operation in the optimal field of view. Irrigation at a brisk rate helps to keep the field from being obscured by blood. The bleeding that occurs with biopsy is usually minor, but if excessive hemorrhage occurs, this can be controlled by electrocautery.

Because these procedures require a larger cystoscope sheath (larger than 22 French) and may cause some patient discomfort, anesthesia is recommended. Intravesical instillation of anesthetic is often sufficient but can be augmented by a bladder pillar block. For bladder installation, the bladder is catheterized and drained; 50 ml of 4% Lidocaine solution is instilled and left in place for 5 minutes. The bladder pillar block can be placed before the Lidocaine is drained from the bladder. The block is performed by injecting 5 ml of 1% Lidocaine solution 5 mm submucosally at the bladder pillars. After placement of a bivalve speculum, the bladder pillars are located in the lateral fornices at 2 and 10 o'clock with respect to the cervix.

## CYSTOURETHROSCOPIC FINDINGS
### Normal Findings

The urethral mucosa is normally pink and smooth, with a posterior longitudinal ridge called the urethral crest. The UVJ is typically round or an inverted horseshoe shape and is completely coapted until the irrigant opens the lumen. The UVJ normally closes briskly and has minimal mobility with Valsalva maneuver.

In its normal state, the bladder mucosa has a smooth surface with a pale pink to glistening white hue. The translucent mucosa affords easy visualization of the branched submucosal vasculature. As the mucosa of the dome gives way to the trigone, it thickens and develops a granular texture. The reddened granular surface of the trigone is commonly covered by a thickened white membrane with a villous contour. Histologic evaluation of the layer reveals squamous metaplasia (Fig. 10-6). The trigone is triangular in shape, with the inferior apex directed toward the UVJ and the ureteral orifices forming the superior apices. As the cystoscope is advanced past the UVJ, the trigone is apparent at the bottom of the field. The interureteric ridge is a visible elevation that forms the superior boundary of the trigone and runs between the ureteral orifices. The intramural portions of the ureters can often be seen as they course from the lateral aspect of the bladder toward the trigone and ureteral orifices. There is marked variation in the ureteral orifices, but they are generally circular or slitlike openings at the apex of a small mound. With efflux of urine, the slit opens and the mound retracts in the direction of the intramural ureter.

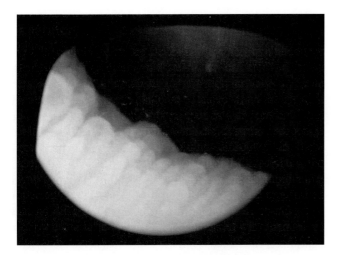

**Fig. 10-6**  Trigone demonstrating squamous metaplasia.

When distended, the bladder is roughly spherical in shape but numerous folds of mucosa are evident in the empty or partially filled bladder. The uterus and cervix can usually be seen indenting the posterior wall of the bladder, which creates posterolateral pouches where the bladder drapes over the uterus into the paravaginal spaces. At times visualization of the bowel peristalsis is possible through the vesical wall.

## Pathologic Findings
### Urethroscopic Pathology

In the urethral syndrome, also known as chronic urethritis, the urethra is reddened, and exudate sometimes can be expressed from the posterior urethral glands. Chronic urethritis may also be associated with fronds or polyps, both of which can be seen in the proximal urethra or at the UVJ. Urethral diverticula appear as ostia, usually along the lateral or posterior surface of the urethra, which may have expressed exudate on palpation (Fig. 10-7).

A stricture is a narrowing of the urethra that typically occurs at the meatus, although proximal or mid-urethral narrowing may also result from prior urethral surgery. Hypoestrogenism results in pale urothelium. A urethral lumen that is pale and rigid and is unresponsive to commands indicates fibrosis and may result in intrinsic sphincter deficiency. During dynamic urethroscopy the patient with genuine stress incontinence cannot close the UVJ to the "hold" and "squeeze" commands, and the UVJ generally opens and descends in response to coughs and Valsalva maneuvers. The patient with intrinsic sphincter deficiency may have a rigid, immobile urethra, with the UVJ unresponsive to commands. In severe cases, the urethral lumen may be visualized from meatus to bladder neck.

### Cystoscopic Pathology

Pathology affecting the bladder can be categorized as mucosal lesions or structural variations. Mucosal lesions are

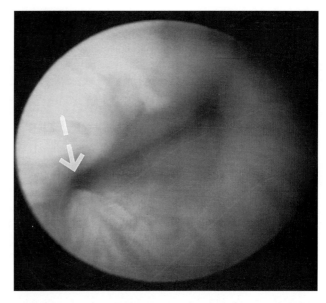

**Fig. 10-7**  Urethroscopic view of the orifice of a suburethral diverticulum *(arrow)*. The proximal urethral orifice is at the upper right side.

either inflammatory or neoplastic, although their coexistence is not uncommon.

Despite its common use to describe infection of the bladder, *cystitis* in its broadest definition refers to inflammation of the bladder mucosa, of which there are several varieties. Cystoscopy should be avoided in the presence of active infectious cystitis, but if performed inadvertently may provide variable findings. In its mildest form, bacterial cystitis can be rather inconspicuous, with little more than pink or peach-colored macules or papules. With increasing severity, mucosal edema and hypervascularity are evident, with loss of the submucosal vascular pattern and marked vascular dilation. In hemorrhagic cystitis, this can progress to individual or confluent mucosal hemorrhages and may be associated with hematuria in addition to irritative voiding symptoms.

The symptoms of hematuria and irritative voiding are typical of several other less common inflammatory conditions that can often be distinguished at cystoscopy. The hemorrhagic cystitis that follows bladder infusion with toxins such as cyclophosphamide is characterized by diffuse mucosal hemorrhage. In radiation cystitis, areas of hemorrhage are surrounded by pale mucosa, which may be fibrotic and hypovascular. A chronic indwelling urethral or suprapubic catheter produces an inflammatory reaction of the mucosa directly in contact with the catheter. Mucosal changes range from pseudopapillary edema and submucosal hemorrhage to vesical fibrosis.

Interstitial cystitis, another form of chronic inflammation, is often associated with hematuria and fibrosis. The pathognomonic lesions appear on refilling the bladder, after initially filling to maximum cystometric capacity. General anesthesia is usually required to fill to maximum cystometric capacity because the associated fibrosis often makes filling intolerable. Glomerulations are the primary finding in very mild cases. These petechial hemorrhages are small red dots that may coalesce to form larger hemorrhagic areas. Rare petechiae are seen in normal patients, especially on the posterior wall and trigone, caused by cystoscope trauma. In contrast, interstitial cystitis patients have at least 10 to 20 glomerulations per field of vision. The classic Hunner ulcer is seen in more severe cases of interstitial cystitis. These ulcers appear as velvety red patches or linear cracks with a granulating base and surrounding vascular congestion.

Recurrent or chronic inflammation can produce characteristic lesions as well. Inflammatory polyps are often identified at the UVJ if the cystoscope is retracted into the proximal urethra and the infusion interrupted to allow them to float into the field of view. They are usually translucent with a villous appearance but can become large enough to partially fill the urethral lumen. Cystitis cystica consists of clear mucosal cysts usually found in multiple areas over the bladder base. The cysts are formed by single layers of subepithelial transitional cells, which degenerate with central liquefaction. Cystitis glandularis has a similar appearance to cystitis cystica, but the cysts are not clear and have a less uniform contour. As in cystitis glandularis, the mechanism of formation is a glandular metaplasia. In cystitis glandularis, however, there is involvement of multiple layers, including the mucus-producing glandular epithelium. Both lesions are associated with chronic irritation of the bladder mucosa and are commonly surrounded by marked inflammation. The association of cystitis glandularis with adenovillous carcinoma of the bladder has led to the belief that cystitis glandularis may be a precursor of adenocarcinoma. A proposed metaplastic transformation from epithelial hyperplasia through cystitis glandularis and finally to adenocarcinoma is based on a case presented by Shaw et al. (1958) of a gradual transition of cystitis glandularis to adenocarcinoma over a 5-year period. There have been two subsequent reports of transformation of cystitis glandularis to adenocarcinoma.

Although it is twice as common in men, bladder cancer is the most common genitourinary neoplasm in women. The vast majority of cases occur past the fifth decade. Transitional cell carcinoma is the most common histologic type, followed by adenocarcinoma and squamous cell carcinoma. Transitional cell carcinoma is usually carcinogen induced. Tobacco, dyes, and organic chemicals are known carcinogens for the transitional epithelium. Adenocarcinoma is more common with bladder extrophy. Squamous cell carcinoma has been reported with chronic indwelling catheters. Cystoscopic appearance is variable, depending on histologic type and grade, but usually reveals a raised lesion with a villous feathery or papillary appearance. Circumferential inflammation is ubiquitous. Superficial transitional cell carcinoma may be multicentric or may have associated carcinoma in situ. Carcinoma in situ can be disturbingly

inconspicuous, often mimicking the macules or plaques of infectious cystitis.

Vesical and ureteral structural variations may be anatomic or functional anomalies. Auxiliary ureteral orifices are examples of rare anatomic anomalies, which are indicative of renal collecting anomalies. When present, they often enter the vesical wall slightly superior to the trigone in near proximity to the other ureteral orifice. Ureteroceles are caused by laxity of the distal ureteral lumen, with herniation into the vesical cavity during efflux.

Trabeculations are considerably more common than auxiliary ureteral orifices or ureterocele. These smooth ridges become evident with distention of the bladder to volumes approaching maximum cystometric capacity. They appear as interlaced cords of different diameters with intervening sacculations. They represent hypertrophied detrusor musculature associated with detrusor instability and functional or anatomic bladder obstruction. A bladder diverticulum can occur when high intravesical pressure produces an enlargement of the intervening sacculations. The thick muscular band that creates the neck varies in diameter and gives way to outpouchings of bladder mucosa. The interior of the diverticulum has been reported to be the site of neoplasm in approximately 7% of cases.

Fistulas may also be encountered at cystoscopy. Approximately 75% are vesicovaginal fistulas (Fig. 10-8) that result from abdominal hysterectomies. They may also occur after vaginal hysterectomies, urologic procedures, radiation, foreign bodies, cancer, and obstetric trauma. Posthysterectomy fistulas are usually located in the bladder base superior to the interureteric ridge, corresponding to the level of the vaginal cuff. The fistulous openings range from small to several centimeters in diameter. In the immediate postoperative state, the surrounding mucosa is edematous and hyperemic; in later stages the mucosa has a smooth appearance. In contrast, vesicoenteric fistulas uniformly have surrounding inflammatory reaction often with bulbous edema, and the fistulous tract is not discernible in two thirds of cases.

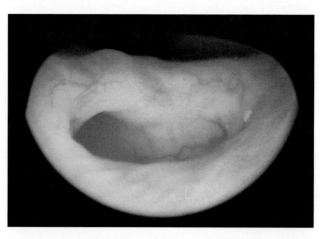

**Fig. 10-8** Vesicovaginal fistula *(bottom)*.

Bladder calculi may result from urinary stasis or the presence of a foreign body, or an inflammatory exudate may coalesce and serve as a nidus for stone formation. Stones have extremely variable cystoscopic appearance in terms of color, size, and shape but generally have an irregular surface. Foreign bodies and stones are usually accompanied by varying degrees of general or localized inflammatory reaction.

## BIBLIOGRAPHY
### Historical Perspective

Gunning JE, Rosenzweig BA: Evolution of endoscopic surgery. In White RA, Klein SR, eds: *Endoscopic surgery,* St Louis, 1991, Mosby.

Hopkins HH, Kopany NS: A flexible fiberscope, using static scanning, *Nature* 179:39, 1954.

Kelly HA: The direct examination of the female bladder with elevated pelvis: the catheterization of the ureters under direct inspection, with and without elevation of the pelvis, *Am J Obstet Dis Wom Child* 25:1, 1894.

Ridley JH: Indirect air cystoscopy, *South Med J* 44:114, 1951.

Robertson JR: Office cystoscopy: substituting the culdescope for the Kelly cystoscope, *Obstet Gynecol* 28:219, 1966.

Robertson JR: Air cystoscopy, *Obstet Gynecol* 32:328, 1968.

Robertson JR: Gynecologic urethroscopy, *Am J Obstet Gynecol* 115:986, 1973.

### Instrumentation

Aso Y, Yokoyama M, Fukutani K, et al: New trial for fiberoptic cystourethroscopy: the use of metal sheath, *J Urol* 115:99, 1976.

Bagley DH, Huffman JL, Lyon ES: *Urologic endoscopy: a manual and atlas,* Boston, 1985, Little, Brown.

Clayman RV, Reddy P, Lange PH: Flexible fiber optic and rigid-rod lens endoscopy of the lower urinary tract: a prospective controlled comparison, *J Urol* 131:715, 1984.

Figueroa TE, Thomas R, Moon TD: A comparison of rigid with flexible instruments, *J Louisiana St Med Soc* 139:26, 1987.

Fowler CG: Fiberscope urethrocystoscopy, *Br J Urol* 56:304, 1984.

Fowler CG, Badenoch DF, Thakar DR: Practical experience with flexible fiberscope cystoscopy in out-patients, *Br J Urol* 56:618, 1984.

Hargreave TB: Practical urological endoscopy, Oxford, 1988, Blackwell Scientific Publications.

Matthews PN, Bidgood KA, Woodhouse RJ: $CO_2$ cystoscopy using a flexible fiberoptic endoscopy, *Br J Urol* 56:188, 1984.

Matthews PN, Skewes DG, Kothari JJ, et al: Carbon dioxide versus water for cystoscopy: a comparative study, *Br J Urol* 55:364, 1983.

### Cystourethroscopic Technique

Aldridge CW, Beaton JH, Nanzig RP: A review of office urethroscopy and cystometry, *Am J Obstet Gynecol* 131:432, 1978.

Clark KR, Higgs MJ: Urinary infection following out-patient flexible cystoscopy, *Br J Urol* 66:503, 1990.

Cundiff GW, Bent AE: The contribution of urethrocystoscopy to a combined urodynamic and urethrocystoscopic evaluation of urinary incontinence in women, *Int J Urogynecol* 7:307, 1996.

Denholm SW, Conn IG, Newsam JE, et al: Morbidity following cystoscopy: comparison of flexible and rigid techniques, *Br J Urol* 66:503, 1990.

Fozard JB, Green DF, Harrison GS, et al: Asepsis and out-patient cystoscopy, *Br J Urol* 55:680, 1983.

Green LF, Khan AU: Cystourethroscopy in the female, *Urology* 10:451, 1977.

Manson AL: Is antibiotic administration indicated after out-patient cystoscopy? *J Urol* 140:316, 1988.

Marier R, Valenti AJ, Madri JA: Gram-negative endocarditis following cystoscopy, *J Urol* 119:134, 1978.

O'Donnell P: Water endoscopy. In Raz S, ed: *Female urology,* Philadelphia, 1983, WB Saunders.

Richards B, Bastable JR: Bacteriuria after outpatient cystoscopy, *Br J Urol* 49:561, 1977.

Robertson JR: Gas endoscopy. In Raz S, ed: *Female urology,* Philadelphia, 1983, WB Saunders.

Robertson JR: Dynamic urethroscopy. In Ostergard DR, ed: *Gynecologic urology and urodynamics,* ed 2, Baltimore, 1985, Williams & Wilkins.

Romero RE, Hicks TH, Galindo GH, et al: Evaluation of the importance of cystoscopy in staging gynecologic carcinomas, *J Urol* 121:64, 1979.

Rosenzweig BA, Bhatia NN: The use of carbon dioxide laser in female urology, *J Gynecol Surg* 7:11, 1991.

Sand PK, Hill RC, Ostergard DR: Supine urethroscopic and standing cystometry as screening methods for the detection of detrusor instability, *Obstet Gynecol* 70:57, 1987.

Scotti RJ, Ostergard DR, Guillaume AA, et al: Predictive value of urethroscopy as compared to urodynamics in the diagnosis of genuine stress incontinence, *J Reprod Med* 35:772, 1990.

Uehling DT: The normal caliber of the adult female urethra, *J Urol* 120:176, 1978.

Worth PH: Cystourethroscopy. In Stanton SL, ed: *Clinical gynecologic urology,* St Louis, 1984, Mosby.

### Cystourethroscopic Findings

Anderson MJ: The incidence of diverticula in the female urethra, *J Urol* 98:96, 1967.

Bergman A, Karram M, Bhatia NN: Urethral syndrome: a comparison of different treatment modalities, *J Reprod Med* 34:157, 1989.

Davis BL, Robinson DG: Diverticula of the female urethra: assay of 120 cases, *J Urol* 104:850, 1970.

Edwards PD, Hurm RA, Jaesehke WH: Conversion of cystitis glandularis to adenocarcinoma, *J Urol* 108:568, 1972.

Hunner GL: A rare type of bladder ulcer in women: report of cases, *Trans South Surg Gynecol Assoc* 27:247, 1914.

Lee RA: Diverticulum of the urethra. Clinical presentation, diagnosis and management, *Clin Obstet Gynecol* 27:490, 1984.

Lyon RP, Smith DR: Distal urethral stenosis, *J Urol* 89:414, 1963.

MacDermott JP, Charpied GC, Tesluk H, et al: Can histological assessment predict the outcome in interstitial cystitis? *Br J Urol* 67:44, 1991.

Marshall FC, Uson AC, Melicow MM: Neoplasm and caruncles of the female urethra, *Surg Gynecol Obstet* 110:723, 1960.

Messing EM, Stamey TA: Interstitial cystitis: early diagnosis, pathology, and treatment, *Urology* 12:381, 1978.

Mufson MA, Belshe RB, Horrigan TJ, et al: Cause of acute hemorrhagic cystitis in children, *Am J Dis Child* 126:605, 1973.

Numazaki Y, Kumasaka T, Yano N, et al: Further study on acute hemorrhagic cystitis due to adenovirus type II, *N Engl J Med* 289:344, 1973.

Richardson FH: External urethroplasty in women: technique and clinical evaluation, *J Urol* 101:719, 1969.

Scotti RJ, Ostergard DR: The urethral syndrome, *Clin Obstet Gynecol* 27:515, 1984.

Shaw JL, Gislason GJ, Imbriglia: Transition of cystitis glandularis to primary adenocarcinoma of the bladder, *J Urol* 79:815, 1958.

Summary of the National Institute of Arthritis, Diabetes, Digestive and Kidney Diseases workshop on interstitial cystitis, National Institute of Health. Bethesda, Maryland, August 28-29, 1987, *J Urol* 140:203, 1988.

Susmans D, Rubenstein AB, Dakin AR, et al: Cystitis glandularis and adenocarcinoma of the bladder, *J Urol* 105:671: 1971.

Walsh A: Interstitial cystitis. In Harrison JH, Gittes RF, Perlmutter AD, et al, eds: *Campbell's urology,* ed 4, Philadelphia, 1979, WB Saunders.

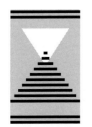

CHAPTER **11**
# Radiologic Studies of the Lower Urinary Tract

Eddie H.M. Sze

Plain Film of the Abdomen
Intravenous Pyelogram
Cystography
Voiding Cystourethrography
Positive-Pressure Urethrography
Ultrasound
  *Doppler sonography*
  *Endoluminal sonography*
Videocystourethrography
Computed Tomography
Magnetic Resonance Imaging

Radiologic studies are an integral part of the evaluation of lower urinary tract dysfunction and abnormalities. Historically, plain radiography and intravenous pyelogram (IVP) were the radiographic tests performed to diagnose urologic problems. More recently, new technological developments in sonography, computed tomography (CT), and magnetic resonance imaging (MRI) have allowed clinicians more versatility to diagnose a variety of urologic and urogynecologic disorders. The focus of this chapter is on the radiologic diagnostic techniques used in clinical urogynecology.

## PLAIN FILM OF THE ABDOMEN

The flat plate of the abdomen, taken as a scout film for IVP or a plain radiograph, can screen for urinary calculi. In addition, it may also reveal masses, bony lesions, abnormal gas patterns in the gastrointestinal tract, and calculi in suburethral diverticula.

## INTRAVENOUS PYELOGRAM

Despite the emergence of other imaging techniques, IVP has remained the modality of choice for visualizing the urinary tract. It is safe, inexpensive, and readily available. It gives detailed anatomic and functional information about the urinary tract. IVP is used to evaluate suspected ureteral obstruction, fistula, urolithiasis, and congenital anomalies.

In addition, the postvoid film can detect bladder and suburethral diverticula, as well as residual urine in the bladder. In acute ureteral obstruction, opacification of the urinary tract is often delayed for several hours or more because of the decreased glomerular filtration rate and increased water and sodium reabsorption in the proximal convoluted tubules. In addition, calyceal dilation may not appear for 24 to 48 hours after the patient becomes symptomatic. A disadvantage is that some abnormalities detected by IVP, such as radiolucent filling defects, are nonspecific in appearance, necessitating the use of other imaging modalities for further characterization.

Some gynecologists use IVP to delineate the course of the pelvic ureters when evaluating large pelvic masses. However, studies have shown that radiologic knowledge of the course of the ureters does not decrease the risk of operative injury to the urinary tract. IVP can identify preexisting abnormalities of the urinary tract, such as hydronephrosis from a pelvic mass or a nonfunctioning kidney from a previous ureteral ligation. It also can detect unsuspected anomalies of the urinary tract (Fig. 11-1), thus allowing surgeons to avoid injury to these structures during surgical dissection.

Women with uterovaginal prolapse are often screened with a preoperative IVP or ultrasonography to detect possible hydronephrosis. The association between uterovaginal prolapse and obstructive uropathy was first reported in the English literature by Brettauer and Rubin in 1923. Several small studies have subsequently shown that up to 100% of women with genital prolapse have hydronephrosis. However, in a recent study from the Cleveland Clinic, Beverly et al. (1997) found that only 0.9% of 323 women with various degrees of uterovaginal prolapse had severe bilateral hydronephrosis. In addition, the presence of hydronephrosis did not alter the surgical treatment of these patients. These investigators concluded that routine preoperative renal evaluation in women undergoing surgery for uterovaginal prolapse is not indicated.

The main contraindications to IVP are a history of severe reaction to contrast media and moderate to severe renal failure. Patients with renal insufficiency may not be able to excrete a sufficient amount of contrast medium to opacify

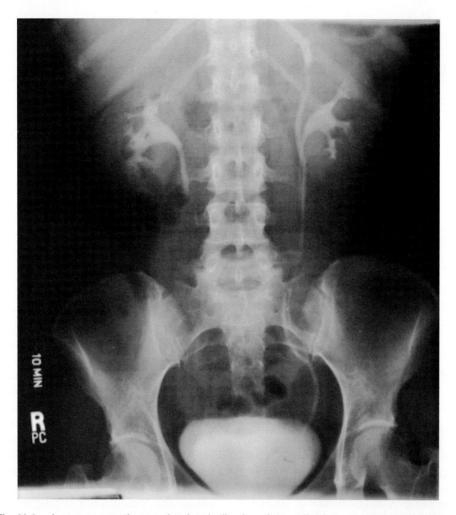

**Fig. 11-1**    Intravenous pyelogram showing duplication of the collecting system of the left kidney.

the urinary tract. In addition, the contrast may also exacerbate the existing renal insufficiency. Relative contraindications include congestive heart failure and mild renal insufficiency.

If the pelvicaliceal or ureteric anatomy is not adequately visualized with IVP or if there is a contraindication to IVP, an alternative approach is to perform a retrograde pyelogram. This is especially useful if there is a coexisting indication for cystoscopy. In retrograde pyelogram, the contrast medium is injected into the upper urinary tract through a cone-tipped catheter placed at cystoscopy under fluoroscopic guidance (Fig. 11-2). This approach is associated with a higher infection rate than antegrade pyelography and may be contraindicated in women with known allergic reaction to contrast media or very recent lower urinary tract trauma or surgery. The large amount of contrast medium injected and the pressure applied during retrograde pyelogram may result in anastomotic leak and extravasation, with systemic absorption of the contrast.

Like the retrograde pyelogram, antegrade pyelography can provide excellent opacification of the renal collecting system. Because this approach involves placing a small-gauge needle into the renal pelvis, it is rarely performed for diagnostic indications only. Antegrade pyelography is usually performed only when there is another indication for percutaneous puncture. To perform an antegrade pyelography, the patient is placed in a prone position. A flexible 20- or 22-gauge needle is inserted into the collecting system under ultrasound or fluoroscopic control after administration of intravenous contrast medium. An obstructed collecting system should be decompressed before contrast medium is injected in order to avoid overdistention and urosepsis. Additional procedures can then be performed to relieve the obstruction temporarily or permanently.

## CYSTOGRAPHY

The primary indication for cystography is to detect possible bladder injury from trauma and surgical procedures. It is also used to investigate possible fistulas between the bladder and adjacent organs and the presence of bladder diverticula. In the past, this study was used extensively to measure the

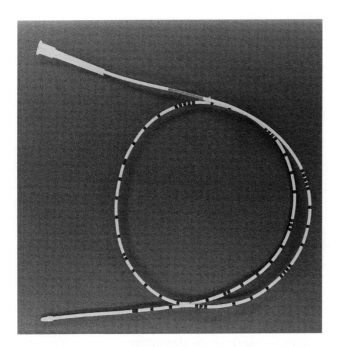

**Fig. 11-2** Ureteral catheter used to perform retrograde pyelography.

posterior urethrovesical angle and its relationship to the symphysis pubis as part of the evaluation for urinary incontinence. However, Drutz et al. (1978) and other investigators found that there is little correlation between these radiographic findings and the underlying functional disturbance based on urodynamic results. Furthermore, the position of the bladder at rest and during straining is more accurately determined by clinical examination. These latter indications are primarily of historical interest and are no longer valid reasons for ordering a cystogram.

To perform a cystogram, a postvoid residual urine is drained and measured. After a plain abdominal film is taken, the bladder is filled via a suprapubic or urethral catheter with contrast medium under low pressure to capacity. Images of the distended bladder and related abnormalities are documented with spot films taken in different views. After the bladder is drained, a postvoid film is obtained to evaluate for extravasated contrast medium.

Contrast from *extra*peritoneal leakage usually forms an irregularly shaped mass around the injured site and remains there for a relatively long time. Contrast medium leaked from an *intra*peritoneal defect diffuses into the entire abdominal cavity and is rapidly absorbed through the peritoneum. Vesicovaginal, vesicouterine, and vesicoenteric fistulas are diagnosed when contrast material from the bladder enters and opacifies the adjacent viscera (Fig. 11-3). Small fistulas may not allow passage of a sufficient amount of contrast to be seen radiographically. Bladder diverticula appear as blind sacs protruding from the bladder or as opacified sacs in an empty bladder on postvoid film. Diverticula are best visualized in the oblique view.

The primary contraindication for cystography is acute urinary tract infection, which is also the most common complication associated with this procedure. Prophylactic antibiotics are usually recommended. The other complication associated with cystography is that some contrast media, such as sodium acetrizoate (Cystokon), can irritate the bladder, resulting in bladder and urethral spasm, mucosal irregularities, vesicoureteral reflux, or uncontrolled urine loss. These iatrogenic causes of lower urinary tract abnormalities may interfere with the interpretation of the cystogram.

## VOIDING CYSTOURETHROGRAPHY

Voiding cystourethrography (VCUG) is a dynamic radiologic study used primarily to evaluate the bladder and the urethra. This diagnostic test is often used to investigate suspected suburethral diverticula (Fig. 11-4), vesicoureteral reflux, increased bladder volume, and congenital abnormalities such as ureterocele and primary megaureter. VCUG involves retrograde filling of the bladder with a dilute water-soluble contrast medium. After the catheter is removed, the patient is instructed to void under fluoroscopic control. With this technique, anatomy of the bladder and urethra can be evaluated in conjunction with assessment of bladder function and capacity. Vesicoureteral reflux and other abnormalities are documented by spot radiographs. An occasional difficulty associated with this test is that the patient may not be able to void on command, especially in a laboratory setting.

## POSITIVE-PRESSURE URETHROGRAPHY

Positive-pressure urethrography was first described and used by Davis and Cian in 1956 to evaluate the female urethra. Today, the primary indication for this diagnostic test is to search for possible suburethral diverticula not visualized on VCUG. The study requires a Trattner catheter, which has two balloons, with an opening in the lumen of the catheter between the two balloons for contrast injection (see Chapter 29). The distal balloon is placed into the bladder, and the proximal (sliding) balloon is positioned just outside the external urethral meatus. The two inflated balloons create a temporary closed system and allow the contrast injected into the urethra to opacify the diverticulum (Fig. 11-5). This radiologic test is often performed in conjunction with VCUG to maximize the diagnostic accuracy.

## ULTRASOUND

The use of ultrasound for the evaluation of the urinary tract has evolved from merely using the bladder as a coupling medium to scanning pelvic structures. Recently, major technical advances in ultrasonic instrumentation have facilitated the establishment of ultrasound as an important diagnostic tool in the management of urinary tract disorders. Compared to the conventional radiologic studies, ultrasound is noninvasive and inexpensive, does not require contrast media, and does not expose the patient and the sonographer to ionizing radiation. The main disadvantage of ultrasound is that the quality of the study depends on the operator to a greater extent than in other imaging techniques.

Transabdominal ultrasound is used to assess adynamic changes in the urinary tract. In the upper tract, ultrasound can detect hydronephrosis, renal stones, and renal parenchymal abnormalities. In the lower tract, ultrasound is used to assess postvoid residual volume, suburethral diverticula, and bladder tumor.

Although abdominal ultrasound is very sensitive in detecting pelvicaliceal dilation, it cannot diagnose the degree of obstruction or indicate whether the hydronephrosis is obstructive or nonobstructive. Unilateral hydronephrosis is not always caused by acute obstruction; it may be caused by ureteral reflux, residual hydronephrosis from a previously relieved obstruction, or prominent renal vasculature. There is also poor correlation between the extent of dilation on ultrasound and the degree of obstruction because severe obstruction may result in mild pelvicaliceal dilation. Furthermore, the dilation may not become evident for up to 48 hours after the onset of symptoms. Localization of the obstruction below the ureteropelvic junction is also limited because abdominal ultrasound often cannot trace the ureter through its retroperitoneal course because of patient size or overlying loops of bowel. Only stones or tumors in the renal pelvis or the ureterovesical junction can sometimes be seen in adult patients. Radiologic studies are usually needed to confirm the location and the cause of obstruction, confirm acute ureteral obstruction before the onset of hydrone-phrosis, and distinguish obstructive from nonobstructive hydronephrosis.

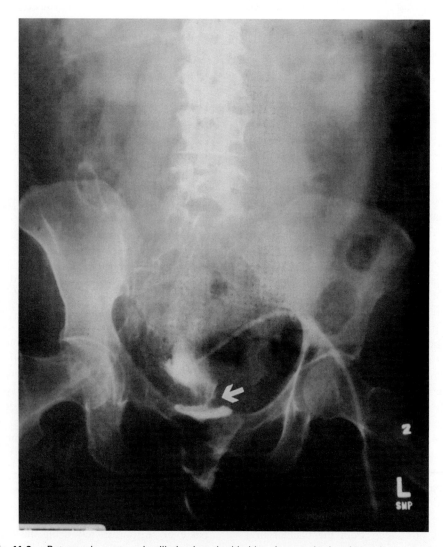

**Fig. 11-3** Retrograde contrast instillation into the bladder via a urethral catheter demonstrating a vesicovaginal fistula.

Transabdominal ultrasound can be used to measure the bladder and postvoid residual volumes. This method requires three diameters (height, width, and depth) measured in two perpendicular planes (transverse and sagittal). Height and depth are measured in the sagittal plane scan; height corresponds to the greatest superoinferior diameter, and depth corresponds to the greatest anteroposterior diameter. Width corresponds to the greatest transverse diameter measured in transverse plane scan. These measurements are not reliable when the bladder volume is less than 50 ml. The bladder volume is estimated by using the formula: Volume (ml) = (H × W × D) × (0.7). The correction factor 0.7 is needed because the shape of the bladder is not circular until it is almost completely full. This formula has an error rate of approximately 21%. Portable ultrasonic devices have been developed specifically to measure residual urine volumes. These units can automatically make three-dimensional measurements of the bladder and calcu-

late the residual urine volume. The scan-predicted volume correlates very well with catheterized volume. Studies have shown that the scan volumes underestimate catheterized volumes by an average of 17 to 20 ml.

Transabdominal ultrasound and, more recently, transvaginal, transperineal, and transrectal approaches have been used to detect anatomic alterations associated with urge and stress incontinence, to select appropriate surgical procedures, and to assess postoperative surgical results and failures. Because this information can be obtained more accurately from clinical examination and urodynamic testing, the definitive value of these sonographic findings remains unproven.

In addition to delineating the anatomy of the lower urinary tract, vaginal ultrasound can be used to measure bladder volume and diagnose suburethral diverticula. Haylen (1989) showed that transvaginal ultrasound can measure bladder volume with a mean accuracy rate of 24%

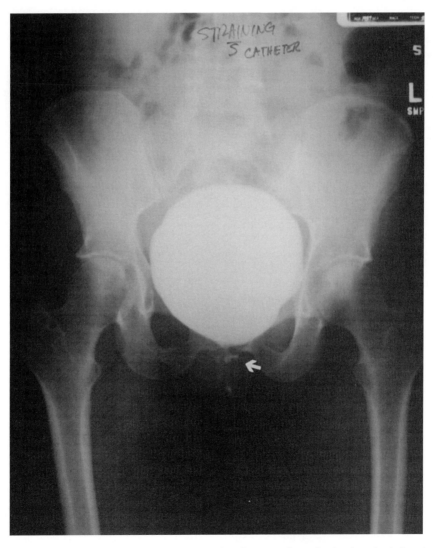

**Fig. 11-4**  Voiding cystourethrogram demonstrating three small proximal suburethral diverticula.

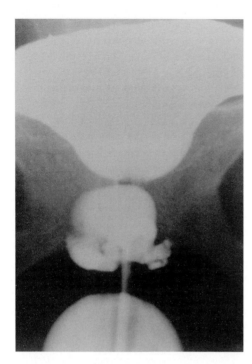

**Fig. 11-5** Positive-pressure urethrogram showing a large, multiloculated suburethral diverticulum.

and an optimum range of 50 to 200 ml. Using the largest transverse and vertical diameters, the bladder volume can be accurately calculated using the formula: Bladder volume (ml) = $5.9 \times H \times D - 14.6$. Vaginal and perineal ultrasound is a useful imaging modality for diagnosing suburethral diverticula. Because the probe can be placed in close proximity to the urethra, vaginal and perineal ultrasound can clearly visualize the position of the ostium and diverticula, its relationship to the urethra and the external sphincter, and diverticular stone.

## Doppler Sonography

One of the limitations of traditional ultrasound is that it does not provide physiologic information about the structures imaged. The use of Doppler sonography has added an element of physiologic investigation to an otherwise anatomic examination. One of the applications of Doppler ultrasound is to diagnose ureteral obstruction. In acute ureteral obstruction, increased collecting system pressure leads to a decrease in renal diastolic pressure and an elevated resistive index. Initial clinical and laboratory studies showed that Doppler ultrasound can detect these changes even before the onset of pelvicaliceal dilation. However, Deyoe et al. (1995) showed that Doppler ultrasound had an 87.5% accuracy in diagnosing acute ureteral obstruction, compared with IVP, and was more tedious and required greater operator experience. This dichotomy of study outcomes and associated technical problems has tempered the high expectations for Doppler ultrasound as a noninvasive modality for diagnosing

ureteral obstruction. Despite these shortcomings, resistive index may be used as an adjunct to traditional ultrasound for diagnosing ureteral obstruction in patients with contraindications to contrast media or radiation and for differentiating obstructive from nonobstructive pyelocaliectasis.

An alternative approach to detect possible ureteral occlusion with Doppler ultrasound is to demonstrate the presence or absence of urine entering the bladder (i.e., ureteric jet phenomenon). Investigators have shown that transvaginal color Doppler can easily detect the echoes created in the ureterovesical junction when a stream of higher-density urine is expelled from the ureteral orifice into the more dilute urine of the bladder. Although ureteric jets are usually absent in complete obstruction, patients with partial occlusion may have a continuous low-level jet pattern that is asymmetric to the contralateral ureter. The only disadvantage of this imaging technique is that asymmetric moment-to-moment fluctuations in jet frequency may result in a prolonged or a falsely positive study. Color Doppler can also be used to locate the channel between the urethra and a diverticulum.

## Endoluminal Sonography

More recently, endoluminal sonography using an ultrasound transducer contained within a small-diameter catheter has been used to evaluate a variety of lumina, including the urethra, ureter, and renal pelvis. The catheter can be passed into the upper urinary tract via a retrograde or antegrade approach. The single-crystal ultrasound transducers within the catheter can produce a cross-sectional image with a radius of approximately 1.5 to 2 cm. These images can then be reconstructed by computer into three-dimensional images. Endoluminal sonography has been used to image stones, neoplasms, strictures, obstruction, and normal anatomic variations of the upper urinary tract.

## VIDEOCYSTOURETHROGRAPHY

Videocystourethrography combines a fluoroscopic voiding cystourethrogram with simultaneous recording of intravesical, intraurethral, and intraabdominal pressures and urine flow rate (see Chapter 6). This technique allows visual assessment of urethral sphincters and bladder function while synchronously recording urodynamic data provided by a double-channel cystometric examination. It is generally considered the gold standard of urodynamic investigation. Common indications include complex cases with equivocal results after routine cystometric studies, failed incontinence surgery, voiding disorders, and neurologic disease. Both Bates et al. (1970) and Stanton et al. (1988) reviewed over 400 videocystourethrograms. Their data showed that this study can conclusively differentiate cough-induced stress incontinence from cough-induced urge incontinence. In addition, it can also diagnose suburethral diverticula and vesicoureteral reflux. One of the main technical difficulties associated with this examination is that approximately 15% of the women cannot void in the standing position, as required by videocystourethrography. Other disadvantages include the radiation exposure and high cost of the test.

Recently, Schaer et al. (1998) used remote control perineal ultrasound with simultaneous urodynamic recordings to evaluate the bladder and the urethra. The examination was performed with the patient in a sitting position. They were able to visualize the bladder neck, the bladder base, and the upper two-thirds of the urethra in all the women. This innovative technique was as informative as videocystourethrography while avoiding radiation exposure and the evaluation of lower urinary tract function in a nonphysiologic position.

## COMPUTED TOMOGRAPHY

The presence and the cause of ureteral obstruction can often be diagnosed by various combinations of IVP, sonography, retrograde pyelography, and antegrade pyelography. However, when these techniques are unable to identify the cause of obstruction, CT can be used to determine the underlying cause. This imaging modality allows direct cross-sectional visualization of the entire urinary tract. With the availability of the modern helical CT scanner, rapid sequence imaging can be performed with excellent time resolution. The urinary tract can be imaged in several planes and the recorded images reconstructed in three dimensions for review. Helical CT provides superior anatomic detail of the upper and lower urinary tract as well as of structures both immediately adjacent to and remote from the ureter.

Recently, Smith and other investigators (1995, 1996, 1998) used non-contrast-enhanced helical CT to evaluate acute flank pain of uncertain cause. They showed that this imaging technique takes about 5 minutes to perform and can accurately characterize intraluminal and extrinsic causes of ureteral obstruction as well as nonrenal causes of acute flank pain.

Urolithiasis is one of the most common causes of acute flank pain and ureteral obstruction. Approximately 90% of renal and ureteral stones contain calcium and are radiopaque. However, it is often difficult to differentiate on plain radiograph whether a calcific density in the pelvis is a stone within the ureter or a phlebolith because both can have a similar location and appearance when the ureter is not visualized. Up to 10% of the renal and ureteral stones are composed of uric acid or xanthine. These stones are radiolucent on abdominal radiographs and appear as nonspecific filling defects on IVP. Non-contrast-enhanced helical CT can determine precisely the location and size of the stone regardless of its composition. Even when the stone is not visualized directly, the presence of both unilateral

ureteral dilatation and perinephric stranding on CT have a high positive predictive value (96%) for diagnosing stone disease. Likewise, the absence of these two secondary CT signs of ureteral obstruction has a high negative predictive value (93%) for excluding stone disease.

## MAGNETIC RESONANCE IMAGING

MRI has evolved into an important diagnostic tool for the evaluation of urogenital abnormalities. Because of its superb soft-tissue contrast, direct multiplanar imaging capability, and high sensitivity in fluid detection, MRI is an ideal technique for evaluating abnormalities not readily imaged with other modalities. It is noninvasive, does not require iodinated contrast media, and does not expose the patient to ionizing radiation.

Fast gradient echo MRI has been used for the dynamic evaluation of pelvic floor anatomy in women with urogenital prolapse and stress urinary incontinence. Images obtained with patients at rest and during Valsalva maneuver can display urethral hypermobility, cystocele, rectocele, enterocele, and vaginal vault prolapse. Unfortunately, it tends to overdiagnose pelvic organ prolapse. MRI can also demonstrate urethral sphincter and levator ani deficiency in women with stress urinary incontinence and genital prolapse. Because this information can also be obtained from clinical examination and multichannel cystometry, the role of this rather expensive imaging modality in the diagnosis and management of incontinence and prolapse remains investigative.

MRI is very accurate in detecting ureterohydronephrosis. The half Fourier acquisition single-shot turbo spin echo (HASTE) technique can determine precisely the level and the degree of obstruction. However, the intrarenal collecting system and the ureters must have sufficient dilation to be completely visualized. The main disadvantage of MRI is its frequent inability to determine the cause of obstruction. Stones, blood clots, and acute hemorrhage may all appear as a filling defect. In addition, MRI may not have sufficient resolution to identify small ureteral calculi in a nondistended collecting system. At present, the use of MRI in evaluating upper urinary tract obstruction should be reserved for patients with contraindications to use of iodinated contrast media or ionizing radiation.

Because of its ability to delineate clearly the urethra and periurethral anatomy without the need for micturition, MRI is ideal for evaluating the presence, location, and complications of suburethral diverticula. In addition, it can demonstrate the relationship between the bladder neck and urethral diverticulum preoperatively in order to help avoid injuring the urethral continence mechanism during surgical resection. Although MRI has limitations for visualizing the ostium, it is still superior to other diagnostic techniques for detecting and characterizing diverticular disease. The only disadvantage is its high cost.

# CONCLUSION

A variety of radiologic studies are available to diagnose urogynecologic and urologic disorders. Clinicians should be aware of the sensitivity, specificity, cost, and limitations of each test in order to select the radiologic study that can accurately diagnose the condition with minimal risk to the patient and at a reasonable cost.

## BIBLIOGRAPHY
### Radiographic Studies

Bates CP, Whiteside CG, Turner-Warwick R: Synchronous cine/pressure/flow/cystourethrography with special reference to stress and urge incontinence, *Br J Urol* 42:714, 1970.

Beverly CM, Walters M, Weber AM, et al: Prevalence of hydronephrosis in patients undergoing surgery for pelvic organ prolapse, *Obstet Gynecol* 90:37, 1997.

Brettauer J, Rubin IC: Hydroureter and hydronephrosis: a frequent secondary finding in cases of prolapse of the uterus and bladder, *Am J Obstet Gynecol* 6:696, 1923.

Churchill DN, Afridi S, Dow D, et al: Uterine prolapse and renal dysfunction, *J Urol* 124:899, 1980.

Davis JH, Cian LG: Positive pressure urethrography: a new diagnostic method, *J Urol* 75:753, 1956.

Dawson P: Intravenous urography revisited, *Br J Urol* 66:561, 1990.

Downing J, Mannion R, Sanchez J: Voiding cystourethrography under anesthesia, *J Urol* 103:357, 1970.

Drutz HP, Shapiro BJ, Mandel F: Do static cystourethrograms have a role in the investigation of female incontinence? *Am J Obstet Gynecol* 130:516, 1978.

Elkin M, Goldman SM, Meng CH: Ureteral obstruction in patients with uterine prolapse, *Radiology* 110:289, 1974.

Goldfarb S, Mieza M, Leiter E: Postvoid film of intravenous pyelogram in diagnosis of ureteral diverticulum, *Urology* 17:390, 1981.

Greenberg M, Stone D, Cochran ST, et al: Female urethral diverticula: double-balloon catheter study, *AJR* 136:259, 1981.

Hadar H, Meiraz D: Total uterine prolapse causing hydroureteronephrosis, *Surg Gynecol Obstet* 150:711, 1980.

Hodgkinson CP: Relationships of the female urethra and bladder in urinary stress incontinence, *Am J Obstet Gynecol* 65:560, 1953.

Hutch JA, Shopfner CE: The lateral cystogram as an aid to urologic diagnosis, *J Urol* 99:292, 1968.

Jones JB, Evison G: Excretion urography before and after surgical treatment of procidentia, *Br J Obstet Gynaecol* 84:304, 1977.

Lang EK, Davis HJ: Positive pressure urethrography: a roentgenographic diagnostic method for urethral diverticula in the female, *Radiology* 72:401, 1959.

Osboren ED, Sutherland CG, Scholl AJ, et al: Roentgenography of urinary tract during excretion of sodium iodide, *JAMA* 80:368, 1923.

Piscitelli JT, Simel DL, Addison WA: Who should have intravenous pyelograms before hysterectomy for benign disease? *Obstet Gynecol* 69:541, 1987.

Sack RA: The value of intravenous urography prior to abdominal hysterectomy for gynecologic disease, *Am J Obstet Gynecol* 134:208, 1979.

Shopfner CE: Cystourethrography: an evaluation of method, *Am J Obstet Gynecol* 95:468, 1965.

Shopfner CE: Clinical evaluation of cystourethrographic contrast media, *Radiology* 88:491, 1967.

Shopfner CE, Hutch JA: The normal urethrogram, *Radiol Clin North Am* 6:165, 1968.

Simel DL, Matchar DB, Piscitelli JT: Routine intravenous pyelograms before hysterectomy in cases of benign disease: possibly effective, definitely expensive, *Am J Obstet Gynecol* 159:1049, 1988.

Smith RC, Rosenfield AT, Choe KA, et al: Acute flank pain: comparison of non-contrast-enhanced CT and intravenous urography, *Radiology* 194:789, 1995.

Stanton SL, Krieger M, Ziv E, et al: Videocystourethrography: its role in assessment of incontinence in the female, *Neurourol Urodyn* 7:712, 1988.

Tanagho EA: Simplified cystography in stress urinary incontinence, *Br J Urol* 46:295, 1974.

Van Nagel JR, Roddick JW: Vaginal hysterectomy, the ureter and excretory urography, *Obstet Gynecol* 39:784, 1972.

### Ultrasound

Asrat T, Roossin MC, Miller EI: Ultrasonographic detection of ureteral jets in normal pregnancy, *Am J Obstet Gynecol* 178:1194, 1998.

Bagley DH, Liu JB: Endoureteral sonography to define the anatomy of the obstructed ureteropelvic junction, *Urol Clin North Am* 25:271, 1998.

Benson JT, Sumners JE: Ultrasound evaluation of female urinary incontinence, *Int Urogynecol J* 1:7, 1990.

Bent AE, Nahhas DE, McLennan MT: Portable ultrasound determination of urinary residual volume, *Int Urogynecol J* 8:200, 1997.

Bhatia NN, Ostergard DR: Use of ultrasound in management of stress incontinence, *Clin Diagn Ultrasound* 15:73, 1984.

Bhatia NN, Ostergard DR, McQuown D: Ultrasonography in urinary incontinence, *Urology* 29:90, 1987.

Burge HJ, Middleton WD, McClennan MT, et al: Ureteral jets in healthy subjects and in patients with unilateral ureteral calculi: comparison with color Doppler US, *Radiology* 180:437, 1991.

Cox IH, Erickson SJ, Foley WD, et al: Ureteric jets: evaluation of normal flow dynamics with color Doppler sonography, *AJR* 158:1051, 1992.

Creighton SM, Pearce JM, Stanton SL: Perineal video-ultrasonography in the assessment of vaginal prolapse: early observations, *Br J Obstet Gynaecol* 99:310, 1992.

Debaere C, Rigauts H, Steyaert L, et al: MR imaging of a diverticulum in a female urethra, *J Belge Radiol* 78:345, 1995.

Deyoe LA, Cronan JJ, Breslaw BH, et al: New techniques of ultrasound and color Doppler in the prospective evaluation of acute renal obstruction. Do they replace the intravenous urogram? *Abdom Imaging* 20:58, 1995.

Dubbins PA, Kurtz AB, Darby J, et al: Ureteric jet effect: the echographic appearance of urine entering the bladder, *Radiology* 140:513, 1981.

Goldberg BB, Bagley D, Liu JB, et al: Endoluminal sonography of the urinary tract: preliminary observations, *AJR* 156:99, 1991.

Griffiths CJ, Murray A, Ramsden PD: Accuracy and repeatability of bladder volume measurement using ultrasonic imaging, *J Urol* 136:808, 1986.

Haylen BT: Verification of the accuracy and range of transvaginal ultrasound in measuring bladder volumes in women, *Br J Urol* 64:350, 1989.

Ireton RC, Krieger JN, Cardenas DD, et al: Bladder volume determination using a dedicated, portable ultrasound scanner, *J Urol* 143:909, 1990.

Koelbl H, Hanzal E, Bernaschek G: Sonographic urethrocystography: methods and application in patients with genuine stress incontinence, *Int Urogynecol J* 2:25, 1991.

Lee TG, Keller FS: Urethral diverticulum: diagnosis by ultrasound, *AJR* 128:690, 1997.

Mainprize TC, Drutz MP: Accuracy of total bladder volume and residual measurements: comparison between real-time ultrasonography and catheterization, *Am J Obstet Gynecol* 160:1013, 1989.

Marks LS, Dorey FJ, Macairan ML, et al: Three-dimensional ultrasound device for rapid determination of bladder volume, *Urology* 50:341, 1997.

Martensson O, Duchek M: Translabial ultrasonography with pulsed colour-Doppler in the diagnosis of female urethral diverticula, *Scand J Urol Nephrol* 28:101, 1994.

Orgaz RE, Gomez AZ, Ramirez CT, et al: Applications of bladder ultrasonography. I. Bladder content and residue, *J Urol* 125:174, 1981.

Ostrzenski A, Osborne NG, Ostrzenska K: Method for diagnosing paravaginal defects using contrast ultrasonographic technique, *J Ultrasound Med* 16:673, 1997.

Platt JF: Duplex doppler evaluation of acute renal obstruction, *Semin Ultrasound CT MRI* 18:147, 1997.

Platt JF: Advances in ultrasonography of urinary tract obstruction, *Abdom Imaging* 23:3, 1998.

Poston GJ, Joseph AE, Riddle PR: The accuracy of ultrasound in the measurement of changes in bladder volume, *Br J Urol* 55:361, 1983.

Quinn MJ, Beynon J, Mortensen NN, et al: Vaginal endosonography in the postoperative assessment of colposuspension, *Br J Urol* 63:295, 1989.

Reuter KL, Young SB, Colby J: Transperineal sonography in the assessment of a urethral diverticulum, *J Clin Ultrasound* 20:221, 1992.

Richmond DH, Sutherst JR: Burch colposuspension or sling for stress incontinence? A prospective study using transrectal ultrasound, *Br J Urol* 64:600, 1989.

Schaer GN, Siegwart R, Perucchini D, et al: Examination of voiding in seated women using a remote-controlled ultrasound probe, *Obstet Gynecol* 91:297, 1998.

Siegel CL, Middleton WD, Teeley SA, et al: Sonography of the female urethra, *AJR* 170:1269, 1998.

Tal Z, Jaffe H, Rosenak D, et al: Ureteric jet examination by color Doppler ultrasound versus IVP for the assessment of ureteric patency following pelvic surgery, *Eur J Obstet Gynecol Reprod Biol* 54:119, 1994.

Timor-Tritsch IE, Haratz-Rubinstein N, Monteagudo A, et al: Transvaginal color Doppler sonography of the ureteral jets: a method to detect ureteral patency, *Obstet Gynecol* 89:113, 1997.

Townsend RR, Meacham RB, Drose JA: Color doppler evaluation of urethral diverticulum, *J Ultrasound Med* 13:309, 1994.

Tublin ME, Dodd GD, Verdile VP: Acute renal colic: diagnosis with duplex Doppler US, *Radiology* 193:697, 1994.

## Computed Tomography

Fielding JR, Steele G, Fox LA, et al: Spiral computerized tomography in the evaluation of acute flank pain: a replacement for excretory urography, *J Urol* 157:2071, 1997.

Neitlich JD, Foster HE, Glickman MG, et al: Detection of urethral diverticula in women: comparison of a high-resolution fast spin echo technique with double balloon urethrography, *J Urol* 159:408, 1998.

Siegel CL, McDougall EM, Middleton WD, et al: Preoperative assessment of ureteropelvic junction obstruction with endoluminal sonography and helical CT, *AJR* 168:623, 1997.

Singal RK, Lee TY, Razvi HA, et al: Evaluation of Doppler ultrasonography and dynamic contrast-enhanced CT in acute and chronic renal obstruction, *J Endourol* 11:5, 1997.

Smith RC, Dalrymple NC, Neitlich J: Noncontrast helical CT in the evaluation of acute flank pain, *Abdom Imaging* 23:10, 1998.

Smith RC, Rosenfield AT, Choe KA, et al: Acute flank pain: comparison of non-contrast-enhanced CT and intravenous urography, *Radiology* 194:789, 1995.

Smith RC, Verga M, Dalrymple N, et al: Acute ureteral obstruction: value of secondary signs on helical unenhanced CT, *AJR* 167:1109, 1996.

## Magnetic Resonance Imaging

Butler H, Bryan PJ, LiPuma JP, et al: Magnetic resonance imaging of the abnormal female pelvis, *AJR* 143:1259, 1984.

Khati NJ, Javitt MC, Schwartz AM, et al: MR imaging diagnosis of a urethral diverticulum, *Radiographics* 18:517, 1998.

Kim B, Hricak H, Tanagho E: Diagnosis of urethral diverticula in women: value of MR imaging, *AJR* 161:809, 1993.

Klutke C, Golomb J, Barbaric Z, et al: The anatomy of stress incontinence: magnetic resonance imaging of the female bladder neck and urethra, *J Urol* 143:563, 1990.

Li W, Chavez D, Edelman RR, et al: Magnetic resonance urography by breath-hold contrast-enhanced three-dimensional FISP, *J Magn Reson Imaging* 7:309, 1997.

Mostafavi MR, Saltzman B, Prasad PV: Magnetic resonance imaging in the evaluation of ureteropelvic junction obstructed kidney, *Urology* 50:601, 1997.

Ozasa H, Mori T, Togashi K: Study of uterine prolapse by magnetic resonance imaging: topographical changes involving the levator ani muscle and the vagina, *Gynecol Obstet Invest* 34:43, 1992.

Regan F, Bohlman ME, Khazan R, et al: MR urography using HASTE imaging in the assessment of ureteric obstruction, *AJR* 167:1115, 1996.

Regan F, Petronis J, Bohlman M, et al: Perirenal MR high signal: a new and sensitive indicator of acute ureteric obstruction, *Clin Radiol* 52:445, 1997.

Reuther G, Kiefer B, Wandl E: Visualization of urinary tract dilatation: value of single-shot MR urography, *Eur Radiol* 7:1276, 1997.

Roy C, Saussine C, Guth S, et al: MR urography in the evaluation of urinary tract obstruction, *Abdom Imaging* 23:27, 1998.

Siegelman ES, Banner MP, Ramchandani P, et al: Multicoil MR imaging of symptomatic female urethral and periurethral disease, *Radiographics* 17:349, 1997.

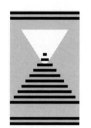

PART III
*Management of Genuine Stress Incontinence and Pelvic Organ Prolapse*

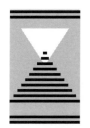

CHAPTER **12**

# Pathophysiology and Obstetric Issues of Genuine Stress Incontinence and Pelvic Floor Dysfunction

Mark D. Walters and Edward R. Newton

---

The female continence mechanism and factors contributing to its failure are not completely understood. Past theories of the mechanisms of stress urinary incontinence tended to focus on single factors to explain bladder neck and urethral incompetence. The last decade has seen remarkable advances in our knowledge of the histology, biochemistry, and neurophysiology that control bladder neck and urethral support and function. We now believe that multiple physiologic factors make up the female continence mechanism. Defects in any of these factors can contribute to the presence and severity of stress incontinence in women.

This chapter reviews the anatomic and physiologic mechanisms of urinary continence and the pathophysiology of stress incontinence in women. The issues of urethral support defects and pelvic floor denervation are summarized to develop the current model of the mechanisms of urethral sphincteric incompetence. Finally, we discuss extensively obstetric factors as they affect pelvic floor, anal, and urethral function.

## MECHANISMS OF URINARY CONTINENCE

The two functions of the lower urinary tract are the storage of urine in the bladder and the timely expulsion of urine from the urethra. The mechanisms that control urinary continence and voiding are complex. Normal function of the central and peripheral nervous systems, bladder wall, detrusor muscle, urethra, and pelvic floor musculature is required. Dysfunction can occur at any of these levels, resulting in various types of lower urinary tract dysfunction.

### Bladder

During physiologic bladder filling, little or no increase in intravesical pressure is observed, despite large increases in urine volume. This process, called accommodation, is caused primarily by passive elastic and viscoelastic properties of the smooth muscle and connective tissue of the bladder wall. As filling increases to a critical intravesical pressure, detrusor muscle contractility is probably inhibited by activation of a spinal sympathetic reflex, which results in inhibition of parasympathetic ganglionic transmission and stimulation of beta-adrenergic receptors in the bladder body. The net effect of these actions is filling and storage of urine within the bladder cavity, with little increase in intravesical pressure relative to volume. Abnormalities in the bladder wall, the detrusor muscle, or bladder innervation can result in incontinence (primarily detrusor instability or hyperreflexia) or voiding dysfunction.

### Urethra
#### *Resting Intraurethral Pressure*

For a patient to remain continent, intraurethral pressure must be greater than intravesical pressure under both resting and stress conditions. At rest urethral resistance is generated by the interaction of urethral smooth muscle, urethral wall elasticity and vascularity, and periurethral striated muscle. Each of these components contributes about one third of overall intraurethral pressure. The smooth muscle and vascular elastic tissue provide a constant amount of tension along the urethra; the periurethral striated urogenital sphincter muscles function prominently in the distal one half of the urethra. Multiple clinical factors, such as age and obstetric history, can affect the function of these urethral components (Fig. 12-1).

### *Urethral Support*

On the basis of extensive work of Jeffcoate and Roberts (1952), Hodgkinson (1953), and others, it appears that intact support of the bladder neck and proximal urethra in a retropubic position is important for maintenance of urinary

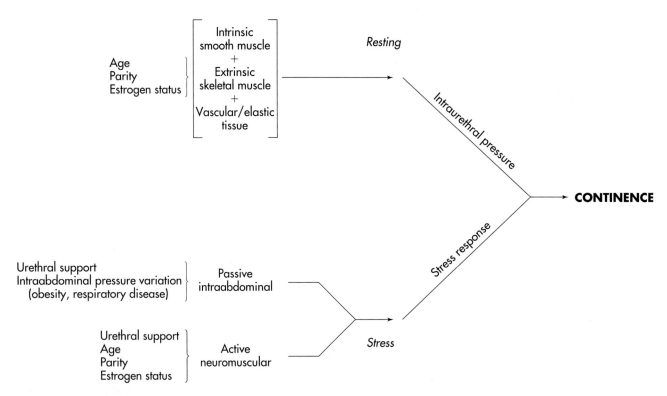

**Fig. 12-1** Factors contributing to the female continence mechanism under resting and stress conditions.

continence under stress. The proximal urethra and bladder neck are supported in a slinglike fashion by the anterior vaginal wall, which is attached bilaterally to the pelvic diaphragm. The vagina thus provides a stable base onto which the urethra and bladder neck rest. With increases in intraabdominal pressure, as with coughing, pressure increases are transmitted equally to the bladder and urethra, maintaining urethral closure and thus continence (Fig. 12-2, *A*). This occurs, at least in part, because the stable suburethral layer of vaginal wall and endopelvic fascia prevents urethral and bladder neck descent and causes urethral compression with straining (Fig. 12-3). According to DeLancey (1994), the underlying stability of the suburethral layer is more important for effective urethral closure than is the position of the urethra relative to the pelvis. In addition, intact bladder neck and urethral support may allow for an efficient reflex pelvic muscle contraction with stress.

### Urethral Innervation

Intact innervation of the urethra and periurethral muscles is important in maintaining continence. With bladder filling, outlet resistance is increased by reflex stimulation of alpha-adrenergic receptors within the smooth muscle of the bladder neck and urethra. Voluntary and reflex stimulation of the muscles of the pelvic diaphragm and the striated urogenital sphincter also occurs, resulting from increased efferent pudendal nerve activity.

### Periurethral Musculature

The levator ani and periurethral striated muscles have a dual role in maintaining urinary continence: they provide resting urethral tone and assist in support (slow-twitch fibers), and they contract rapidly with increased intraabdominal pressure (fast-twitch fibers). The contributions to urethral resistance at rest were already discussed.

Rapid voluntary and reflex periurethral striated muscle contraction, predominantly in the mid- and distal urethra, augments urethral pressure during rapid increases in intraabdominal pressure and interruption of urination. Using cinefluorography, Lund et al. (1959) observed two actions when a woman is asked to interrupt her urine stream. The first is a prompt constriction of the voluntary musculature, which immediately interrupts the urine stream in the mid-urethra. The urine distal to the constriction is voided but the contents of the proximal urethra are forced back into the bladder. Simultaneously, the base of the bladder is seen to rise and is drawn cephalad. Both of these actions are quick and decisive and are characteristic of voluntary fast-twitch muscle contraction. Rapid intraabdominal pressure rises reflexedly induce these same actions. Continence occurs primarily at the level of the bladder base; the mid-urethral periurethral muscles act as a backup mechanism by stopping and "milking back" urine that has entered the proximal urethra.

This concept was supported by Constantinou and Govan (1982), who showed that urethral pressure spikes precede,

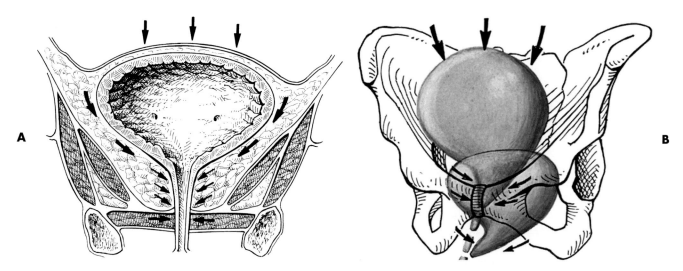

**Fig. 12-2**   Pressure transmission concept for stress continence and incontinence. **A,** In continent women, rises in intraabdominal pressure are transmitted equally to the bladder and urethra. **B,** In women with anterior vaginal support defects, the bladder base descends and the urethra rotates during increases in intraabdominal pressure. This can lead to decreased pressure transmission to the urethra relative to the bladder, which then results in stress urinary incontinence.

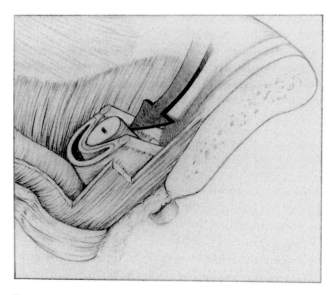

**Fig. 12-3**   Hammock hypothesis for stress continence. Lateral view of pelvic floor with urethra, vagina, and fascial tissues at level of bladder neck indicating compression of urethra by downward force *(arrow)* against supportive tissues, indicating influence of abdominal pressure on urethra.

From DeLancey JOL: *Am J Obstet Gynecol* 170:1718, 1994.

and are often greater than, intravesical pressure spikes during coughing in continent women. The area of greatest pressure increase was in the distal half of the urethra. Heidler et al. (1987) noted that pressure increases in the distal urethra with sneezing in dogs decrease after transecting the pelvic muscles from the urethra. Koelbl et al. (1989)

showed that the diameter of fast-twitch levator ani muscles on biopsy correlated significantly with urethral closure pressure with stress.

### Urethral Coaptation

The urethra is a pliable structure whose lumen must be completely sealed or coapted to maintain continence. The urethral wall must be sufficiently soft so that external forces can act on it to effect closure. Several studies by Zinner et al. (1980, 1983) using mechanical models showed higher resistance to water flow when a softer lumen and a lubricating filler were used within the outflow tube. This finding makes clinical sense because a rigid urethra, as results from multiple surgeries or mucosal atrophy, has poor closure properties. Because clinical scientific studies rarely address this issue, however, the actual importance of urethral softness and mucosal seal as they pertain to continence remains uncertain.

## PATHOPHYSIOLOGY OF GENUINE STRESS INCONTINENCE
### Genuine Stress Incontinence With Urethral Hypermobility

Genuine stress incontinence results when the bladder neck and urethra fail to maintain a watertight seal at rest and under conditions of increased intraabdominal pressure. By definition, the central nervous system and bladder wall function normally in this condition. Failure of urethral closure results when any of the factors that maintain continence become abnormal.

Adequate resting intraurethral resistance appears to be important for continence. Urethral pressure can be viewed as a threshold level, below which urine loss occurs in women with incomplete transmission of pressure to the urethra with stress. Compared to continent controls, mean resting urethral pressures are lower and vascular pulsations generally absent in women with genuine stress incontinence. In addition, maximum urethral pressure tends to be lower with increasing severity of incontinence.

Descent and mobility of the proximal urethra and bladder base with stress are generally regarded as an important etiologic component of urethral sphincter incompetence. The basic anatomic defect appears to be the loss of integrity of the vaginal musculofascial attachments that support the bladder neck and urethra in a retropubic position. Hypermobility and descent of these structures with increased intraabdominal pressure lead to impaired pressure transmission to the urethra (see Fig. 12-2, *B*), ineffective compression caused by an unstable suburethral layer (Fig. 12-4), and possibly an inefficient periurethral skeletal muscle response.

Damage to the nerves that control the pelvic floor and periurethral muscles probably contributes to the genesis of genuine stress incontinence. Damage to the pudendal nerve, as may occur during childbirth, can cause weakness and atrophy of the medial portions of the levator ani muscles as well as the voluntary muscles of the perineum. This damage can predispose to vaginal support defects and to decreased fast-twitch reflex pelvic muscle contraction, a factor that is believed to aid in continence during stress. Obstetric issues, as they relate to pelvic muscle denervation, are discussed more thoroughly later in the chapter.

Simultaneous measurement of urethral, bladder, and abdominal pressures, as with multichannel urethrocysto-

metry, has provided a better understanding of the mechanisms of continence and stress incontinence. In a large, controlled study of urodynamic findings in women with genuine stress incontinence using microtransducer catheters to measure resting and stress urethral pressure profiles, Hilton and Stanton (1983) found that subjects with genuine stress incontinence had significantly lower total urethral length, maximum urethral pressure, and pressure transmission ratios along the urethra than did continent controls. The total urethral length and maximum pressure decreased progressively with increasing severity of incontinence. Deficient pressure transmission ratios were noted in incontinent subjects, but not in continent controls, and did not correlate with severity. These investigators concluded that the main pathophysiologic event causing genuine stress incontinence is deficient pressure transmission to the urethra. The severity of incontinence is determined by the degree of abnormalities in resting maximum urethral pressure, urethral and intraabdominal pressure variations, and urethral response to sustained stress. Because no attempt was made to correlate pressure transmission ratios with measures of urethral mobility, it is unknown whether deficient pressure transmission results from urethral hypermobility, abnormal reflex urethral muscle contraction, or other undefined factors.

The amplitude of rapid increases in intraabdominal pressure can influence the severity of stress incontinence. This relationship makes clinical sense because many women who are not incontinent normally still leak small amounts of urine with a full bladder during episodes of strong coughing or with aerobic exercise. Large amplitude rises can be seen with obesity, acute and chronic pulmonary problems, exercise, and occupational factors.

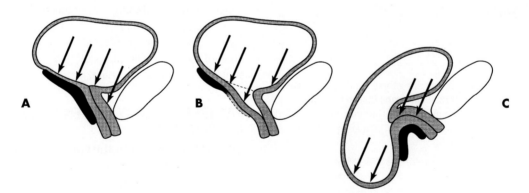

**Fig. 12-4** Hammock hypotheses for stress continence and incontinence. **A,** Abdominal pressure *(arrows)* forces urethra against stable supportive layer *(black)* and compresses urethra closed. **B,** Unstable supportive layer *(shaded)* is ineffective in providing resistant backstop against which urethra can be compressed. **C,** Despite low, extraabdominal position of urethra and presence of cystourethrocele, supportive layer is firm and provides adequate backstop against which urethra may be compressed closed.

From DeLancey JOL: *Am J Obstet Gynecol* 170:1719, 1994.

## Intrinsic Sphincter Deficiency

When the urethra no longer functions as a sphincter and cannot maintain a watertight seal even at rest, the condition is called *intrinsic sphincter deficiency* (ISD). The bladder neck and urethra can be hypermobile or fixed and nonmobile. The causes of ISD are not completely known but are probably related to neuromuscular changes and damage (as with aging and vaginal delivery) or trauma (as with prior bladder neck surgery). The muscles involved in urethral closure can be very lax, or the urethral wall can be rigid and scarred. Either mechanism can lead to failure of urethral coaptation and explains the radiologic finding of an open bladder neck at rest. Patients with ISD are often severely incontinent; leaking can occur with standing or with minimal exertion. Urodynamically, these patients tend to have lower maximal urethral closure and leak point pressures. Cases of "low-pressure urethra" and "lead-pipe urethra" fit into this category.

## OBSTETRIC DELIVERY AND PELVIC FLOOR DYSFUNCTION

For years, circumstantial evidence has supported a relationship between obstetric trauma and urinary and fecal stress incontinence. The evidence includes higher rates of incontinence among parous women than among nulliparous women and an association between anatomic pelvic floor abnormalities and incontinence. Unfortunately, obstetricians have introduced many interventions to prevent birth-related stress incontinence with neither an adequate evaluation of their efficacy nor an understanding of the pathologic mechanisms of incontinence. Examples of obstetric interventions include episiotomy, forceps operations, perineal massage, alternative birth positions, epidural anesthesia, and cesarean delivery.

A complete understanding of the problem requires review of the mechanism of birth, the onset of stress incontinence, the injuries associated with childbirth, and the efficacy of interventions designed to prevent perineal trauma.

## Vaginal Delivery and Pelvic Floor Damage

In a classic review, Power (1946) described the mechanism by which the fetus negotiates the birth canal and is expelled through the pelvic diaphragm. In brief, as the flexed occiput anterior fetal head strikes the pelvic floor, the levator ani muscle segments are funneled from behind forward. The ischiococcygeus muscle is the first to receive the impact, but the head is often preceded by a dilating wedge of amniotic fluid and membranes that transfers most of the pressure onto the front of the pubococcygeus muscle. The anococcygeal raphe is pushed down until it becomes vertical. The ischiococcygeus assumes a vertical plane and acts as a deflecting surface for the descending head, which is deflected downward and forward onto the iliococcygeus.

After the resistance of the ischiococcygeus is overcome,

the head is shunted onto the pubococcygeus segment, which is stretched anteroposteriorly and peripherally. The perineal membrane is pulled upward as it is attached to the peripherally dilating vagina. The perineal body is pushed downward as the head is propelled along the axis of the pelvic outlet. The deep transverse perineus muscle is flattened peripherally and stretched vertically. The rectovaginal septal fibers are stretched peripherally and longitudinally and often torn. As the sphincter group of muscles—the bulbocavernosus, ischiocavernosus, transverse perinei and periurethral muscles—are dilated, they are converted into a short muscular tube along the axis of the pelvic outlet.

As the biparietal diameter of the fetal head reaches the transverse diameter of the pelvic outlet, the uterovaginal canal is converted into one continuous hiatus. The lateral ligaments of the cervix uteri (endopelvic fascia) are flattened peripherally and stretched vertically. The vagina is dilated spherically and the pelvic diaphragm is changed from an oblique to a vertical plane. At this point—"crowning"—episiotomy and outlet forceps are often used to "prevent" pelvic injury; this moment is well after maximum stretching and possible injury have occurred to the levator ani muscles and endopelvic fascia supporting the uterus and vagina.

This sequence describes the process in an occiput anterior position. The shape of the pelvis, preexisting pelvic muscle mass and strength, strength of fascial supports, fetal presentation, position, and size all contribute to different strains, stresses, and locations of particular injuries to the pelvic floor and perineum. Childbirth injuries may involve disruption of anatomic relationships and subsequent loss of mechanical advantage, denervation of the pelvic floor muscles through injury to the pudendal nerve or its branches, or a combination of the two.

In a classic paper, Delee (1920) described the anatomic injuries as they occur. The fetal head advancing through the hiatus genitalis rips the vagina off its fascial anchorings, sliding it downward and outward. Likewise, the rectum is torn from its attachment to the levator ani muscles and fascia. The head tears or overstretches the levator muscles, causing their diastasis. Anteriorly, the fascia between the vagina and bladder is stretched in a radial and downward fashion. This motion may tear the vagina and bladder off their anchorage to the upper surface of the endopelvic fascia or the levator ani and posterior surface of the pubic symphysis.

Between 1945 and 1955, Gainey (1955) systematically evaluated 2000 patients for evidence of postpartum pelvic tissue damage. Table 12-1 describes the frequency of pelvic tissue damage. Episiotomy appeared to protect the patient from pelvic tissue damage; however, the data did not control for maternal and fetal size, socioeconomic status, fetal presentation, or maternal parity. A total of 92 (4.6%) patients complained of stress incontinence at postpartum evaluation. Examination of these patients with regard to pelvic tissue

**Table 12-1** Incidence of Postpartum Pelvic Injury

| | Percentage of patients | |
| | No episiotomy | Mediolateral |
| Pelvic finding | (*N* = 1000) | (*N* = 1000) |
|---|---|---|
| Detached urethra | 18 | 9 |
| Vaginal relaxation | 14 | 3 |
| Levator atrophy | 31 | 12 |
| Cystocele | 26 | 10 |
| Rectocele | 12 | 2 |
| Detached rectovaginal septum | 24 | <1 |
| Anal sphincter damage | <1 | <1 |
| Uterine descensus | 1 | 3 |

From Gainey HL: *Am J Obstet Gynecol* 70:800, 1955.

**Table 12-2** Predictors of Posterior Vaginal Trauma After Vaginal Delivery

| Risk factors | Adjusted odds ratios* |
|---|---|
| Midline episiotomy | 4.9-16.5 |
| Nulliparity | 2.5-4.0 |
| Operative delivery | 2.5-3.5 |
| Birthweight ≥4000 g | 1.5-2.5 |
| Occiput posterior | 1.2-1.8 |

*Numbers represent the minimum and maximum adjusted odds ratios reported in the medical literature.

damage shows a statistically significant association between stress incontinence and both levator atrophy and urethral detachment.

The descriptions by Powers, Delee, Gainey, and others relied on personal observation of the birth process, as measured through serial rectal examinations or radiographic pelvimetry, and a superior knowledge of pelvic anatomy obtained through autopsy study. Most obstetric labors that they observed were heavily medicated. Current labor management and patient demographics are quite different. Vaginal examinations and ultrasound provide different, more objective measurements of soft tissue anatomy. The current use of epidural anesthesia paralyzes the voluntary pelvic muscle groups, radically changing their ability to resist and direct the position of the fetal head. Patients are having fewer children and many more are avoiding perineal trauma altogether by cesarean birth. Thus, the classic descriptions must be confirmed using modern methodology and obstetric management.

## Vaginal Delivery and Perineal Damage

Recently, interest in perineal trauma has been renewed through retrospective multivariate analyses and prospective randomized trials. However, the evaluations and outcome variables usually relate to the severity of posterior perineal trauma (i.e., does the injury extend to or include the rectal sphincter or rectal mucosa?). The average incidence of third-degree (anal sphincter only) or fourth-degree (anal sphincter and rectal mucosa) lacerations in the literature is 6.5% (0.4% to 23.9%) in patients with midline episiotomy, 1.3% (0.5% to 2.0%) in patients with mediolateral episiotomy, and 1.4% (0% to 6.4%) in patients without episiotomy.

Posterior vaginal and perineal injury is an important cause of anal incontinence and rectovaginal fistula; however, its relationship with urinary incontinence is unclear. Most studies have neither defined clearly nor ascertained systematically the frequency of anterior vaginal or periurethral injury. Labial, periclitoral, and periurethral injury usually are classified together and were reported in only

two recent studies. The incidence was reported to be 12.7% and 21.9%.

Study of risk factors for perineal trauma has been limited to predictors of third- and fourth-degree lacerations. Table 12-2 describes the typical adjusted odds ratios for predictors of posterior vaginal trauma on multivariate analyses. Other risk factors for posterior trauma are reported in some studies and include Asian race, black race, second stage of labor greater than 90 minutes, physician (versus midwife) delivery, and lithotomy position.

The positive association between episiotomy and posterior trauma has been supported by large cohort and randomized, controlled trials. In a retrospective study of 4200 deliveries by Helwig et al. (1993), deliveries involving episiotomy were more than twice as likely to result in third- or fourth-degree perineal lacerations (relative risk 2.4). Harrison et al. (1984) randomized 181 primigravid women to routine mediolateral episiotomy or to restricted use of mediolateral episiotomy. The episiotomy group sustained rectal injury in 5 of 89 cases (5.6%), compared to no cases of rectal injury in the restricted group. Sleep et al. (1984) randomized 1000 women to liberal use of mediolateral episiotomy (51% of patients) or restricted mediolateral episiotomy (10% of patients). A liberal policy toward episiotomy resulted in significantly more maternal vaginal trauma and more suturing.

The association between operative delivery and perineal trauma has also been studied in a randomized fashion. Yancey et al. (1991) randomly assigned uncomplicated, term gestations at 2+ station in occiput-anterior position to routine outlet forceps or to spontaneous delivery. Among patients delivered by outlet forceps, the incidence of third- or fourth-degree laceration was 30 of 165 (18%) versus 12 of 168 (7%) in women who delivered spontaneously. Midline episiotomy and outlet forceps were the only factors significantly associated with rectal trauma on multivariate analysis.

Sleep and Grant (1987) performed a postal questionnaire of the 1000 patients who participated in the randomized clinical trial 3 years earlier. No apparent differences were noted between nonresponders and responders in 674 subjects. Among women with no more children (*n* = 401), 129

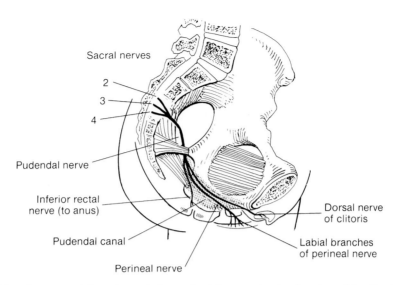

**Fig. 12-5** Course and branches of the pudendal nerve in the female pelvis. Shaded area represents section of nerve that is sometimes damaged with childbirth.

(32%) described stress incontinence, 51 (12.7%) had urge incontinence, and 53 (13.2%) had dyspareunia. Thirty-nine (9.7%) of the women had urinary incontinence severe enough to require a pad. These symptoms were reported with equal frequency in the episiotomy and no-episiotomy groups. These results were not correlated with the presence or absence of acute injuries in the original study. More important, they were not correlated with the presence or absence of levator injury or detached urethra at follow-up examination.

Anal sphincter rupture during vaginal delivery is an important predictor of anal incontinence. Sphincter disruption can be occult (without perineal laceration) or overt (after third- and fourth-degree lacerations) and can result in lower resting and squeeze anal pressures. Fecal incontinence is common in these women, although some studies note that it is equally common in women without sphincter disruption, suggesting that other factors, such as nerve damage and altered muscle function, may be important.

## Vaginal Delivery and Pudendal Nerve Damage

Primary obstetric injury is believed to occur to the innervation of the pelvic floor muscles, especially the pudendal nerve. Damage to the pudendal nerve is thought to occur distal to the ischial spine in the pudendal canal and to the perineal branches of the pudendal nerve (Fig. 12-5). Nerve damage may result from longitudinal stretching with perineal descent or from direct compression. This injury leads to abnormalities in neurologic control, resulting in pelvic muscle and striated urogenital sphincter atrophy. The denervation and muscle atrophy exacerbate the mechanical disadvantages that result from childbirth-related perineal stretching and subsequent repair.

Pudendal nerve terminal motor latency (PNTML) and single-fiber electromyography (EMG) of the external anal sphincter muscle have been used to test this theory. An increase in the terminal motor latency implies damage to or loss of a population of rapidly conducting, large myelinated motor fibers in the distal portion of the nerve or conduction block representing damage to these motor fibers between the point of stimulation and the muscle itself. Single-fiber EMG fiber density measurements can be used as a sensitive index of reinnervation (by collateral axial sprouting) after nerve damage has occurred.

Snooks et al. (1986) studied 122 pregnant women antepartum, 24 to 72 hours after delivery, and 2 months after delivery. Thirty-four nulliparous women were controls. Pudendal nerve terminal motor latency and fiber density in the external anal sphincter muscle were increased significantly at 48 to 72 hours postpartum and at 2 months postpartum, respectively. These changes were associated with multiparity, forceps delivery, increased duration of second stage of labor, anal sphincter tear, and high birthweight. Epidural anesthesia and cesarean delivery did not increase the likelihood of abnormal results. Although cesarean delivery is usually considered to be protective against pudendal nerve injury, Fynes et al. (1998) demonstrated that cesarean delivery performed in late labor, even in the absence of attempted vaginal delivery, sometimes results in changes consistent with neurologic injury to the anal sphincter mechanism.

Using single-fiber EMG, Anderson (1984) demonstrated higher motor unit fiber density of the external anal sphincter in women with genuine stress incontinence than in continent controls. The changes were independent of age, uterovaginal prolapse, or a history of surgery for incontinence. In a later study using similar methodology, Smith et al. (1989) showed that partial denervation of pelvic floor muscles with subsequent reinnervation is a normal accompaniment of aging and is increased by childbirth. Women with stress urinary incontinence, fecal incontinence, or pelvic organ prolapse have significantly greater denervation of the pelvic floor than do asymptomatic women. These studies suggest that peripheral denervation causes the periurethral, anal, and pelvic striated muscles to be mechanically less efficient. Abnormal function of these muscles could then result in lower resting urethral pressure, lower reflex striated muscle response with stress, descent of the bladder base and urethra with stress, and lower anal squeeze pressures.

In 1990, Snooks et al. reported a 5-year follow-up in 14 of 24 multiparous women who participated in the original study. All 14 women were delivered without the assistance of forceps. Five of 14 (38%) developed stress incontinence. Both fiber density and PNTML were increased in all five women who complained of stress incontinence.

Pudendal neuropathy may affect continence indirectly through a loss of muscle strength with neurogenic atrophy or directly by disruption of neurologic control mechanisms. Decreased pelvic muscle tone secondary to denervation can lead to absent or weak fast-twitch skeletal muscle contractions with stress. Widening of the levator hiatus also results, which probably contributes to the development of pelvic organ prolapse. Anal sphincter weakness can result in anal incontinence.

A decrease in pelvic muscle and anal sphincter strength after vaginal delivery is well documented using vaginal or anal pressure transducers or standardized digital measurement. Snooks et al. (1986) measured maximum anal pressure in 14 multiparous women during pregnancy, 24 to 72 hours after delivery, and 2 months and 5 years postpartum. Twenty nulliparous women were controls. At 5 years, maximum anal canal pressure (50 cm $H_2O$) remained depressed from antepartum values in the same women (74 cm $H_2O$) and from nulliparous controls (105 cm $H_2O$). These results were similar to values found at 24 to 72 hours and 2 months postpartum.

Sampselle et al. (1990) studied 20 nulliparous women at 32 to 36 weeks' gestation and at 6 weeks' postpartum. Measurements included digital muscle score, observed incontinence, and urine flow interruption time. Mean pelvic muscle strength scores were correlated inversely with observed standing stress incontinence and reported stress incontinence. Vaginal birth was associated with a highly significant loss in strength, whereas cesarean delivery was not. In another study, Gordon and Logue (1985) measured vaginal squeeze pressure with a pressure transducer. At 1 year post-delivery, neither perineal damage nor episiotomy influenced squeeze pressures, but when the data were stratified by no exercise, pelvic muscle exercises, and general exercise, highly significant improvement in pressure was noted in the exercise groups. This and other studies suggest that, when performed regularly and consistently, pelvic muscle exercises are effective in strengthening pelvic muscles.

The existence of an inherently weak urethral sphincter mechanism in women is apparent in epidemiologic studies of the onset of stress urinary incontinence. Five percent to 13% of young nulliparas suffer frequent stress incontinence. When pregnancy occurs, by 32 weeks' gestation, 30% to 53% of primiparas and 40% to 85% of multiparas experience occasional stress urinary incontinence. Postpartum, 6% to 11% of women have stress incontinence. Retrospectively, Beck and Hsu (1965) noted that 65% of their patients with stress incontinence first complained of incontinence when pregnant and 14% developed incontinence in the puerperium. Theories that evoke anatomic or pudendal nerve injury at birth as a cause of urinary incontinence must incorporate and explain the common occurrence of incontinence before and during pregnancy.

## CONCLUSION

Multiple physiologic factors, only one of which is urethral support, make up the female urinary continence mechanism. Other important factors include resting intraurethral pressure, pressure transmission to the urethra with increases in intraabdominal pressure, and the magnitude of rises in intraabdominal pressure. Abnormal urethral support and pelvic muscle denervation probably lead to deficient transmission of abdominal pressure to the urethra, ineffective compression caused by an unstable suburethral layer, and inefficient pelvic muscle contractions with stress. These factors result in genuine stress incontinence in some women.

The etiology of stress urinary incontinence is more complex than the simple theories that evoke anatomic or neurologic injury during childbirth. Most likely, maternal characteristics, fetal size and position, labor characteristics, and obstetric management define the likelihood of anatomic or nerve injury. These injuries unmask a susceptibility to stress incontinence, which is defined genetically (tissue strength, mechanical and anatomic relationships) and behaviorally (nutrition, smoking, and exercise).

For years obstetricians intervened at delivery to prevent perineal trauma and subsequent stress incontinence. The failure to systematically define and ascertain the frequency of perineal injuries at delivery and the failure to correlate those injuries with documented stress incontinence are surprisingly persistent deficiencies in the literature. Without the support of clinical trials with randomization of treatment, interventions such as midline episiotomy and outlet forceps have persisted for years. Recently, appropriately conducted trials not only have failed to show a benefit to episiotomy and outlet forceps, but have actually shown more posterior vaginal trauma with forceps and midline episiotomy. On the other hand, if urinary stress incontinence is the outcome variable of interest, then the incidence of posterior trauma may not be a proxy for that injury. Measures of postpartum urinary tract performance are a necessary part of future outcome analyses.

The massive social, medical, and financial impact of urinary and fecal incontinence in women warrants a major commitment to the understanding of the pathophysiology of the disease. The relationship between pregnancy, childbirth, and incontinence will require longitudinal studies of the lower urinary tract and anal sphincter before, during, and after pregnancy in a large, heterogenous group of primiparous women. Unbiased subject selection and standardized ascertainment of history, physical examination, and diagnostic testing (cystometrogram, urethral pressure studies, endoanal ultrasound, studies of pudendal nerve function, and others) are critical. Results then could be correlated in multivariate analyses with demographic, morphometric, and obstetric variables.

## BIBLIOGRAPHY
### Mechanisms of Urinary Continence and Incontinence

Awad SA, Downie JW: Relative contributions of smooth and striated muscles to the canine urethral pressure profile, *Br J Urol* 48:347, 1976.

Bazeed MA, Thuroff JW, Schmidt RA, et al: Histochemical study of urethral striated musculature in the dog, *J Urol* 128:406, 1982.

Bernstein IT: The pelvic floor muscles: muscle thickness in healthy and urinary-incontinent women measured by perineal ultrasonography with reference to the effect of pelvic floor training. Estrogen receptor studies, *Neurourol Urodyn* 16:237, 1997.

Blaivas JG: Classification of stress urinary incontinence, *Neurourol Urodyn* 2:103, 1983.

Blaivas JG, Olsson CA: Stress incontinence: classification and surgical approach, *J Urol* 139:727, 1988.

Bunne G, Obrink A: Urethral closure pressure with stress: a comparison between stress incontinent and continent women, *Urol Res* 6:127, 1978.

Constantinou CD, Govan DE: Spatial distribution and timing of transmitted and reflexly generated urethral pressures in healthy women, *J Urol* 127:964, 1982.

DeLancey JOL: Structural support of the urethra as it relates to stress urinary incontinence: the hammock hypothesis, *Am J Obstet Gynecol* 170:1713, 1994.

Enhorning G: Simultaneous recording of intravesical and intraurethral pressure, *Acta Chir Scand* (suppl) 276:1, 1961.

Gosling JA, Dixon JS, Critchley HO: A comparative study of the human external sphincter and periurethral levator ani muscles, *Br J Urol* 53:35, 1981.

Heidler H, Casper F, Thuroff JW: Urethral closure under stress conditions: contribution and relative share of intraurethral and periurethral striated muscles, *Neurourol Urodyn* 6:151, 1987.

Hilton P, Stanton SL: Urethral pressure measurement by microtransducer: the results in symptom-free women and in those with genuine stress incontinence, *Br J Obstet Gynaecol* 90:919, 1983.

Hodgkinson CP: Relationships of the female urethra and bladder in urinary stress incontinence, *Am J Obstet Gynecol* 65:560, 1953.

Jeffcoate TN, Roberts H: Observations on stress incontinence of urine, *Am J Obstet Gynecol* 64:721, 1952.

Koebl H, Strassegger H, Riss PA, et al: Morphological and functional aspects of pelvic floor muscles in patients with pelvic relaxation and genuine stress incontinence, *Obstet Gynecol* 74:789, 1989.

Lund CJ, Fullerton RE, Tristan TA: Cinefluorographic studies of the bladder and urethra in women, *Am J Obstet Gynecol* 78:706, 1959.

McGuire EJ, Lytton B, Pepe V, et al: Stress urinary incontinence, *Am J Obstet Gynecol* 47:255, 1976.

Muellner SR: The physiology of micturition, *J Urol* 65:805, 1951.

Petros P, Ulmsten U: An integral theory of female urinary incontinence, *Acta Obstet Gynecol Scand* 153(suppl):7, 1990.

Rud T, Andersson KE, AsmussenM, et al: Factors maintaining the intraurethral pressure in women, *Invest Urol* 17:343, 1980.

Walters MD: Mechanisms of continence and voiding, with International Continence Society classification of dysfunction, *Obstet Gynecol Clin North Am* 16:773, 1989.

Walters MD, Jackson GM: Urethral mobility and its relationship to stress incontinence in women, *J Reprod Med* 35:777, 1990.

Wein AJ, Barrett DM: *Voiding function and dysfunction,* Chicago, 1988, Year Book Medical Publishers.

Zinner NR, Sterling AM, Ritter RC: Role of inner urethral softness in urinary incontinence, *Urology* 16:115, 1980.

Zinner NR, Sterling AM, Ritter RC: Evaluation of inner urethral softness, *Urology* 22:446, 1983.

### Obstetric Issues

Anderson RS: A neurogenic element to urinary genuine stress incontinence, *Br J Obstet Gynaecol* 91:141, 1984.

Avery MD, Van Arsdale L: Perineal massage: effect on the incidence of episiotomy and laceration in a nulliparous population, *J Nurse Midwifery* 37:18, 1987.

Beck RP, Hsu N: Pregnancy, childbirth and the menopause related to the development of stress incontinence, *Am J Obstet Gynecol* 91:820, 1965.

Borgata L, Dieming SL, Cohen WR: Association of episiotomy and delivery position with deep perineal laceration during delivery in nulliparous women, *Am J Obstet Gynecol* 160:294, 1989.

Crawford LA, Quint EH, Pearl ML, et al: Incontinence following rupture of the anal sphincter during delivery, *Obstet Gynecol* 82:527, 1993.

Delee JB: The prophylactic forceps operation, *Am J Obstet Gynecol* 1:34, 1920.

Donnelly V, Fynes M, Campbell D, et al: Obstetric events leading to anal sphincter damage, *Obstet Gynecol* 92:955, 1998.

Dougherty MC, Bishop KR, Abrams RM, et al: The effect of exercise on the circumvaginal muscles in postpartum women, *J Nurse Midwifery* 34:8, 1989.

Fischer SR: Factors associated with the occurrence of perineal lacerations, *J Nurse Midwifery* 24:18, 1979.

Fornell EKU, Berg G, Hallböök O, et al: Clinical consequences of anal sphincter rupture during vaginal delivery, *J Am Coll Surg* 183:553, 1996.

Francis WJ: Disturbances in bladder function in relation to pregnancy, *J Obstet Gynaecol Br Emp* 67:353, 1960.

Francis WJ: The onset of stress incontinence, *J Obstet Gynaecol Br Emp* 67:899, 1960.

Fynes M, Donnelly VS, O'Connell PR, et al: Cesarean delivery and anal sphincter injury, *Obstet Gynecol* 92:496, 1998.

Gainey HL: Postpartum observation of pelvic tissue damage: further studies, *Am J Obstet Gynecol* 70:800, 1955.

Gordon H, Logue M: Perineal muscle function after childbirth, *Lancet* 2:123, 1985.

Green JR, Soohoo SL: Factors associated with rectal injury in spontaneous delivery, *Obstet Gynecol* 73:732, 1989.

Handa VL, Harris TA, Ostergard DR: Protecting the pelvic floor: obstetric management to prevent incontinence and pelvic organ prolapse, *Obstet Gynecol* 88:470, 1996.

Harrison RF, Brennan M, North PM, et al: Is routine episiotomy necessary? *BMJ* 288:1971, 1984.

Heidkamp MC, Leong FC, Brubaker L, et al: Pudendal denervation affects the structure and function of the striated, urethral sphincter in female rats, *Int Urogynecol J* 9:88, 1998.

Helwig JT, Thorp JM, Bowes WA: Does midline episiotomy increase the risk of third- and fourth-degree lacerations in operative vaginal deliveries? *Obstet Gynecol* 82:276, 1993.

Homsi R, Daikoku NH, Littlejohn J, et al: Episiotomy: risks of dehiscence and rectovaginal fistula, *Obstet Gynecol Surv* 49:803, 1994.

Meyer S, Schreyer A, deGrandi P, et al: The effect of birth on urinary continence mechanisms and other pelvic-floor characteristics, *Obstet Gynecol* 92:613, 1998.

Nodine P, Roberts J: Factors associated with perineal outcome during childbirth, *J Nurse Midwifery* 32:123, 1987.

Nygaard IE, Rao SS, Dawson JD: Anal incontinence after anal sphincter disruption: a 30-year retrospective cohort study, *Obstet Gynecol* 89:896, 1997.

Power RM: The pelvic floor during parturition, *Surg Gynecol Obstet* 83:296, 1946.

Rieger N, Schloithe A, Saccone G, et al: The effect of a normal vaginal delivery on anal function, *Acta Obstet Gynecol Scand* 76:769, 1997.

Sampselle CM, Brink CA, Wells JJ: Digital measurement of pelvic muscle strength in childbearing women, *Nurs Res* 38:134, 1989.

Sampselle CM: Changes in pelvic muscle strength and stress urinary incontinence associated with childbirth, *J Obstet Gynecol Neonatal Nurs* 19:371, 1990.

Schuessler B, Hesse V, Dimpfel T, et al: Epidural anesthetic and avoidance of postpartum stress urinary incontinence, *Lancet* 1:762, 1988.

Scott JC: Stress incontinence in nulliparous women, *J Reprod Med* 2:96, 1969.

Shiono P, Klebanoff MA, Carey JC: Midline episiotomies: more harm than good? *Obstet Gynecol* 76:765, 1990.

Sleep J, Grant A: West Bershire perineal management trial: three year follow up, *BMJ* 295:749, 1987.

Sleep J, Grant A, Garcia J, et al: West Berkshire perineal management trial, *BMJ* 289:587, 1984.

Smith AR, Hosker GL, Warrell DW: The role of partial denervation of the pelvic floor in the aetiology of genitourinary prolapse and stress incontinence of urine. A neurophysiological study, *Br J Obstet Gynaecol* 96:24, 1989.

Snooks SJ, Swash M: Abnormalities of the innervation of the urethral striated sphincter musculature in incontinence, *Br J Urol* 56:401, 1984.

Snooks SJ, Swash M: Perineal nerve and transcutaneous spinal stimulation: new methods for investigation of the urethral striated sphincter musculature, *Br J Urol* 56:406, 1984.

Snooks SJ, Swash M, Henry MM, et al: Risk factors in childbirth causing damage to the pelvic floor innervation, *Int J Colorect Dis* 1:20, 1986.

Snooks SJ, Swash M, Mathers SE: The effect of vaginal delivery on the pelvic floor: a five-year follow-up, *Br J Surg* 70:1358, 1990.

Stanton SL, Kerr-Wilson R, Harris VG: The incidence of urological symptoms in normal pregnancy, *Br J Obstet Gynaecol* 87:897, 1980.

Sultan AH, Kamm MA, Hudson CN, et al: Anal-sphincter disruption during vaginal delivery, *N Engl J Med* 329:1905, 1993.

Swash M, Snooks SJ, Henry MW: Unifying concept of pelvic floor disorders and incontinence, *J R Soc Med* 78:906, 1985.

Tetzschner T, Sørensen M, Lose G, et al: Pudendal nerve function during pregnancy and after delivery, *Int Urogynecol J* 8:66, 1997.

Thorp JM, Bowes WA: Episiotomy: can its routine use be defended? *Am J Obstet Gynecol* 160:1027, 1989.

Thorp JM, Bowes WA, Braune RG, et al: Selected use of midline episiotomy: effect on perineal trauma, *Obstet Gynecol* 70:260, 1987.

Walker MP, Farine D, Rolbin SH, et al: Epidural anesthesia, episiotomy and obstetric laceration, *Obstet Gynecol* 77:688, 1991.

Wilcox LS, Strobino DM, Baruffi G, et al: Episiotomy and its role in the incidence of perineal laceration in a maternity center and a tertiary hospital obstetric service, *Am J Obstet Gynecol* 160:1047, 1989.

Wynne JM, Myles JL, Jones I, et al: Disturbed anal sphincter function following vaginal delivery, *Gut* 39:120, 1996.

Yancey MK, Herpolsheimer A, Jordan GD, et al: Maternal and neonatal effects of outlet forceps delivery compared with spontaneous vaginal delivery in term pregnancies, *Obstet Gynecol* 78:646, 1991.

Zacharin RF: "A Chinese anatomy": the pelvic supporting tissues of the Chinese and Occidental female compared and contrasted, *Aust NZ J Obstet Gynaecol* 17:1, 1977.

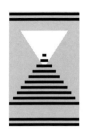

CHAPTER 13

# Genuine Stress Incontinence and Pelvic Organ Prolapse
## Nonsurgical Treatment

Ingrid Nygaard and Molly C. Dougherty

---

Behavioral Modification
   *Fluid intake and voiding pattern*
   *Bowel care*
   *Weight loss*
   *Removal of transient causes*
Bladder Training
Physiotherapy
   *Pelvic floor muscle exercises*
   *Vaginal cones*
   *Formal biofeedback*
   *Electrical stimulation*
Pharmacologic Therapy
   *Estrogen*
   *Alpha-adrenergic stimulating agents*
   *Other*
Mechanical Devices

---

Surgery has long been considered the mainstay of treatment for urinary incontinence and pelvic organ prolapse. However, nonsurgical treatment can alleviate or improve symptoms for a substantial number of women. Based on a wide body of evidence, it is recommended that unless extenuating circumstances exist, nonsurgical treatment for urinary incontinence should be undertaken before surgical treatment is considered. Although it is true that the complete cure rate of nonsurgical treatments is lower than for surgical treatment, the satisfaction rate can be quite high, given the lack of significant risk and morbidity of such treatment. Many researchers are actively exploring questions about nonsurgical treatment; thus, it is anticipated that in the future, clinicians will have more information about which modalities to use for specific patients.

## BEHAVIORAL MODIFICATION

Before embarking on formal treatment, the clinician and patient should review possible behavioral contributions to incontinence.

## Fluid Intake and Voiding Pattern

The voiding diary is a very important tool (Fig. 13-1). By reviewing a 3- to 7-day record of the patient's intake and output, the patient and clinician can discuss whether decreasing the fluid intake or increasing the voiding interval is appropriate. There is no need to decrease fluid intake in women with normal urinary output, but women who drink excessive volumes can benefit by restructuring their intake. The clinician should evaluate women with severe thirst and polydipsia for diabetes and hypercalcemia before simply decreasing intake. Restricting fluids after 6 PM often results in fewer nocturnal voids and may be particularly helpful to those with restricted mobility. Certain professions are associated with more infrequent voiding than professions with easier bathroom access. When a woman becomes aware of the connection between her daily stress incontinence and concomitant very full bladder, she usually finds the time to void once in the middle of the working day.

Review of the voiding diary also provides an opportunity to discuss the association for some patients between caffeinated and carbonated beverages and incontinence or frequency. Advise women who report a high caffeine intake (more than 3 cups per day) to slowly taper down to 1 to 2 cups per day. Making this change gradually over 3 to 4 weeks helps to minimize the caffeine withdrawal headaches experienced by many.

Managing stress urinary incontinence requires the woman to change other habitual behaviors as well. Rushing to the toilet tends to increase abdominal pressure and contribute to poor muscle coordination. When faced with possible urine loss, the woman should be taught to stop the activity she is engaged in, to sit down if possible until the urge passes, and to proceed slowly to the toilet.

## Bowel Care

Many women report an association between their bowel status and urinary incontinence. Therefore, women who do not have regular bowel habits should be instructed on appropriate fluid and fiber intake to maintain more healthy gastrointestinal function.

**145**

## BLADDER CHART INSTRUCTIONS

Having a record of your voiding pattern will help us to diagnose and treat your specific problem. Please fill out the diary for 3 days (they don't have to be back-to-back). Try to pick days in which you can conveniently measure your urine volumes. A large measuring cup can be used to collect and measure the amount of urine voided. You can measure in CCs or ounces.

If you use pads for your incontinence problem, please record how many pads you used each day.

A sample bladder chart for a morning is shown below.

| Urinated in toilet (time and amount) | Small accident (time) | Large accident (time) | Activity during accident | Fluid intake (time, amount, type of fluid) |
|---|---|---|---|---|
| 7:00 AM      400 cc | | | | |
| | | | | 7:15 AM<br>Orange juice   100 cc<br>Coffee             100 cc |
| | 8:45 AM | | Coughed | |
| 8:50 AM      100 cc | | | | |
| | 10:15 AM | | Heard running water | |
| | | | | 11:00 AM<br>Water     300 cc<br>Cola       240 cc |
| | | 11:25 AM | Sneezed three times | |
| | | | | |

**Fig. 13-1**   Voiding diary.

In the nursing home population, fecal impaction is associated with urinary incontinence, and disimpaction is therapeutic.

## Weight Loss

Many studies have found obesity to be an independent risk factor for stress incontinence. However, only a few studies reported a decrease in incontinence in women who lost weight; these studies were limited to morbidly obese women undergoing bariatric surgery. Bump et al. (1992) reported that 9 of 12 women became continent after losing a mean of 43 kg (mean preoperative weight 131 kg). Similarly, Deitel et al. (1988) found that only 11% of 138 women had symptoms of stress incontinence after bariatric surgery, compared to 61% preoperatively. There is currently no information about whether women who are slightly or moderately obese benefit from weight loss.

## Removal of Transient Causes

Although it is widely known that certain medications may exacerbate urge incontinence, fewer clinicians are aware that alpha-adrenergic blocking medications (such as prazosin) can precipitate stress incontinence. Women whose incontinence is temporally correlated with such medications might present for evaluation and consideration of surgery; the leakage resolves when the antihypertensive medication is discontinued or changed to a different type. Along a related track, Julian (1987) reported on a series of women undergoing treatment for "stress incontinence." The cough stress test was negative, and the women were ultimately diagnosed with excessive vaginal discharge caused by unopposed estrogen. This highlights the importance of documenting stress incontinence before proceeding with surgical treatment.

An acute urinary tract infection can cause transient stress

**Box 13-1**
## INCONTINENCE ORGANIZATIONS

National Association for Continence (NAFC)
PO Box 8306
Spartanburg, SC 29305

The Simon Foundation
Box 815
Wilmette, IL 60091

incontinence as well as urgency and urge incontinence. Some strains of *Escherichia coli* can inhibit the periurethral alpha-adrenergic fibers; incontinence resolves once the infection is treated.

Some women report that their stress incontinence is related only to certain provocations. A common precipitator is coughing. On occasion, nonsmoking women with chronic coughing may have complete resolution of the incontinence after treatment for sinusitis, allergic rhinitis, or other treatable conditions. Although the patient will still have stress incontinence if she coughs vigorously, treatment of the cough can make her condition less symptomatic, rendering surgery for the incontinence unnecessary.

Books and pamphlets often help women learn that they are not alone with their problems and reinforce information provided in the office or clinic setting. The clinician should review published materials carefully to avoid confusion resulting from discrepancies in various publications. Organizations dedicated to public education and self-help for urinary incontinence are an important source of information (see Box 13-1) and may be helpful to women undertaking behavioral management. Several organizations for professionals also generate and disseminate information on urinary incontinence.

## BLADDER TRAINING

Scheduling regimens, including bladder training, are often used to manage urge and stress incontinence. Using an approach based on behavior modification that included patient education and scheduled voiding, Fantl et al. (1991) reported a 57% reduction in incontinence episodes and a 54% reduction in amount of fluid lost. The effect was similar for both detrusor instability and genuine stress incontinence (GSI). The voiding schedule is based on the woman's daytime voiding interval, derived from the bladder diary. During the first week, the voiding interval is 30 or 60 minutes. The woman is encouraged to void on schedule, even if the desire to void is not present. Relaxation and distraction techniques are used to suppress urge sensations. However, when urgency cannot be suppressed and leakage is imminent, the woman may void to prevent leakage.

The woman meets with the clinician for 6 consecutive weeks, and the bladder diaries are reviewed. A decrease in the number of leak episodes and tolerance of the prescribed interval without interruptions signal readiness to increase the voiding interval by 30 minutes. During visits, the clinician provides positive reinforcement and optimism. The goal is to reach a 3-hour voiding interval. After 6 weeks, the woman is encouraged to assume a comfortable voiding schedule. Bladder training does not impose fluid modifications.

## PHYSIOTHERAPY

Because the bladder and other pelvic organs are supported by muscles (the pelvic floor, or levator ani muscles), various forms of physiotherapy are often helpful in the treatment of stress incontinence. Common forms of physiotherapy include Kegel exercises, exercising with the aid of biofeedback, and electrical stimulation therapy. It is helpful for the clinician to have a good understanding of the anatomy of the muscles involved (see Chapter 1). It is unclear whether physiotherapy is successful because it reeducates muscle action or because it strengthens muscles. Recently, Bernstein (1997) measured the muscle width ultrasonographically and found no correlation between increased muscle thickness and decreased incontinence after a course of pelvic muscle exercises.

### Pelvic Floor Muscle Exercises

It is essential to physically assess the levator muscles before commencing with therapy. During a pelvic examination, feel the muscles while they are at rest and while the woman is attempting an active contraction. Note areas of muscle that are absent or atrophied. Assess the tone by the degree of resistance to the finger during contraction. One third of women perform the exercises incorrectly, given simply the verbal instruction to "squeeze as if you are trying to stop your flow of urine." However, after appropriate training, most women are able to contract correctly.

There are many recommended pelvic muscle exercise regimens, but several measures are essential:
1. Ascertain that the patient is correctly contracting the levator muscles.
2. Encourage discrete exercise sessions each day, or at least 4 days per week.
3. Schedule frequent follow-up visits with your team.
4. Do not encourage patients to stop their flow of urine. This is counterproductive to the mission of voiding, and whether or not patients are able to interrupt their flow is not correlated with treatment success.
5. Once you have determined that the muscles are stronger on examination, teach the patient to make a conscious effort to precontract the muscles during times of increased abdominal strain.

**Box 13-2**

## PELVIC MUSCLE EXERCISE INSTRUCTIONS

The muscles that surround the vagina, the pelvic muscles, help support the pelvic organs. Pelvic muscle exercise (PME) was popularized by Dr. Arnold Kegel and often is called Kegel exercises. Most health professionals agree that PME is beneficial to women. Weakened pelvic muscles (PM) often result in loss of urine during an increase in abdominal pressure, which can occur when laughing, coughing, or jogging.

Begin by emptying your bladder. Adjust your clothing so that you can be comfortable and relaxed. Lie down with your head slightly elevated (at a 20-degree angle), your knees bent and comfortable.

Try tensing your fist into a tight ball, to a count of five. Now completely relax your fist. Can you feel the difference between the two states? It is important that you are able to do so. When you contract or tighten your PM, it is important but often difficult to keep your abdominal, buttock, and thigh muscles relaxed. Should you note a problem with tightening too many muscles, take a deep breath and focus on relaxing your whole body before proceeding.

Isolating and tightening a specific muscle, as you did with your fist, may help you learn to concentrate and focus on the PM. Try to think about the area around your vagina. Draw the muscles together quickly as though you are trying to stop urinating or a bowel movement. When you have pulled the muscles together quickly and deliberately, actively hold the contraction for 10 seconds. Relax completely after the contraction subsides. Relax approximately 15 seconds before beginning another PM contraction.

When you begin to exercise these muscles, you may note that your muscles tire easily or that you are not able to hold the contraction for 10 seconds. As you continue to exercise, this problem will become less common. In addition, a short 30-second break at these points may be helpful. If you think that you are no longer tightening or contracting your muscles, it is important not to tighten them during the remainder of the 10-second count. What you are trying to do is gain control and strength in the muscles. By retightening, or "flicking" the muscle, you will not be as successful in gaining control and strength.

### Directions for a PM Exercise Contraction

To the count of 10 seconds:
1. Contract deliberately, quickly, and hard.
2. Actively hold the contraction, hard and firm.
3. Hold it, hard and firm.
4. Hold it, hard and firm.
5. Hold it, hard and firm.
6. Hold it, hard and firm.
7. Hold it, hard and firm.
8. Hold it, hard and firm.
9. Hold it, hard and firm.
10. Relax completely.

Begin by doing 15 of these contractions each session (day) three times a week every other day. Add 10 contractions at the end of each month until you build up to 35 contractions in a session. Good luck!

Adapted from Dougherty M, Bishop K: *Circumvaginal muscle (CVM) exercise instructions*, 1987.

6. Consult physical therapy colleagues when available. They have greater insight into muscle biomechanics and techniques to improve your patients' outcomes.

Women who can effectively and correctly contract the pelvic muscles on their own generally do not require formal biofeedback. They can be instructed on the technique and on an exercise program to do at home. However, studies have shown that the more frequent the follow-up with the health care provider, the more successful the outcome. Follow-up intervals must be decided within the confines of each practice; common intervals are monthly for 3 to 4 months and then periodically for maintenance. One example of an exercise program is shown in Box 13-2. Many women with stress incontinence are initially unable to contract the muscles for longer than a few seconds and may require 6 to 8 weeks to work up to a 10-second contraction. Women with weak muscles should begin exercising supine. As they gain strength, they should progress to sitting and finally standing. Women should be counseled to relax completely between contractions. If relaxation is not attained, a generalized muscular tonus in the pelvis may occur, making it more difficult for the woman to sense the intensity of her efforts.

Some women find that keeping a log of their exercise progress allows them to follow changes in muscle strength,

which generally occur before improvement in incontinence. Although one group of researchers found that compliance and success increased in women who exercised with the aid of a specially designed audiocassette, another group found no difference between women who exercised with and without such an aid.

It is easy for women who are comfortable with their bodies to learn to monitor their pelvic muscle contractions. Tact and urging are needed with others. Nevertheless, self-monitoring techniques have a place in behavioral management and provide women with a way to feel independent in tracking their progress. By encouraging improved compliance, these techniques may contribute to the success of behavioral management. To monitor one's own progress, the woman places her index finger intravaginally and contracts the pelvic muscle. The pressure of the contraction against her finger provides some information about the quality of her contraction.

## Vaginal Cones

Exercising with the aid of weighted vaginal cones is sometimes more helpful than exercising without such aids, but generally, results are similar. Vaginal weights (or cones) provide a form of biofeedback at home. The woman inserts the cone with the least weight into her vagina, as she would a tampon. As she goes about her activities, the weight of the cone causes it to slip out unless she contracts the pelvic muscles firmly and consistently to keep the cone in place. She is instructed to retain the cone for 15 minutes twice a day. When successful with a specific cone on two successive occasions, she graduates to the next heavier cone.

## Formal Biofeedback

Biofeedback is widely used to facilitate behavior change and to manage incontinence. Some clinicians report good results with the use of a physiograph, which provides a visual recording of abdominal, bladder, and vaginal pressures.

Biofeedback is usually an intensive therapy, with sessions occurring weekly or more often. Gains from biofeedback are seen quickly. Dougherty et al. (unpublished) found that an average of 5.5 sessions scheduled two to three times per week was sufficient for women to develop control of abdominal pressure, attain characteristic pelvic muscle pressure curves, and achieve improvement in leakage episodes and urine loss. Burgio et al. (1990) also reported significant improvement in leak episodes, with one to eight sessions spaced 2 to 4 weeks apart.

Biofeedback requires equipment that monitors signals representing relevant physiologic processes (i.e., from the abdomen and pelvic muscles) and provides the woman with auditory or visual information that varies with the signal produced. Ideally, a permanent record is obtained for review later. Sensors for monitoring may be surface electrodes or intravaginal or rectal probes. Many equipment systems dedicated to or adaptable for biofeedback are available.

One advantage of biofeedback is that the procedures are individualized and focus on elements that contribute to incontinence. Although no single pattern for biofeedback has emerged in the literature, it may be organized around specific steps, as described in Box 13-3.

An important step in biofeedback is learning to control abdominal pressure. Some women, attempting to inhibit leakage, inspire and contract the abdominal muscles. This increases abdominal pressure (and bladder pressure) and contributes to leakage. With biofeedback, women learn to control behaviors that increase abdominal pressure.

A second step in biofeedback is mastering voluntary contractions of the pelvic muscles. Women, both continent and incontinent, vary widely in the force with which they are able to contract these muscles. A woman who cannot produce a palpable contraction on examination will benefit from biofeedback to help her produce contractions that she can monitor and enhance. Increasing the intensity of a muscle contraction and then gradually relaxing is a technique used in biofeedback generally and, when applied to the pelvic muscles, also may play a role in continence.

Another important step is to duplicate events in the office or clinic that reflect everyday activities that lead to

**Box 13-3**
## GUIDELINES FOR BIOFEEDBACK

Guideline 1: Plan for approximately 20-min sessions.
Guideline 2: Review woman's experience since last session.
Guideline 3: Review and record woman's progress toward goals at each session.

**Biofeedback Routine: Progression of Activity**

*Step 1: Abdominal (ABD) pressure*
Experiment with maneuvers to increase ABD pressure.
Cough, laugh. Head lift (hands on abdomen).
Head lift with inspiration and hold.
Conscious tightening of abdomen.
Extend abdomen by voluntary extension of abdominal muscles.
OBJECTIVE: Learn and control increases in abdominal pressure.

*Step 2: Quick, intense pelvic muscle (PM) contraction of short duration*
Contract quickly, briefly. Helps to get an initial feel for contraction. Relax to baseline. Work toward PM contractions without increasing ABD activity.
OBJECTIVE: PM contraction without ABD activity.

*Step 3: 10-second PM contraction*
Contract firmly and quickly, hold. Relax to baseline. Work toward PM contractions without increasing ABD activity.
OBJECTIVE: PM contraction sustained for 10 seconds with ABD activity controlled.

*Step 4: Slow, deliberate PM contraction*
Focus on slow, deliberate increases in PM activity and a controlled return to baseline.
Maintain stable, low ABD activity.
OBJECTIVE: To promote sensations associated with subtle changes in PM contraction and relaxation of PM.

*Step 5: Individualized biofeedback sessions*
Use sitting and standing positions. Perform PM biofeedback session with full bladder. Perform activities that provoke leakage at home (coughs, laughs) and practice control with PM contractions.
OBJECTIVE: Duplicate events in office or clinic that provoke leaks at home and practice control.

leakage. In these sessions, the woman practices relaxing her abdominal muscles and contracting the pelvic muscles to overcome imminent leaks while monitoring the effect of her efforts with the biofeedback equipment. Patients are instructed to drink 250 to 500 ml fluid an hour before the session to make the practice realistic. The woman may sit or stand as she duplicates behavior that provokes leaks (coughs, laughs) while monitoring her behavior on the biofeedback equipment.

## Electrical Stimulation

Functional electrical stimulation is another physiotherapy modality, used with some frequency by physical therapists around the world. The first stimulators were implanted surgically with radio-linked electrodes adjacent to the urethral musculature. Various types of incontinence were treated with an overall success rate of about 50%. Because of the risks of surgical implantation and various technical failures requiring reoperation, implantable electrical devices generally were replaced by removable external devices. However, implantable sacral anterior root nerve stimulators still are available for detrusor hyperreflexia and neuropathic voiding disorders.

Automatic integrated functional electrical stimulation systems in the form of anal and vaginal plugs (independent or connected to a portable battery-operated stimulator) were then developed. Different designs and sizes of electrodes have been used, such as the vaginal ring pessary, the elliptical Hodge's pessary, and cylindrical anal and vaginal plug electrodes.

In research settings, intravaginal electrical stimulation augments urethral sphincteric function and inhibits bladder contractility. It is theorized that pelvic muscle stimulation is achieved by direct electrical stimulation of afferent fibers in the pudendal nerve, which results in polysynaptic reflex responses. This mechanism activates a number of muscles from a single stimulation site. The electrical impulse runs along the afferent limb of the pudendal nerve to the sacral nerve roots and by efferent pathways to the pelvic floor muscles. Pelvic muscle contraction occurs and results in increased urethral closure pressure.

Intravaginal electrical stimulation also causes bladder inhibition. At low intravesical volumes, the hypogastric (sympathetic) nerves mediate bladder inhibition. At higher volumes, inhibition of the pelvic nerve (parasympathetic) completes the reflexogenic bladder inhibition. Both reflex arcs (pudendal to hypogastric and pudendal to pelvic) are activated by stimulation of pudendal nerve afferents.

Based on their observations, Godec and Kralj (1976) predicted favorable results from the application of electrical stimulation for urinary incontinence when (1) the morphology of the urinary tract is preserved, (2) the spinal center for micturition is preserved, (3) there is a low degree of peripheral denervation of the muscles of the pelvic floor, (4) urodynamic and neurophysiologic responses to electrical stimulation are positive, and (5) any lesion of the medulla spinalis is between T6 and T12. The clinical indications and contraindications of electrical stimulation are presented in Box 13-4.

Intravaginal electrodes are available as independent systems or attached to external stimulating devices. Complete independent systems consist of a battery and an electronic circuit placed in a waterproof housing made of plexiglass with electrodes made of stainless steel. This system is automatically turned on when the electrodes come in contact with the walls of the vagina and turned off when the contact is broken by their removal. The device contains a microvibrator from which a continuous train of monophasic rectangular pulses of different frequencies and pulse

**Box 13-4**

## INDICATIONS AND CONTRA-INDICATIONS OF FUNCTIONAL ELECTRICAL STIMULATION

**Indications**

Genuine stress incontinence (GSI)
Detrusor instability
Mixed GSI and detrusor instability
Sensory urgency
Detrusor hyperreflexia
Neuropathic voiding dysfunction

**Contraindications**

*Extraurinary*

Severe vaginal prolapse
Pregnancy
Vaginal infections
Heavy menstruation or other vaginal bleeding
History of cardiac arrhythmia
Demand cardiac pacemaker

*Urinary*

Urinary retention, elevated residual urinary volumes caused by incomplete bladder emptying
Extraurethral incontinence
Urinary infection
Vesicoureteral reflux

widths is delivered. Intravaginal electrodes that are used with an external stimulator can be connected to office stimulators for periodic acute maximal stimulation or to home stimulators for daily stimulation. The stimulators have switches to adjust device characteristics, including current intensity, character of stimulation (continuous or intermittent), and frequency. Several devices are available for use in the United States and Canada; a typical device is shown in Fig. 13-2.

In clinical use, a maximal response with minimal energy consumption is desired. This response requires two types of electrical characteristics: alternating pulses and intermittent stimulation. Intermittent rather than constant stimulation circumvents the problem of muscle fatigue without sacrificing effectiveness. A stimulation frequency of 20 to 50 Hz and a pulse duration of 1 to 5 ms is most effective for urethral closure; a stimulation frequency of 10 Hz is most effective for bladder inhibition.

Because of the various devices that have been used and the many variations in their electrical characteristics, clinical results are difficult to compare among studies. Eriksen (1990) reported on the treatment of 121 women with stress and motor urge incontinence with an integrated, automatic electrical anal stimulator, which was worn for most of each day. Twenty-three patients discontinued treatment because of various side effects, most notably anal discomfort and

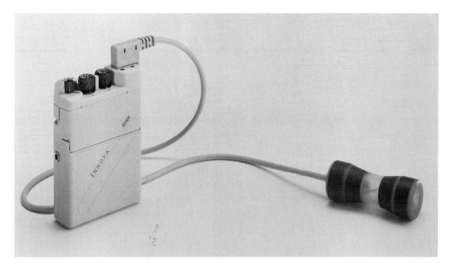

**Fig. 13-2** Innova electrical stimulation unit (Empi, Minneapolis, MN).

pain. The remaining 98 women were treated with anal stimulation for an average of 9 months. Continence was achieved in 64% of the patients with stress incontinence, 65% of those with motor urge incontinence, and 53% of those with mixed stress and motor urge incontinence. Urodynamic changes after treatment included increased bladder volume measured at first desire to void, increased maximum cystometric capacity, and fewer detrusor contractions. In 45% of patients with detrusor instability, a stable bladder with normal sensation and capacity was found after therapy. In patients with stress incontinence, a significant increase was observed in functional urethral length.

In a prospective study of 55 women with stress incontinence awaiting surgical repair, Eriksen (1990) prescribed electrical stimulation for at least 2 months. Surgical treatment was avoided in 56% of these patients. A cost-benefit analysis showed that the total cost of stress incontinence therapy could be reduced by 40% with long-term use of electrical stimulation.

At the time of this writing, two randomized placebo-controlled clinical trials that address the efficacy of electrical stimulation have been published. Sand et al. (1995) treated 52 women with GSI: 35 used an active vaginal probe and 17 used a sham device for 12 weeks. The number of incontinent episodes decreased by at least 50% in 48% of women using the active device and in 13% of those using the sham device. Whether this result was clinically significant is unclear because the average number of incontinent episodes per week decreased from 14 to 10 in the active group. A second trial by Smith (1996) randomized 18 women with stress incontinence to either electrical stimulation via a vaginal probe or pelvic floor muscle exercises, and 38 women with detrusor instability to either electrical stimulation or anticholinergic therapy. All treatments decreased incontinence frequency, and there was no difference between treatments. Women with stress incontinence who

used the electrical stimulator decreased the mean daily number of incontinent episodes from 3.0 to 1.4, whereas women with detrusor instability decreased from 3.4 to 1.4.

Susset et al. (1995) evaluated variables predictive of a good response to electrical stimulation therapy. The most significant factors predictive of a reduction in incontinent episodes included lower patient age, presence of estrogen, absence of detrusor instability and intrinsic sphincter deficiency, low urethral hypermobility, and compliance with treatment. Obesity, severity of incontinence, parity, and previous surgery had no predictive effects.

Physiotherapy of various forms has limitations. It is time consuming and requires considerable commitment from the woman. Not all women benefit from such management of GSI. In fact, across studies of all behavioral interventions for multiple problems, approximately 12% of patients drop out and 30% do not improve at all. The number of women who are totally dry after treatment is small (10% to 20%), but many women may be satisfied with improved, rather than total, urinary control. Little is known about what characteristics of the woman or her situation predict "cure" versus minimal to moderate improvement. Keeping abreast of the literature permits the clinician to use research-based statements to place the potential outcomes of behavioral management in perspective for women.

## PHARMACOLOGIC THERAPY

See Table 13-1 for a review of pharmacologic therapy available to treat stress incontinence.

### Estrogen

The urethra and bladder contain a rich supply of estrogen receptors, and it is therefore biologically feasible that estrogen replacement affects postmenopausal urogenital symptoms. Estrogen does promote vaginal cellular maturation

**Table 13-1**  Pharmacologic Therapy for Genuine Stress Incontinence

| Classification of drug | Name of drug | Minimum/maximum dosage | Potential side effects |
|---|---|---|---|
| Hormone | Conjugated estrogen (or comparable estrogen preparation) | Oral: 0.3 mg QD/1.25 mg QD cyclically or continuously<br>Vaginal: 2 g QD/4 g QD then weekly for maintenance | Increased risk of endometrial carcinoma (unless opposed with cyclic progestin), irregular vaginal bleeding |
| Alpha-sympathomimetic | Pseudoephedrine hydrochloride | 15 mg BID/30 mg QID | Drowsiness, dry mouth, hypertension |
| | Phenylpropanolamine hydrochloride | 50 mg QD/75 mg BID | Drowsiness, dry mouth, hypertension |
| Tricyclic antidepressant | Imipramine hydrochloride | 25 mg QD/75 mg BID | Anticholinergic effects, orthostatic hypotension, hepatic dysfunction, mania, cardiovascular effects (especially in the elderly); MAO inhibitors prohibited |
| Beta-sympathetic blocker | Propranolol hydrochloride | 10 mg BID/40 mg TID | Fatigue, lethargy, cardiovascular effects |

and beneficial vaginal flora; clinically, estrogen improves symptoms of atrophy such as vaginal dryness, irritation, and burning. Whether it also improves urinary incontinence is controversial. Earlier nonrandomized studies with subjective outcome measures reported often dramatic improvement in symptoms of both urge and stress incontinence. However, randomized studies examining stress incontinence specifically report mixed results. Samsioe et al. (1985) found no difference in stress incontinence symptoms in patients randomly assigned to receive oral estriol or placebo. Wilson et al. (1987) reported greater subjective improvement in stress incontinent women taking estrogen than those taking placebo, but no objective difference was found in either urethral pressure profile or volume of urine lost. Cardozo (1990) reported no greater subjective improvement in women with stress incontinence symptoms randomized to estrogen implants, but video-urethrography revealed a significant improvement in bladder base descensus in women who received estrogen. In a double-blind, placebo-controlled study of the effect of estrogen on urge incontinence in postmenopausal women, Walter et al. (1978) described significant improvement in sensory and motor urgency after estrogen treatment compared to placebo. Nevertheless, there were no statistically significant changes in the maximal urethral closure pressure or functional urethral length between estrogen- and placebo-treated groups.

In a more recent randomized, double-blind, placebo-controlled study, Walter et al. (1990) noted cure or improvement in incontinence complaints in 43% of women given estriol, compared to no improvement in the placebo group. Significant improvement was noted in 1-hour pad test results, but not in the number of leakage episodes per 24 hours. Most recently, Fantl et al. (1996) examined the efficacy of estrogen replacement therapy in 83 hypoestrogenic women with urinary incontinence and found no differences between the placebo and treatment groups in the number of

incontinent episodes, volume of urine loss, standardized quality of life outcomes, or subjective improvement.

Cardozo et al. (1998) assessed the efficacy of estrogen on relief of various urogenital symptoms, including urinary frequency, nocturia, urgency, and dysuria. In this meta-analysis, urinary incontinence was not addressed. The authors found that there was a statistically significant benefit of estrogen therapy for all outcomes.

## Alpha-Adrenergic Stimulating Agents

The bladder neck and proximal urethra in women contain predominantly alpha-adrenoreceptors. Stimulation of these receptors produces smooth muscle contraction, causing increased bladder outlet resistance.

Treatment of patients with stress incontinence with alpha-adrenergic stimulating drugs improves symptoms in some patients. Drugs that have been studied include ephedrine, phenylephrine, midodrine, norfenefrine, and phenylpropanolamine (PPA). Ephedrine is a noncatecholamine sympathomimetic agent that owes part of its peripheral action to the release of noradrenaline, which also directly stimulates alpha- and beta-adrenergic receptors.

Studies using norephedrine chloride have shown an increase in maximal urethral closure pressure, but not functional urethral length. In a 14-week, double-blind crossover study that compared the effects of norephedrine chloride with placebo, Ek et al. (1978) showed reduction of urinary leakage with the drug in 12 of 22 patients. Diokno and Taub (1975) reported good to excellent results in 27 of 38 patients with GSI treated with ephedrine sulfate. In general, effects are most notable in patients with mild to moderate symptoms but do not sufficiently improve severe symptoms of stress incontinence to offer an alternative to surgical treatment. PPA shares the pharmacologic properties of ephedrine and is approximately equal in peripheral potency, while causing less central stimulation. Several placebo-controlled studies have evaluated PPA in the treatment of women with GSI. Using the dosage of 50 mg twice daily, improvement is noted in 60% to 70% of patients, mainly in those with less severe disease. Although modest increases in maximum urethral pressure were noted, these did not correlate with either serum concentration or subjective urinary symptom response.

PPA is a component of numerous prescription and over-the-counter medications that are marketed for the treatment of nasal and sinus congestion and appetite suppression. Pharmacologic studies of PPA at these dosages revealed few clinically significant adverse effects. Nevertheless, reports of serious complications, including seizures, stroke, and death, with over-the-counter preparations containing PPA suggest that these drugs must be used with care. Alpha-adrenergic stimulating drugs are usually used for the temporary, intermittent, or seasonal relief of stress incontinence symptoms. If long-term cure is desired, other treatments are probably more appropriate.

Estrogen and alpha-sympathetic agonist medications may have an additive effect in the treatment of stress incontinence. Studies of combined therapy generally show an improvement in symptoms; however, the objective effects on urethral pressure are less consistent. Ahlström et al. (1990) treated 29 women with stress incontinence with either estriol alone or combined estriol and phenylpropanolamine. Those receiving the combined therapy had a better clinical response and more significant improvements in maximum urethral closure pressure. However, other studies have found no significant differences in objective results in women on combined therapy.

Based on these results and the low risk of short-term estrogen use, it seems reasonable to recommend a 6- to 8-week course of estrogen therapy in atrophic women with urinary incontinence. If clear-cut improvement is not reported after this trial period and the woman has no other reason to be on estrogen replacement therapy, treatment can then be discontinued. At this time, there is no information about whether estrogen therapy improves the effectiveness of physiotherapy in the treatment of stress incontinence.

## Other

Imipramine hydrochloride, an antidepressant with alpha-adrenergic agonist and anticholinergic effects, appears to improve symptoms in some women with stress urinary incontinence. Gilja et al. (1984) reported a 71% cure rate in 21 women after treatment with imipramine hydrochloride. These investigators documented an increase in functional urethral length and maximum urethral pressure after a daily dose of 75 mg imipramine hydrochloride.

Theoretically, beta-adrenergic blocking agents might be expected to potentiate an alpha-adrenergic effect, thereby increasing resistance in the urethra. Gleason et al. (1974) reported success in treating stress incontinent patients with the beta-adrenergic blocking agent propranolol in oral doses of 10 mg four times daily. Although such treatment has been suggested as alternative drug therapy in patients with sphincteric incompetence and hypertension, no reports of such efficacy have appeared. Other reports have noted no significant changes in urethral pressure profile measurements in normal women after beta-adrenergic blockade.

## MECHANICAL DEVICES

With the advent of modern surgical techniques, pessaries were considered a relic of the past and for a period of time were rarely offered or used. Recently, there has been a resurgence of interest in this therapeutic modality. Physicians are becoming more conscious of the long-term risks and failure rates of surgical procedures, and patients are becoming more interested in considering all options for their problem.

Some patients choose to wear a pessary as the final therapy for their pelvic floor dysfunction, whereas others use a pessary to temporize before considering surgery and many more wear such a device only when undertaking an activity that results in urine loss, such as exercise. We believe that offering appropriate candidates the choice of expectant management, a pessary or other device, or surgery constitutes good informed consent. A pessary also can be a useful diagnostic tool for the clinician. By reducing prolapse for several weeks with a pessary, the patient and clinician can obtain a clue about whether similar surgical reduction of prolapse will resolve symptoms of pelvic and back pain, urinary urgency and frequency, or voiding dysfunction, or precipitate symptoms of stress incontinence. This in turn will help to ensure that the patient has reasonable expectations of postoperative results. It has been suggested, although not yet established, that wearing a mechanical device that mimics the postoperative results of a retropubic urethropexy, such as the Introl prosthesis (UroMed, Needham, MA), will predict the odds of surgical success for a given woman.

Today, many pessaries and vaginal devices are available to treat incontinence or prolapse. Some are easier for a woman to manage herself than others. Our approach is to begin a fitting session with one of the more inexpensive, user-friendly devices before proceeding to pessaries that are more expensive or more difficult for the patient to manage. In our experience, adverse outcomes from wearing a pessary, such as vaginal abrasions or ulcerations, are rare if a patient is able to insert and remove the pessary on her own and thus remove it overnight at least once per week. We currently follow the steps in Box 13-5 in the pessary-fitting process for each diagnostic condition.

Visiting nurses can be an invaluable resource for women unable to care for pessaries on their own. They are usually able to visit the woman at home, remove the pessary in the evening, and return in the morning to replace it. Excessive

**Box 13-5**
## SUGGESTED SEQUENCE FOR FITTING PESSARIES FOR PROLAPSE

**Apical Prolapse: Vaginal Vault, Uterus**

1. Ring with support
2. Incontinence dish with support
3. Donut
4. Inflatoball
5. Gelhorn (for uterine prolapse only)
6. Cube (rarely used; see text)

**Cystocele**

1. Ring with support
2. Incontinence dish or dish with support
3. Contraceptive diaphragm (Ortho Pharmaceuticals, Raritan, NJ)
4. Gehrung
5. Donut

**Rectocele**

1. Ring with support
2. Gehrung

Devices made by Mylex Products, Chicago, except as noted.

foul-smelling discharge or bleeding signals a need to arrange medical follow-up.

Before a pessary-fitting session, all women with even slight vaginal atrophy are pretreated for 6 weeks with estrogen cream. Women are instructed to come to the fitting session with a moderately full bladder. For women with stress incontinence, this allows testing of the efficacy of the pessary, and for women with prolapse, this determines whether reduction of the prolapse is accompanied by incontinence. In addition, all women attempt to void with the pessary in place before leaving the office. Women are instructed to mimic vigorous activity in the clinic area (such as brisk walking, jumping jacks, straining), and the patient is then sent home with the best fit. Vaginal devices commonly used to treat stress incontinence are shown in Fig. 13-3; the fitting sequence is shown in Box 13-6. Once home, the best fit in the office fails for approximately one fourth of women, who then return for further fitting. Our recommendation for follow-up care is shown in Box 13-7. Because women in our practice generally remove the pessary at least once a week, they rarely encounter excessive or malodorous vaginal discharge and thus have little use for creams other than estrogen.

We present a special word of caution about the cube pessary. The suction cups on each side of the cube allow this

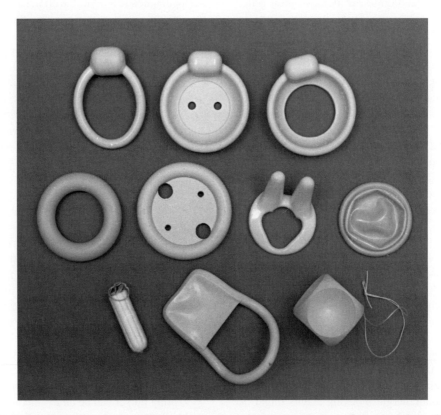

**Fig. 13-3** Vaginal devices useful for treatment of stress incontinence. *Top row, left to right:* incontinence ring, incontinence dish with support, incontinence dish. *Middle row:* Suarez continence ring, ring with support, Introl, diaphragm. *Bottom row:* tampon, Hodge pessary, cube. (See text for manufacturer information.)

pessary to retain its intravaginal position when other pessaries fall out; the same suction cups can cause significant ulceration in the vagina. We have seen several postmenopausal women who developed large, weeping ulcers after wearing the cube pessary for only 2 or 3 days. Therefore, we now reserve the use of this type of pessary for women with extremely healthy vaginal tissue who are able to remove it nightly. Patients and clinicians must take care to release the suction by sweeping a finger between the pessary and the upper vaginal wall before attempting removal.

Three newer devices for stress incontinence include the urethral insert (or plug), the urethral patch, and the urethral meatus suction cap. At the time of this writing, the FDA has approved the Reliance Urinary Control Insert (UroMed Corporation, Needham, MA), and other companies are testing alternative urethral inserts. A sterile insert is placed into the urethra by the patient; it is removed before a void, after which a new sterile insert is reinserted. Such inserts are appropriate for women with pure stress incontinence, no history of recurrent urinary tract infections, and no serious contraindications to bacteriuria (such as artificial heart valves). Although many women do develop bacteriuria and transient hematuria secondary to insert use, this is often not clinically significant. However, because the inserts are not completely without risk, their use should be supervised by a physician versed in the expected findings and management of problems.

The urethral patch (Impress Softpatch, UroMed, Needham, MA) appears to be appropriate for women to try without physician guidance. A new patch must be reapplied after each void. Preliminary study of this modality found that the patch dislodged during detrusor contractions; this finding alleviates concerns that a woman with detrusor instability who wears the patch may be at risk for ureteral reflux because of outlet obstruction. Two different soft external patches that mimic suction caps are also now available (Fem Assist, Insight Medical, Bolten, MA, and CapSure, Bard, Covington, GA). These caps can be reapplied after voids and reused for up to a week.

## CONCLUSION

Unfortunately, no treatment exists that cures all women with stress incontinence and pelvic organ prolapse 100% of the time. Surgery, long considered the gold standard for treating these conditions, loses some effectiveness with time, such that the 80% to 90% cure rate seen 2 to 5 years postoperatively decreases to 50% to 60% 10 years later. In addition, about a third of women experience problems such as de novo detrusor instability, enterocele, or voiding dysfunction postoperatively, driving the satisfaction rate further down. Although conservative management cures far fewer women than surgery, the decreased risk and expense combined with the reasonable improvement rates associated with conservative therapy make this approach attractive as a first treatment option for most women.

---

**Box 13-7**

### PESSARY CARE INSTRUCTIONS

**Initial Pessary Use**

Estrogen cream, if needed
Pessary fitting
Vigorous activity in office
Void in office
Home with pessary

**First Follow-Up Visit (1 Week; 1 to 3 Days for Cube)**

Examine vagina
Adjust type and size as needed
Teach insertion and removal
Visiting nurse referral(?) (see text)

**Long-Term Follow-Up**

***Woman can insert and remove***
Return visits: 2 weeks, 3 months later, every 6 to 12 months
Remove pessary each night or at least once per week
Leave out overnight
Use estrogen cream on pessary as lubricant
***Woman cannot insert and remove***
Return visits: 2 weeks, 4 weeks later, 6 weeks later, etc., up to
   3 months
Determine appropriate pessary removal interval
Optimal: remove and have nurse reinsert in morning (or vice
   versa)
Estrogen: systemic or cream 3 times per week
Triple sulfa cream or acigel may decrease discharge

---

**Box 13-6**

### SUGGESTED SEQUENCE FOR FITTING VAGINAL DEVICES FOR STRESS INCONTINENCE

1. Incontinence ring (no cystocele)
   Incontinence dish (mild to moderate cystocele)
   Incontinence dish with support (moderate or severe cystocele or concomitant vault prolapse)
2. Suarez Continence Ring (Cook Urologic, Spencer, IN)
3. Mylex Ring with support
4. Introl (UroMed, Needham, MA)
5. Cook Continence Ring (Cook Urologic, Spencer, IN)
6. Tampon (for mild stress incontinence only)
7. Hodge pessary
8. Contraceptive diaphragm (Ortho Pharmaceuticals, Raritan, NJ)
9. Cube pessary

---

Devices made by Mylex Products, Chicago, except as noted.

## BIBLIOGRAPHY
### Behavioral Modification

Basmajian JV, ed: *Biofeedback principles and practice for clinicians,* Baltimore, 1989, Williams & Wilkins.

Bump RC, Sugerman HJ, Fantl JA, et al: Obesity and lower urinary tract function in women: effect of surgically induced weight loss, *Am J Obstet Gynecol* 167:392, 1992.

Burgio KL, Whitehead WE, Engel BT: Urinary incontinence in the elderly, *Ann Intern Med* 103:507, 1985.

Cardozo LD, Stanton SL, Hefner J, et al: Idiopathic bladder instability treated by biofeedback, *Br J Urol* 40:250, 1978.

Deitel M, Stone E, Kassam HA, et al: Gynecologic-obstetric changes after loss of massive excess weight following bariatric surgery, *J Am Coll Nutr* 7:147, 1988.

Diokno AC, Brown MD, Brock BM, et al: Prevalence and outcome of surgery for female incontinence, *Urology* 33:285, 1989.

Dwyer PL, Lee ETC, Hay DM: Obesity and urinary incontinence in women, *Br J Obstet Gynaecol* 95:91, 1988.

Dwyer PL, Teele JS: Prazosin: a neglected cause of genuine stress incontinence, *Obstet Gynecol* 79:117, 1992.

Julian TM: Pseudoincontinence secondary to unopposed estrogen replacement in the surgically castrate premenopausal female, *Obstet Gynecol* 70:382, 1987.

### Bladder Training

Fantl JA, Wyman JF, McClish DK, et al: Efficacy of bladder training in older women with urinary incontinence, *JAMA* 265:609, 1991.

Hadley EC: Bladder training and related therapies for urinary incontinence in older people, *JAMA* 256:372, 1986.

McClish DK, Fantl JA, Wyman JF, et al: Bladder training in older women with urinary incontinence: relationship between outcome and changes in urodynamic observations, *Obstet Gynecol* 77:281, 1991.

Wyman JF, Fantl JA: Bladder training in ambulatory care management of urinary incontinence, *Urol Nurs* 11:11, 1991.

### Physiotherapy

Bernstein IT: The pelvic floor muscles: muscle thickness in healthy and urinary-incontinent women measured by perineal ultrasonography with reference to the effect of pelvic floor training. Estrogen receptor studies, *Neurourol Urodyn* 16:237, 1997.

Bø K, Hagen RH, Kvarstein B, et al: Pelvic floor muscle exercise for the treatment of female stress urinary incontinence, *Neurourol Urodyn* 9:489, 1990.

Bø K, Larsen S: Pelvic floor muscle exercise for the treatment of female stress urinary incontinence: classification and characterization of responders, *Neurourol Urodyn* 11:497, 1992.

Burgio KL: Behavioral training for stress and urge incontinence in the community, *Gerontology* 36 (suppl 2):27, 1990.

Burns PA, Pranikoff K, Nochajski T, et al: Treatment of stress incontinence with pelvic floor exercises and biofeedback, *J Am Geriatr Soc* 38:341, 1990.

Caputo RM, Benson JT, McClellan E: Intravaginal maximal electrical stimulation in the treatment of urinary incontinence, *J Reprod Med* 38:667, 1993.

Dougherty MC, Bishop KR, Mooney RA, et al: The effect of circumvaginal muscle exercise, *Nurs Res* 38:331, 1989.

Dougherty MC, Bishop KR, Mooney RA, et al: Graded exercise: effect of pressures developed by the pelvic muscles. In Funk SG, Tornquist EM, Champagne MT, et al, eds: *Key aspects of elder care: managing falls, incontinence, and cognitive impairment,* New York, 1992, Springer.

Eriksen BC: Electrostimulation of the pelvic floor in female urinary incontinence, *Acta Obstet Gynecol Scand* 69:359, 1990.

Eriksen BC, Bergmann S, Mjølnerød OK: Effect of anal electrostimulation with the "Incontan" device in women with urinary incontinence, *Br J Obstet Gynaecol* 94:147, 1987.

Eriksen BC, Eik-Nes SH: Long-term electrostimulation of the pelvic floor: primary therapy in stress incontinence? *Urol Int* 44:90, 1989.

Eriksen BC, Mjølnerød OK: Changes in urodynamic measurements after successful anal electrostimulation in female urinary incontinence, *Br J Urol* 59:45, 1987.

Erlandson BE, Fall M: Intravaginal electrical stimulation in urinary incontinence. An experimental and clinical study, *Scand J Urol Nephrol* 44 (suppl):1, 1977.

Fall M, Ahlstrom K, Carlsson CA, et al: Contelle: pelvic floor stimulator for female stress-urge incontinence, *Urology* 27:282, 1986.

Fall M, Erlandson C, Carlsson A, et al: Effects of electrical intravaginal stimulation on bladder volume. An experimental and clinical study, *Urol Int* 33:440, 1978.

Ferguson KL, McKey PL, Bishop KR, et al: Stress urinary incontinence: effect of pelvic muscle exercise, *Obstet Gynecol* 75:671, 1990.

Fossberg E, Sørensen S, Ruutu M, et al: Maximal electrical stimulation in the treatment of unstable detrusor and urge incontinence, *Eur Urol* 18:120, 1990.

Gallo ML, Staskin DR: Cues to action: pelvic floor muscle exercise compliance in women with stress urinary incontinence, *Neurourol Urodyn* 16:167, 1997.

Godec C, Fravel R, Cass AS: Optimal parameters of electrical stimulation in the treatment of urinary incontinence, *Invest Urol* 18:239, 1981.

Godec C, Kralj B: Selection of patients with urinary incontinence for application of functional electrical stimulation, *Urol Int* 31:124, 1976.

Klarskov P, Belving D, Bischoff N, et al: Pelvic floor exercise versus surgery for female urinary stress incontinence, *Urol Int* 41:129, 1986.

Kondo A, Yamada Y, Niijima R: Treatment of stress incontinence by vaginal cones: short- and long-term results and predictive parameters, *Br J Urol* 76:464, 1995.

Kralj B: The treatment of female urinary incontinence by functional electrical stimulation. In Ostergard DR, Bent AE, eds: *Urogynecology and urodynamics,* ed 3, Baltimore, 1991, Williams & Wilkins.

Lamhut P, Jackson TW, Wall LL: The treatment of urinary incontinence with electrical stimulation in nursing home patients: a pilot study, *J Am Geriatr Soc* 40:48, 1992.

Lindstrom S, Fall M, Carlsson CA, et al: The neurophysiological basis of bladder inhibition in response to intravaginal electrical stimulation, *J Urol* 129:405, 1983.

Nygaard IE, Kreder KJ, Lepic MM, et al: Efficacy of pelvic floor muscle exercises in women with stress, urge, and mixed urinary incontinence, *Am J Obstet Gynecol* 174:120, 1996.

Peattie AB, Plevnik S, Stanton SL: Vaginal cones: a conservative method of treating genuine stress incontinence, *Br J Obstet Gynaecol* 95:1049, 1988.

Petersen T, Just-Christensen JE, Kousgaard P, et al: Anal sphincter maximum functional electrical stimulation in detrusor hyperreflexia, *J Urol* 152:1460, 1994.

Plevnik S: Electrical therapy. In Stanton SL, ed: *Clinical gynecologic urology,* St Louis, 1984, Mosby.

Sampselle CM, Brink CA, Wells TJ: Digital measurement of pelvic muscle strength in childbearing women, *Nurs Res* 38:134, 1990.

Sand PK, Richardson DA, Staskin DR, et al: Pelvic floor electrical stimulation in the treatment of genuine stress incontinence: a multicenter, placebo-controlled trial, *Am J Obstet Gynecol* 173:72, 1995.

Schiøtz HA: One month maximal electrostimulation for genuine stress incontinence in women, *Neurourol Urodyn* 13:43, 1994.

Smith JJ: Intravaginal stimulation randomized trial, *J Urol* 155:127, 1996.

Sundin T, Carlsson CA: Reconstruction of several dorsal roots innervating the urinary bladder: an experimental study in cats. I. Studies on the normal afferent pathways in the pelvic and pudendal nerves, *Scand J Urol Nephrol* 6:176, 1972.

Sundin T, Carlsson CA, Koch NG: Detrusor inhibition induced from mechanical stimulation of the anal region and from electrical stimulation of the pudendal nerve afferents, *Invest Urol* 11:374, 1974.

Susset J, Galea G, Manbeck K, et al: A predictive score index for the outcome of associated biofeedback and vaginal electrical stimulation in the treatment of female incontinence, *J Urol* 153:1461, 1995.

Tanagho EA, Schmidt RA, Orvis BR: Neural stimulation for control of voiding dysfunction: a preliminary report in 22 patients with serious neuropathic voiding disorders, *J Urol* 142:340, 1989.

Tapp AJS, Hills B, Cardozo LD: Randomized study comparing pelvic floor physiotherapy with the Burch colposuspension, *Neurourol Urodyn* 8:356, 1989.

Tries J: Kegel exercises enhanced by biofeedback, *J Enterostomal Ther* 17:67, 1990.

Trontelj JV, Janko M, Godec C, et al: Electrical stimulation for urinary incontinence, *Urol Int* 29:213, 1974.

Wall LL, Davidson TG: The role of muscular re-education by physical therapy in the treatment of genuine stress urinary incontinence, *Obstet Gynecol Surv* 47:322, 1992.

Wells TJ: Pelvic (floor) muscle exercise, *J Am Geriatr Soc* 38:333, 1990.

Wells TJ, Brink CA, Diokno AC, et al: Pelvic muscle exercise for stress urinary incontinence in elderly women, *JAMA* 39:785, 1991.

**Pharmacologic Treatment: Estrogen**

Abrams R, Stanley H, Carter R, et al: Effect of conjugated estrogens on vaginal blood flow in surgically menopausal women, *Am J Obstet Gynecol* 13:374, 1982.

Ahlström K, Sandahl B, Sjöberg B, et al: Effect of combined treatment with phenylpropanolamine and estriol, compared with estriol treatment alone, in postmenopausal women with stress urinary incontinence, *Gynecol Obstet Invest* 30:37, 1990.

Bergman A, Karram M, Bhatia N: Changes in urethral cytology following estrogen administration, *Gynecol Obstet Invest* 29:211, 1990.

Beisland HO, Fossberg E, Moer A, et al: Urethral sphincteric insufficiency in postmenopausal females: treatment with phenylpropanolamine and estriol separately and in combination, *Urol Int* 39:211, 1984.

Bhatia NN, Bergman A, Karram MM: Effects of estrogen on urethral function in women with urinary incontinence, *Am J Obstet Gynecol* 160:176, 1989.

Bump RC, Friedman CI: Intraluminal urethral pressure measurements in the female baboon: effects of hormonal manipulation, *J Urol* 136:508, 1986.

Cardozo L: Role of estrogens in the treatment of female urinary incontinence, *J Am Geriatr Soc* 38:326, 1990.

Cardozo L, Bachmann G, McClish D, et al: Meta-analysis of estrogen therapy in the management of urogenital atrophy in postmenopausal women: second report of the Hormones and Urogenital Therapy Committee, *Obstet Gynecol* 92:722, 1998.

Faber P, Heidenreich J: Treatment of stress incontinence with estrogen in postmenopausal women, *Urol Int* 32:221, 1977.

Fantl JA, Bump RC, Robinson D, et al: Efficacy of estrogen supplementation in the treatment of urinary incontinence, *Obstet Gynecol* 88:745, 1996.

Fantl JA, Cardozo L, McClish DK, et al: Estrogen therapy in the management of urinary incontinence in postmenopausal women: a meta-analysis. First report of the Hormones and Urogenital Therapy Committee, *Obstet Gynecol* 82:12, 1994.

Hilton P, Stanton SL: The use of intravaginal oestrogen cream in genuine stress incontinence, *Br J Obstet Gynaecol* 90:940, 1983.

Hilton P, Tweddel AL, Mayne C: Oral and intravaginal estrogens alone and in combination with alpha-adrenergic stimulation in genuine stress incontinence, *Int Urogynecol J* 1:80, 1990.

Kinn AC, Lindskog M: Estrogens and phenylpropanolamine in combination for stress urinary incontinence in postmenopausal women, *Urology* 32:273, 1988.

Miodrag A, Castleden CM, Vallance TR: Sex hormones and the female urinary tract, *Drugs* 36:491, 1988.

Molander U, Milsom I, Ekelund P, et al: Effect of oral oestriol on vaginal flora and cytology and urogenital symptoms in postmenopause, *Maturitas* 12:113, 1990.

Onuoro CO, Ardoin JA, Dunnihoo DR, et al: Vaginal estrogen therapy in the treatment of urinary tract symptoms in postmenopausal women, *Int Urogynecol J* 2:3, 1991.

Rud T: The effects of estrogens and gestagens on the urethral pressure profile in urinary continent and stress incontinent women, *Acta Obstet Gynecol Scand* 59:265, 1980.

Samsioe G, Jansson I, Mellström D, et al: Occurrence, nature and treatment of urinary incontinence in a 70-year-old female population, *Maturitas* 7:335, 1985.

Schreiter F, Fuchs P, Stockamp K: Estrogenic sensitivity of α-receptors in the urethra musculature, *Urol Int* 31:13, 1976.

Semmens JP, Wagner G: Estrogen deprivation and vaginal function in postmenopausal women, *JAMA* 248:445, 1982.

Ulmsten U, Stormby N: Evaluation of the urethral mucosa before and after oestrogen treatment in postmenopausal women with a new sampling technique, *Gynecol Obstet Invest* 24:208, 1987.

Versi E, Cardozo L, Studd J: Long-term effects of estradiol implants on the female urinary tract during the climacteric, *Int Urogynecol J* 1:87, 1990.

Walter S, Kjaergaard B, Lose G, et al: Stress urinary incontinence in postmenopausal women treated with oral estrogen (estriol) and alpha-adrenoreceptor-stimulating agent (phenylpropanolamine): a randomized double blind placebo-controlled study, *Int Urogynecol J* 1:74, 1990.

Walter S, Wolf H, Barlebo H, et al: Urinary incontinence in postmenopausal women treated with estrogens, *Urol Int* 33:135, 1978.

Wilson PD, Faragher B, Butler B, et al: Treatment with oral piperazine oestrone sulphate for genuine stress incontinence in postmenopausal women, *Br J Obstet Gynaecol* 94:568, 1987.

**Pharmacologic Treatment: Nonhormonal**

Awad SA, Downie JW, Kiruluta HG: Alpha-adrenergic agents in urinary disorders of the proximal urethra. I. Sphincteric incontinence, *Br J Urol* 50:332, 1978.

Bernstein E, Diskant BM: Phenylpropanolamine: a potentially hazardous drug, *Ann Emerg Med* 11:311, 1982.

Collste L, Lindskog M: Phenylpropanolamine in treatment of female stress urinary incontinence, *Urology* 30:398, 1987.

Diokno A, Taub M: Ephedrine in treatment of urinary incontinence, *Urology* 5:624, 1975.

Donker P, van der Sluis C: Action of beta adrenergic blocking agents on the urethral pressure profile, *Urol Int* 31:6, 1976.

Ek A, Andersson KE, Gullberg B, et al: The effects of long-term treatment with norephedrine on stress incontinence and urethral closure pressure profile, *Scand J Urol Nephrol* 12:105, 1978.

Fossberg E, Beisland HO, Lundgren RA: Stress incontinence in females: treatment with phenylpropanolamine, *Urol Int* 38:293, 1983.

Gilja I, Radej M, Kovacic M, et al: Conservative treatment of female stress incontinence with imipramine, *J Urol* 132:909, 1984.

Gleason D, Reilly R, Bottaccini M, et al: The urethral continence zone and its relation to stress incontinence, *J Urol* 112:81, 1974.

Lehtonen T, Rannikko S, Lindell O, et al: The effect of phenylpropanolamine on female stress urinary incontinence, *Ann Chir Gynaecol* 75:236, 1986.

Liebson I, Bigelow G, Griffiths R, et al: Phenylpropanolamine effects on subjective and cardiovascular variables at recommended over-the-counter dose levels, *J Clin Pharmacol* 27:685, 1987.

Lose G, Diernæs E, Rix P: Does medical therapy cure female stress incontinence? *Urol Int* 44:25, 1989.

Montague DK, Stewart BH: Urethral pressure profiles before and after Ornade administration in patients with stress urinary incontinence, *J Urol* 122:198, 1979.

Öbrink A. Bunne G: The effect of alpha-adrenergic stimulation in stress incontinence, *Scand J Urol Nephrol* 12:205, 1978.

Stewart BH, Banowsky LHW, Montague DK: Stress incontinence: conservative therapy with sympathomimetic drugs, *J Urol* 115:558, 1978

Wein AJ: Pharmacologic treatment of incontinence, *J Am Geriatr Soc* 38:317, 1990.

## Mechanical Devices

Abu-Sitta MK, Kapur G, Enhorning G: Stress incontinence alleviated by an intravaginal device, *Int Urogynecol J* 6:95, 1995.

Bhatia N, Bergman A, Gunning J: Urodynamic effects of a vaginal pessary in women with stress urinary incontinence, *Am J Obstet Gynecol* 147:876, 1983.

Davila GW: Vaginal prolapse: management with nonsurgical techniques, *Postgrad Med* 99:171, 1996.

Davila GW, Ostermann KV: The bladder neck support prosthesis: a nonsurgical approach to stress incontinence in adult women, *Am J Obstet Gynecol* 171:206, 1994.

Miller JL, Bavendam T: Treatment with the Reliance urinary control insert: one-year experience, *J Endourol* 10:287, 1996.

Nygaard I: Prevention of exercise incontinence with mechanical devices, *J Reprod Med* 40:89, 1995.

Realini JP, Walters MD: Vaginal diaphragm rings in the treatment of stress urinary incontinence, *J Am Board Fam Pract* 3:99, 1990.

Staskin D, Bavendam T, Miller J, et al: Effectiveness of a urinary control insert in the management of stress urinary incontinence: early results of a multicenter study, *Urology* 47:629, 1996.

Suarez GM, Baum NH, Jacobs J: Use of standard contraceptive diaphragm in management of stress urinary incontinence, *Urology* 37:119, 1991.

Sulak PJ, Kuehl TJ, Shull BL: Vaginal pessaries and their use in pelvic relaxation, *J Reprod Med* 38:919, 1993.

Versi E, Griffiths DJ, Harvey M: A new external urethral occlusive device for female urinary incontinence, *Obstet Gynecol* 92:286, 1998.

## Self-Help Guides

Burgio KL, Pearce KL, Lucco AJ: *Staying dry. A practical guide to bladder control,* Baltimore, 1989, Johns Hopkins.

Chalker R, Whitmore KE: *Overcoming bladder disorders,* New York, 1990, Harper & Row.

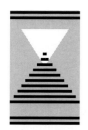

CHAPTER **14**

# Retropubic Operations for Genuine Stress Incontinence

Mark D. Walters

Since 1949, when Marshall et al. first described retropubic urethrovesical suspension for the treatment of stress urinary incontinence, retropubic procedures have emerged as consistently curative. Although numerous terminologies and variations of retropubic repairs have been described, the basic goal remains the same: to suspend and to stabilize the anterior vaginal wall, and thus the bladder neck and proximal urethra, in a retropubic position. This prevents their descent and allows urethral compression against a stable suburethral layer. Selection of a retropubic approach (versus a vaginal approach) depends on many factors, such as the need for laparotomy for other pelvic disease, the amount of pelvic organ relaxation, the status of the intrinsic urethral sphincter mechanism, the age and health status of the patient, and the preference and expertise of the surgeon.

Few data differentiate one retropubic procedure from another, although all have advantages and disadvantages. This chapter describes the surgical techniques for the three most studied and popular retropubic procedures: the Burch colposuspension, the Marshall-Marchetti-Krantz (MMK) procedure, and the paravaginal defect repair. The surgical techniques described herein are contemporary modifications of the original operations: Tanagho (1976) described the modified Burch colposuspension, and Krantz (1986) described the MMK technique. The paravaginal defect repair has been described by Richardson et al. (1981) and Shull and Baden (1989) (paravaginal repair) and by Turner-Warwick (1986) and Webster and Kreder (1990) (vaginal obturator shelf repair). Although less critically studied, this technique is regionally popular and widely performed in the United States. The operations described do not represent one correct technique but a commonly used and proven method.

This chapter describes only retropubic suspension procedures that use an abdominal wall incision for direct access into the space of Retzius. The use of laparoscopy and miniincision laparotomy to enter the retropubic space and perform these and similar procedures is expanding, both in terms of clinical experience and in research. The reader is encouraged to see Chapter 16 for a thorough critique of the use of operative laparoscopy for urinary incontinence and prolapse.

## INDICATIONS FOR RETROPUBIC PROCEDURES

Retropubic urethrovesical suspension procedures are indicated for women with the diagnosis of genuine stress incontinence (GSI) and a hypermobile proximal urethra and bladder neck. These procedures yield the best results when the urethral sphincter is capable of maintaining a watertight seal at rest but cannot withstand the unequal transmission of abdominal pressure to the proximal urethra, relative to the bladder, with straining. This situation corresponds to types I and II GSI as described by McGuire (1981). Although retropubic procedures can be used for intrinsic sphincter deficiency with urethral hypermobility, other more obstructive operations probably yield better long-term results (see Chapter 15).

To diagnose GSI, clinical and urodynamic (simple or complex) tests must be performed to evaluate bladder filling, storage, and emptying. Clinically, the urethra is shown to be incompetent by visually observing loss of urine simultaneous with increases in intraabdominal pressure. Urodynamic or radiologic methods may also be used for diagnosis.

Abnormalities of bladder-filling function, such as detrusor instability, can coexist with urethral sphincter incompetence in up to 30% of patients and may be associated with a lower cure rate after retropubic surgery.

Women with GSI should generally have a trial of conservative therapy before corrective surgery is offered. Conservative treatment comes in the form of pelvic muscle exercises, bladder retraining, pharmacologic therapy, functional electrical stimulation, and mechanical devices, such as pessaries. Eligible postmenopausal patients with atrophic urogenital changes should be prescribed estrogen before surgery is considered.

## SURGICAL TECHNIQUES
### Operative Setup and General Entry into the Retropubic Space

The patient is supine, with the legs supported in a slightly abducted position, allowing the surgeon to operate with one hand in the vagina and the other in the retropubic space. The vagina, perineum, and abdomen are sterilely prepped and draped in a fashion that permits easy access to the lower abdomen and vagina. A three-way 16- or 20-French Foley catheter with a 20- to 30-ml balloon is inserted sterilely into the bladder and kept in the sterile field. The drainage port of the catheter is left to gravity drainage, and the irrigation port is connected to sterile water with or without blue dye. One perioperative intravenous dose of an appropriate antibiotic should be given as prophylaxis against infection.

A Pfannenstiel or Cherney incision is made. During intraperitoneal surgery, the peritoneum is opened, the surgery is completed, and the cul-de-sac is plicated, if necessary. The retropubic space is then exposed. Staying close to the back of the pubic bone, the surgeon's hand is introduced into the retropubic space and the bladder and urethra gently moved downward. Sharp dissection is not usually necessary in primary cases. To aid visualization of the bladder, 100 ml sterile water with methylene blue or indigo carmine dye may be instilled into the bladder after the catheter drainage port is clamped.

If previous retropubic or needle suspension procedures have been performed, dense adhesions from the anterior bladder wall and urethra to the symphysis pubis are often present. These adhesions should be dissected sharply from the pubic bone until the anterior bladder wall, urethra, and vagina are free of adhesions and are mobile. If identification of the urethra or lower border of the bladder is difficult, one may perform a cystotomy, which, with a finger inside the bladder, helps to define the bladder's lower limits for easier dissection, mobilization, and elevation.

### Burch Colposuspension

After the retropubic space is entered, the urethra and anterior vaginal wall are depressed. No dissection should be performed in the midline over the urethra or at the ure-

throvesical junction, thus protecting the delicate musculature of the urethra from surgical trauma. Attention is directed to the tissue on either side of the urethra. The surgeon's nondominant hand is placed in the vagina, palm facing upward, with the index and middle fingers on each side of the proximal urethra. Most of the overlying fat should be cleared away, using a swab mounted on a curved forceps. This dissection is accomplished with forceful elevation of the surgeon's vaginal finger until glistening white periurethral fascia and vaginal wall are seen (Fig. 14-1). This area is extremely vascular, with a rich, thin-walled venous plexus that should be avoided, if possible. The position of the urethra and the lower edge of the bladder is determined by palpating the Foley balloon and by partially distending the bladder to define the rounded lower margin of the bladder as it meets the anterior vaginal wall.

Once dissection lateral to the urethra is completed and vaginal mobility is judged to be adequate by using the vaginal fingers to lift the anterior vaginal wall upward and forward, sutures are placed. No. 0 or 1 delayed absorbable or nonabsorbable sutures are placed as far laterally in the anterior vaginal wall as is technically possible. We apply two sutures of No. 0 braided polyester on an SH needle (Ethibond; Ethicon, Inc., Somerville, NJ) bilaterally, using double bites for each suture. The distal suture is placed approximately 2 cm lateral to the proximal third of the urethra. The proximal suture is placed approximately 2 cm

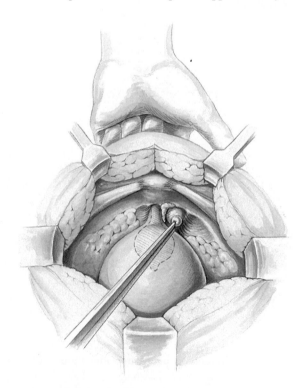

**Fig. 14-1** Dissection of the lateral retropubic space. After forceful elevation of the surgeon's vaginal finger, the fat overlying the glistening white periurethral fascia is cleared in preparation for suture placement.

lateral to the bladder wall at or slightly proximal to the level of the urethrovesical junction. In placing the sutures, one should take a full thickness of vaginal wall, excluding the epithelium, with the needle parallel to the urethra (Fig. 14-2, *inset*). This maneuver is best accomplished by suturing over the surgeon's vaginal finger at the appropriate selected sites. On each side, after the two sutures are placed, they are passed through the pectineal (Cooper's) ligament so that all four suture ends exit above the ligament (Fig. 14-2). Before the sutures are tied, a 1 × 4 cm strip of Gelfoam may be placed between the vagina and obturator fascia below Cooper's ligament to aid adherence and hemostasis.

As noted previously, this area is extremely vascular, and visible vessels should be avoided if possible. When excessive bleeding occurs, it can be controlled by direct pressure, sutures, or vascular clips. Less severe bleeding usually stops with direct pressure and after tying the fixation sutures.

After all four sutures are placed in the vagina and through the Cooper's ligaments, the assistant ties first the distal sutures and then the proximal ones, while the surgeon elevates the vagina with the vaginal hand. In tying the sutures, one does not have to be concerned about whether the vaginal wall meets Cooper's ligament, so one should not place too much tension on the vaginal wall. A suture bridge may be placed between the two points without causing complications. After the sutures are tied, one can easily insert two fingers between the pubic bone and the urethra, thus preventing compression of the urethra against the pubic bone. Vaginal fixation and urethral support depend more on fibro-sis and scarring of periurethral and vaginal tissues over the obturator internus fascia than on the suture material itself.

## Marshall-Marchetti-Krantz Procedure

The retropubic space is exposed and the urethra and bladder base palpated with the Foley catheter in place. The surgeon's nondominant hand is placed into the vagina and the index and middle fingers are placed at the urethrovesical neck on either side of the urethra. Gentle dissection of periurethral fat is made at the urethrovesical junction on each side over the vaginal fingers. This area is extremely vascular, having a rich, thin-walled venous plexus that should be avoided, if possible. Some surgeons perform a cystotomy routinely to aid periurethral dissection and suture placement.

Delayed absorbable sutures are usually used and are placed at right angles to the urethra and parallel to the vesical neck. A single suture is placed bilaterally at the urethrovesical junction. A double bite is taken over the surgeon's finger, incorporating full thickness of the vaginal wall but excluding the vaginal epithelium. After placement of the sutures, the point of fixation of the urethra to the symphysis pubis can be determined by elevating the two vaginal fingers to the point where the vesical neck comes in contact with the pubic symphysis and noting the position at which the sutures will be placed into the pubic periosteum. The needle is placed medially to laterally against the periosteum and turned with a simple wrist action. It may involve the cartilage in the midline, depending on the width, thickness, and availability of the periosteum. The sutures on each

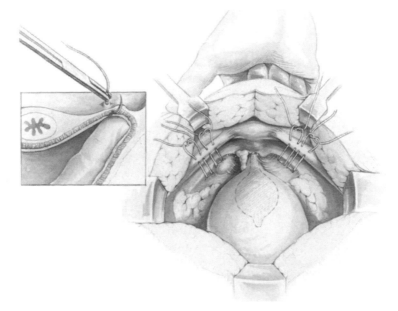

**Fig. 14-2** Technique of Burch colposuspension. After the two sutures are placed on each side, they are passed through the pectineal (Cooper's) ligament, so that all four suture ends exit above the ligament to facilitate knot tying. *Inset:* In placing the sutures, one should take a full thickness of vaginal wall, excluding the epithelium, with the needle parallel to the urethra. This maneuver is best achieved by suturing over the vaginal finger.

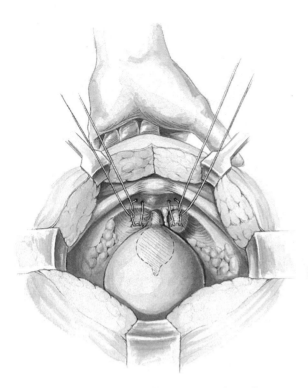

**Fig. 14-3** Marshall-Marchetti-Krantz procedure. One suture is placed bilaterally at the level of the bladder neck and then into the periosteum of the pubic symphysis.

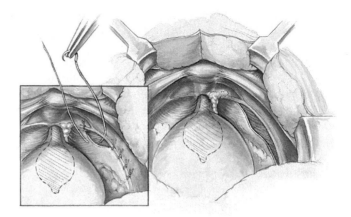

**Fig. 14-4** Lateral paravaginal defect and technique of paravaginal repair. Five or six sutures are placed, first through the full thickness of the vagina (excluding the vaginal epithelium), and then into the obturator internus fascia or arcus tendineus fasciae pelvis, 3 to 4 cm below the obturator fossa.

side are placed accordingly and tied, with the vaginal finger elevating the urethrovesical junction (Fig. 14-3). Venous bleeding is usually controlled by tying the sutures or with direct pressure.

## Paravaginal Defect Repair

The object of the paravaginal defect repair is to reattach, bilaterally, the anterolateral vaginal sulcus with its overlying endopelvic fascia to the pubococcygeus and obturator internus muscles and fascia at the level of the arcus tendineus fasciae pelvis. The retropubic space is entered, and the bladder and vagina are depressed and pulled medially to allow visualization of the lateral retropubic space, including the obturator internus muscle, and the fossa containing the obturator neurovascular bundle. Blunt dissection can be carried dorsally from this point until the ischial spine is palpated. The arcus tendineus fasciae pelvis is often visualized as a white band of tissue running over the pubococcygeus and obturator internus muscles from the back of the lower edge of the symphysis pubis toward the ischial spine. A lateral paravaginal defect representing avulsion of the vagina off the arcus tendineus fasciae pelvis or of the arcus tendineus fasciae pelvis off the obturator internus muscle may be visualized (Fig. 14-4).

The surgeon's nondominant hand is inserted into the vagina. While gently retracting the vagina and bladder medially, the surgeon elevates the anterolateral vaginal sulcus. Starting near the vaginal apex, a suture is placed, first through the full thickness of the vagina (excluding the vagi-

nal epithelium) and then into the obturator internus fascia or arcus tendineus fasciae pelvis, 1 to 2 cm anterior to its origin at the ischial spine. After this first stitch is tied, additional (four or five) sutures are placed through the vaginal wall and overlying fascia and then into the obturator internus at about 1-cm intervals toward the pubic ramus (Fig. 14-4, *inset*). The most distal suture should be placed as close as possible to the pubic ramus, into the pubourethral ligament. No. 2-0 or 3-0 nonabsorbable suture on a medium-sized, tapered needle is usually used for the paravaginal repair.

The vaginal obturator shelf procedure enters the retropubic space as noted previously, but does not continue dissection to the ischial spine. Three interrupted No. 0 or 1 nonabsorbable or delayed absorbable sutures are placed bilaterally at 1-cm intervals through the paravaginal fascia and vaginal wall (excluding the vaginal epithelium), beginning at the urethrovesical junction and continuing proximally toward the bladder base. These sutures are then passed horizontally through the adjacent obturator fascia and underlying muscle and tied. To fill the retropubic dead space, the peritoneum is opened and an omental pedicle is brought down into the retropubic space.

These procedures leave free space between the symphysis pubis and the proximal urethra but secure support so that rotational descent of the proximal urethra and bladder base is prevented with sudden increases in intraabdominal pressure. According to Turner-Warwick (1986), these procedures avoid overcorrection and fixation of the periurethral fascia, which might compromise the functional movements of the urethra and bladder base and lead to obstruction and voiding difficulty. This principle may explain why the paravaginal defect repair usually results in spontaneous voiding on the first or second postoperative day. In fact, the vaginal obturator shelf repair has been used to correct patients with dysfunctional voiding symptoms after previous retropubic surgery.

## General Intraoperative and Postoperative Procedures

If the surgeon is concerned that intravesical suture placement or ureteral obstruction may have occurred, cystoscopy—either transurethrally or through the dome of the bladder—or cystotomy may be performed to document ureteral patency and absence of intravesical sutures after retropubic procedures.

Closed suction drains in the retropubic space are used only as necessary when hemostasis is incomplete and there is concern about postoperative hematoma. The bladder is routinely drained with a suprapubic or transurethral catheter for 1 to 2 days. After that time, the patient is allowed to begin voiding trials and postvoid residual urine volumes are checked, either with the suprapubic catheter or by intermittent self-catheterization.

## CLINICAL RESULTS

Many studies report clinical experiences with retropubic urethral suspension procedures for stress urinary incontinence. Although most of these studies are methodologically flawed, increasing numbers of high-quality studies, including prospective randomized trials, are being conducted. Currently, however, few prospective studies are available comparing the results of the various procedures for GSI.

Mainprize and Drutz (1988) summarized 56 articles reporting results of MMK procedures up to 1988. Few of these articles used preoperative diagnostic urodynamic tests and only Milani et al. (1985) reported postoperative urodynamic data after 1 year. Of 2712 cases, 2334 (86.1%) succeeded, 73 (2.7%) improved, and 305 (11.2%) failed. The success rate of primary MMK procedures was 92.1%; the success rate was 84.5% when the MMK procedure was used for recurrent incontinence.

In the study by Milani et al. (1985), the rate of continence confirmed by urodynamic studies was 71% after 1 year. After MMK procedures, the recurrence of stress incontinence increases over time: the longer the observation period, the more cases of recurrence are seen. Using a self-reported interview, Park and Miller (1988) showed that 86% of patients treated with primary MMK procedures were cured during the first 3 years after surgery and only 66% were still continent after 3 to 10 years.

Only a few studies have been done assessing the paravaginal defect repair for GSI. Early studies using subjective outcome measures reported that over 90% of women were continent after this procedure. However, in a prospective randomized trial, Columbo et al. (1996) found that only 61% of women were continent 3 years after a paravaginal defect repair compared with 100% of women continent after a Burch colposuspension. We currently believe that the paravaginal defect repair should be used for anatomic correction of anterior vaginal wall prolapse but not as primary treatment of GSI.

The Burch colposuspension is the best-studied retropubic

procedure. From 1980 to 1990, at least 18 studies reported using the Burch colposuspension in women with urodynamically proved GSI with objective measures of cure. Follow-up times ranged from 3 months to 7 years. At 3 to 24 months after surgery, 59% to 100% of patients became continent, for an overall average cure rate of 84%. At 3 to 7 years, continence rates range from 63% to 89%, for an average rate of 77%. Although objectively incontinent, a small percentage of additional patients were judged to be improved and satisfied with their surgical results. The overall reported absolute failure rate is 13.6% at 3 to 24 months and 14% at 5 to 7 years.

In an excellent study, Eriksen et al. (1990) reported 91 women with urodynamically proved GSI, with or without bladder stability, who had undergone Burch colposuspension. Urodynamic evaluation was done on 76 patients after 5 years. Stress incontinence was cured in 71% of the patients with stable bladders preoperatively and in 57% of those with stress incontinence and detrusor instability, a nonsignificant difference. After 5 years, only 52% of the study group was completely dry and free of complications; about 30% needed further incontinence therapy.

Several studies have been done that assessed women more than 10 years after undergoing a Burch procedure. Alcalay et al. (1995) followed a cohort of 109 women (out of a group of 366 eligible women) who underwent Burch colposuspension between 1974 and 1983. The mean follow-up interval was 13.8 years. Both subjective and objective outcome measures were collected during the follow-up period. The cure of incontinence was found to be time-dependent, with a decline for 10 to 12 years and then a plateau at 69% (Fig. 14-5). Cure rates were significantly lower in woman who had had previous bladder neck surgery. Approximately 10% of patients required at least one additional surgery to cure her stress incontinence.

Several review articles have been published comparing the cure rates of retropubic procedures with those of other procedures for the treatment of GSI. In 1994, Jarvis reviewed the studies after 1970 that addressed surgical treatment of GSI using objective outcome measures. As has been shown with other studies, the cure rates for surgical treatment of recurrent incontinence are generally somewhat lower than for first procedures. Jarvis noted that only the MMK procedure, the Burch colposuspension, endoscopic bladder neck suspension, and sling procedures produce mean continence rates above 85% for primary procedures and above 80% for repeat procedures. He also noted that the average cure rates of only colposuspension and sling procedures have tight confidence intervals, implying that studies describing these procedures have yielded the most consistent results.

Black and Downs published an excellent systematic review in 1996 describing the effectiveness of surgery for stress incontinence in women. The methodological quality of studies was assessed, including all of the randomized controlled trials to that time. Only two randomized con-

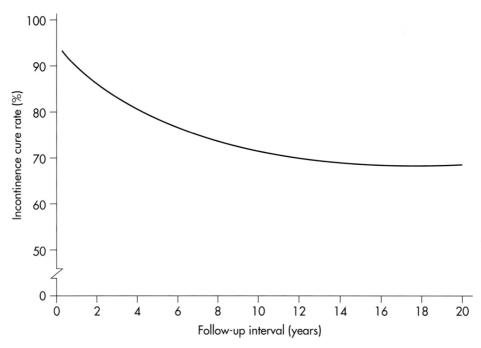

**Fig. 14-5**   Long-term cure rate after Burch colposuspension for genuine stress incontinence (after Alcalay et al. [1995]).

trolled trials of colposuspension were available. The study noted that different methods of performing colposuspension (e.g., Burch colposuspension and MMK procedure) have not been shown to be associated with significant differences in outcome. There is preliminary evidence that laparoscopic colposuspension and open paravaginal defect repair may have somewhat lower cure rates than open Burch procedures. Colposuspension appears to be more effective than anterior colporrhaphy and needle urethropexy procedures in curing and improving stress incontinence. About 85% of women can expect to be continent 1 year after colposuspension, compared to 50% to 70% after anterior colporrhaphy and needle suspension. Primary procedures are generally more effective than repeat procedures. The benefit of Burch colposuspension is maintained for at least 5 years, whereas the benefits from anterior colporrhaphy and needle suspension diminish quite rapidly. Of the four prospective studies comparing Burch colposuspension and sling procedures, none report a difference in cure, however defined, regardless of whether the operations were carried out as primary or secondary operations.

The American Urological Association convened the Female Stress Urinary Incontinence Clinical Guidelines Panel to analyze the literature up to 1993 regarding surgical procedures for treating stress urinary incontinence. The data from this meta-analysis indicate that after 48 months, retropubic suspensions and sling procedures seem to be more efficacious than transvaginal needle suspension procedures or anterior colporrhaphy. The panel's opinion also noted that retropubic suspensions and sling procedures are associated

with slightly higher complication rates, including longer convalescence and postoperative voiding dysfunction.

Clinical conditions that increase the risk of surgical failure for retropubic urethropexy are shown in Box 14-1. They include obesity, menopause, prior hysterectomy, and prior antiincontinence procedures. Advanced age does not appear to be associated with lower rates of cure after colposuspension, although one study described a somewhat higher mean age in patients who failed incontinence surgery. Urodynamic findings that increase the risk of surgical failure include signs of intrinsic urethral sphincter deficiency, abnormal perineal electromyography, and concurrent detrusor instability. Patients with intrinsic sphincter deficiency probably are better treated with a more obstructive operation, such as a sling procedure, if the urethra is hypermobile, or with periurethral injections of a bulking agent if the urethra is nonmobile.

Detrusor instability or urge incontinence may coexist in up to 30% of patients with GSI. The term *mixed incontinence* has been used to describe this condition. In addition, about 15% of patients with GSI who preoperatively have a stable cystometrogram develop de novo detrusor instability after a colposuspension procedure. The course of the detrusor instability after a retropubic repair in patients with mixed incontinence is unpredictable. Interestingly, some studies demonstrate that 50% to 60% of patients with mixed incontinence are cured of their detrusor instability by surgical support of the bladder neck. A much smaller percentage (approximately 5% to 10%) have worsening of their instability, with the remainder (20% to 30%) having

**Box 14-1**

**CONDITIONS THAT DECREASE THE CHANCE OF CURE OF INCONTINENCE AFTER RETROPUBIC BLADDER NECK SUSPENSION**

**Clinical**

Advanced age (?)
Hypoestrogenic state
Obesity
Prior hysterectomy
Prior procedures to correct GSI

**Urodynamic**

Detrusor instability (preoperative or postoperative)
Intrinsic urethral sphincter deficiency
    Lower maximal urethral pressure
    Lower leak point pressure
    Lower functional urethral length
    Open bladder neck at rest on video-urodynamics
    Nonmobile bladder neck
Abnormal perineal electromyography

**Surgical**

Intraoperative blood loss greater than 1000 ml

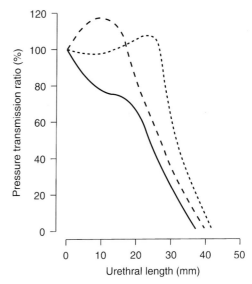

**Fig. 14-6** Pressure transmission profiles in stress incontinent women before (—) and after (– – –) successful colposuspensions, compared with a group of 20 symptom-free women (---).
From Hilton P, Stanton SL: *Br J Obstet Gynaecol* 90:934, 1983.

persistence. Unfortunately, no preoperative urodynamic parameters have been identified that can accurately predict the course of detrusor instability after incontinence surgery. For this reason, we believe that women with mixed incontinence should initially receive nonsurgical therapy. Karram and Bhatia (1989) found that 32% of women with mixed incontinence became dry after nonsurgical therapy. These data suggest that initial nonsurgical therapy will save up to one third of patients the cost and morbidity of incontinence surgery.

## MECHANISMS OF CURE

Retropubic suspension procedures elevate and stabilize the bladder neck and proximal urethra in a high retropubic position. This results, at least partially, in mechanical compression of the urethra against the stable, elevated anterior vaginal wall or the posterosuperior aspect of the symphysis pubis during episodes of increased abdominal pressure. The principal urodynamic change in urethrovesical function postoperatively is increased pressure transmission to the urethra, relative to the bladder, during elevations in intraabdominal pressure. Resting urethral pressure and functional urethral length are unchanged, suggesting that the intrinsic function of the urethra is not altered appreciably by this type of surgery. The greater the difference in preoperative and postoperative pressure transmission ratios, the more likely the patient will be continent after Burch

colposuspension. If the retropubic procedure fails to elevate and stabilize the urethra and postoperative pressure transmission ratios remain less than 100%, the patient may continue to have stress incontinence postoperatively. Appropriate elevation of the bladder neck and urethra, accompanied by pressure transmission ratios near 100%, result in continence in most patients. This concept is supported by a study by Penttinen et al. (1989b), who noted a significant negative correlation between postoperative bladder neck mobility and pressure transmission ratios, indicating that correction of the urethrovesical anatomic disorder eliminates the functional disorder and restores continence.

MMK and perhaps Burch procedures probably tend to overelevate and fix the urethra in a retropubic position. Hilton and Stanton (1983) found that pressure transmission profiles after successful Burch colposuspensions differed from those of continent control subjects, with pressure transmission ratios in the proximal half of the urethra significantly higher than 100% (Fig. 14-6). This observation suggests that an additional mechanism, probably partial outflow obstruction, results. Bump et al. (1988) determined that patients with postoperative voiding abnormalities and detrusor instability had pressure transmission ratios significantly greater than 100%, supporting the hypothesis that obstruction may play a role in post-continence-surgery voiding dysfunction and detrusor instability. Paravaginal defect repair procedures do not tend to overelevate the bladder neck and proximal urethra; thus they may have somewhat lower cure rates for stress incontinence but with fewer postoperative problems, such as urgency and voiding dysfunction.

# COMPLICATIONS
## Short-Term Postoperative

Of the retropubic procedures, the MMK procedure is the most extensively studied with regard to complications. In a thorough review of the literature, Mainprize and Drutz (1988) summarized the postoperative complications (excluding urinary retention) of MMK procedures (Table 14-1). Wound complications and urinary infections are the most common surgical complications. Direct surgical injury to the urinary tract occurs rarely. Bladder lacerations occurred in 0.7% of patients; sutures through the bladder and urethra and catheters sewn into the urethra occurred in 0.3% of patients. Ureteral obstruction occurred in 0.1% of patients. Accidental placement of sutures into the bladder during Burch colposuspension or paravaginal repair, resulting in vesical stone formation, painful voiding, recurrent cystitis, or fistula, can occur but is rare.

Ureteral obstruction occurs rarely after Burch colposuspension and results from ureteral stretching or kinking after elevation of the vagina and bladder base. One study reported three unilateral ureteral obstructions and three bilateral ureteral obstructions in 483 Burch colposuspensions (1.2%). All patients were treated successfully with removal of sutures and ureteral stenting. No cases of transected ureters have been reported. Ericksen et al. (1990) found that 1 of 75 patients (1.3%) followed for 5 years after Burch procedures had absent unilateral renal function caused by presumed complete ureteral obstruction. This patient had developed only transient postoperative fever.

Lower urinary tract fistulas are uncommon after retropubic procedures, with various types occurring after 0.3% of MMK procedures. Fistulas are probably less common after Burch and paravaginal repairs because the sutures are placed several centimeters lateral to the urethra.

**Table 14-1**  Postoperative Complications in 2712 Marshall-Marchetti-Krantz Procedures

| Type of complication | Percent |
| --- | --- |
| Wound, total | 5.5 |
|   Infection or hematoma | 3.4 |
|   Hernia or dehiscence | 1.8 |
|   Other | 0.3 |
| Urinary tract infection | 3.9 |
| Osteitis pubis | 2.5 |
| Direct surgical injury to the urinary tract | 1.6 |
|   Bladder tears | 0.7 |
|   Urethral obstruction | 0.5 |
|   Sutures through bladder or urethra with or without catheter sewn in | 0.3 |
| Ureteral obstruction or hydronephrosis | 0.1 |
| Fistula | 0.3 |
| Death | 0.2 |

Modified from Mainprize TC, Drutz HP: *Obstet Gynecol Surv* 43:724, 1988.

## Postoperative Voiding Difficulties

The incidence of voiding difficulties after colposuspension varies widely, although patients rarely have urinary retention after 30 days. Eriksen et al. (1990) found that only 2 of 91 patients had delayed spontaneous micturition after Burch colposuspension when the catheter was removed the third day postoperatively. Fifteen percent of these patients had residual urine volumes of 100 to 300 ml the fifth day after surgery. In contrast, Korda et al. (1989) had a mean postoperative catheter drainage of 10 days (range 5 to 60 days) for 174 patients after colposuspension. Twenty-five percent of these patients required catheter drainage for more than 10 days.

Lose et al. (1987) found that colposuspension can change the original micturition pattern and introduce an element of obstruction that can disturb the balance between voiding forces and outflow resistance, resulting in immediate postoperative as well as late voiding difficulties. Urodynamic findings that may occur after colposuspension include decreased flow rate, increased micturition pressure, and increased urethral resistance.

Urodynamic tests may be used to predict early postoperative voiding difficulties. Bhatia and Bergman (1984) found that all patients with adequate detrusor contraction and flow rates preoperatively were able to resume spontaneous voiding by the seventh postoperative day after Burch colposuspension. One third of patients who voided without detrusor contraction required bladder drainage for 7 days or longer. No patients with decreased flow rates and absent detrusor contraction during voiding were able to void in less than 7 days postoperatively. The use of a Valsalva maneuver during voiding may further lead to postoperative voiding difficulties, perhaps by intensifying obstruction at the bladder neck. In another study, these authors (Bhatia and Bergman, 1986) found that preoperative uroflowmetry and postvoid residual urine volumes were not predictive of postoperative voiding difficulties after Burch procedures.

## Detrusor Instability

Detrusor instability is a recognized postoperative complication of retropubic procedures. Unstable bladders as demonstrated on cystometrogram have been reported in 7% to 27% of patients with GSI and stable bladders preoperatively, with follow-up of up to 5 years after Burch colposuspension. Postoperative detrusor instability is more common in patients with previous bladder neck surgery and in those with mixed detrusor instability and GSI preoperatively. In a study of 148 patients with GSI and stable bladders preoperatively, Steel et al. (1986) reported that 24 (16.2%) patients had postoperative detrusor instability on cystometrogram 6 months after surgery. Ten of the 24 patients with detrusor instability were completely asymptomatic. Of the 14 symptomatic patients, four were improved with drugs aimed at correcting the instability. The remaining 10 patients (6.8%) remained symptomatic with detrusor instability 3 to 5 years after surgery.

The mechanism for this phenomenon is unknown. Some authors have suggested that postoperative onset of detrusor instability may be caused by disruption of the autonomic innervation of the bladder, although this relationship has not been proved. As noted previously, excessive urethral elevation or compression can lead to partial outflow obstruction and resulting detrusor instability. Whatever the mechanism, postoperative detrusor instability predictably occurs in a small but significant number of patients. Patients undergoing retropubic urethropexy should understand that the operation may cause urinary incontinence caused by detrusor instability, even if it cures their sphincteric incontinence.

## Osteitis Pubis

Osteitis pubis is a painful inflammation of periosteum, bone, cartilage, and ligaments of structures of the anterior pelvic girdle. It is a recognized postoperative complication of urologic and radical gynecologic procedures involving the prostate gland or urinary bladder. In urogynecology, osteitis pubis occurs after 0.74% to 2.5% of MMK procedures; the incidence is partially related to the diagnostic criteria used. It also can occur, although rarely, after placement of artificial urinary sphincters and after radical pelvic surgery for gynecologic malignancies.

The cause of osteitis pubis is unclear. It may result from infection, from trauma to the periosteum, or from impaired circulation in the vessels around the symphysis pubis. The disease typically occurs 2 to 12 weeks postoperatively. Osteitis pubis is characterized by suprapubic pain radiating to the thighs and exacerbated by walking or abduction of the lower extremities, marked tenderness and swelling over the symphysis pubis, and radiographic evidence of bone destruction with separation of the symphysis pubis. The clinical course varies from prolonged, progressive debilitation over several months to spontaneous resolution after several weeks. Suggested conservative treatments include rest, physical therapy, steroids, and nonsteroidal antiinflammatory agents. Whatever the therapy, however, noninfectious osteitis pubis tends to be self-limiting.

Recalcitrant cases may be due to pubic osteomyelitis. Diagnosis is made by bone biopsy and bacterial culture. Kammerer-Doak et al. (1998) found positive cultures in 71% of patients with clinical osteitis pubis who failed to respond to conservative therapy. Treatments are antibiotics, incision and drainage if abscess formation occurs, or symphyseal wedge resection or debridement.

## Enterocele and Rectocele

Burch (1968) first reported that enteroceles occurred in 7.6% of cases after the Burch procedure, but only two thirds of these patients required surgical correction. Langer et al. (1988) reported that 13.6% of patients who had undergone Burch procedures, but no hysterectomy or cul-de-sac obliteration, developed an enterocele 1 to 2 years postoperatively. Alcalay et al. (1995) noted that 26% of patients during a 10- to 20-year follow-up period after Burch colposuspension underwent a rectocele repair and 5% underwent an enterocele repair. Whenever possible, a cul-de-sac obliteration in the form of uterosacral plication, Moschcowitz procedure, or McCall culdeplasty should be performed at the time of retropubic suspension to prevent enterocele formation, although the true efficacy of this prophylactic maneuver is unknown. Rectocele repair should be done as indicated for symptomatic or large rectoceles.

## ROLE OF HYSTERECTOMY IN THE TREATMENT OF INCONTINENCE

Gynecologists often perform hysterectomies at the time of retropubic or vaginal surgery for GSI. Although it was generally believed that the presence of a uterus somehow contributed to the genesis of sphincteric incompetence, few data support this theory. Langer et al. (1988) assessed the effect of concomitant hysterectomy during Burch colposuspension on the cure rate of GSI. Forty-five patients were randomly assigned to receive colposuspension only or colposuspension plus abdominal hysterectomy and cul-de-sac obliteration. Using urodynamic investigations 6 months after surgery, the rate of cure for stress incontinence between the two groups did not differ statistically (95.5% and 95.7% for the no-hysterectomy and hysterectomy groups, respectively). This study clearly showed that hysterectomy adds little to the efficacy of Burch colposuspension in curing GSI. In general, hysterectomies should be performed only for specific uterine pathology or for the treatment of uterovaginal prolapse.

## PREGNANCY AFTER RETROPUBIC SURGERY

Most physicians suggest that the patient finish her childbearing before surgical correction of stress incontinence is attempted. Few data demonstrate the continence status when pregnancy or vaginal delivery occurs after a retropubic repair. Only eight pregnancies have been reported after MMK procedures. Seven patients delivered vaginally, and one delivered by cesarean section because she also had undergone a vesicovaginal fistula repair. All of the patients were reportedly continent after delivery, although no long-term follow-up is available. Thus, although surgical treatment for stress incontinence generally should be reserved for women who have finished their childbearing, no data convincingly demonstrate that a pregnancy and vaginal delivery would not be satisfactory for women after retropubic surgery.

## BIBLIOGRAPHY

### Surgical Technique

Bhatia NN, Karram MM, Bergman A: Role of antibiotic prophylaxis in retropubic surgery for stress urinary incontinence, *Obstet Gynecol* 74:637, 1989.

Blaivas JG, Olsson CA: Stress incontinence: classification and surgical approach, *J Urol* 139:727, 1988.

Burch JC: Urethrovaginal fixation to Cooper's ligament for correction of stress incontinence, cystocele, and prolapse, *Am J Obstet Gynecol* 81:281, 1961.

Gleason DM, Reilly RJ, Pierce JA: Vesical neck suspension under vision with cystotomy enhances treatment of female incontinence, *J Urol* 115:555, 1976.

Korda A, Ferry J, Hunter P: Colposuspension for the treatment of female urinary incontinence, *Aust NZ J Obstet Gynaecol* 29:146, 1989.

Krantz KE: The Marshall-Marchetti-Krantz procedure. In Stanton SL, Tanagho EA, eds: *Surgery of female incontinence,* ed 2, New York, 1986, Springer-Verlag.

Linder A, Golomb J, Korczak D: Endoscopic control during colposuspension procedure for the treatment of stress urinary incontinence, *Eur Urol* 16:372, 1989.

Marshall VF, Marchetti AA, Krantz KE: The correction of stress incontinence by simple vesicourethral suspension, *Surg Gynecol Obstet* 88:509, 1949.

McGuire EM: Urodynamic findings in patients after failure of stress incontinence operations. In Zinner NR, Sterling AM, eds: *Female incontinence,* New York, 1981, Alan R Liss.

McGuire EJ, Lytton B, Pepe V, et al: Stress urinary incontinence, *Obstet Gynecol* 47:255, 1976.

Richardson AC, Edmonds PB, Williams NL: Treatment of stress urinary incontinence due to paravaginal fascial defect, *Obstet Gynecol* 57:357, 1981.

Shull BL: How I do the abdominal paravaginal repair, *J Pelvic Surg* 1:43, 1995.

Shull BL, Baden WF: A six-year experience with paravaginal defect repair for stress urinary incontinence, *Am J Obstet Gynecol* 160:1432, 1989.

Tanagho EA: Colpocystourethropexy: the way we do it, *J Urol* 116:751, 1976.

Timmons MC, Addison WA: Suprapubic teloscopy: extraperitoneal intra-operative technique to demonstrate ureteral patency, *Obstet Gynecol* 75:137, 1990.

Turner-Warwick R: Turner-Warwick vagino-obturator shelf urethral repositioning procedure. In Debruyne FMJ, van Kerrebroeck EVA, eds: *Practical aspects of urinary incontinence,* Dordrecht, The Netherlands, 1986, Martinus Nijhoff.

Webster GD, Kreder KJ: Voiding dysfunction following cystourethropexy: its evaluation and management, *J Urol* 144:670, 1990.

### Results and Mechanism of Cure

Alcalay M, Monga A, Stanton SL: Burch colposuspension: a 10-20 year follow up, *Br J Obstet Gynaecol* 102:740, 1995.

Bergman A, Ballard CA, Koonings PP: Comparison of three different surgical procedures for genuine stress incontinence: prospective randomized study, *Am J Obstet Gynecol* 160:1102, 1989.

Bergman A, Elia G: Three surgical procedures for genuine stress incontinence: five-year follow-up of a prospective randomized study, *Am J Obstet Gynecol* 173:66, 1995.

Bergman A, Koonings PP, Ballard CA: Primary stress urinary incontinence and pelvic relaxation: prospective randomized comparison of three different operations, *Am J Obstet Gynecol* 161:97, 1989.

Bhatia NN, Bergman A: Modified Burch versus Pereyra retropubic urethropexy for stress urinary incontinence, *Obstet Gynecol* 66:255, 1985.

Black NA, Downs SH: The effectiveness of surgery for stress incontinence in women: a systematic review, *Br J Urol* 78:497, 1996.

Bump RC, Fantl JA, Hurt WG: Dynamic urethral pressure profilometry pressure transmission ratio determinations after continence surgery: understanding the mechanism of success, failure, and complications, *Obstet Gynecol* 72:870, 1988.

Burton G: A randomized comparison of laparoscopic and open colposuspension, *Neurourol Urodynam* 4:497, 1994.

Columbo M, Milani R, Vitobello D, et al: A randomized comparison of Burch colposuspension and abdominal paravaginal defect repair for female stress urinary incontinence, *Am J Obstet Gynecol* 175:78, 1996.

Columbo M, Scalambrino S, Maggioni A, et al: Burch colpopsuspension versus modified Marshall-Marchetti-Krantz urethropexy for primary genuine stress urinary incontinence: a prospective, randomized clinical trial, *Am J Obstet Gynecol* 171:1573, 1994.

Enhorning G: Simultaneous recording of intravesical and intraurethral pressure, *Acta Chir Scand* (suppl) 276:1, 1961.

Eriksen BC, Hagen B, Eik-Nes SH, et al: Long-term effectiveness of the Burch colposuspension in female urinary stress incontinence, *Acta Obstet Gynecol Scand* 69:45, 1990.

Feyereist J, Dreher E, Haenggi W, et al: Long-term results after Burch colposuspension, *Am J Obstet Gynecol* 171:647, 1994.

Gillon G, Stanton SL: Long-term follow-up of surgery for urinary incontinence in elderly women, *Br J Urol* 56:478, 1984.

Henriksson L, Ulmsten U: A urodynamic evaluation of the effects of abdominal urethrocystopexy and vaginal sling urethroplasty in women with stress incontinence, *Am J Obstet Gynecol* 131:77, 1978.

Herbertsson G, Iosif CS: Surgical results and urodynamic studies 10 years after retropubic colpourethrocystopexy, *Acta Obstet Gynecol Scand* 72:298, 1993.

Hertogs K, Stanton SL: Mechanism of urinary continence after colposuspension: barrier studies, *Br J Obstet Gynaecol* 92:1184, 1985.

Hilton P, Stanton SL: A clinical and urodynamic assessment of the Burch colposuspension for genuine stress incontinence, *Br J Obstet Gynaecol* 90:934, 1983.

Jarvis GJ: Surgery for genuine stress incontinence, *Br J Obstet Gynaecol* 101:371, 1994.

Karram MM, Bhatia NN: Management of coexistent stress and urge urinary incontinence, *Obstet Gynecol* 73:4, 1989.

Koonings PP, Bergman A, Ballard CA: Low urethral pressure and stress urinary incontinence in women: risk factor for failed retropubic surgical procedure, *Urology* 36:245, 1990.

Kujansuu E: Urodynamic analysis of successful and failed incontinence surgery, *Int J Gynaecol Obstet* 21:353, 1983.

Langer R, Golan A, Ron-El R, et al: Colposuspension for urinary stress incontinence in premenopausal and postmenopausal women, *Surg Gynecol Obstet* 171:13, 1990.

Langer R, Ron-El R, Neuman N, et al: The value of simultaneous hysterectomy during Burch colposuspension for urinary stress incontinence, *Obstet Gynecol* 72:866, 1988.

Laursen H, Farlie R, Rasmussen KL, et al: Colposuspension Burch: an 18 year follow-up study, *Neurourol Urodynam* 13:445, 1994.

Leach GE, Dmochowski RR, Appell RA, et al: Female stress urinary incontinence clinical guidelines panel summary report on surgical management of female stress urinary incontinence, *J Urol* 158:875, 1997.

Mainprize TC, Drutz HP: The Marshall-Marchetti-Krantz procedure: a critical review, *Obstet Gynecol Surv* 43:724, 1988.

Milani R, Scalambrino S, Quadri G, et al: Marshall-Marchetti-Krantz procedure and Burch colposuspension in the surgical treatment of female urinary incontinence, *Br J Obstet Gynaecol* 92:1050, 1985.

Mundy AR: A trial comparing the Stamey bladder neck suspension procedure with colposuspension for the treatment of stress incontinence, *Br J Urol* 55:687, 1983.

Park GS, Miller EJ: Surgical treatment of stress urinary incontinence: a comparison of the Kelly plication, Marshall-Marchetti-Krantz, and Pereyra procedures, *Obstet Gynecol* 71:575, 1988.

Penttinen J, Käär K, Kauppila K: Colposuspension and transvaginal bladder neck suspension in the treatment of stress incontinence, *Gynecol Obstet Invest* 28:101, 1989a.

Penttinen J, Lindholm EL, Käär K, et al: Successful colposuspension in stress urinary incontinence reduces bladder neck mobility and increases pressure transmission to the urethra, *Arch Gynecol Obstet* 244:233, 1989b.

Richmond DH, Sutherst JR: Burch colposuspension or sling for stress incontinence? A prospective study using transrectal ultrasound, *Br J Urol* 64:600, 1989.

Rydhström H, Iosif CS: Urodynamic studies before and after retropubic colpourethrocystopexy in fertile women with stress urinary incontinence, *Arch Gynecol Obstet* 241:201, 1988.

Sand PK, Bowen LW, Ostergard DR, et al: Hysterectomy and prior surgery as risk factors for failed retropubic cystourethropexy, *J Reprod Med* 33:171, 1988.

Sand PK, Bowen LW, Panganiban R, et al: The low pressure urethra as a factor in failed retropubic urethropexy, *Obstet Gynecol* 69:399, 1987.

Stanton SL, Cardozo L, Williams JE, et al: Clinical and urodynamic features of failed incontinence surgery in the female, *Obstet Gynecol* 51:515, 1978.

Thunedborg P, Fischer-Rasmussen W, Jensen SB: Stress urinary incontinence and posterior bladder suspension defects, *Acta Obstet Gynecol Scand* 69:55, 1990.

van Geelen JM, Theeuwes AGM, Eskes TKAB, et al: The clinical and urodynamic effects of anterior vaginal repair and Burch colposuspension, *Am J Obstet Gynecol* 159:137, 1988.

Weil A, Reyes H, Bischoff P, et al: Modifications of the urethral rest and stress profiles after different types of surgery for urinary stress incontinence, *Br J Obstet Gynaecol* 91:46, 1984.

Wheelan JB: Long-term results of colposuspension, *Br J Urol* 65:329, 1990.

## Complications

Applegate GB, Bass KM, Kubik CJ: Ureteral obstruction as a complication of the Burch colposuspension procedure: case report, *Am J Obstet Gynecol* 156:445, 1987.

Bhatia NN, Bergman A: Urodynamic predictability of voiding following incontinence surgery, *Obstet Gynecol* 63:85, 1984.

Bhatia NN, Bergman A: Use of preoperative uroflowmetry and simultaneous urethrocystometry for predicting risk of prolonged postoperative bladder drainage, *Urology* 28:440, 1986.

Burch JC: Cooper's ligament urethrovesical suspension for stress incontinence, *Am J Obstet Gynecol* 100:764, 1968.

Cardozo LD, Stanton SL, Williams JE: Detrusor instability following surgery for genuine stress incontinence, *Br J Urol* 51:204, 1979.

Ferriani RA, Silva de MF, Dias de Moura M, et al: Ureteral blockage as a complication of Burch colposuspension: report of 6 cases, *Gynecol Obstet Invest* 29:239, 1990.

Galloway NTM, Davies N, Stephenson TP: The complications of colposuspension, *Br J Urol* 60:122, 1987.

Kammerer-Doak DN, Cornella JL, Magrina JF, et al: Osteitis pubis after Marshall-Marchetti-Krantz urethropexy: a pubic osteomyelitis, *Am J Obstet Gynecol* 179:586, 1998.

Langer R, Ron-El R, Newman M, et al: Detrusor instability following colposuspension for urinary stress incontinence, *Br J Obstet Gynaecol* 95:607, 1988.

Lose G, Jorgensen L, Mortensen SO, et al: Voiding difficulties after colposuspension, *Obstet Gynecol* 69:33, 1987.

Maulik TG: Kinked ureter with unilateral obstructive uropathy complicating Burch colposuspension, *J Urol* 130:135, 1983.

Rebenack P, Thompson RJ, Wilf LH: Osteomyelitis pubis following a Burch retropubic urethropexy, *J Gynecol Surg* 6:205, 1990.

Rosenthal RE, Spickard WA, Markham RD, et al: Osteomyelitis of the symphysis pubis: a separate disease from osteitis pubis, *J Bone Joint Surg* 64:123, 1982.

Sand PK, Bowen LW, Ostergard DR, et al: The effect of retropubic urethropexy on detrusor stability, *Obstet Gynecol* 71:818, 1988.

Sauoberg B: Hydrodynamics of micturition following Marshall-Marchetti-Krantz procedure for stress urinary incontinence, *Scand J Urol Nephrol* 16:11, 1982.

Steel SA, Cox C, Stanton SL: Long-term follow-up of detrusor instability following the colposuspension operation, *Br J Urol* 58:138, 1986.

Turner-Warwick RT: The pathogenesis and treatment of osteitis pubis, *Br J Urol* 32:464, 1960.

Wiskind AK, Creighton SM, Stanton SL: The incidence of genital prolapse after the Burch colposuspension, *Am J Obstet Gynecol* 167:399, 1992.

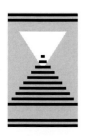

CHAPTER 15

# Surgery for Genuine Stress Incontinence
## Vaginal Procedures, Injections, and the Artificial Urinary Sphincter

Neeraj Kohli and Mickey M. Karram

The vaginal approach to surgical treatment of genuine stress incontinence (GSI) comprises a wide variety of procedures based on different surgical principles to correct GSI associated with urethral hypermobility and intrinsic sphincter deficiency (ISD). Compared to retropubic procedures, advantages include the ability to readily perform concurrent vaginal prolapse repair, decreased perioperative

and postoperative morbidity, and shorter hospitalization and recovery. However, when compared with retropubic procedures, some vaginal procedures have lower long-term cure rates. This chapter reviews the indications, techniques, complications, and results of anterior colporrhaphy with suburethral plication, transvaginal needle suspension, suburethral sling, injection of bulk-enhancing agents, and the artificial urinary sphincter.

## ANTERIOR COLPORRHAPHY WITH SUBURETHRAL PLICATION

Anterior colporrhaphy is one of the oldest and most revered operations in gynecology. At one time, suburethral (Kelly) plication was the mainstay of surgical treatment for GSI. First described by Kelly in 1914, anterior colporrhaphy with suburethral plication corrected anterior vaginal prolapse (distention-type cystocele) while stabilizing the suburethral fascia to prevent urethral descent. The Kelly-Kennedy modification, described by Kennedy in 1937, involved dissection of the urethra from the vaginal wall with plication of the injured sphincter muscle at the urethrovesical junction. The objective was to provide preferential support to the proximal urethra and bladder neck and create some posterior urethral angulation when compared to the bladder base.

The following is a discussion of the Kelly-Kennedy suburethral plication for surgical correction of GSI. Anterior colporrhaphy for anterior vaginal prolapse is presented in Chapter 17.

### Indications

The use of suburethral plication for GSI has declined over recent years as a result of a better understanding of the pathophysiology of urinary incontinence, development of new surgical techniques, and studies indicating higher failure rates with this procedure. Suburethral plication is not usually used as a first-line surgical treatment for GSI. Nevertheless, it is a useful procedure in selected clinical situations such as GSI, usually coexistent with advanced prolapse, in elderly or medically fragile patients who are either unable to undergo extensive or lengthy abdominal procedures or are at high risk for significant voiding

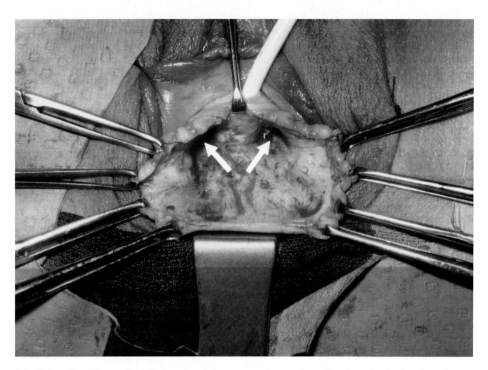

**Fig. 15-1** Anterior vaginal wall opened for cystocele repair and suburethral plication. Arrows depict dissection to inferior pubic ramus before placement of suburethral sutures.

dysfunction or retention if other procedures are performed. If significant GSI persists or develops postoperatively, bulking agents can be injected.

The appropriate role of prophylactic suburethral plication in continent women with anterior vaginal prolapse and urethral hypermobility is controversial. Some subjectively continent women with advanced prolapse demonstrate urinary leakage only after the prolapse is reduced (occult or potential incontinence). However, currently used reduction maneuvers probably overestimate the true prevalence of potential incontinence, so the need for an antiincontinence procedure is uncertain. Suburethral plication is as successful as transvaginal needle suspension in preventing the development of GSI after prolapse repair, with fewer complications.

## Technique

Deep venous thrombosis prophylaxis and preoperative antibiotics are recommended for all patients. With the patient in the dorsal lithotomy position, the vagina and perineum are sterilely prepped and draped. A Foley catheter with a 10-ml balloon is inserted in the bladder to allow identification of the bladder neck. A weighted speculum is placed in the vagina for easy visualization of the anterior vaginal wall. Submucosal injection of saline or hemostatic solution may decrease bleeding and facilitate dissection in the proper plane. A midline incision is made through the vaginal mucosa from the base of the cystocele to the mid-urethra. The mucosal edges are grasped with Allis or T clamps and drawn laterally. Vaginal flaps are dissected

and the anterior vagina mobilized using a scalpel or Metzenbaum scissors, with care taken to preserve the fascial tissue at its attachment over the bladder. Entry into a white-appearing avascular space confirms the proper plane of dissection. The spaces lateral to the urethrovesical junction are sharply and bluntly dissected toward the inferior pubic ramus (Fig. 15-1).

Once the vaginal flaps have been developed, the urethrovesical junction is identified by gentle traction on the Foley catheter and palpation of the catheter balloon. Surgical repair begins at the urethrovesical junction using delayed absorbable or permanent suture. The first plicating stitch is placed into the periurethral endopelvic fascia at the urethrovesical junction on one side and then on the other side. One or two stitches are placed proximal and distal to the initial stitch. When these sutures are tied, tissue pulled to the midline creates a suburethral shelf that provides posterior urethral support (Fig. 15-2). The main goal of a suburethral plication procedure is to provide preferential support to the proximal urethra and bladder neck and create some posterior urethral angulation when compared to the support provided at the bladder base. The remaining anterior vaginal prolapse is repaired as described in Chapter 17.

Postoperative bladder drainage is recommended, and voiding trials are begun 24 to 48 hours after surgery.

## Results

The literature reporting the success rate of suburethral plication for GSI varies from 34% to 91%. The extent of preoper-

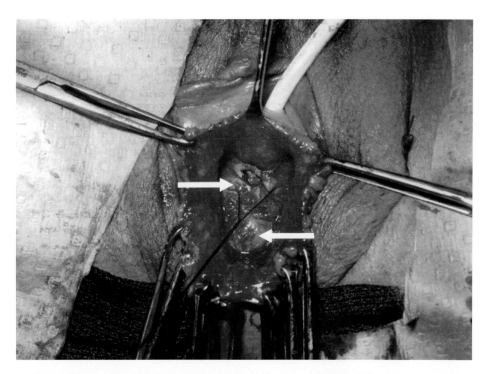

**Fig. 15-2** Upper arrow demonstrates suburethral plication of endopelvic fascia at the bladder neck. Lower arrow depicts mild cystocele caused by a midline fascial defect.

**Table 15-1** Recently Published Studies Reporting Outcome of Anterior Colporrhaphy With Suburethral Plication for the Correction of GSI

| Author | Study design | Outcome measure | Number of patients and procedure(s) performed | Postoperative follow-up (mo) | Success rates (%) |
|---|---|---|---|---|---|
| Harris et al. (1995) | Retrospective | Subjective | 50 AR<br>26 RU | 66 | AR 46<br>RU 75 |
| Liapis et al. (1996) | Prospective | Objective | 41 AR<br>40 RU | 36 | AR 57<br>RU 88 |
| Bergman and Elia (1995) | Prospective | Objective | 30 AR<br>30 TVNS<br>33 RU | 60 | AR 37<br>TVNS 43<br>RU 82 |
| Tamussino et al. (1995) | Retrospective | Objective | 186 AR and RU | 60 | AR 46<br>RU 86 |
| Beck et al. (1991) | Retrospective | Objective | 72 AR<br>122 revised AR | 6-60+ | AR 75<br>Revised AR 91 |
| Vahlensieck and Schander (1985) | Retrospective | Subjective | 200 AR | 24-96 | AR 70 |

*AR*, Anterior repair; *RU*, retropubic urethropexy; *TVNS*, transvaginal needle suspension.

ative evaluation, including diagnostic assessment of incontinence, is often poorly described in reports on suburethral plication. In addition, length of follow-up and outcome measures (subjective versus objective) are often highly variable and inconsistent, even within studies. In many reports, the main indication for anterior colporrhaphy with suburethral plication is anterior vaginal prolapse repair; the effects on GSI are often incidental and poorly documented.

The results of recently published reports of suburethral plication for GSI are listed in Table 15-1. In a meta-analysis of 11 studies on anterior repair for GSI, 957 patients had an overall cure rate of 65% (range 31% to 91%) and a cure or improvement rate of 74% (range 31% to 98%); the complication rates averaged 14%. The variation in reported success rates may result from different surgical techniques, including the extent of endopelvic fascial dissection, location and depth of stitch placement, and use of permanent versus absorbable suture. It probably also relates to differences in patient populations and selection bias in study design. Because very few studies used random assignment to treatment, patients having suburethral plication probably differ from patients having retropubic procedures or suburethral slings. The poor long-term results of suburethral plication are probably explained by the nature of periurethral endopelvic fascia, which lacks the durability required to adequately support the bladder neck over time. Because of these poor long-term results, in most cases suburethral plication is no longer recommended for surgical correction of GSI.

## TRANSVAGINAL NEEDLE SUSPENSION PROCEDURES

Transvaginal needle suspension procedures stabilize the bladder neck by anchoring vaginal tissue to the rectus fascia or, more recently, the pubic bone. First described by Pereyra in 1959, the needle urethropexy has undergone more than 30 modifications in an attempt to improve cure rates and minimize complications. The original Pereyra technique included bilateral passage of a special needle carrier through an abdominal stab incision into the unopened vagina. Extension of a stylet resulted in a Y-shaped double vaginal penetration. Suture placement (No. 30 steel wire) followed by withdrawal of the needle back through the abdominal incision resulted in vaginal wall elevation. Many modifications advocating varied amounts of dissection and different anchoring tissues have since been described.

### Indications

Like retropubic procedures, needle suspensions are indicated for the surgical treatment of anatomic GSI with urethral hypermobility. The primary goal is to support the bladder neck and prevent descent during rises in abdominal pressure.

Needle suspensions may be chosen over other antiincontinence procedures based on the patient's age and medical condition, associated pelvic organ prolapse, and the surgeon's skill and training. Although still commonly performed, needle suspensions have become less popular because of lower long-term cure rates compared with suburethral slings and retropubic operations.

### Techniques

The procedures can be performed under general, spinal, epidural, or local anesthesia, with the patient in the dorsal lithotomy position. Deep venous thrombosis prophylaxis and preoperative antibiotics are recommended. The lower abdomen, vagina, and perineum are cleansed and draped in a sterile fashion, and a Foley catheter is inserted into the bladder for bladder drainage and to identify the location of the urethrovesical junction. The following is a brief description of the commonly performed needle suspension procedures.

### *Modified Pereyra Procedure*

A small transverse skin incision 2 cm above the pubic symphysis is taken down to the anterior rectus fascia. The anterior vaginal epithelium is incised in the midline at the level of the proximal urethra and bladder neck. Using Metzenbaum scissors, dissection is extended laterally to the inferior pubic ramus on each side. Anterolateral attachments of periurethral tissue are released using blunt or sharp dissection (Figs. 15-3 and 15-4). The surgeon's fingertip is

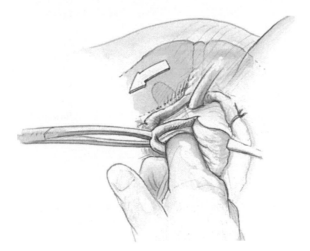

**Fig. 15-3** Technique of blunt dissection into retropubic space. With tip of index finger flexed anteriorly against posterior symphysis, paraurethral attachment to pubic bone is perforated downward toward ischial spine, completely detaching endopelvic fascia.

From Karram MM: In Hurt WG, ed: *Urogynecologic surgery,* Gaithersburg, Md, 1992, Aspen.

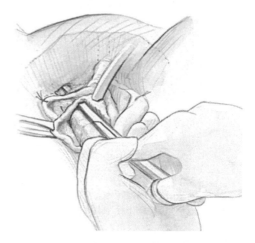

**Fig. 15-4** Technique of vaginal entrance using Metzenbaum scissors. Endopelvic fascia is perforated at inferior margin of pubic bone as guided by surgeon's index finger. Blades of scissors are separated and dissection is completed by inserting a finger into space created as in Fig. 15-3.

From Karram MM: In Hurt WG, ed: *Urogynecologic surgery,* Gaithersburg, Md, 1992, Aspen.

flexed medially to hook the edges of the detached fascia, which are grasped and brought down into the vaginal field (Fig. 15-5). A No. 0 polypropylene suture is passed in a helical fashion several times through this detached fascia. Traction on this suture confirms correct placement in strong supportive tissue. The Pereyra ligature carrier is introduced through the lateral aspect of the abdominal skin incision and advanced through the retropubic space into the vaginal incision by direct finger guidance (Fig. 15-6). Each suspension suture is transferred from the vagina to the suprapubic incision. Cystoscopy is performed to assess for bladder injury or stitch penetration. The sutures are tied above the anterior rectus fascia.

### Stamey Procedure

Two small transverse suprapubic incisions are made 5 cm above the pubic symphysis on each side of the midline and taken down until the anterior rectus fascia is exposed. A T-shaped incision is made on the anterior vaginal mucosa, and the vaginal wall is dissected off the underlying urethra and bladder, exposing the bladder neck. One of three special needles (Fig. 15-7), each at a different angle, is passed blindly through the retropubic space along the vesical neck, which is identified by gentle traction on the Foley balloon. A 70-degree cystoscope is inserted into the bladder to observe that lateral motion of the needle produces indenta-

tion or movement of the vesical wall at the bladder neck. Once proper placement is confirmed, the tip of the needle is advanced into the vagina, threaded with No. 2 monofilament nylon suture, and withdrawn through the suprapubic incision. The needle is again passed through the same incision 1 to 2 cm lateral to the original entry to exit in the vagina approximately 1 cm distal to the previous needle exit site. The vaginal end of the nylon suture is passed through a 1-cm tube of 5-mm knitted Dacron arterial graft to buttress the vaginal tissue, threaded through the needle, and pulled out through the suprapubic incision. This procedure is repeated on the opposite side. The vaginal incision is irrigated with antibiotic solution and closed, burying the Dacron buttresses. Gentle traction is placed on the suspension sutures, which are tied loosely on each side.

### Raz Procedure

The Raz modification differs from the Pereyra procedure in its use of vaginal wall in addition to endopelvic fascia as anchoring tissue to stabilize the bladder neck (Fig. 15-8). The technique begins with an inverted U-shaped incision of the anterior vaginal wall and vaginal dissection lateral to the urethra and bladder neck. The retropubic space is entered and dissected as previously described. Monofilament suture, typically No. 1 polypropylene, is placed in a helical fashion through the detached endopelvic fascia and full-thickness

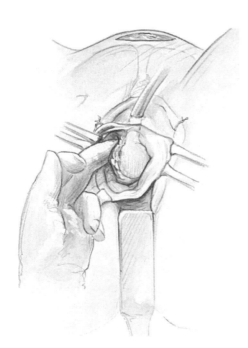

**Fig. 15-5** Finger is placed behind detached endopelvic fascia, mobilizing it into vaginal field, to facilitate placement of helical suture.

From Karram MM: In Hurt WG, ed: *Urogynecologic surgery,* Gaithersburg, Md, 1992, Aspen.

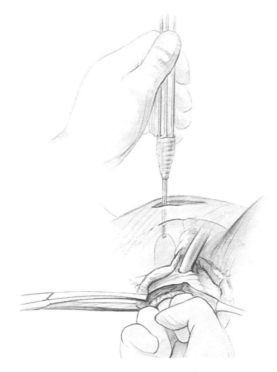

**Fig. 15-6** Passage of needle is under direct finger guidance. Vaginal finger is inserted to posterior aspect of rectus muscle.

From Karram MM: In Hurt WG, ed: *Urogynecologic surgery,* Gaithersburg, Md, 1992, Aspen.

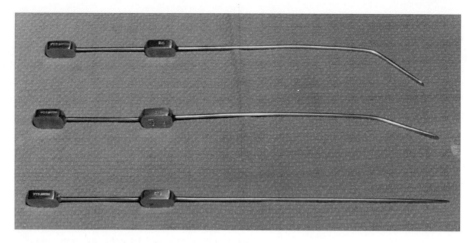

**Fig. 15-7**    A series of Stamey needles *(bottom to top):* a straight needle, a 15-degree angled needle, and a 30-degree angled needle.

Courtesy Pilling Company, Fort Washington, Pennsylvania.

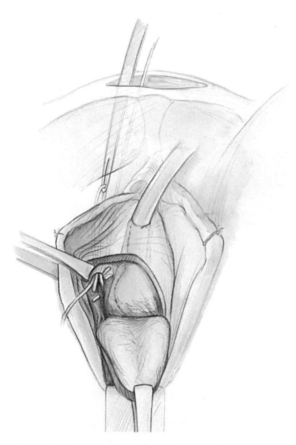

**Fig. 15-8**    Raz procedure. Helical suture is taken through detached endopelvic fascia and anchored in full-thickness vaginal wall, excluding epithelium.

From Karram MM: In Hurt WG, ed: *Urogynecologic surgery,* Gaithersburg, Md, 1992, Aspen.

vaginal wall, excluding epithelium. The suprapubic transfer and tying of the suspension sutures are identical to those of the modified Pereyra procedure.

## Muzsnai Procedure

Muzsnai developed his modification after observing that the integrity and strength of the detached endopelvic fascia were weak and unpredictable. The dissection is identical to that of the modified Pereyra procedure. Two permanent sutures are placed on each side through the inside of the vaginal wall, excluding the epithelium, lateral to the bladder neck. Sutures are then transferred to the suprapubic incision. With a hand elevating the anterior vagina, the sutures are tied, creating a dimple in the lateral area of the vaginal fornix on each side, as in an abdominal colposuspension.

## Gittes Procedure

The Gittes procedure is similar to the original Pereyra procedure in that no vaginal incision is made. A small puncture is made through the suprapubic skin and subcutaneous tissue, 2 cm superior to the pubic bone and 5 cm lateral to the midline on each side. A 30-degree Stamey needle is introduced into this incision, passed through the rectus fascia, and carefully advanced along the posterior aspect of the pubic bone. With the surgeon's other hand elevating the anterior vaginal wall lateral to the bladder neck, identified by palpation of the Foley balloon, the tip of the needle is popped through the unopened vagina. A No. 2 nylon suture is threaded through the eye of the needle, which is then withdrawn. A second pass is made through a different site on the rectus fascia, with the vaginal exit point of the needle selected by touch and sight to be 2 cm cephalad to the original vaginal penetration. Using a free needle, the suture is anchored to the vaginal wall between the first and second penetration in a helical fashion and then

**Table 15-2**   Differences Among Various Suspension Procedures

| Procedure | Vaginal incision | Needle passage | Anchoring tissue | Use of cystoscopy |
|---|---|---|---|---|
| Modified Pereyra | Midline | Direct finger guidance | Pubourethral ligament and endopelvic fascia | Rule out injury |
| Stamey | T-shaped | Blind | Pubocervical fascia | Confirm suture placement |
| Raz | Inverted U | Direct finger guidance | Endopelvic fascia and vaginal wall | Rule out injury |
| Gittes | None | Blind | Full thickness of vaginal wall | Confirm suture placement |
| Percutaneous bone fixation | None | Blind | Full thickness of vaginal wall | Rule out injury |

transferred to the suprapubic region. Cystourethroscopy is performed during passage of the sutures to identify any inadvertent bladder injury or suture penetration. The sutures are tied tightly into the stab incision, resulting in elevation of the anterior vagina and bladder neck.

### Bone Fixation Procedures

To provide a stable anchoring point not dependent on patient position or fascial integrity and to reduce postoperative discomfort and the pulling sensation caused by attaching sutures to the rectus fascia, Leach described the bone fixation technique for transvaginal needle suspension in 1988. One modification of this technique, described by Benderev (1994), uses special instrumentation and bone anchors to perform it as a percutaneous procedure.

A 3- to 4-cm midline suprapubic skin incision is made to expose the periosteum of the pubic tubercle. Using a bone locator to establish the direct symmetric position over the pubic tubercle, a titanium bone anchor with attached No. 1 permanent monofilament suture is drilled or pushed into the cortex of the symphysis bilaterally. One end of the suspension suture is threaded through a special ligature carrier that is used to perforate two sites in the unopened anterior vagina 1 cm lateral to the bladder neck on each side. The suture passer, operated with a thumb lever and three-position toggle, is guided through the retropubic space directly behind the pubic bone to perforate the vaginal wall.

Cystoscopy is performed to identify bladder injury. The passer is withdrawn into the retropubic space above the endopelvic fascia and then passed again, slightly cephalad to the first vaginal exit point. This series of steps is repeated, resulting in a Z-shaped suture configuration. Cystoscopy is again performed to assess bladder and urethral integrity. The procedure is repeated on the opposite side. After both sides are completed, traction is placed on the free end of the suture to confirm adequate strength and location at the bladder neck. The sutures are tied to the bone anchors, using the suture spacer to prevent excessive tension on the suspension sutures. The suprapubic skin incision is irrigated and closed.

Table 15-2 and Fig. 15-9 review the differences between the various modifications of the transvaginal needle suspension procedures.

### Results

Published results of transvaginal needle suspensions report cure rates varying from 40% to 100% depending on the method of postoperative assessment and duration of follow-up. In one review of more than 2000 patients, the success rate was 85% with variable follow-up. However, most reports are observational studies with limited sample size and nonstandardized follow-up. Few define the severity of incontinence or use objective measures of cure. Some modifications have few or no objective long-term data available regarding success rates.

In a randomized trial of 289 patients with primary GSI and coexisting pelvic relaxation treated with anterior colporrhaphy, modified Pereyra procedure, or retropubic urethropexy, Bergman et al. (1989b) reported significantly better results with the retropubic approach. Although objective cure rates were comparable on short-term follow-up, 1-year cure rates were significantly higher with Burch colposuspension (87%) than with Pereyra needle suspension (70%) or anterior colporrhaphy (69%). At 5 years, Burch colposuspension maintained its durability (82%), whereas the results of needle suspension (37%) and anterior colporrhaphy (43%) continued to deteriorate (Bergman and Elia, 1995). These data indicate that needle procedures are no more successful than suburethral plication in the surgical treatment of GSI.

Based on a review of all relevant articles published since 1970, Jarvis (1994) reported a meta-analysis of 213 studies comparing outcomes of antiincontinence procedures. The cure rate for transvaginal needle suspensions was considerably lower than for retropubic approaches or suburethral slings on both objective and subjective assessment. The Agency for Health Care Policy and Research (AHCPR) Urinary Incontinence Update Panel reviewed more than 40 studies comprising 3015 patients who had needle suspensions and found a 74% cure rate, with variable follow-up for the combined series (Fantl et al., 1996). Table 15-3 reviews studies comparing different needle suspensions to other antiincontinence procedures. Because of the lower surgical cure rate when compared to retropubic urethropexy or suburethral sling, needle suspensions continue to undergo modifications with the hope of improving surgical outcomes.

## SUBURETHRAL SLING PROCEDURES

The first sling operation was reported by von Giordano in 1907 using the gracilis muscle flap in a patient with epispadias (Hohenfellner and Petrie, 1986). Since that time, numerous modifications of the surgical approach and the

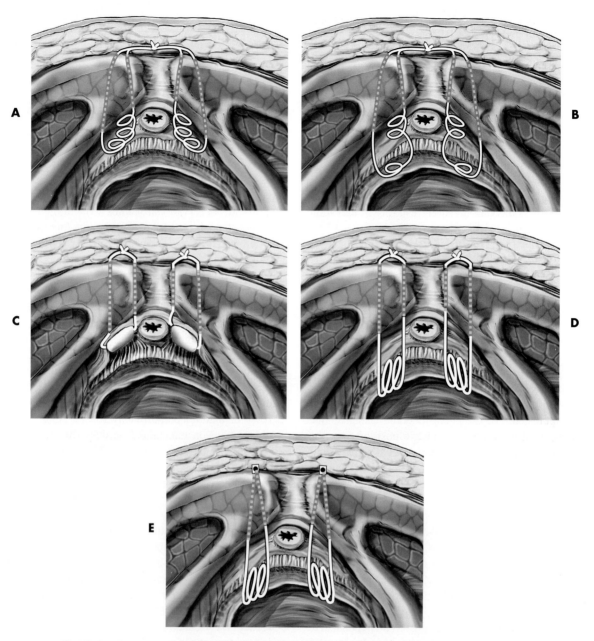

**Fig. 15-9** Transvaginal needle suspension modifications. **A,** Modified Pereyra procedure. **B,** Raz procedure. **C,** Stamey procedure. **D,** Gittes procedure. **E,** Percutaneous bone fixation procedure.

materials used for slings have been published, but all adhere to the principle of supporting the urethra and bladder neck in a hammock that provides static stabilization of the urethra at rest and dynamic compression of the urethra with increased abdominal pressure.

Muscular slings were eventually abandoned because of difficulty in maintaining the muscle's blood supply and mechanical problems associated with incorporating bulky tissue beneath the urethra. In 1917, the Goebell-Frankenheim-Stoekel procedure was described, which secured the pyramidalis muscle and rectus fascia beneath the urethra after plication of the periurethral fascia. Aldridge (1942)

reported the use of two strips of rectus fascia sutured in the midline below the urethra via a separate vaginal incision.

To overcome the limitations of organic slings, such as poor quality of fascial tissue, inadequate length of fascia, and need for additional harvesting procedures, inorganic materials have been used for the sling graft. In 1956, Bracht first reported the use of nylon for a sling. Clear superiority of organic over synthetic materials for slings has not been demonstrated. However, there is a potentially increased rate of infection and erosion with synthetic materials.

Suburethral slings can be performed using a variety of techniques, including a full-length strip of tissue anchored

**Table 15-3**  Published Studies Comparing Needle Suspension Procedures With Other Antiincontinence Procedures

| | No. of patients | Outcome analysis | Cure rate by procedure (%) | | | | Length of follow-up |
|---|---|---|---|---|---|---|---|
| | | | Needle suspension | Anterior colporrhaphy | Retropubic urethropexy | Suburethral sling | |
| Mundy (1983) | 51 | Subjective | 76 S | 40 S | 89 BC | 73 BC | 12 mo |
| | | Objective | | | | | |
| Riggs (1986) | 204 | Mixed | 77 P | | 86 MMK | | 5-10 yr |
| Spencer et al. (1987) | 95 | Subjective | 61 S | | 57 MMK | | 2-10 yr |
| English and Fowler (1988) | 45 | Objective | 58 S | | | | 6 mo |
| Bergman et al. (1989a) | 107 | Objective | 72 P | 65 | 91 BC | | 12 mo |
| Hilton (1989) | 21 | Objective | 80 S | | | 90 | 6 mo |
| Bergman et al. (1989b) | 289 | Objective | 70 P | 69 | 87 BC | | 12 mo |
| Karram et al. (1992) | 93 | Subjective | 82 P | | | | 12 mo |
| | | Objective | 63 P | | | | |
| Korman et al. (1994) | 106 | Subjective | 47 S | | | | 9-45 mo |
| Trockman et al. (1995) | 125 | Subjective | 20 P | | | | 5-13 yr |
| Bergman and Elia (1995) | 93 | Objective | 43 P | 37 | 82 BC | | 5 yr |

*S*, Stamey; *P*, Pereyra; *BC*, Burch colposuspension; *MMK*, Marshall-Marchetti-Krantz.

to the rectus fascia, a half-length strip of tissue anchored to the rectus fascia using suture, a patch sling procedure using a small patch anchored to the rectus fascia via a modified needle suspension approach, an in situ vaginal sling, a suburethral sling sutured or screwed into the descending pubic rami or fascia over the levator muscle, and a tension-free vaginal tape (TVT). There are few randomized prospective studies comparing these modifications.

## Indications

Traditionally, a suburethral sling has been recommended for stress urinary incontinence caused by ISD (or Type III incontinence), that is, failure of the urethral sphincter to maintain a watertight seal regardless of bladder neck position. These patients present with severe stress incontinence, decreased vaginal pliability, low resting urethral closure pressure, and low Valsalva leak point pressures. Endoscopic or radiographic studies commonly reveal an open bladder neck at rest.

There are probably two mechanisms of continence after the suburethral sling. First, the sling restores normal urethrovesical junction support at rest. Second, the sling functions as a backboard against which the urethra is compressed during increased abdominal pressure. Increased outflow resistance is created by upward displacement of the sling, with rectus muscle shortening during stress. These forces combine to produce closure of the bladder neck and functional continence.

Given this dual mode of action and good long-term outcomes, indications for suburethral slings have broadened over the last decade. They are used as a primary procedure in patients with urethral hypermobility and coexisting ISD; other indications include recurrent incontinence or coexisting medical or social conditions that increase the risk of failure (e.g., chronic pulmonary disease, obesity, athleti-

cism, and congenital tissue weakness). Recently, advocates of the suburethral sling have proposed its use as a primary surgical treatment in women with anatomic GSI, arguing that slings have good long-term outcomes with or without ISD. Others maintain that slings are associated with a higher incidence of complications, specifically synthetic graft erosion or infection, and postoperative voiding dysfunction, compared with other antiincontinence procedures. The role of suburethral slings in the primary treatment of GSI and urethral hypermobility is currently controversial and requires ongoing investigation.

This operation should be used with caution in patients with incomplete bladder emptying secondary to detrusor dysfunction. Patients who void by Valsalva maneuver on preoperative evaluation with minimal or no detrusor contraction may be at increased risk of transient or permanent postoperative voiding dysfunction. All patients undergoing sling procedures should be taught intermittent self-catheterization preoperatively. History of pelvic radiation and presence of a urinary fistula should also be considered relative contraindications because they may predispose the operative site to tissue breakdown, especially if synthetic sling material is used.

## Techniques

Most variations of the suburethral sling are performed in a similar manner. However, the surgeon must choose among several options in planning the operation. First, the choice of sling material must be considered preoperatively. Most organic materials require some type of harvesting operation, through either a vaginal incision (vaginal patch), an abdominal incision (rectus fascia), or an incision in the lower extremity (fascia lata). Recently, the use of cadaver fascia or dermal allograft as sling material has been reported with good surgical outcomes and few associated complications.

We routinely use cadaver fascia because it provides a strong organic material without the need for harvesting procedures. Synthetic material should be prepared and soaked in an antibiotic solution before use.

The optimal route and surgical technique of the suburethral sling must also be considered preoperatively. Most surgeons perform sling procedures via a combined abdominal-vaginal route, with a major portion of the dissection performed vaginally. The procedure can also be performed entirely via an abdominal approach with tunneling of the sling between the urethra and the vagina; however, this approach increases the likelihood of urethral trauma. A separate vaginal incision does not seem to increase the infectious morbidity of the operation or the incidence of sling erosion.

Choice of sling material, approach, and operative technique is at the discretion of the surgeon. To date, no randomized trials have compared these variations. The indications for each variation are identical.

### Harvesting of Autologous Fascia

If the use of autologous fascia lata or rectus fascia is planned, the graft is harvested before the vaginal dissection.

For a fascia lata graft, a 3- to 4-cm transverse skin incision is made about 8 cm above the mid-patella, lateral to the knee in the lower thigh. Blunt dissection exposes the underlying fascia lata. A 4- by 6-cm piece of fascia lata is removed if a patch sling is to be performed. Subcutaneous tissue is reapproximated, the skin is closed, and a pressure bandage is placed. If a full sling is preferred, a long strip of fascia lata can be obtained using a Wilson fascial stripper or a vein stripper (Fig. 15-10). In either case, closure of the fascial defect is not necessary.

To obtain anterior rectus fascia, a low transverse abdominal incision is made about 4 cm above the pubic symphysis. Blunt dissection is performed until the underlying rectus fascia is visualized. An appropriately sized piece of rectus fascia is harvested in the transverse direction using sharp dissection or electrocautery. The fascial incision is closed

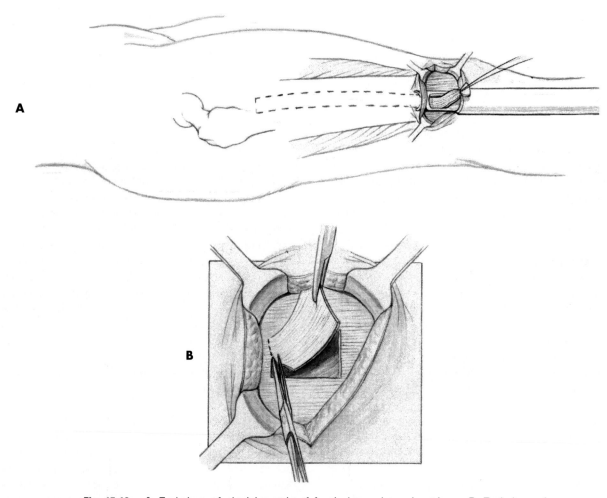

**Fig. 15-10**  **A,** Technique of obtaining strip of fascia lata using vein stripper. **B,** Technique of obtaining patch of fascia lata.

using delayed absorbable suture. The abdominal incision is packed until the vaginal portion of the procedure is completed.

### Operative Details of the Various Sling Modifications

The patient is placed in stirrups in the dorsal lithotomy position. The vagina and lower abdomen are appropriately prepped and draped. Saline or dilute epinephrine solution can be injected beneath the epithelium of the anterior vagina to facilitate dissection. A midline or inverted U-shaped anterior vaginal incision is made. The vaginal epithelium is carefully dissected off the underlying periurethral and paravesical fascia using blunt and sharp dissection. This dissection is extended bilaterally to the inferolateral aspect of the pubic rami. The retropubic space is entered under direct visualization using blunt or sharp dissection, as previously described for transvaginal needle suspensions (see Figs. 15-3 and 15-4).

At this time, suburethral plication and anterior colporrhaphy should be performed if necessary. The bladder neck is identified by gentle traction on the Foley catheter and palpation of the inflated balloon. The sling material is brought into the vaginal field and may be fixed to the posterior aspect of the proximal urethra in the midline with delayed absorbable suture.

For the full-length sling, two small transverse incisions are made in the rectus fascia via the abdominal incision just lateral to the midline. A long clamp is inserted through the incision and passed down through the space of Retzius under direct finger guidance, similar to the needle passage during a Pereyra procedure. The strap of fascia or synthetic material is grasped at one end, and the clamp is pulled up through the space of Retzius, pulling the graft end through the abdominal incision to the rectus fascia, where it is sewn into place. This procedure is repeated on the opposite side, adjusting for adequate tension at the bladder neck (Fig. 15-11).

For the half-sling and patch sling techniques, permanent sutures are placed at the lateral surfaces of the sling graft. The sutures are transferred with a needle ligature carrier under direct finger guidance to above the anterior rectus fascia (Fig. 15-12). For patch slings, some surgeons do not enter the retropubic space and thus transfer the sutures with blind passage of the ligature carrier. Care is taken to preserve an adequate tissue bridge of rectus fascia between the sutures on each side. Cystourethroscopy is performed to identify inadvertent bladder or urethral injury. Tension on the sling should result in closure of the internal urethral meatus, confirming the correct position of the sling at the bladder neck. The suspension sutures on the sling material are tied on each side to the rectus fascia, with care taken to prevent excessive tension at the bladder neck.

Various methods of determining correct tension have been described, but no consensus exists for an objective method of assessing the tension necessary to achieve continence yet prevent postoperative voiding dysfunction. McGuire and O'Connell (1995) tie the sling to increase urethral pressure beneath the sling by 6 to 10 cm $H_2O$. Others fill the bladder with fluid and then adjust sling tension so that compression of the full bladder does not cause leakage. Use of a cotton swab at the bladder neck to tie the sling until the Q-tip angle is 0 to +10 degrees to the horizontal and endoscopic visualization of partial coaptation at the bladder neck has been reported. The proper amount of tension placed on sutures or the sling remains a matter of experience. We routinely place a right-angle clamp between the urethra and the sling graft during tying, with the goal of maintaining zero tension at rest. The compressive mechanism of the suburethral sling should ideally be activated only during increases in abdominal pressure.

After the sutures are tied, the anterior vaginal incision is closed. A suprapubic catheter is commonly placed, and the vagina is packed with a sterile dressing.

For the in situ vaginal wall sling, a patch of full-thickness vaginal wall with mucosa, approximately 2 cm deep and 3 cm wide, is circumscribed and left attached under the proximal urethra and bladder neck. A No. 1 permanent monofilament suture is fixed to the right and left sides of the patch using full-thickness bites in a mattress or running

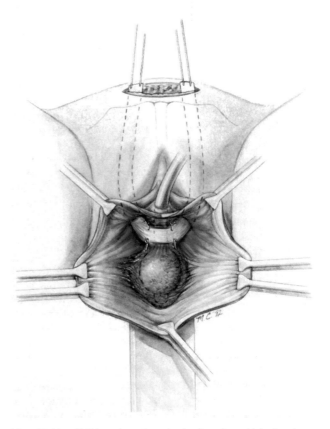

**Fig. 15-11** Full-length suburethral sling in which fascia or synthetic material is passed and tied above the anterior rectus fascia.

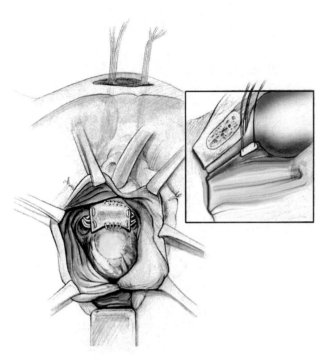

**Fig. 15-12** Patch sling using combined needle suspension sling procedure in which a suburethral patch of fascia or synthetic material is suspended to the anterior rectus fascia with permanent suture.

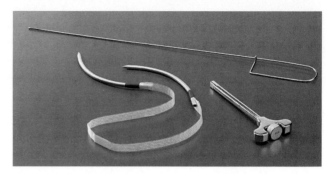

**Fig. 15-13** Tension-free vaginal tape instrumentation including *(clockwise from top)* a Foley catheter guide, needle introducer/ handle, and specially designed needles attached to a synthetic suburethral sling tape.

Courtesy Ethicon Inc., Somerville, New Jersey.

technique. The surgeon does not break into the retropubic space. A small suprapubic skin incision is extended to the fascia near the top of the pubic bone. A needle ligature carrier transfers the sutures above the rectus fascia, where they are sutured to the rectus fascia or periosteum of the pubic symphysis.

Recently, tension-free vaginal tape (TVT) has been described as an ambulatory surgical procedure for the treatment of GSI. The procedure aims to restore the pubourethral ligament and suburethral vaginal hammock by using specially designed needles attached to a synthetic sling material (Fig. 15-13). It can be performed under local anesthesia. Although long-term data are unavailable, initial results are encouraging. Local anesthetic is injected in the abdominal skin just above the pubic symphysis and downward along the back of the pubic bone into the space of Retzius. A small incision is made on each side just medial to the pubic tubercle at the superior rim of the pubic bone. The vaginal mucosa overlying the urethra and bladder neck is injected with a hemostatic agent. A 1.5-cm incision is made along the anterior vaginal mucosa beginning approximately 0.5 cm from the external urethral meatus. Tissue on either side of the urethra is minimally dissected with scissors. The needle tip is inserted into the vaginal incision, and the endopelvic fascia is perforated under the inferior ramus of the pubic bone. The needle is then guided along the inside of the pubic bone until the tip of the needle has pierced the anterior rectus fascia and reached the abdominal

skin incision. The procedure is repeated on the opposite side. In this way, the sling material, a prolene tape (Ethicon Inc., Somerville, New Jersey) covered by a plastic sheath, is placed in a U-shape around the mid-urethra. Cystoscopy is performed to identify bladder or urethral injury. The plastic sheath is then removed, and the sling material is not fixed to the endopelvic fascia or rectus fascia but simply cut on each side at the level of the skin. The vaginal and abdominal incisions are closed.

Other modifications include vaginally placed synthetic or autologous sling material that is sutured or screwed into the descending pubic rami or fascia over the levator muscle. Fig. 15-14 shows a cross-section of the various sling modifications previously discussed.

## Results

Cure rates of slings for stress incontinence vary from 70% to 95%. Some of this variation results from lack of consistent outcome parameters, variable length of follow-up, and variations in the techniques and materials used for the sling procedure. Cure rates using inorganic sling materials are similar to those with autologous grafts. Table 15-4 reviews reported complication rates with synthetic and autologous slings.

Several large studies summarizing surgical results (Black and Downs, 1996; Haab et al., 1996) of treatment of GSI show that the cure rates after sling procedures are similar to that after Burch colposuspension. However, populations of patients studied may not be comparable in that Burch colposuspension is usually done for primary GSI, whereas slings, until recently, have been reserved for recurrent incontinence and ISD. Very few studies provide objective outcome data, and many are biased by differences in sling technique and operator experience. In addition, few studies report untoward effects of these procedures. Complications of voiding dysfunction, recurrent infection, and irritative bladder symptoms may be more disturbing to the patient than her preoperative stress incontinence. Given the fre-

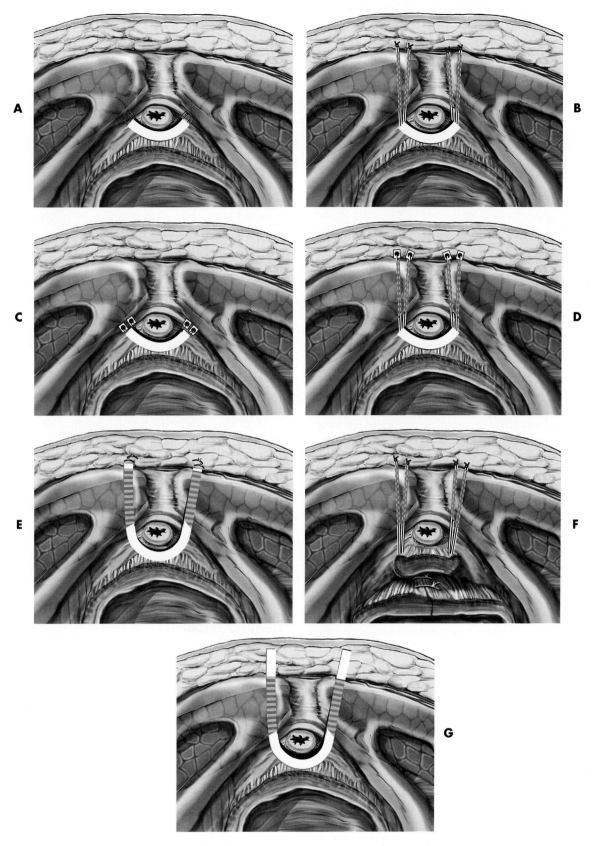

**Fig. 15-14** Suburethral sling modifications. **A,** Mini sling: attachment of sling material to endopelvic fascia bilaterally. **B,** Patch sling: attachment of sling material to anterior rectus fascia by permanent suture. **C,** Bone fixation sling: attachment of sling material to inferior aspect of pubic rami. **D,** Percutaneous bone fixation patch sling: attachment of sling material via permanent sutures to bone anchors in pubic symphysis. **E,** Full-length sling: attachment of sling material to anterior rectus fascia. **F,** In situ vaginal wall sling: full-thickness vaginal wall attached to anterior rectus fascia by permanent suture. **G,** Tension-free vaginal tape: suburethral synthetic tape passed above anterior rectus fascia without suture attachment.

**Table 15-4** Review of Literature Noting Incidence of Complications After Suburethral Sling Operations

| Complications | Autologous sling (%) (*N* = 493) | Synthetic sling (%) (*N* = 616) | Total (%) (*N* = 1109) |
|---|---|---|---|
| Urinary retention | 3.8 | 10.2 | 7.4 |
| Detrusor instability | 7.9 | 1.5 | 4.3 |
| Urgency and frequency | 3.6 | 2.9 | 3.2 |
| Wound infection | 2.4 | 1.8 | 3.0 |
| Urinary tract infection | 4.4 | 1.6 | 2.9 |
| Urethral and bladder injury | 3.8 | 1.3 | 2.4 |
| Sling revision/removal | 1.6 | 2.4 | 2.1 |
| Fistula | 0.8 | 0.8 | 0.8 |
| Poor vaginal healing | — | 1.5 | 0.8 |
| Sling erosion | — | 1.0 | 0.5 |
| Wound abscess | — | 0.6 | 0.4 |
| Sinus tract formation | — | 0.8 | 0.4 |
| Other | 1.8 | — | 0.8 |

From Horbach NS: Suburethral sling procedures. In Ostergard D, Bent A, ed: *Urogynecology and urodynamics: theory and practice,* ed 3, Baltimore, 1991, Williams & Wilkins.

quency with which sling operations are performed currently, randomized trials reporting surgical outcome and complications are needed.

## COMPLICATIONS OF VAGINAL PROCEDURES FOR GSI
### Lower Urinary Tract Injury

Injury to the bladder or urethra can result from any of the vaginal procedures previously described for stress incontinence. This can occur during the dissection of the vaginal epithelium off the underlying fascia or during the lateral dissection below the inferior pubic ramus, which is performed for certain needle procedures and suburethral sling procedures. Injury to the urethra and bladder are more common in patients who have had previous anterior vaginal wall or bladder neck surgery. Cystotomy and urethrotomy should be repaired in layers at the time of the injury and continuous bladder drainage instituted postoperatively for 7 to 14 days to allow adequate healing.

Needle suspension–related injury to the bladder can occur during needle insertion or suprapubic transfer of suspension sutures. Inadvertent stitch penetration into the bladder lumen is more common in modifications such as the Stamey or Gittes procedures, which entail blind passage of the needle ligature through the retropubic space. Intraoperative cystoscopy is mandatory and should identify bladder injury or inadvertent stitch penetration. If an intravesical suture is noted, it should be removed and passed again under direct finger guidance. Unrecognized injury or suture penetration in the bladder lumen may result in postoperative detrusor instability, persistent uri-

nary tract infection, or formation of a bladder calculi. Injury to the ureter during vaginal operations for stress incontinence is rare.

## Voiding Dysfunction and Retention

Voiding difficulty and even retention rarely occur in patients after various antiincontinence surgeries. No consistent preoperative findings successfully predict which patients will develop postoperative voiding dysfunction. Patients with preoperative voiding dysfunction demonstrated by high postvoid residual urine volume, abnormal uroflowmetry, or absent or weak detrusor contraction on pressure flow study may be more likely to develop postoperative voiding dysfunction or retention, although this has not been substantiated consistently in published reports. In our opinion, extensive dissection required for advanced anterior vaginal wall prolapse and the aggressiveness of the repair probably prolong the time to normal voiding. It is our opinion that needle suspension procedures are associated with a higher incidence of postoperative voiding dysfunction and irritative bladder symptoms than are retropubic procedures.

Because suburethral sling procedures can significantly increase urethral outlet resistance, most complications related to these procedures are secondary to obstruction and result in various forms of voiding difficulty and even permanent retention. The exact incidence of retention after sling procedures is unknown but is quoted in the literature as 2% to 10%. If severe voiding dysfunction or retention results from any antiincontinence procedure, the surgeon and the patient must decide whether it would be best to undergo a second operation to take down the repair or loosen the sling in the hope of allowing spontaneous normal voiding. If it is decided to take down a procedure or loosen the sling material, this can be accomplished via vaginal or retropubic approach and is discussed in Chapter 26.

### Detrusor Instability and Irritative Bladder Symptoms

Postoperative detrusor instability with urgency, frequency, or urge incontinence occurs in anywhere from 2% to 50% of patients after various operations for stress incontinence. This may be because of preexisting detrusor instability, now unmasked, with increased bladder volumes caused by a return of outflow resistance, or de novo (new onset) instability related possibly to infection, foreign body reaction, denervation, or anatomic urethral obstruction. De novo detrusor instability is usually transient and responds well to bladder retraining and anticholinergic therapy.

Two recent studies note that up to 50% of patients who have undergone suburethral sling procedures develop irritative bladder symptoms such as urgency, frequency, nocturia, and dysuria (Staskin, 1997; Owens et al., 1999). These are subjective complaints that are often not documented on postoperative cystometric testing. Whether these symptoms relate to the amount of periurethral dissection or sling tension is unknown. Management is similar to that for patients with postoperative detrusor instability.

## Recurrent or Persistent Incontinence

Postoperative incontinence after a vaginal antiincontinence procedure may be caused by immediate surgical failure, development of de novo or worsening of preexisting detrusor instability, ISD, overflow incontinence, or fistula formation. The most common cause of recurrent or persistent incontinence after transvaginal needle suspension procedures is recurrence or worsening of the GSI caused by failure to provide adequate urethral support or development of ISD. This results from weakening of the anchoring tissues or inaccurate placement of the suspension sutures. Webster et al. (1984) and Lockhart et al. (1982) report that more than 50% of women with persistent urinary leakage following various antiincontinence procedures have urge incontinence and detrusor instability. It is always difficult to determine whether postoperative instability developed de novo or was present preoperatively and either persisted or worsened.

## Development of Prolapse

Because GSI and symptomatic pelvic organ prolapse very often coexist, it is important to discuss potential untoward effects of the incontinence procedure on the results of various prolapse repairs. Recent data seem to indicate that the rate of recurrent prolapse may be increased when needle suspensions are performed with other reconstructive vaginal procedures. In a randomized trial of 88 women undergoing either vaginal or abdominal reconstructive pelvic surgery for advanced prolapse, Benson et al. (1996) found that patients undergoing abdominal repair had significantly better surgical outcome and required fewer reoperations for recurrent incontinence or prolapse. Forty-two percent of the patients in the vaginal group underwent needle suspension. The reoperation rate was 33% of the vaginal group and 16% in the abdominal group. Kohli et al. (1996) report the incidence of recurrent cystocele following transvaginal needle suspension with concurrent anterior colporrhaphy to be as high as 33% on 1-year follow-up, compared to 7% when anterior colporrhaphy alone was performed. In a study of 96 women undergoing sacrospinous ligament fixation with and without transvaginal needle suspension, Sze et al. (1997) found that the incidence of recurrent prolapse was significantly higher in patients undergoing concurrent needle procedures (33%) than in those undergoing sacrospinous fixation with or without anterior colporrhaphy (19%). Finally, in a recent prospective randomized trial, Bump et al. (1996) compared the outcome of anterior colporrhaphy with endopelvic suburethral plication to that of transvaginal needle suspension in conjunction with other reconstructive vaginal procedures. They note that the outcome of prolapse, as well as incontinence and voiding dysfunction, was much better in the endopelvic suburethral plication group than in the needle suspension group. Although the reason for these findings is uncertain, possibilities include pelvic neuropathy produced by vaginal dissection, iatrogenic paravaginal defects created during retropubic mobilization, and significant alteration in normal vaginal axis.

## Hemorrhage

Bleeding complications can occur after all of the vaginal operations for incontinence mentioned in this chapter. Excessive bleeding and hematoma formation are more common after procedures that require vaginal entry into the retropubic space (i.e., invasive needle operations and suburethral sling procedures). Excessive intraoperative bleeding may occur during mobilization of the perivesical venous plexus and may be controlled with suture ligation, elevation of the bladder neck resulting in tamponade, or vaginal packing. When excessive bleeding occurs from high up in the retropubic space, a technique described by Katske and Raz (1987) is the placement of a sponge-wrapped Foley catheter with 30-ml balloon into the bleeding space to achieve transvaginal tamponade. Meticulous surgical technique and knowledge of surgical anatomy are essential for the prevention and management of vascular injuries during these procedures.

## Infection and Erosion

A subset of complications including erosion, infection, and sinus formation occur more commonly when synthetic materials are used for sling placement or buttresses are placed during needle suspension operations. A small proportion of patients may require removal of an eroded permanent suture. These problems sometimes are complicated further by coexisting infection. Although few cases can be managed conservatively, the majority of the patients require removal of the foreign body or sling material. Because of complications specific to synthetic material, there is a growing trend toward the use of autologous or donor-directed organic materials for suburethral sling procedures.

## Nerve Damage

These operations are performed with the patient in the dorsal lithotomy position, which can result in nerve damage from compression or stretch injuries. The nerve most often involved is the common peroneal nerve, but injury to the obturator, sciatic, tibia, fibula, or saphenous nerves can also occur (Table 15-5). These injuries usually resolve spontaneously over time. Early recognition and appropriate neurologic and physical medicine consultations are recommended.

Surgical injury to the ilioinguinal nerve can occur during placement and tying of sling material or suspension sutures during transvaginal needle procedures. These patients present with characteristic complaints of pain in the medial groin and inner thigh. Miyazaki and Shook (1992) reported seven cases of ilioinguinal nerve entrapment in their series of 402 needle suspensions. Three patients were treated with

**Table 15-5** Nerves Susceptible to Injury During Needle Suspension Procedures

| Nerve | Location of injury | Mechanism of injury | Clinical presentation |
| --- | --- | --- | --- |
| Common peroneal | Fibular neck | Compression against brace | Footdrop |
| Sciatic | Sciatic notch | Compression or stretching during hip flexion | Weakness during knee flexion or loss of common peroneal or tibial nerve function |
| Obturator | Pubic ramus | Compression | Weakness of ipsilateral thigh on adduction |
| Femoral | Inguinal ligament | Compression during hyperflexion of hips | Quadriceps weakness, gait impairment, decreased sensation over anterior thigh and medial calf |
| Saphenous | Medial aspect of knee | Stretching during hyperflexion of hips | Burning or aching pain in medial calf |
| Ilioinguinal | Lateral to pubic tubercle | Nerve entrapment by suspension sutures | Pain in medial groin, labia, or inner thigh |

surgical suture removal, whereas the remaining four had spontaneous resolution of their symptoms. Because the nerve is most vulnerable to injury near its exit from the superficial inguinal ring, sutures or sling material should be attached and tied medial to the pubic tubercle or body of the symphysis pubis to prevent nerve entrapment.

## INJECTION OF BULK-ENHANCING AGENTS

Injection of bulking agents is a minimally invasive technique for restoring the continence mechanism at the bladder neck and increasing outflow resistance. The technique was first described by Murless in 1938, followed in 1955 by the use of paraffin wax (Quackels) and sclerosing agents in 1963 (Sachse). However, this technique was not widely used until the recent development of more suitable materials for injection, such as polytetrafluoroethylene (PTFE or Teflon; Berg, 1973) and collagen (Shortliffe et al., 1989). Advantages of injections include the ability to perform the procedure in the office with minimal complications. In addition, the injection's effect can be assessed immediately by having the patient perform provocative maneuvers such as Valsalva and coughing. Despite tremendous growth of interest recently in injectable agents, few published randomized trials have compared different agents or techniques with other treatments for stress incontinence.

### Indications

The mechanism of action of intraurethral injections is to coapt the urethral lumen at the bladder neck to recreate normal sphincteric competence. Thus, bulking agents are best used for patients with urinary incontinence secondary to a poorly functioning urethral sphincter (ISD) in the absence of urethral hypermobility. Injections are especially well suited to patients whose coexisting medical conditions make major operative procedures unacceptably risky. The procedure is also attractive for patients who have had previous pelvic radiation because these patients are at higher risk for infection or erosion after placement of an artificial sphincter or suburethral sling.

The use of bulking injectables for GSI associated with urethral hypermobility with or without coexisting ISD is controversial. Most clinicians would recommend the use of traditional antiincontinence procedures such as retropubic

urethropexy or suburethral sling. Although several authors report suboptimal results in patients with stress incontinence and urethral hypermobility, a study by Herschorn and Radomski (1997) reported equal success rates among patients with anatomic GSI (Type II) and ISD (Type III); however, patients with anatomic GSI required more injections and more material per injection.

For evaluation of complex and severe forms of incontinence, complete urodynamic testing should be performed before the procedure. Patients with incomplete bladder emptying should be cautioned that they are at increased risk for postoperative urinary retention. Patients with urgency symptoms caused by detrusor instability should be treated before injection therapy. The only absolute contraindications to injectable therapy are uncontrollable detrusor overactivity and known hypersensitivity to the injectable agents.

### Injectable Materials

The ideal material for periurethral injection is easily injected, is biocompatible, causes little or no inflammatory reaction, and is associated with minimal complications with respect to tolerance and immunogenic response. To achieve long-term success, the agent should have limited biodegradability or propensity for migration. Because none of the available agents are ideal, new agents continue to be developed.

#### *Collagen*

Glutaraldehyde cross-linked (GAX) bovine collagen (Contigen) is a biocompatible and biodegradable product composed of sterile, nonpyrogenic bovine dermocollagen cross-linked with glutaraldehyde and disbursed in a phosphate-buffered physiologic saline solution. The cross-linking process improves the integrity of the material for injection. It is associated with minimal inflammatory response and no foreign body reaction. Time analysis studies have reported that collagen begins to degrade in about 12 weeks but is replaced by neovascularization and deposition of host collagen by fibroblasts. In the pilot multicenter trial, 4% of female patients exhibited hypersensitivity during skin testing. GAX collagen is the only injection material currently approved by the FDA for injection in women with GSI.

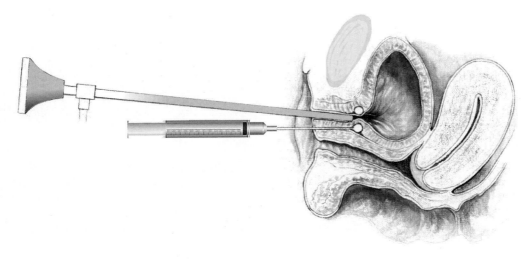

**Fig. 15-15**    Technique used for injection of periurethral bulk-enhancing agents.

### Polytetrafluoroethylene

PTFE paste is a sterile mixture of PTFE micropolymer particles, glycerin, and polysorbate. These particles stimulate ingrowth of fibroblasts at the injection site and eventually become encapsulated, producing a permanent bolstering effect. Unfortunately, animal and human studies have shown that PTFE particles migrate to distant sites, including the brain, lungs, kidney, and spleen and can induce chronic foreign body reaction and granuloma formation. Therefore, its use is controversial. Although not approved for the treatment of stress incontinence in the United States, PTFE has been approved in Canada and Europe.

### Autologous Fat

Autologous fat is a biocompatible injectable that is readily available and easily obtainable. Harvest of autologous fat can be performed with a variety of techniques, ranging from aspiration with a large-bore needle to liposuction. Fat integrates as a graft, but a significant portion of it is absorbed and replaced by inflammation or fibrosis, with connective tissue producing the final bulk effect. Unfortunately, the high degree of absorption limits the usefulness of fat as an effective injectable agent for long-term cure.

### New Materials

A variety of new injectable materials, including silicone polymers, carbon particles, and injectable, inflatable balloons, are currently under development. The basic mechanisms of these agents are similar in that they produce a primary bulk response followed by secondary inflammation and collagen deposition.

## Techniques

Injection techniques are the same, regardless of the material chosen. Intraurethral injection of bulking agents can be performed via the transurethral or periurethral approach. In the transurethral approach, a needle is inserted below the urothelium at the bladder neck under direct cystoscopic vi-

sualization. With the periurethral approach, a spinal needle is inserted percutaneously along the wall of the urethra while injection of the material in the correct location is confirmed by urethroscopy. The transurethral technique allows more accurate placement of the needle with reduced operative time, but this can be offset by loss of collagen from the urethral puncture site, bleeding into the operative field, or infection. Although the periurethral approach minimizes intraurethral bleeding and extravasation of the injectable substance, it requires greater operator experience for exact determination of the location and amount of injected material. The choice of method depends on the operator's experience and available instrumentation. Most investigators prefer a transvaginal periurethral approach, but recent advances in instrumentation have made the transurethral technique easier and more effective. Unfortunately, there are few data comparing the efficacy of the two techniques.

### Periurethral Injection

With the patient in the dorsal lithotomy position, the periurethral area is covered with 2% lidocaine jelly. Plain 1% lidocaine is injected periurethrally at the 3 and 9 o'clock positions, using 2 to 4 ml on each side. A 0- or 30-degree endoscope is placed into the urethra. A 22-gauge spinal needle is positioned periurethrally at the 4 or 8 o'clock position, with the bevel of the needle directed toward the urethral lumen (Fig. 15-15). The needle is slowly advanced periurethrally in a suburothelial plane under direct cystoscopic vision. Bulging of the tip of the needle against the lining of the urethra is observed and confirms proper position of the needle. Only tissue at the tip of the needle should move; if the whole urethra moves, the needle is too deep in the muscular portion of the urethra. When the needle is at the bladder neck, the agent is injected until swelling creates the appearance of occlusion of the urethral lumen. Once the urethra is approximately 50% occluded, the needle is removed and reinserted on the opposite side, where the procedure is repeated.

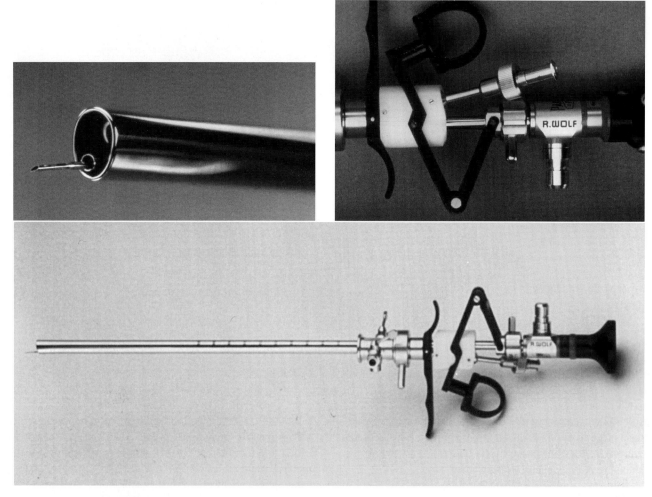

**Fig. 15-16** Instrumentation used for transurethral injection of bulk-enhancing agents. The specially designed endoscopic system has an advancing needle at the distal end, which allows direct injection below the urothelium at the bladder neck.

Courtesy Wolf Medical Systems, Vernon Hills, Illinois.

Recently, Neal et al. (1995) introduced a technique that facilitates periurethral needle placement using methylene blue mixed with local anesthetic, enabling the surgeon to place the implant more accurately.

### Transurethral Injection

Patient positioning and preparation are identical to those in the periurethral approach, except without the periurethral injection of local anesthetic. After the urethra is anesthetized with topical 2% lidocaine jelly, urethroscopy with a 0-degree lens is performed. A specially designed cystoscopic needle or attachment is used to advance a needle transurethrally directly into the mucosa of the urethra just below the internal urethral meatus. Alternatively, a specialized endoscopic delivery system can be used to visualize the bladder neck and inject the bulking agent (Wolf Medical Systems; Fig. 15-16). Once the bevel of the needle has been fully inserted below the urothelium, injection of the agent is completed, with resulting bulging of the urethral lumen (Figs. 15-17 and 15-18). Slight extravasation of the injection material is normal. This procedure is performed at the 4 o'clock position and then repeated on the opposite side at the 8 o'clock position.

After completion of the periurethral or transurethral technique, the patient is asked to stand and perform various provocative maneuvers to assess whether urinary continence has been achieved. The patient is asked to void, and a postvoid residual urine volume is checked via catheterization or bladder ultrasound. Patients with incomplete bladder emptying should be taught intermittent self-catheterization and reassured that this is probably temporary.

## Complications

Perioperative complications associated with intraurethral injections are uncommon. The incidence of immediate urinary retention following intraurethral injection ranges

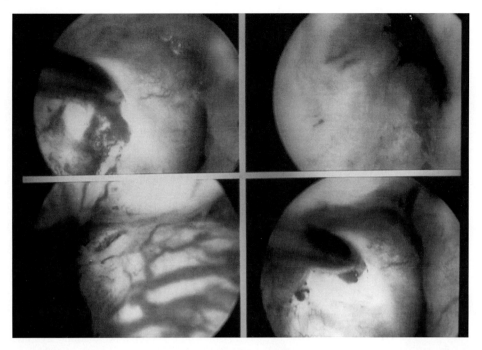

**Fig. 15-17**   Endoscopic appearance of successful transurethral collagen injection. Note bulging of the urothelium, leading to coaptation of the urethral lumen at the bladder neck.

from 15% to 25% of patients. This usually resolves within 24 to 48 hours. Patients with incomplete bladder emptying should be taught intermittent self-catheterization. The use of an indwelling urethral catheter should be avoided to prevent molding of the bulking agent around the catheter.

Irritative voiding symptoms occur in 1% to 20% of patients following collagen injection, and 5% develop urinary tract infections. We routinely place patients on a 3-day course of oral antibiotics after the procedure. A preoperative catheterized specimen of urine for culture is recommended to assess baseline status.

In general, complications associated with bulk-enhancing agents are minor and self-limited. Serious long-term complications have not been reported.

## Results

Intraurethral injection of bulking agents improves or cures 70% to 100% of patients, depending on type and length of follow-up. In 137 women with ISD participating in the multicenter North American study group, 96.4% were dry 1 year later. Each patient required an average of 2.5 injections with an average of 24.3 ml total collagen injected per patient during the study period. In an AHCPR meta-analysis of 15 studies with 528 patients followed for up to 2 years, 49% of patients were cured and 67% were cured or improved. Variations in cure rates may be caused by differences in technique of injection, type of injectable material, definition of outcomes, length of follow-up, or type of incontinence treated.

Table 15-6 compares the outcomes of studies using collagen, PTFE, and autologous fat. No randomized trials comparing the effectiveness of different agents have been performed to date. Studies of new injectable agents are under way.

## IMPLANTATION OF THE ARTIFICIAL URINARY SPHINCTER

Another method of therapy for the female patient with severe stress incontinence secondary to urethral damage is implantation of an artificial urinary sphincter. Theoretically, this is an attractive mode of therapy because it can be considered a controlled obstruction. Only implantation of an artificial sphincter allows for urethral obstruction to be voluntarily relieved at the time of voiding. The use of this mode of therapy has not gained wide acceptance, probably because of lack of experience among urogynecologic surgeons, technical difficulties encountered during placement of the cuff, and fear of mechanical difficulties with the device.

The first artificial sphincter implanted in a woman was in 1972 by Scott et al. This model (AS721) consisted of a set of valves that controlled the direction of fluid flow within the system, as well as the pressure of the urethra and bladder neck, by means of a cuff placed around it. Since then, numerous modifications of the original device have been made. Currently, the most sophisticated artificial sphincter available is the AMS 800.

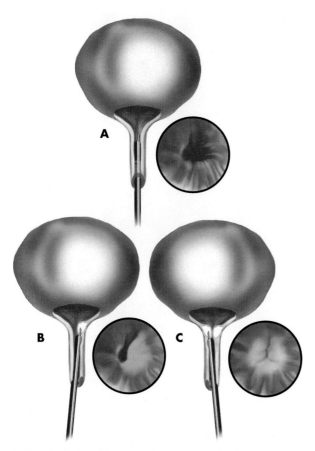

**Fig. 15-18** Urethroscopic view of transurethral injection of a bulk-enhancing agent. **A,** Note bladder neck is open before injection. **B,** Submucosal placement of needle results in partial closure of bladder neck. **C,** Injection is completed when bladder neck is completely closed.

## Description of the AMS 800 Prosthesis

The AMS 800 artificial urinary sphincter consists of a cuff, a pressure-regulating balloon, a control pump, and tubing (Fig. 15-19). The control pump assembly is placed subcutaneously in the labia majora (Fig. 15-20). It contains one-way valves, resistors, and a poppet valve. The poppet valve controls the flow of fluid from the balloon to the cuff. The position of the poppet valve is easily palpated through the skin because of a nipple in the plastic of the pump control assembly. Pressure on the nipple prevents the cuff from filling, thus deactivating the device. Activation of the device requires a firm squeeze over the pump, which allows primary deactivation and delayed activation without a second operation.

The cuff is placed around the bladder neck and consists of an inner pliable leaflet attached to a firm Dacron backing. The cuff is available in various sizes. The smallest have a diameter of 4 to 5 cm, with increments of 0.5 cm up to 8 cm, and then 1-cm increments up to 11 cm.

The balloon is placed in the retropubic space, where it is subjected to the effects of changes in intraabdominal

pressure. Balloon pressures range from 51 to 60 cm $H_2O$ to 71 to 80 cm $H_2O$ in 10-cm-$H_2O$ increments.

Unlike that of earlier models, the tubing is now "resistant" and color coded for easy intraoperative identification. The balloon pump tubing is black, and the cuff pump tubing is white.

When the patient feels the urge to urinate, she squeezes the pump through the labia, which transfers fluid to the balloon. When she releases the pump, fluid is sucked from the cuff into the pump. The process is repeated until the pump goes flat, signifying that the cuff is deflated. The patient is then able to void. The balloon automatically begins repressurization. About 3 minutes are required for the cuff to refill, thus allowing adequate time to complete urination.

## Indications and Preoperative Preparation

The artificial urinary sphincter has been implanted in both men and women for various types of incontinence, including postprostatectomy incontinence, stress incontinence, epispadias, and neuropathic bladder dysfunction secondary to meningomyelocele, spinal cord injury, multiple sclerosis, sacral agenesis, and spinal cord tumors.

Specifically with regard to incontinence in women, the AMS 800 is most suitable for patients with stress incontinence secondary to poor urethral sphincteric function. The preoperative evaluation of candidates is aimed at excluding patients who have underlying disease that would result in a high risk of device failure or who would be at risk for upper urinary tract injury once the device was implanted. This evaluation should include urine culture and sensitivity, intravenous urography, voiding cystourethrography, cystourethroscopy, and urodynamic evaluation.

Patients with urinary tract infections must be treated before implantation to reduce the risk of device contamination. Patients with an overactive detrusor should be controlled medically before implantation. Patients with poor urinary flow and excessive postvoid residual urine can still undergo implantation if they accept the possibility that permanent intermittent self-catheterization will be required. Previous surgery, radiation, or trauma in the region of the urethrovaginal septum can make cuff placement difficult and increase the possibility of cuff erosion and urethral damage.

Patient motivation is the foremost consideration when selecting patients for artificial sphincter implantation. They must have adequate manual dexterity, mental capacity, and motivation to manipulate the pump mechanism each time they need to urinate. The only two absolute contraindications for implanting an artificial sphincter are uncontrollable detrusor instability or hyperreflexia and high-grade vesicoureteral reflux.

Because this is a synthetic device inserted into a closed space, precautions must be taken preoperatively to reduce the chance of infection. Thus, the device and instruments are

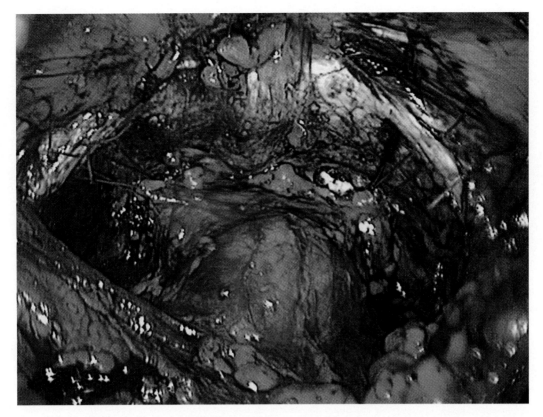

**Plate 1**   Laparoscopic panoramic view of a completed Burch colposuspension.

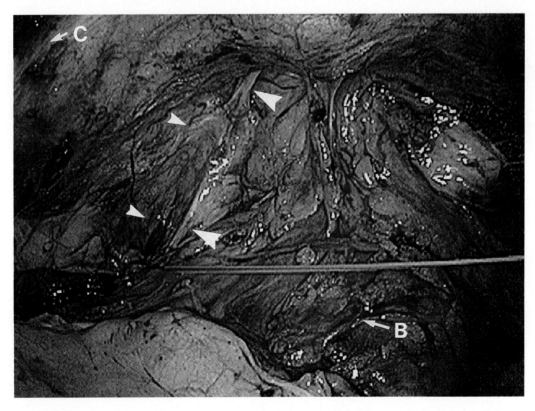

**Plate 2**   Laparoscopic view of apical suture during paravaginal defect repair. Arrows show left arcus tendineus fasciae pelvis. *B,* Bladder; *C,* Cooper's ligament.

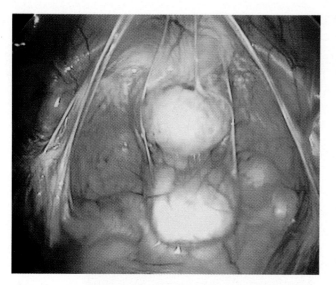

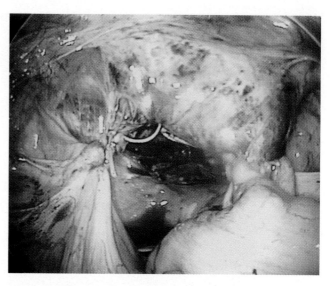

**Plate 3** Laparoscopic view before a uterosacral vaginal vault suspension preparing for dissection of the pubocervical and rectovaginal fasciae. Spongesticks have been placed in the vagina (above) and rectum (below).

**Plate 4** Laparoscopic uterosacral vaginal vault suspension. Uterosacral ligaments have been stitched into the pubocervical and rectovaginal fasciae.

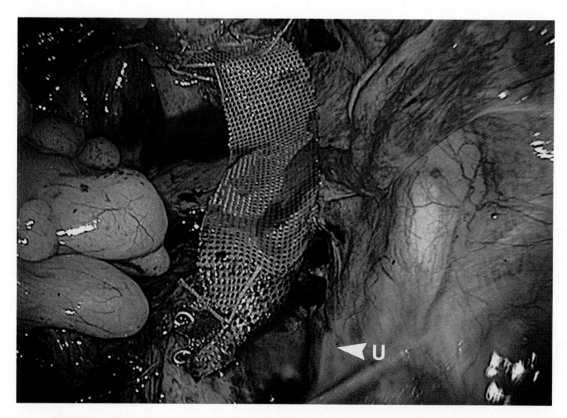

**Plate 5** Laparoscopic sacral colpopexy. Mesh extends from the vagina to the sacral promontory. Arrow shows position of right ureter.

**Table 15-6**    Comparative Studies of Bulk-Enhancing Agents for Urinary Stress Incontinence

| Study | Number of patients | Type of incontinence | Average follow-up (mo) | Number cured (%) | Number improved (%) | Number failed (%) |
|---|---|---|---|---|---|---|
| **Collagen** | | | | | | |
| Stricker and Haylen (1993) | 50 | ISD | 11 | 21 (42) | 20 (40) | 7 (14) |
| McGuire and Appell (1994) | 13 | ISD | >12 | 63 (46) | 47 (34) | 29 (19) |
| | 7 | Hypermobile | >12 | 8 (47) | 3 (17) | 6 (35) |
| | 17 | | | | | |
| O'Connell et al. (1995) | 42 | ISD | 1-2 | 20 (45) | 8 (18) | 16 (37) |
| Monga et al. (1995) | 60 | Mixed | 12 (N = 54) | 22 (40) | 20 (37) | 12 (22) |
| | | | 24 (N = 29) | 14 (48) | 6 (20) | 4 (14) |
| Herschorn and Radomski (1997) | 18 | ISD: 60 | >24 | 27 (43) | 29 (47) | 6 (10) |
| | 1 | Hypermobile: 121 | >36 | 13 (52) | 8 (32) | 4 (16) |
| Swami et al. (1997) | 10 | Mixed | 24 | 27 (25) | 43 (40) | 37 (35) |
| | 7 | | | | | |
| **Polytetrafluoroethylene** | | | | | | |
| Politano (1982) | 51 | — | 6 | (51) | (20) | (29) |
| Beckingham et al. (1992) | 26 | — | 36 | (7) | (20) | (73) |
| Harrison et al. (1993) | 36 | — | 61 | (11) | (22) | (67) |
| Lopez et al. (1993) | 74 | — | 31 | (56) | (20) | (24) |
| **Autologous Fat** | | | | | | |
| Trockman and Leach (1995) | 32 | — | 6 | 4 (12) | 14 (44) | 14 (44) |
| Haab et al. (1997) | 45 | — | 7 | 6 (13) | 13 (29) | 26 (58) |
| Su et al. (1998) | 26 | — | 17 | 13 (50) | 4 (15) | 9 (35) |

*ISD,* Intrinsic sphincter deficiency.

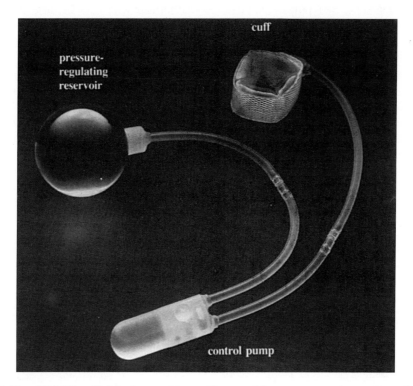

**Fig. 15-19**    AMS 800 artificial urinary sphincter. Note small button on control pump for activation and deactivation of the device.

Courtesy American Medical Systems, Minnetonka, Minnesota.

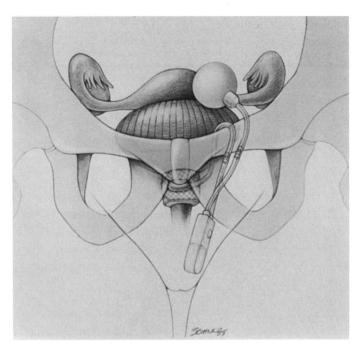

**Fig. 15-20**   Implanted artificial urinary sphincter.
Courtesy American Medical Systems, Minnetonka, Minnesota.

soaked in antimicrobial solutions, and proper antibiotic levels are achieved in all tissues before implantation.

## Techniques for Implantation

Implantation of the artificial urinary sphincter has historically been via an abdominal approach to minimize infection and contamination. More recently, however, a transvaginal approach has also been described. Regardless of the route of cuff placement, certain precautions must always be taken. Excessive handling of the device should be avoided. All components of the device except the control assembly are composed of silicone rubber and are thus vulnerable to puncture from needles or sharp instruments. Silicone-shod hemostats to clamp the tubing are used to avoid damage to the device. Blood must not enter the tubing because it will block the one-way valves in the pump assembly and result in device malfunction.

If an abdominal approach is elected, a low transverse muscle-cutting incision allows for the best exposure of the retropubic space. A urethral catheter with a 30-ml balloon is placed for easy identification of the bladder neck. The retropubic space is entered, and dissection is carried down to the level of the bladder neck. If the patient has undergone previous retropubic surgery, excessive scar tissue may be encountered and one should not hesitate to open the bladder to facilitate the dissection. A small incision is made in the endopelvic fascia on each side of the bladder neck. Dissection between the urethra and the vagina must be

performed with care because there is no anatomic plane between these two structures.

Caution must be taken to make sure that the plane of dissection is distal to the ureteral orifices. A cutter clamp or right-angle scissors is helpful for this dissection. The placing of a finger in the vagina and the elevation of the urethra with a Babcock clamp will help delineate the correct plane. Once created, the suburethral tunnel is gently dilated with a right-angle clamp so that it will accept a 2-cm cuff.

A cuff sizer is then passed to measure the circumference of the bladder neck. The adult female bladder neck generally requires a 7- to 9-cm cuff. With the use of a right-angle clamp, the appropriately sized cuff is slid into position. The tubing is routed through the layers of the anterior abdominal wall to emerge in the subcutaneous position near the left side of the incision. The pressure-regulating balloon is placed in the prevesical space and its tubing routed in a manner similar to that described for the cuff.

A Hegar dilator is bluntly dissected into one labium majora to create a space for the pump. The pump is then placed in the dissected space so that it rests immediately beneath the skin to allow for easy palpation and manipulation. All tubing from the three components is passed to the subcutaneous space, and filling of the system and connections are made according to the published instructions from the manufacturers.

The device is then left in a deactivated mode for approximately 6 weeks to allow adequate tissue healing. A

Foley catheter is left in place for 24 to 48 hours. If the bladder or urethra was opened, drainage should be continued for 7 to 10 days.

More recently, Appell (1988) advocated a transvaginal approach for insertion of the cuff. The goal is to decrease the chance of injury to the proximal urethra and bladder neck, which can easily occur with the abdominal route. An inverted U-shaped incision is made in the anterior vaginal wall, and the vaginal mucosa is dissected away from the posterior urethra and bladder neck. At the level of the bladder neck, the dissection is extended laterally and the retropubic space is sharply or bluntly entered between the pubic bone and the endopelvic fascia. Sharp and blunt dissection is used to completely mobilize the proximal urethra and bladder neck. The catheter is removed, and the cuff sizer is passed circumferentially around the bladder neck. The appropriate-sized cuff is inserted and snapped in place.

A 6-cm transverse skin incision is then made approximately one finger-breadth above the symphysis pubis. The rectus muscle on one side is transected to allow access to the retropubic space. Using a tubing passer, the tubing from the cuff is passed superiorly to exit through the lower abdominal incision. The vaginal incision is then closed with a 2-0 absorbable suture, and a vaginal packing is placed.

If there is concern about the integrity of the vaginal wall, interposition of a Martius fat pad from the labium not containing the pump may be considered. A space is bluntly created in the retropubic space to accommodate the pressure-regulating balloon. The remainder of the connections and implantation of the pump are performed as previously described.

## Results and Complications

The artificial urinary sphincter has been shown to be effective in restoring continence in appropriately selected female patients. Diokno et al. (1987) reported a 91% success rate in 32 women who had the device implanted abdominally. Mechanical complications requiring surgical repair occurred in 21% of these patients. These complications included two loose cuffs, two cuff leaks, two tubing kinks, and one connector leak. All of these complications were successfully corrected. Two nonmechanical complications were reported: One pelvic abscess occurred, which required removal of the device, and one superficial wound dehiscence developed. More recently, Appell (1988) reported 34 women who underwent implantation via a combined vaginal and abdominal approach; he achieved a 100% cure rate for incontinence with no case of erosion or infection. Other studies by Scott (1985), Donovan et al. (1985), Mundy and Stephenson (1984), and Stanton (1985) have also reported good results.

## CONCLUSION

Vaginal operations for GSI include a wide variety of surgical procedures. Goals of preoperative assessment are to objec-

tively demonstrate GSI, assess for urethral hypermobility and ISD, and determine whether any detrusor abnormalities are contributing to the patient's symptoms. Surgical therapy should be individualized based on the patient's presentation and coexisting modifying factors, including age, concurrent medical conditions, and need for additional vaginal surgery. Every pelvic reconstructive surgeon should be familiar with these procedures with respect to surgical technique, cure rates, and diagnosis and management of postoperative complications. Future trends seem to indicate an expanded role for suburethral slings and bulk-enhancing agents while needle suspension procedures become less popular.

## BIBLIOGRAPHY
### Anterior Colporrhaphy With Suburethral Plication
Beck RP, McCormick S, Nordstrom L: A 25-year experience with 519 anterior colporrhaphy procedures, *Obstet Gynecol* 78:1011, 1991.

Bergman A, Elia G: Three surgical procedures for genuine stress incontinence: five-year follow-up of a prospective randomized trial, *Am J Obstet Gynecol* 173:66, 1995.

Fantl JA, Newman DK, Colling J, et al: Urinary incontinence in adults: acute and chronic management. *Clinical practice guideline, no 2, 1996 update*, Rockville, Md, US Department of Health and Human Services, Public Health Services, Agency for Health Care Policy and Research, 1996.

Harris RL, Yancey CA, Wiser WL, et al: Comparison of anterior colporrhaphy and retropubic urethropexy for patients with genuine stress urinary incontinence, *Am J Obstet Gynecol* 173:167, 1995.

Jarvis GJ: Surgery for genuine stress incontinence, *Br J Obstet Gynaecol* 101:371, 1994.

Kelly HA, Dunn W: Urinary incontinence in women without manifest injury to the bladder, *Surg Gynecol Obstet* 18:444, 1914.

Kennedy WT: Incontinence of urine in the female, the urethral sphincter mechanism, damage of function and restoration of control, *Am J Obstet Gynecol* 34:576, 1937.

Kohli N, Karram MM: Transvaginal needle suspension procedures. In Lentz G, ed: *Urogynecology: diagnosis and treatment of female incontinence,* New York, 1998, Chapman-Hall.

Liapis A, Pyrgiotis E, Kontoravdis A, et al: Genuine stress incontinence: prospective randomized comparison of two operative methods, *Eur J Obstet Gynecol Reprod Biol* 64:69, 1996.

Ostergard DR, Bent AE, eds: The evaluation of different surgical procedures. In *Urogynecology and urodynamics: theory and practice,* Baltimore, 1991, William & Wilkins.

Park GS, Miller EJ: Surgical treatment of stress urinary incontinence: a comparison of the Kelly plication, Marshall-Marchetti-Krantz, and Pereyra procedures, *Obstet Gynecol* 71:575, 1988.

Tamussino K, Zivkovic F, Pieber D, et al: Funfo-Jabres-Ergebnisse nach Inkontinenzoperation, *Gynakol Geburtschilfliche Rundsch* 35:175, 1995.

Vahlensieck WK, Schander K: Long-term results of the operative treatment of stress incontinence by anterior colporrhaphy with diaphragmplasty, *Geburtshilfe Frauenheilkd* 45:887-890, 1985.

VanGeelen JM, Theeuwes AG, Eskes TK, et al: The clinical and urodynamic effects of anterior vaginal repair and Burch colposuspension, *Am J Obstet Gynecol* 159:137, 1988.

### Transvaginal Needle Suspension Procedures
Ashken MH, Abrams PH, Lawrence WT: Stamey endoscopic bladder neck suspension for stress incontinence, *Br J Urol* 56:629, 1984.

Benderev TV: A modified percutaneous outpatient bladder neck suspension system, *J Urol* 153:2316, 1994.

Benson JT, Lucente V, McClellan E: Vaginal versus abdominal reconstructive surgery for the treatment of pelvic support defects: a prospective randomized study with long term outcome evaluation, *Am J Obstet Gynecol* 175:1418, 1996.

Bergman A, Ballard CA, Koonings PP: Comparison of three different surgical procedures for genuine stress incontinence: prospective randomized study, *Am J Obstet Gynecol* 160:1102, 1989a.

Bergman A, Kooning PP, Ballard CA: Primary stress urinary incontinence and pelvic relaxation: prospective randomized comparison of three different operations, *Am J Obstet Gynecol* 161:91, 1989b.

Bhatia NN, Bergman A: Modified Burch versus Pereyra retropubic urethropexy for stress urinary incontinence, *Obstet Gynecol* 66:255, 1985.

Bhatia NN, Bergman A: Use of preoperative uroflowmetry and simultaneous urethrocystometry for predicting risk of prolonged postoperative bladder drainage, *Urology* 28:440, 1986.

Cardoza LD, Stanton SL, Williams JE: Detrusor instability following surgery for genuine stress incontinence, *Br J Urol* 51:204, 1979.

English PJ, Fowler JW: Videourodynamic assessment of the Stamey procedure for stress incontinence, *Br J Urol* 62(6):550, 1988.

Gittes RF, Loughlin KR: No incision pubovaginal suspension for stress incontinence, *J Urol* 138:568, 1987.

Griffith-Jones MD, Abrams PH: The Stamey endoscopic bladder neck in the elderly, *Br J Obstet Gynecol* 65:170, 1990.

Hilton P: A clinical and urodynamic study comparing the Stamey bladder neck suspension and suburethral sling procedures in the treatment of genuine stress incontinence, *Br J Obstet Gynecol* 96:213, 1989.

Karram MM, Angel O, Koonings P, et al: The modified Pereyra procedure. A clinical and urodynamic review, *Br J Obstet Gynecol* 99:655, 1992.

Karram MM, Bhatia NN: Management of coexistent stress and urge urinary incontinence, *Obstet Gynecol* 73:4, 1989.

Karram MM, Bhatia NN: Transvaginal needle bladder neck suspension procedures for stress urinary incontinence: a comprehensive review, *Obstet Gynecol* 73:906, 1989.

Katske FA, Raz S: Use of Foley catheter to obtain transvaginal tamponade, *Urol Urotech* May 1987, p 8.

Kelly MJ, Knielsen K, Bruskewitz R, et al: Symptom analysis of patients undergoing modified Pereyra bladder neck suspension for stress urinary incontinence. Preoperative and postoperative findings, *Urology* 28:213, 1991.

Kelly MJ, Zimmern PE, Leach GE: Complications of bladder neck suspension procedures, *Urol Clin North Am* 18:342, 1991.

Kohli N, Sze EHM, Karram MM: Incidence of recurrent cystocele after transvaginal needle suspension procedure with and without concomitant anterior colporrhaphy, *Am J Obstet Gynecol* 175:1476, 1996.

Koonings PP, Bergman A, Ballard CA: Low urethral pressure and stress urinary incontinence in women: risk factor for failed retropubic surgical procedure, *Urology* 36:245, 1990.

Korman HJ, Sirls LT, Kirkemo AK: Success rates by modified Peyera bladder neck suspension determined by outcomes analysis, *J Urol* 152(5):1453, 1994.

Leach GE: Bone fixation technique for transvaginal needle suspension, *Urology* 31:388, 1988.

Leach GE, Yip CM, Donovan BJ: Mechanism of continence after modified Pereyra bladder neck suspension, *Urology* 29:328, 1987.

McGuire EJ, Savastano JA: Stress incontinence and detrusor instability/urge incontinence, *Neurourol Urodyn* 4:313, 1985.

Miyazaki F, Shook G: Ilioinguinal nerve entrapment during needle suspension for stress incontinence, *Obstet Gynecol* 80:246, 1992.

Mundy AR: A trial comparing the Stamey bladder neck suspension procedure with colposuspension for the treatment of stress incontinence, *Br J Urol* 55:687, 1983.

Muzsnai D, Carrillo E, Dubin C, et al: Retropubic vaginopexy for correction of urinary stress incontinence, *Obstet Gynecol* 59:113, 1982.

Peattie AB, Stanton SL: The Stamey operation for correction of genuine stress incontinence in the elderly woman, *Br J Obstet Gynecol* 96:983, 1989.

Pereyra AJ: A simplified surgical procedure for the correction of stress incontinence in women, *West J Surg* 67:223, 1959.

Pereyra AJ, Lebherz TB: Combined urethral vesical suspension vaginal urethroplasty for correction of urinary stress incontinence, *Obstet Gynecol* 30:537, 1967.

Pereyra AJ, Lebherz TB: The revised Pereyra procedure. In Buchsbaum H, Schmidt JD, eds: *Gynecologic and obstetric urology,* Philadelphia, 1978, WB Saunders.

Raz S: Modified bladder neck suspension for female stress incontinence, *Urology* 17:82, 1981.

Riggs JA: Retropubic cystourethropexy: a review of two operative procedures with long-term follow-up, *Obstet Gynecol* 68:98, 1986.

Spencer JR, O'Connor VJ, Schaeffer AJ: A comparison of endoscopic suspension of the vesical neck with suprapubic vesicourethropexy for treatment of stress urinary incontinence, *J Urol* 137:411, 1987.

Spencer JR, O'Connor VJ, Schaeffer AJ: Comparison of procedures for stress urinary incontinence, *AJA Update Series* 6:1, 1987.

Stamey TA: Endoscopic suspension of the vesical neck for urinary incontinence in females, *Ann Surg* 192:465, 1980.

Stamey TA, Schaffer AJ, Condy M: Clinical and roentgenographic evaluation of endoscopic suspension of the vesical neck for urinary incontinence, *Surg Gynecol Obstet* 140:355, 1975.

Sze EHM, Miklos JR, Partol L, et al: Sacrospinous ligament fixation with transvaginal needle suspension for advanced pelvic organ prolapse and stress incontinence, *Obstet Gynecol* 89:94, 1997.

Trockman BA, et al: Modified Peyera bladder neck suspension: 10-year mean follow-up using outcomes analysis in 125 patients, *J Urol* 154(5):1041, 1995.

Webster GD, Sihelnik SA, Stone AR: Female urinary incontinence: the incidence, identification and characterization of detrusor instability, *Neurourol Urodyn* 3:235, 1984.

Zimmern PE, Schmidbauer CP, Leach GE, et al: Vesicovaginal and urethrovaginal fistulae, *Semin Urol* 424, 1986.

## Suburethral Slings

Aldridge AH: Transplantation of fascia for relief of urinary stress incontinence, *Am J Obstet Gynecol* 44:398, 1942.

Barns HH: Round ligament sling operation for stress incontinence, *J Obstet Gynaecol Br Emp* 57:404, 1950.

Beck RP: The sling operation. In Buchsbaum HJ, Schmidt JD, eds: *Gynecologic and obstetric urology,* ed 2, Philadelphia, 1982, WB Saunders.

Beck RP, McCormick RN, Nordstrom L: The fascia lata sling procedure for treating recurrent genuine stress incontinence of urine, *Obstet Gynecol* 72:699, 1988.

Black NA, Downs SH: The effectiveness of surgery for stress incontinence in women: a systematic review, *Br J Urol* 78(4):497, 1996.

Blaivas JG: Pubovaginal sling. In Kursh ED, McGuire EJ, eds: *Female urology,* Philadelphia, 1994, Lippincott.

Bracht E: Eine besondere form der zügelplastik, *Geburtshilfe Und Frauenheilkund* 16:782, 1956.

Breen JM, Geer BM, May GE: The fascia lata suburethral sling for treating recurrent urinary stress incontinence, *Am J Obstet Gynecol* 177(6):1363, 1997.

Bryans FE: Marlex gauze hammock sling operation with Cooper's ligament attachment in the management of recurrent urinary incontinence, *Am J Obstet Gynecol* 133:292, 1979.

Bump RC, Hurt WG, Theofrastous JP, et al: Randomized prospective comparison of needle culposuspension versus endopelvic fascia plication for potential stress incontinence prophylaxis in women undergoing vaginal reconstruction for stage III or IV pelvic organ prolapse, *Am J Obstet Gynecol* 175:325: 1996.

Goebell R: Zur operativen beseitigung der angeborenen, *Incontinentia Vesicae Z Gynakol Urol* 2:187, 1910.

Haab F, Zimmern PE, Leach GE: Female stress urinary incontinence due to intrinsic sphincter deficiency: recognition and management, *J Urol* 156(1):3, 1996.

Hadley RH, Zimmern PE, Staskin DR, et al: Transvaginal needle bladder neck suspension, *Urol Clin North Am* 12:299, 1985.

Hilton P: A clinical and urodynamic study comparing the Stamey bladder neck suspension and suburethral sling procedures in the treatment of genuine stress incontinence, *Br J Obstet Gynaecol* 96:213, 1989.

Hilton P, Stanton SL: Clinical and urodynamic evaluation of the polypropylene (Marlex) sling for genuine stress incontinence, *Neurol Urodyn* 2:145, 1983.

Hodgkinson CP, Kelly W: Urinary incontinence in the female. III. Round ligament technique for retropubic suspension of the urethra, *Obstet Gynecol* 10:493, 1957.

Hohenfellner R, Petrie E: Sling procedures in surgery. In Stanton SL, Tanagho E, eds: *Surgery of female incontinence,* ed 2, Berlin, 1986, Springer-Verlag, pp 105-113.

Horbach NS: Suburethral sling procedures. In Ostergard D, Bent A, eds: *Urogynecology and urodynamics: theory and practice,* ed 3, Baltimore, 1991, Williams & Wilkins.

Horbach NS, Blanco JS, Ostergard DR, et al: A suburethral sling procedure with polytetrafluoroethylene for the treatment of genuine stress incontinence in patients with low urethral closure pressure, *Obstet Gynecol* 71:648, 1988.

Jarvis GJ, Fowlie A: Clinical and urodynamic assessment of the porcine dermis bladder sling in the treatment of genuine stress incontinence, *Br J Obstet Gynaecol* 92:1189, 1985.

Karram MM, Bhatia NN: Patch procedure: modified transvaginal fascia lata sling for recurrent or severe stress urinary incontinence, *Obstet Gynecol* 75:461, 1990.

Kersey J: The gauze hammock sling operation in the treatment of stress incontinence, *Br J Obstet Gynaecol* 90:945, 1983.

Lockhart JL, Tirado A, Morillo G, et al: Vesicourethral dysfunction following cystourethropexy, *J Urol* 128:943, 1982.

Low JA: Management of severe anatomic deficiencies of urethral sphincter function by a combined procedure with a fascia lata sling, *Am J Obstet Gynecol* 105:149, 1969.

McGuire EJ: Urodynamic findings in patients after failure of stress incontinence operations, *Prog Clin Biol Res* 78:351, 1981.

McGuire EJ: Abdominal procedures for stress incontinence, *Urol Clin North Am* 12:285, 1985.

McGuire EJ, Bennett CJ, Konnak JA, et al: Experience with pubovaginal slings for urinary incontinence at University of Michigan, *J Urol* 138:525, 1987.

McGuire EJ, Lytton B: Pubovaginal sling procedure for stress incontinence, *J Urol* 119:82, 1978.

McGuire EJ, O'Connell HE: Surgical treatment of intrinsic urethral dysfunction: slings, *Urol Clin North Am* 22(3):657, 1995.

McGuire EJ, Wang CC, Usitalo H, et al: Modified pubovaginal sling in girls with myelodysplasia, *J Urol* 135:94, 1986.

McLaren HC: Fascial slings for stress incontinence, *J Obstet Gynaecol Br Emp* 64:673, 1957.

McLaren HC: Late results from sling operations, *J Gynecol* 75:10, 1968.

McLennan MT, Bent AE: Fascia lata suburethral sling vs. Burch retropubic urethropexy: a comparison of morbidity, *J Reprod Med* 43(6):488, 1993.

Millin T, Read C: Stress incontinence of urine in the female: Millin's sling operation for stress incontinence, *Postgrad Med J* 24:51, 1948.

Morgan JE: A sling operation using Marlex polypropylene mesh for treatment of recurrent stress incontinence, *Am J Obstet Gynecol* 106:369, 1970.

Morgan JE, Farrow GA, Steward FE: The Marlex sling operation for the treatment of recurrent stress urinary incontinence. A 16-year review, *Am J Obstet Gynecol* 151:224, 1985.

Nichols DH: The Mersilene mesh gauze hammock for severe urinary stress incontinence, *Obstet Gynecol* 41:88, 1973.

Obrink A, Bunne G: The margin of incontinence after three types of operation for stress incontinence, *Scand J Urol Nephrol* 12:209, 1978.

Ogundipe A, Rosenzweig BA, Karram MM, et al: Modified suburethral sling procedures for treatment of recurrent or severe stress urinary incontinence, *Surg Obstet Gynecol* 175:173, 1992.

Owens RG, Kohli N, Wynne J, et al: Long-term results of a fascia lata suburethral patch sling for severe stress incontinence, *J Pelvic Surg* (in press, 1999).

Parker RT, Addison WA, Wilson CJ: Fascia lata urethrovesical suspension for recurrent stress urinary incontinence, *Am J Obstet Gynecol* 135:843, 1979.

Poliak A, Daniller AI, Liebling RW: Sling operation for recurrent stress incontinence using the tendon of the palmaris longus, *Obstet Gynecol* 63:850, 1984.

Ridley JG: Appraisal of the Goebell-Frankenheim-Stoekel sling procedure, *Am J Obstet Gynecol* 95:714, 1966.

Stanton SL, Brindley GS, Holmes DM: Silastic sling for urethral sphincter incompetence in women, *Br J Obstet Gynaecol* 92:747, 1985.

Staskin DR, Choe JM, Breslin DS: The Gore-tex sling procedure for female sphincteric incontinence: indications, technique, and results, *World J Urol* 15(5):295, 1997.

Stoeckel W: Uber die verwendung der musculi pyridimale beider operativen behandlung der incontinentia urinae, *Gynakologe* 41:11, 1917.

Stothers L, Chopra A, Raz S: Vaginal wall sling for anatomic incontinence and intrinsic sphincter damage: efficacy and outcome analysis, *J Urol* 153:525, 1995.

Ulmsten V, Henriksson L, Johnson P, et al: An ambulatory surgical procedure under local anesthesia for treatment of female urinary incontinence, *Int Urogynecol J* 7:81, 1996.

Weinberger MW, Ostergard DR: Postoperative catheterization, urinary retention, and permanent voiding dysfunction after polytetrafluoroethylene suburethral sling placement, *Obstet Gynecol* 87(1):50, 1996.

Williams TJ, TeLinde RW: The sling operation for urinary incontinence using Mersilene ribbon, *Obstet Gynecol* 19:241, 1962.

Young SB, Rosenblatt PL, Pingeton DM, et al: The Mersilene mesh suburethral sling: a clinical and urodynamic evaluation, *Am J Obstet Gynecol* 173(6):1719, 1995.

## Injection of Bulk-Enhancing Agents

Appell RA: Injectables for urethral incompetence, *World J Urol* 8:208, 1990.

Appell RA: New developments: injectables for urethral incompetence in women, *Int Urogynecol J* 1:117, 1990.

Beckingham IJ, Wemyss-Holden G, Lawrence WT: Long-term follow-up of women treated with periurethral Teflon injections for stress incontinence, *Br J Urol* 69:580, 1992.

Berg S: Polytef augmentation urethroplasty. Correction of surgically incurable urinary incontinence by injection technique, *Arch Surg* 107:379, 1973.

Berman CJ, Kreder KJ: Comparative cost analysis of collagen injection and fascia lata sling cystourethropexy for the treatment of type III incontinence in women, *J Urol* 157:122, 1997.

Boykin W, Rodriguez FR, Brizzolara JP, et al: Complete urinary obstruction following periurethral polytetrafluoroethylene injection for urinary incontinence, *J Urol* 141:1199, 1989.

Cervigni M, Panei M: Periurethral autologous fat injection for type III stress urinary incontinence, *J Urol* 149:403A, 1993.

Claes H, Stroobants D, van Meerbeek J, et al: Pulmonary migration following periurethral polytetrafluoroethylene injection for urinary incontinence, *J Urol* 142:821, 1989.

Cross CA, English SF, Cespedes RD, et al: A follow-up on transurethral collagen injection therapy for urinary incontinence, *J Urol* 159:106, 1998.

Deane AM, English P, Hehir M, et al: Teflon injection in stress incontinence, *Br J Urol* 140:1101, 1985.

Eckford SD, Abrams P: Para-urethral collagen implantation for female stress incontinence, *Br J Urol* 68:586, 1991.

Faerber GJ: Endoscopic collagen injection therapy in elderly women with type I stress urinary incontinence, *J Urol* 155:512, 1996.

Ford CN, Martin DW, Warren TF: Injectable collagen in laryngeal rehabilitation, *Laryngoscope* 95:513, 1988.

Haab F, Zimmern PE, Leach GE: Urinary stress incontinence due to intrinsic sphincteric deficiency: experience with fat and collagen periurethral injections, *J Urol* 157:1283, 1997.

Harrison SC, Brown C, O'Boyle PJ: Periurethral Teflon for stress urinary incontinence: medium-term results, *Br J Urol* 71:25, 1993.

Harriss DR, Iacovou JW, Lemberger RJ: Peri-urethral silicone microimplants (Macroplastique) for the treatment of genuine stress incontinence, *Br J Urol* 78:722, 1996.

Herschorn S, Radomski SB: Collagen injections for genuine stress urinary incontinence: patient selection and durability, *Int Urogynecol J* 8:18, 1997.

Khullar V, Cardozo LD, Abbott D, et al: GAX collagen in the treatment of urinary incontinence in elderly women: a two-year follow up, *Br J Obstet Gynecol* 104:96, 1997.

Kieswetter H, Fischer M, Wober L, et al: Endoscopic implantation of collagen (GAX) for the treatment of urinary incontinence, *Br J Urol* 69:22, 1992.

Leonard MP, Canning DA, Epstein JI, et al: Local tissue reaction to the subureteric injection of glutaraldehyde cross-linked bovine collagen in humans, *J Urol* 143:1209, 1990.

Lim KB, Ball AJ, Feneley RCL: Periurethral Teflon injection: a simple treatment for urinary incontinence, *Br J Urol* 55:208, 1983.

Lockhart JL, Walker RD, Vorstam B, et al: Periurethral polytetrafluoroethylene injection following urethral reconstruction in female patients with urinary incontinence, *J Urol* 140:51, 1988.

Lopez AE, Padron OF, Patsins G, et al: Transurethral polytetrafluoroethylene injection in female patients with urinary incontinence, *J Urol* 150:856, 1993.

Malizia AA, Reiman MM, Myers RP, et al: Migration and granulation after periurethral injection of Polytef (Teflon), *JAMA* 251:3277, 1984.

McGuire EJ, Appell R: Transurethral collagen injection for urinary incontinence, *Urology* 43:413, 1994.

Mittleman RE, Marraccini JV: Pulmonary Teflon granulomas following periurethral Teflon injection for urinary incontinence (letter), *Arch Pathol Lab Med* 107:611, 1983.

Monga AK, Robinson D, Stanton SL: Periurethral collagen injections for genuine stress incontinence, *Br J Urol* 76:156, 1995.

Moore KN, Chetner MP, Metcalfe JB, et al: Periurethral implantation of glutaraldehyde cross-linked collagen (Contigen) in women with type I or type III stress incontinence: quantitative outcome measures, *Br J Urol* 75:359, 1995.

Murless BC: The injection treatment of stress incontinence, *J Obstet Gynaecol Br Emp* 45:67, 1938.

Neal DE Jr, Lahaye ME, Lowe DC: Improved needle placement technique in periurethral collagen injection, *Urology* 45(5):865, 1995.

O'Connell HE, McGuire EJ, Aboseif S, et al: Transurethral collagen therapy in women, *J Urol* 154:1463, 1995.

Osther PJ, Rohe HF: Female urinary stress incontinence treated with Teflon injections, *Acta Obstet Gynecol Scand* 66:33, 1987.

Palma PC, Riccetto CL, Netto Jr NR: Urethral pseudolipoma: a complication of periurethral lipo-injection for stress urinary incontinence in a woman, *J Urol* 155:646, 1996.

Politano VA: Periurethral Teflon injection for urinary incontinence, *Urol Clin North Am* 5:451, 1978.

Politano VA: Periurethral polytetrafluorethylene injection for urinary urethral incontinence, *J Urol* 172:439, 1982.

Politano VA: Migration of polytetrafluorethylene polytef (letter), *JAMA* 254:1903, 1985.

Politano VA, Small MP, Harper JM, et al: Periurethral Teflon injection: a simple treatment for urinary incontinence, *J Urol* 111:180, 1974.

Quackels R: Deux incontinence après adénectomie guéries par injection de paraffine dans la périnée, *Acta Urol Belg* 23:259, 1955.

Richardson TD, Kennelly MJ, Faerber GJ: Endoscopic injection of glutaraldehyde cross-linked collagen for the treatment of intrinsic deficiency in women, *Urology* 46:378, 1996.

Sachse H: Treatment of urinary incontinence with sclerosing solutions: indications, results, complications, *Urol Int* 15:225, 1963.

Santarosa RP, Blaivas JG: Periurethral injection of autologous fat for the treatment of sphincteric incontinence, *J Urol* 151:607, 1994.

Schulman CC, Simon J, Wespes E, et al: Endoscopic injection of Teflon for female urinary incontinence, *Eur Urol* 9:246, 1982.

Shortliffe LMD, Freiha FS, Kessler R, et al: Treatment of urinary incontinence by the periurethral implantation of glutaraldehyde cross-linked collagen, *J Urol* 141:538, 1989.

Smith DN, Appell RA, Winters JC, et al: Collagen injection therapy for female intrinsic sphincteric deficiency, *J Urol* 157:1275, 1997.

Stricker P, Haylen B: Injectable collagen for type III female stress incontinence: the first 50 Australian patients, *Med J Aust* 158:80, 1993.

Su T-H, Wang K-G, Hsu C-Y, et al: Periurethral fat injection in the treatment of recurrent genuine stress incontinence, *J Urol* 159:411, 1998.

Swami S, Batista JE, Abrams P: Collagen for female genuine stress after a minimum 2-year follow-up, *Br J Urol* 80:757, 1997.

Trockman BA, Leach GE: Surgical treatment of intrinsic urethral dysfunction: injectables (fat), *Urol Clin North Am* 22:665, 1995.

Winters JC, Appell R: Periurethral injection of collagen in the treatment of intrinsic sphincter deficiency in the female patient, *Urol Clin North Am* 22:673, 1995.

**Artificial Urinary Sphincter**

Appell RA: Techniques and results in the implantation of the artificial urinary sphincter in women with type III stress urinary incontinence by vaginal approach, *Neurourol Urodyn* 7:613, 1988.

Diokno AC, Hollander JB, Alderson TP: Artificial urinary sphincter for recurrent female urinary incontinence: indications and results, *J Urol* 137:778, 1987.

Diokno AC, Sonda LP: Compatibility of genitourinary prostheses and intermittent self-catheterization, *J Urol* 125:659, 1981.

Donovan MG, Barrett DM, Furlow WL: Use of the artificial urinary sphincter in the management of severe incontinence in females, *Surg Gynecol Obstet* 161:17, 1985.

Furlow WL: Implantation of a new semiautomatic artificial genitourinary sphincter: experience with primary activation and deactivation in 47 patients, *J Urol* 126:741, 1981.

Hadley HR: The artificial sphincter in the female, *Prob Urol* 5:123, 1991.

Karram MM, Rosenswerg B, Bhatia NN: The artificial urinary sphincter in the management of severe urinary incontinence in women. Urogynecological perspective, *J Reprod Med* 38:791, 1993.

Light JK: Abdominal approach for implantation of the AS-800 artificial urinary sphincter in females, *Neurourol Urodyn* 7:603, 1988.

Mundy AR, Stephenson TP: Selection of patients for implantation of the Brantley Scott artificial urinary sphincter, *Br J Urol* 56:717, 1984.

Perulkar BC, Barrett DM: Application of the AS-800 artificial sphincter for intractable urinary incontinence in females, *Surg Gynecol Obstet* 171:131, 1990.

Scott FB: The use of the artificial sphincter in the treatment of urinary incontinence in the female patient, *Urol Clin North Am* 12:305, 1985.

Scott FB, Bradley WE, Timm GW: Treatment of urinary incontinence by an implantable prosthetic urinary sphincter, *Urology* 1:252, 1973.

Scott FB, Bradley WE, Timm GW: Treatment of urinary incontinence by an implantable prosthetic urinary sphincter, *J Urol* 112:75, 1974.

Stanton SL: Artificial urinary sphincters (letter), *BMJ* 291:413, 1985.

Webster GD, Sihelnik SA: Trouble-shooting the malfunctioning Scott artificial urinary sphincter, *J Urol* 131:269, 1985.

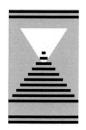

CHAPTER **16**

# *Laparoscopic Surgery for Genuine Stress Incontinence and Pelvic Organ Prolapse*

Marie Fidela R. Paraiso and Tommaso Falcone

---

---

Since laparoscopic retropubic urethropexy was introduced in 1991, the application of laparoscopy to surgical procedures for incontinence has evolved rapidly. The possible advantages of laparoscopic surgery are improved visualization of anatomy of the space of Retzius and peritoneal cavity because of laparoscopic magnification, insufflation effects, and improved hemostasis; shortened hospitalization; decreased postoperative pain and more rapid recovery and return to work; and better cosmetic appearance of smaller incisions. Disadvantages of laparoscopic surgery include technical difficulty of retroperitoneal dissection and in acquiring suturing skills, increased operating time early in the surgeon's experience, and greater hospital cost secondary to increased operating room time and the use of disposable surgical instruments.

Adoption of laparoscopic treatment of vaginal apex and posterior wall support defects has been less rapid, probably because most gynecologic surgeons prefer the vaginal route. There have been few case series on these procedures; however, they are increasing in number in the literature.

## LAPAROSCOPIC RETROPUBIC SURGICAL PROCEDURES

In the first report, Vancaillie and Schuessler (1991) duplicated the conventional Marshall-Marchetti-Krantz (MMK) procedure laparoscopically. Subsequently, Albala et al.

(1992) published a case series of MMK and Burch procedures. Numerous laparoscopic Burch case series have ensued. Many investigators have modified the laparoscopic retropubic colposuspension using mesh, staples, bone anchors, coils, and fibrin sealant. A variety of suturing and needle devices have also been used to simplify laparoscopic suturing and knot-tying, the most difficult skills to acquire.

It is well documented that the Burch procedure can be performed via a small laparotomy incision with good long-term success and minimal morbidity. In order to replace this accepted and effective approach with laparoscopic access, there must be comparable efficacy and an equivalent or better complication rate. If one is to consider performing a laparoscopic retropubic bladder neck suspension, we believe that it should be performed exactly the same as the open procedure. Modifications to the open procedure represent essentially new operations, thus requiring further study and outcome analysis.

### Indications

After the patient has been diagnosed with genuine stress incontinence (GSI) and has opted for surgical management, the choice of laparoscopic versus open retropubic colposuspension depends on numerous factors: history of previous pelvic or antiincontinence surgery; history of severe abdominopelvic infection or known extensive abdominopelvic adhesions; patient age and weight; ability to undergo general anesthesia; need for concomitant abdominal, pelvic, or vaginal surgery; patient preference; and operator experience and preference. To date, most laparoscopic colposuspensions have been done only for primary GSI because of difficulty in dissecting retropubic adhesions. Many patients prefer laparoscopic surgery because of the smaller, more cosmetic incisions, shorter recuperation time, and rapid return to work. We explain to our patients that we perform the same procedure open and laparoscopically and that it is only the route that differs. We also state that the procedure outcomes are still preliminary because reported studies are based on short-term follow-up.

### Anatomy

Thorough knowledge of the anatomy of the anterior abdominal wall is mandatory for safe and effective trocar insertion. The umbilicus is approximately at the L3-L4 level and the aortic bifurcation is at L4-L5. In obese women the umbilicus is caudal to the bifurcation. Thus, the intraumbilical trocar should be introduced at a more acute angle toward the pelvis in thin women and closer to 90 degrees in obese women. The left common iliac vein courses over the lower lumbar vertebrae from the right side and may be inferior to the umbilicus. Common iliac arteries course 5 cm before bifurcating into the internal and external iliac arteries. The ureter crosses the common iliac artery at or above its bifurcation.

The superficial epigastric artery, a branch of the femoral artery, courses cephalad and can be transilluminated. The inferior epigastric artery branches from the external iliac artery at the medial border of the inguinal ligament and runs lateral to and below the rectus sheath at the level of the arcuate line. It is accompanied by two inferior epigastric veins (Fig. 16-1). The median umbilical ligament, the embryonic urachus, is attached to the apex of the bladder and extends to the umbilicus. The urachus remains patent in some women and may be somewhat vascular. The medial umbilical folds, the peritoneum overlying the obliterated umbilical arteries, are the lateral landmarks of dissection of the parietal peritoneum during transperitoneal surgery into the space of Retzius. The upper margin of the dome of the bladder is noted approximately 3 cm above the pubic symphysis when the bladder is filled with 300 ml of fluid. Before distention of the bladder, the upper margin of the dome lies several centimeters above the pubic symphysis.

The important landmarks of the space of Retzius are Cooper's ligaments; the accessory or aberrant obturator veins; the obturator neurovascular bundles, which are 3 to 4 cm above the arcus tendineus fasciae pelvis; the bladder neck, which is delineated by placing traction on the Foley bulb; and the arcus tendineus fasciae pelvis and arcus tendineus levator ani, which insert into the pubic bone (Figs. 16-2 and 16-3).

## Operative Technique
### Operative Setup and Instrumentation

The operating room setup is shown in Fig. 16-4. The monitor screens should be placed lateral to the legs in direct view of the surgeon standing on the opposite side of the table. The scrub nurse should be in the center if two monitor screens are used; otherwise, the scrub nurse is located behind one surgeon and the electrosurgical unit or harmonic scalpel on the opposite side. After the three-way Foley catheter and uterine manipulator (if needed) have been placed, the vaginal tray with cystoscope is set aside, if desired, for later use.

Ideal stirrups for combined laparovaginal cases are the Allen stirrups (Allen Medical, Garfield, Ohio) that have levers that can quickly convert the patient from low to high lithotomy position while preserving sterility of the field. A Mayo stand positioned between the legs or a sterile pouch attached to the thigh is equipped with commonly used instruments such as unipolar scissors, bipolar cautery, graspers, and laparoscopic blunt-tipped dissectors. The irrigation should be set up before making incisions for trocars.

For standard suturing technique, needle holder preference is determined by comfort of the surgeon. The Storz Scarfi needle holder and notched assistant needle holder (Karl Storz Endoscopy, Culver City, California) are most

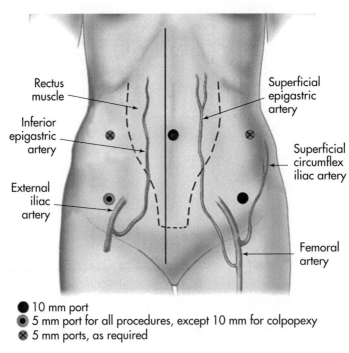

● 10 mm port
◉ 5 mm port for all procedures, except 10 mm for colpopexy
⊗ 5 mm ports, as required

**Fig. 16-1** Anatomy of the anterior abdominal wall and suggested laparoscopic trocar positions.

like conventional needle holders used during laparotomy. Conventional and 90-degree self-righting German needle holders (Ethicon Endo-Surgery, Inc., Cincinnati, Ohio) have ratchet spring handles and the Talon curved needle drivers with spring handles (Cook OB/GYN, Spencer, Indiana) self-right the needle at an angle, either 45 or 90 degrees to the needle driver shaft, depending on the style chosen. Disposable suturing devices have been introduced that include the Endo-stitch (U.S. Surgical Corp., Norwalk, Connecticut) and the Capio (previously known as the

Laurus device; Microvasive Boston Scientific, Inc., Natick, Massachusetts). Extracorporeal knot-tying is preferred because of technical facility and the ability to hold more tension on the suture. The choice of an open-ended or close-ended knot pusher for extracorporeal knot-tying depends on surgeon preference. Our suture of choice is the double-armed No. 0 Ethibond 36-inch suture on a SH or CT-2 needle (Ethicon, Inc., Somerville, New Jersey). Our alternative choice for suture is No. 0 Gore-Tex (W.L. Gore and Associates, Inc., Phoenix, Arizona). Forty-eight-inch suture is preferred when suturing from ports at the level of the umbilicus. Sterile steel thimbles may be used by the surgeon or assistant when elevating the vagina while the surgeon is placing the stitches in the vaginal wall.

### Skin Incisions for Trocar Sites

Intraumbilical or infraumbilical incisions are made depending on the anatomy of the umbilicus. Many variations of the accessory trocar sites have been described. We use two additional trocars: a 10/12-mm disposable trocar with reducer in the right lower quadrant (if knot-tying from the right) lateral to the right inferior epigastric vessels and a reusable 5-mm port in the left lower quadrant lateral to the left inferior epigastric vessels. Trocars are placed lateral to the rectus muscle, approximately 3 cm medial to and above the anterior superior iliac spine. An additional 5-mm port may be placed on the principal surgeon's side so that he or she can operate with two hands. Both reusable and disposable ports may be secured with circumferential screws to prevent port slippage. Port placement is shown in Fig. 16-1.

### Route: Extraperitoneal or Intraperitoneal

The choice of extraperitoneal or intraperitoneal approach depends on whether concomitant intraperitoneal procedures

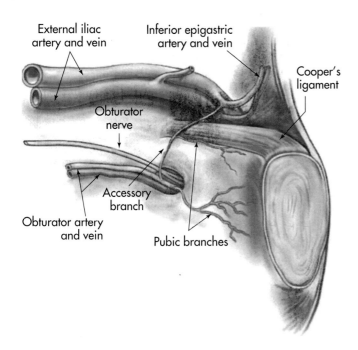

**Fig. 16-2** Anatomy of the pelvic sidewall near Cooper's ligament.

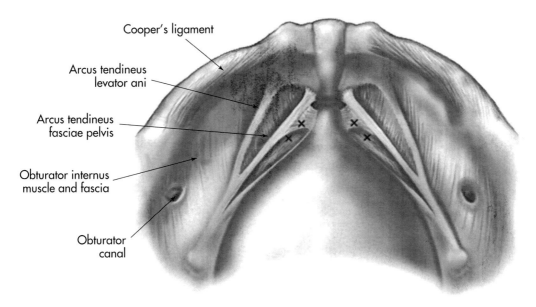

**Fig. 16-3** Retropubic space anatomy. *X* identifies suture placement during Burch procedure.

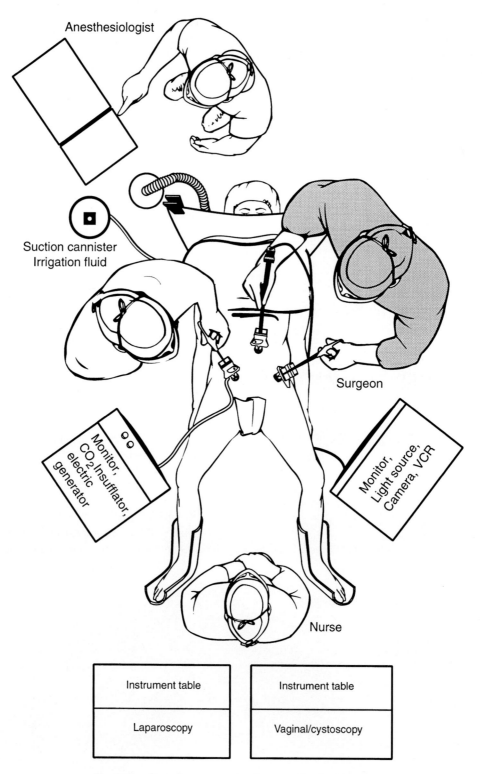

**Fig. 16-4** Operating room setup for operative laparoscopy.

are being performed, on whether the patient has had previous abdominal wall surgery, and on surgeon preference. Previous retropubic surgery is a contraindication for extraperitoneal approach and low transverse or midline incisions make the dissection more difficult and prone to failure. Some surgeons report less operating time, easier dissection, and fewer bladder injuries with the extraperitoneal route. This route is sometimes easier because the balloon performs the majority of the dissection. Others prefer the intraperitoneal approach because it allows a larger operating space for safe, secure, comfortable handling of the suture. Furthermore, a culdeplasty or other intraperitoneal surgery can be performed concomitantly.

The intraperitoneal approach begins with insertion of the zero-degree laparoscope through a 10-mm intraumbilical or infraumbilical cannula followed by intraabdominal insufflation. Inspection of the peritoneal cavity is performed, delineating the inferior epigastric vessels, abdominal and pelvic organs, pelvic adhesions, and coexisting abdominal or pelvic pathology. Two additional trocars (a 5-mm and a 10/12-mm) are placed under direct vision, one on each side, as previously noted.

All trocars are nondisposable except the 10/12-mm trocar through which 5- and 10-mm instruments are introduced. This site is used for introduction of the needles and sutures. Some surgeons backload suture through 5-mm ports and introduce and remove needles through the skin incisions. This is easily accomplished in thinner patients. However, trauma to the subcutaneous tissues and inferior epigastric vessels may result with this technique. Furthermore, it is difficult to use this technique with sutures with double-armed needles.

The bladder is filled with 200 to 300 ml sterile water or saline (indigo carmine or methylene blue is optional). Using sharp dissection with electrocautery or harmonic scalpel, a transverse incision 2 cm above the bladder reflection between the medial umbilical folds is made. Identification of the loose areolar tissue at the point of incision confirms a proper plane of dissection. Blunt and sharp dissection aiming toward the posterior-superior aspect of the pubic symphysis decreases risk of bladder injury. Blunt dissection then is carried out inferolaterally on both sides in order to identify the pubic symphysis, Cooper's ligaments, and bladder neck. Medial dissection over the urethra should be avoided.

The extraperitoneal approach to the space of Retzius is best performed using a balloon dissector (Origin Medsystems, Menlo Park, California; U.S. Surgical Corp., Norwalk, Connecticut). This approach begins with an infraumbilical incision and modified open laparoscopy. After the anterior sheath of the rectus fascia is incised, a finger is swept around the rectus muscle over the posterior rectus sheath and into the preperitoneal space. Lubricated Hagar dilators can aid blunt dissection to the retropubic space. The space of Retzius is dissected by tunneling the tip of the dissector to the posterior superior aspect of the pubic symphysis. The balloon is subsequently inflated under video guidance. A 10-mm Hasson cannula or its modification (some alternatives have inflatable balloons on the shaft to decrease $CO_2$ loss) is then placed, a zero-degree laparoscope is inserted, and $CO_2$ is insufflated into the preperitoneal space.

Further delineation of the retropubic anatomy is achieved with blunt dissection. Two additional ports are placed under direct vision lateral to the inferior epigastric vessels, taking special care to avoid entry into the peritoneal cavity.

## Laparoscopic Burch Colposuspension

After the space of Retzius is exposed, the surgeon places two fingers in the vagina and identifies the urethrovesical junction by placing gentle traction on the Foley catheter. With elevation of the vaginal fingers, the vaginal wall lateral to the bladder neck is exposed by using a laparoscopic blunt-tipped dissector. As recommended by Tanagho (1976), no dissection is performed within 2 cm of the bladder neck to avoid bleeding and damage to the periurethral musculature and nerve supply.

We place stitches in the vaginal wall excluding the vaginal epithelium at the level of, or just proximal to, the midurethra and bladder neck (see Fig. 16-3). No. 0 nonabsorbable suture is placed in a figure-of-eight stitch incorporating the entire thickness of the anterior vaginal wall. The needle is then passed through Cooper's ligament ipsilaterally. If double-armed suture is used, we make two passes through Cooper's ligament and subsequently tie above the ligament. We place gelfoam (Pharmacia Upjohn, Inc., Kalamazoo, Michigan) between the vaginal wall and the obturator fascia before knot-tying in order to promote fibrosis. With simultaneous vaginal elevation, the suture is tied with six extracorporeal square knots. Two granny half-hitches (equivalent to a surgical knot) and a flat square knot secure the stitch. Our technique for laparoscopic Burch procedure is illustrated in Plate 1 (after p. 190).

Sutures are tied as they are placed in order to avoid tangling. Midurethral stitches are placed first, although this is a matter of preference. It is easier to place stitches from the contralateral port. For example, a right-handed surgeon elevates the vagina with his or her left hand while simultaneously placing stitches on the patient's right side through the lower left port. In this circumstance the principal surgeon must switch sides with the assistant. If the lower quadrant ports are placed higher (at or slightly below the level of the umbilicus), placement of ipsilateral stitches is facilitated because the angle to the ipsilateral vaginal wall and Cooper's ligament is less acute. The appropriate level of bladder neck elevation is estimated with the assistant's vaginal hand. The assistant elevates the vaginal wall in order to place the urethra and bladder neck in a high retropubic position, which does not result in kinking or compression of the urethra. The goal is to elevate the vaginal wall to the level of the arcus tendineus fasciae pelvis bilaterally so that the bladder neck is supported and stabilized by the vaginal wall that acts as a hammock between both arcus tendineus fasciae. In tying the sutures, the surgeon should not reapproximate the vaginal wall to Cooper's ligament or place too much tension on the vaginal wall. A suture bridge of 1.5 to 2 cm is common.

## Laparoscopic Marshall-Marchetti-Krantz Procedure

The approach to the space of Retzius is identical to that for the laparoscopic Burch procedure. The surgeon's index and middle fingers of the nondominant hand are placed into the vagina at the bladder neck on each side of the urethra. A laparoscopic blunt-tipped dissector is used to dissect the periurethral fat. A figure-of-eight stitch of No. 0 delayed absorbable, 36-inch suture on a CT-2 needle is placed at the urethrovesical junction at right angles to the urethra and parallel to the vesical neck. The stitch is then placed in the periosteum of the pubic bone. Extracorporeal knot-tying is performed while the assistant maintains the preferred elevation of the urethrovesical junction. A single suture is placed bilaterally.

### Laparoscopic Paravaginal Defect Repair

Laparoscopic approach to the space of Retzius for the paravaginal defect repair is identical to the Burch procedure. The dissection is carried out laterally with a blunt-tipped dissector until the obturator internus muscle, obturator foramen with neurovascular bundle, and arcus tendineus fasciae pelvis are delineated. A vaginal hand is used to elevate the vagina and retract the bladder medially, thus aiding in the dissection of the vagina and lateral landmarks. Blunt dissection is carried out dorsally until vaginal palpation of the ischial spine is visualized laparoscopically.

Starting at the vaginal apex, a No. 2-0 nonabsorbable, 36- or 48-inch suture on a CT-2 needle is used to place a stitch into the full thickness of the vagina (excluding the vaginal epithelium) and then into the arcus tendineus fasciae pelvis, which is 3 to 4 cm below the obturator fossa (Plate 2). This is then tied extracorporeally. An additional three to five sutures are placed through the vaginal wall and into the arcus tendineus or fascia of the obturator internus muscle at 1-cm intervals until the defect is closed. The same procedure is performed on the opposite side.

If this procedure is performed concomitantly with the Burch colposuspension, the paravaginal defect repair should be performed first because exposure of the lateral defect decreases after the Burch sutures are tied. We place the stitch at the level of the ischial spine first and then place subsequent distal stitches as needed.

### General Intraoperative and Postoperative Procedures

The patient is instructed to take one bottle of magnesium citrate or equivalent bowel preparation and limit her diet to clear liquids on the day before surgery. Placing an orogastric or nasogastric tube to decompress the stomach at the time of surgery is also helpful. Patients receive prophylactic intravenous antibiotic therapy 30 minutes before surgery. Pneumatic compression stockings are routinely used. The Burch procedure, MMK, and paravaginal defect repair are performed under general anesthesia in the low lithotomy position. A 16-French three-way Foley catheter with a 20- to 30-ml balloon is attached to continuous drainage, and the irrigation port is connected to sterile water or saline.

After all sutures are placed and tied, transurethral cystos-

copy or suprapubic teloscopy is done to document ureteral patency and absence of sutures in the bladder. A suprapubic catheter is placed, if desired. The surgeon must reinspect the space of Retzius for bleeding while reducing the carbon dioxide insufflation. Routine closure of the peritoneum is not performed. All ports are removed under direct visualization and the peritoneum and fascia of all 10/12-mm incisions are reapproximated with the Endoclose device (U.S. Surgical Corp., Norwalk, Connecticut) or the Grice needle (New Ideas in Medicine, Inc., Clearwater, Florida). The skin is closed in a subcuticular fashion. The fascia and subcutaneous fat are infiltrated with a long-acting local anesthetic, such as bupivacaine hydrochloride 0.5%, if desired.

Postoperative care consists of oral pain medication (intravenous, if needed), rapid diet advancement, ambulation, and continuation of pelvic floor muscle exercises. Voiding trials begin on the first postoperative day. The suprapubic tube is clamped when the patient is awake. The patient voids with urge or every 3 hours. Voids and postvoid residuals are measured and recorded. The patient is allowed to unclamp the suprapubic tube at night and attach it to a catheter bag for drainage. Once the patient has voided 80% of total bladder volume during two serial attempts (voids must be greater than 150 ml), the suprapubic catheter is removed. Many patients are able to go home on the same day if adequately counseled preoperatively. Preoperative teaching includes discussion of postoperative analgesics, the need for a caretaker at home during the immediate recovery period, instruction in catheter care or intermittent self-catheterization, and explanation of goals to be reached before outpatient discharge. Patients are instructed to refrain from sexual intercourse and lifting objects greater than 10 pounds for at least 6 weeks. They are cautioned to heed to these instructions despite rapid recovery.

## Clinical Results and Complications

There have been several case series reporting laparoscopic Burch colposuspension with conventional suturing technique (Table 16-1). Liu (1994) reported one of the largest series; 132 patients were followed for 3 to 27 months with a 97% cure rate (completely dry) and 10% complication rate (four bladder injuries, four patients with urinary retention, one with ureteral obstruction, three with detrusor instability, and one with gross hematuria caused by insertion of a suprapubic catheter). Lobel and Davis (1997) reported decreased success rates with increasing follow-up in their series of 35 patients who underwent a variety of retropubic colposuspensions using needle modifications for suturing. They concluded that the success rate of laparoscopic Burch procedures is similar to that of open Burch at 1 year (86%) but decreases considerably thereafter (69% at 34 months). Ross (1998) reported multichannel urodynamic evaluation and cure rates of laparoscopic Burch colposuspension with suturing technique to be 93% at 1 year and 89% at 2 years.

**Table 16-1**  Review of the Literature: Laparoscopic Burch Colposuspension With Suturing Technique

| Author (year) | No. of patients | Follow-up (mo)* | Subjective data | Objective data | Cure rate (%) | Major complication rate (%) |
|---|---|---|---|---|---|---|
| Albala et al. (1992) | 10 | 7 | Yes | No | 100 | 0 |
| Liu (1994) | 132 | 18 (3-27) | Yes | Yes | 96 | 7.4 |
| Gunn et al. (1994) | 15 | (4-9) | Yes | No | 100 | 0 |
| Nezhat et al. (1994) | 62 | (8-30) | Yes | Yes | 100 | 10 |
| Langebrekke et al. (1995) | 8 | 3 | Yes | Yes | 87.5 | 25 |
| Carter (1995) | 50 | (12-36) | Yes | No | 100 | 6 |
| Radomski and Herschorn (1996) | 34 | 17.3 | No | No | 85 | 11.8 |
| Flax (1996) | 47 | (2-15) | Yes | No | 73 | 12.8 |
| Cooper et al. (1996) | 113 | 8 (1-28) | Yes | No | 87 | 23.8 |
| Lam and Rosen (1997) | 107 | 16 (1.5-36) | Yes | Yes | 98 | 7.4 |
| Papasakelariou and Papasakelariou (1997) | 32 | 24 | Yes | No | 90.6 | 6.3 |
| Lobel and Davis (1997) | 35 | 34 | Yes | No | 68.6 | 22.9 |
| Ross (1998) | 48 | 24 | Yes | Yes | 89 | 6.3 |

*Single value denotes mean. Values in parentheses denote range.

Complication rates vary from 0% to 25% (Table 16-1). Bladder injury is the most common complication but declines with increased experience. Laparoscopic bladder injury is detected by direct observation of urine or fluid in the operating field or by gaseous distention of the urinary bag. Most studies do not differentiate between major and minor complications. Major operative and early postoperative complications include urinary tract and bowel injury, inferior epigastric and other major vessel injury, blood loss requiring transfusion, and abscess formation of the space of Retzius. Long-term problems include failure of the procedure requiring resuspension, new-onset urethral intrinsic sphincter deficiency, de novo detrusor instability requiring long-term medical management, urinary retention requiring permanent catheterization, voiding pain with or without suture material in the bladder, vesicovaginal fistula, ureteral obstruction requiring reoperation, posterior compartment compensatory defects requiring surgery, and incisional hernias. No deaths have been reported.

Continence rates vary from 69% to 100%. Six of 12 studies reported objective data. Total operative time varied from 35 to 330 minutes, with means ranging from 90 to 196 minutes. Most authors reported less blood loss, shorter hospitalization, and less frequent postoperative voiding dysfunction and de novo detrusor instability when compared to the abdominal route. The decreased incidence of urinary retention and detrusor instability associated with laparoscopic Burch is a preliminary observation because there are few prospective comparative trials. Reasons for less frequent postoperative voiding dysfunction are unknown, and possible explanations include sutures not being tied as tightly, which is intentional or unintentional as a result of

technique variables; less dissection of the periurethral and paracolpium tissues by some surgeons; and less postoperative pain associated with smaller incisions.

There are several case series reporting modifications of the retropubic urethropexy. Ou et al. (1993) first reported the use of hernia staples and polypropylene mesh in 40 patients who underwent a modified retropubic colposuspension with a cure rate of 100% at 6 months. Von Theobald et al. (1995) sutured prolene mesh to the vagina and stapled it to Cooper's ligament in 37 patients with 8% of patients experiencing complications (two bladder injuries and one patient with pelvic pain requiring mesh removal 1 year later). Using subjective and objective measures, 70% of patients were completely dry and 16% were highly improved. Hannah and Chin (1996) reported 100 patients in whom mesh and staples or tacks were used. Follow-up ranged from 12 to 24 months, and the cure rate was 91% based on subjective outcome.

Lyons (1995) reported the Nolan-Lyons modification of suturing the vagina and stapling the suture to Cooper's ligament in 38 women with stress incontinence; a 92% cure rate at 12 months was found. Henley (1995) described his modification of using staples to secure permanent suture to the vagina and to Cooper's ligament in 60 patients; however, no follow-up data were reported.

In the French literature, Grossmann et al. (1996) summarized 21 case series, which included a total of 578 patients with follow-up varying from 3 to 21 months (many studies did not include length of follow-up). They found a 96% success rate at 12 months with a laparoconversion rate of 3.6% and average complication rate of 12.5%. There is no report of subjective or objective data or a distinc-

**Table 16-2**   Comparative Studies of Laparoscopic Retropubic Urethropexy

| Author (year) | Follow-up (mo) | No. of patients | Lsc Burch cure (%) | Open Burch cure (%) | Lsc modification cure (%) | Lsc MMK cure (%) | Raz cure (%) |
|---|---|---|---|---|---|---|---|
| Burton (1993)* | 12 | 30/30 | 73 | 97 | | | |
| Polascik et al. (1995) | 20.8/35.6 | 12/10 | 83 | 70 | | | |
| Lyons (1995) | >12 | 10/10/10 | 90 | 90 | 90 | | |
| McDougall et al. (1995) | 12 | 10/8/23 | 78† | | | 75 | 82 |
| Das and Palmer (1995) | 10 | 10/10/10 | | 100 | 90‡ | | 100 |
| Ross (1995) | 12 | 30/32 | 94 | 93 | | | |
| Ross (1996) | 12 | 35/34 | 91 | | 94§ | | |
| Burton (1997)* | 36 | 30/30 | 60 | 93 | | | |
| Su et al. (1997) | >12 | 46/46 | 80† | 96 | | | |
| Miannay et al. (1998) | 24 | 36/36 | 68 | 64 | | | |
| Saidi et al. (1998) | 12.9/16.3 | 70/87 | 91 | 92 | | | |

*Lsc,* Laparoscopic.
*Published in abstract form.
†The single-stitch modified Burch with conventional suturing was performed.
‡In this modification, bone anchors were used with one stitch on each side.
§The staple-mesh modification was used.

tion between cure and improvement rates. The authors divided the patients into three groups, which all had similar success rates: intraperitoneal colposuspensions (304), extraperitoneal colposuspensions (171), and mixed vaginal-laparoscopic colposuspensions (69) in which Stamey or Pereyra needles were often used to place the stitches through Cooper's ligament.

There are ten comparative studies in the literature (Table 16-2). Burton and Su et al. reported randomized trials. Burton (1993, 1997) reported 60 patients randomized to open and laparoscopic colposuspension and published abstracts on subjective data consisting of analog scores and data that included pad tests, urinary diaries, and videocystourethrography. His surgical technique included four polyglycolic sutures (two on each side). The cure rates for laparoscopic colposuspension were considerably worse than open colposuspension and decreased significantly from 1 year (73% versus 97%) to 3 years (60% versus 93%) of follow-up. Su et al. (1997) reported a randomized trial of 92 patients with follow-up of at least 1 year. The cure rate and bladder neck position of laparoscopic colposuspension were significantly lower. Technique and suture differed in the procedures; one stitch of nonabsorbable polyester suture was used on each side in the majority of laparoscopic suspensions compared with three absorbable sutures on each side in the open technique. Laparoscopic colposuspensions were associated with less operative time and fewer complications.

Ross (1995) has reported a prospective cohort comparing laparoscopic and open Burch procedures. Cure rates of 94% for laparoscopic Burch and 93% for open Burch were achieved at 1 year. Ross (1996) compared the staple-mesh modification with laparoscopic Burch using standard suture technique and noted cure rates of 94% and 91%, respectively, at 12 months.

When comparing laparoscopic Burch and MMK with the Raz vaginal needle suspension, McDougall et al. (1995) reported that the laparoscopic procedures were associated with significantly less postoperative parenteral analgesia and shorter time to resume a normal voiding pattern. Polascik et al. (1995) performed a cost analysis that suggested that the laparoscopic approach might be more cost-effective because of shorter hospitalization.

Three investigations evaluated cost of open and laparoscopic Burch colposuspension. Kung et al. (1996) found total charges for the open Burch urethropexy ($5692) to be significantly higher than for the laparoscopic route ($2398). Average hospitalization was significantly higher for the open group (11.2 days) than for the laparoscopic group (3.6 days). However, the prolonged hospital stay in the open group of this Canadian study is not standard care in the United States. Loveridge et al. (1997) reviewed 49 consecutive patients who underwent laparoscopic (26) and open (23) colposuspension and found that overall in-hospital costs were similar because the increase in operative time in the laparoscopic group offset the longer hospital stay in the open group. Kohli et al. (1997) compared open (21 patients) and laparoscopic (17 patients) colposuspension and found that although mean length of stay was significantly different (2.1 days versus 1.3 days), the total hospital charges were significantly higher for the laparoscopic group ($4960) than for the open group ($4079). This difference was attributed to longer operating time.

Ostrzenski (1998) has reported a prospective series of 28 patients who underwent laparoscopic paravaginal defect repair for genuine stress incontinence. Mean operative time was 2 hours and 45 minutes, and all patients were discharged on the same day. The cure rate was 93% based on subjective and objective data for minimum follow-up of 24 months.

## Technical Skill Development for Laparoscopic Colposuspension

Before doing laparoscopic retropubic procedures, the surgeon should have adequate experience in performing these procedures by laparotomy and experience in performing operative laparoscopic procedures (adnexectomy, hysterectomy). The technique of laparoscopic suturing may be learned in a stepwise fashion. A surgeon can begin to develop suturing skills on inanimate models in pelvic trainers. It is optimal to use laparoscopes, cameras, and video monitors to simulate operative conditions and improve depth perception. The next step involves performing laparoscopic retropubic procedures on pigs or goats in animal labs. Cadaver laboratories are ideal but less accessible. A surgeon should perform initial cases of laparoscopic bladder neck suspensions with an experienced advanced laparoscopist who is proctoring and assisting. In our experience, a surgeon gains the most proficiency during the first 20 cases.

## LAPAROSCOPIC SURGERY FOR ENTEROCELE, VAGINAL APEX PROLAPSE, AND RECTOCELE
### Indications

The indications for laparoscopic enterocele, vaginal apex prolapse, and rectocele repairs are identical to those for vaginal and abdominal routes. The choice of laparoscopic route is determined by surgeon and patient preference and the laparoscopic skill of the surgeon. Additional factors that should be considered include history of pelvic or antiincontinence surgery, previous failed sacrospinous colpopexy, short vagina, severe abdominopelvic adhesions, patient age and weight, need for concomitant pelvic surgery, and the patient's ability to undergo general anesthesia.

### Anatomy

When considering the anatomy of the repair of pelvic organ support, a surgeon must keep in mind the three levels of support of the vagina described by DeLancey (1992). The upper fourth of the vagina (level I) is suspended by the cardinal/uterosacral complex, the middle half (level II) is attached laterally to the arcus tendineus fasciae pelvis and the medial aspect of the levator ani muscles, and the lower fourth (level III) is fused to the perineal body. The endopelvic fascia (also referred to as pubocervical fascia anteriorly and rectovaginal fascia posteriorly) contributes to the integrity of the wall of the vagina. All pelvic support defects, whether anterior, apical, or posterior, represent a break in the continuity of the endopelvic fascia and/or a loss of its suspension, attachment, or fusion to adjacent structures. The goals of pelvic reconstructive surgery are to correct all defects, thus reestablishing vaginal support at all three levels, and to maintain or restore normal visceral and sexual function.

The anatomic landmarks during laparoscopic enterocele repair are the pubocervical fascia, the rectovaginal fascia,

the uterosacral ligaments, and the ureter, which courses along the pelvic sidewall and is approximately 1 to 1.5 cm lateral to the uterosacral ligament as it passes underneath the uterine artery. If a uterosacral ligament–vaginal vault suspension is performed, the portion of the uterosacral ligaments proximal to their break from previous attachment to the vagina is delineated. Richardson (1995) describes breaks in the endopelvic fascia and uterosacral/cardinal ligaments rather than attenuation and stretching of tissue as the cause of vaginal apex prolapse. He defines *enterocele* as a condition in which there is peritoneum in contact with vaginal mucosa with no intervening fascia.

The key anatomic landmarks of sacral colpopexy are the middle sacral artery and vein; the sacral promontory with anterior longitudinal ligament; the aortic bifurcation and the vena cava, which are at the L4-L5 level; the right common iliac vessels and right ureter, which are at the right margin of the presacral space; and sigmoid colon, which is at the left margin. The left common iliac vein is medial to the left common iliac artery and can be damaged during dissection or retraction.

The anatomic landmarks of laparoscopic rectocele repair are the rectovaginal septum, made up of Denonvilliers' fascia, and its lateral attachment to the medial aspect of the levator ani muscles. Denonvilliers' fascia is the endopelvic fascia attached to the uterosacral cardinal ligament complex superiorly, the superior fascia of the levator ani muscle laterally, and the perineal body inferiorly. The rectovaginal septum is the posterior point of attachment of the sacral colpopexy mesh. *Rectovaginal fascia, rectovaginal septum,* and *Denonvilliers' fascia* are synonymous. The pubocervical fascia is the anterior point of mesh attachment during sacral colpopexy.

### Operative Technique
#### Laparoscopic Moschcowitz and Halban Procedures

The Moschcowitz procedure is performed laparoscopically exactly as during laparotomy. A No. 0 nonabsorbable 36-inch suture is stitched in the peritoneum around the cul-de-sac in a pursestring fashion and subsequently tied extracorporeally. Additional sutures are placed as needed. The ureters should be carefully examined during and after the Moschcowitz procedure. The peritoneum medial to the ureters may be incised in order to prevent ureteral kinking.

The Halban procedure is performed by suturing No. 0 nonabsorbable suture starting at the posterior vagina and proceeding longitudinally over the cul-de-sac peritoneum and then over the inferior sigmoid serosa. These sutures are tied as they are placed. Sutures should be approximately 1 cm apart. There is little risk of ureteral compromise with this procedure; however, it is important to visualize the ureters after all sutures are tied.

#### Laparoscopic Enterocele Repair

The enterocele sac is dissected laparoscopically or vaginally so that the endopelvic fascial defects are identified and the pubocervical fascia and rectovaginal fascia are delineated. If the enterocele is large, the surgeon excises redundant peritoneum and vagina by the vaginal route, taking care not to foreshorten or narrow the vaginal apex. A vaginal obturator, spongestick, or equivalent vaginal manipulator (EEA sizer by U.S. Surgical Corp., Norwalk, Connecticut, or the CDH by Ethicon Endo-Surgery, Inc., Cincinnati, Ohio) may be used for delineation of the vaginal apex or rectum when performing the dissection laparoscopically. The pubocervical and rectovaginal fascial edges are reapproximated with No. 0 nonabsorbable suture in interrupted stitches until the fascial defect is closed. Extracorporeal knot-tying is performed after each stitch is placed. This is often performed concomitantly with a uterosacral ligament–vaginal vault suspension so that level I suspension is reestablished.

### Laparoscopic Uterosacral Ligament–Vaginal Vault Suspension

To suspend the vaginal apex to the uterosacral ligament, the surgeon must dissect and delineate the pubocervical and rectovaginal fasciae (Plate 3). The surgeon sutures the full thickness of the uterosacral ligament at the proximal portion of its break with No. 0 nonabsorbable suture and reattaches it to the vaginal apex with a full thickness stitch incorporating the uterosacral/cardinal ligament complex and rectovaginal fascia, excluding the vaginal epithelium. This stitch is tied extracorporeally, and the opposite uterosacral ligament is reattached in the same fashion. Two or three additional stitches are taken more proximally in the uterosacral ligaments on each side in order to reattach it to the rectovaginal fascia (Plate 4). Plication of the uterosacral ligaments is not necessary. If concomitant enterocele repair is performed, the uterosacral ligaments may be tagged before dissection of the posterior vagina and rectovaginal septum so that they are easily identified for subsequent suspension. To protect the ureters, peritoneal incisions may be made lateral to the uterosacral ligaments.

The apical vault repair described by Ross (1997a) reestablished the lateral and posterior pericervical rings of endopelvic fascia by bringing the rectovaginal septum and cardinal/uterosacral ligaments together. After the peritoneum is dissected off the vaginal apex and the pubocervical fascia and rectovaginal septum are identified, No. 0 nonabsorbable suture is used to incorporate the left and right uterosacral and cardinal ligaments, the rectovaginal septum, and posterior vaginal wall in pursestring stitches, thus plicating the uterosacral ligaments. The first stitch is placed in the uterosacral ligament approximately 3 to 4 cm proximal to the vaginal apex. Three or more successive stitches are placed until the vaginal apex is reached. The final suture incorporates the pubocervical fascia into the repair. This repair differs from the uterosacral ligament–vaginal vault suspension by placement of pursestring sutures resulting in uterosacral ligament plication.

### Laparoscopic Sacral Colpopexy

In addition to the intraumbilical port, a 10/12-mm trocar should be placed in both lower quadrants for suture introduction. One additional 5-mm port is placed at the level of the umbilicus, lateral to the rectus muscle for retraction (see Fig. 16-1). After the ancillary ports are placed, dissection of the peritoneum off the vaginal apex is performed to delineate the rectovaginal fascia. Anterior dissection is performed (taking care to avoid damage to the bladder) if a Y-shaped or T-shaped mesh is stitched to the pubocervical fascia anteriorly or if enterocele repair is needed. A vaginal obturator, spongestick, or equivalent vaginal manipulator (EEA Sizer by U.S. Surgical Corp., Norwalk, Connecticut, or the CDH by Ethicon Endo-Surgery, Inc., Cincinnati, Ohio) is used for delineation of the vaginal apex or rectum.

If exposure of the sacral promontory and presacral space is not adequate, the patient should be tilted to her left and/or a fan retractor (Origin Medsystems, Menlo Park, California) placed through an ancillary port. The peritoneum overlying the sacral promontory is incised longitudinally and extended to the cul-de-sac. A laparoscopic dissector or hydrodissection is used to expose the periosteum of the sacral promontory. If blood vessels are encountered during the dissection, coagulation or clip placement is used to achieve hemostasis. A Halban procedure or other culdeplasty is usually performed. When a concomitant enterocele repair is performed, this is completed before mesh placement.

A 10- × 2.5-cm autologous fascia lata, freeze-dried nonradiated cadaveric fascia lata, polypropylene, or Dacron mesh is introduced through the 10/12-mm port. When a T-shaped mesh is used, a 4- × 2.5-cm mesh is sutured to the larger piece of mesh with No. 0 nonabsorbable suture. The mesh is sutured to the vaginal apex anteriorly with two pairs of No. 0 nonabsorbable sutures and into the posterior vaginal apex and rectovaginal septum with three similar rows of suture (Plate 5). When using a T-shaped mesh, it is easier to suture the anterior portion first so that the cephalad portion of the mesh may be retracted anteriorly while the posterior rows of sutures are being placed. Another technique used to incorporate a T-shaped mesh includes suturing two pieces of mesh separately. The larger piece of mesh is sutured into the posterior wall of the vagina, and the smaller piece of mesh is sutured to the anterior wall. We then sew both pieces together into the vaginal apex and trim the excess anterior mesh. The sutures are tied extracorporeally as they are placed. Care is taken to place the stitches through the entire thickness of the vaginal wall, excluding the epithelium. The surgeon sutures the mesh to the longitudinal ligament of the sacrum in two rows of two No. 0 nonabsorbable suture (Plate 5). No undue tension is placed on the mesh. Titanium tacks or hernia staples may also be used to attach the mesh to the anterior longitudinal ligament of the sacrum. The redundant portion of the mesh is excised. The peritoneum is reapproximated over the mesh with No. 2-0 polyglactin suture. If the mesh remains exposed, sigmoid epiploic fat may be sutured over it.

A concomitant laparoscopic Burch colposuspension is performed if the patient has urethral hypermobility with GSI. A paravaginal defect repair is performed, if needed, to treat anterior vaginal wall defects. If rectal prolapse is present, a rectopexy can be performed laparoscopically. We perform these combined cases with our colorectal surgery colleagues.

### Laparoscopic Rectocele Repair

The rectovaginal septum is opened using electrocautery, harmonic scalpel, or laser. Blunt dissection with blunt-tipped dissectors or dolphin-tipped dissectors, hydrodissection, or sharp dissection may be used to open the rectovaginal space down to the perineal body. This dissection should follow surgical planes and be bloodless. The perineal body is sutured to the rectovaginal septum. The rectovaginal fascial defects are closed with No. 0 nonabsorbable suture. If the rectovaginal fascia is detached from the iliococcygeus fascia, it is reattached with No. 0 nonabsorbable suture. The medial aspects of the levator ani muscles may also be plicated, but care should be taken to avoid a posterior vaginal ridge. Lyons and Winer (1997) have reported the use of polyglactin mesh in extensive rectocele repairs.

## Clinical Results and Complications

The current gynecologic literature for laparoscopic pelvic reconstruction is sparse and consists of descriptive studies with short-term follow-up. There are several reports of laparoscopic rectopexy in the colorectal surgery literature, which is beyond the scope of this chapter. There are no reports that evaluate clinical results and complications of uterosacral shortening and culdeplasty, although these techniques have been described by a few authors. Lyons and Winer (1995) reported 276 enterocele repairs or prophylaxis with Halban or Moschcowitz procedures and noted no complications other than trocar site infections. Cadeddu et al. (1996) described a modified Moschcowitz procedure, approximating the posterior vaginal fascia with the anterior wall of the rectum. Koninckx et al. (1995) used the carbon dioxide laser for vaporization of the enterocele sac, followed by uterosacral shortening and suspension of the posterior vaginal wall.

Lyons and Winer (1997) evaluated prospectively, at 3-month intervals for 1 year, 20 patients who underwent laparoscopic rectocele repair with polyglactin mesh and concomitant reparative procedures. An objective telephone interviewer asked a series of questions with regard to bowel and sexual function. The mean operative time for rectocele repair was 35 minutes (range 20 to 48 minutes). Estimated blood loss was minimal and hospital stay was less than 24 hours. Eighty percent of patients had symptomatic relief of digital defecation and prolapse at 1 year.

There are a small number of reports of laparoscopic

repair of vaginal apex prolapse. Nezhat et al. (1994) reported a series of 15 patients who underwent laparoscopic sacral colpopexy in whom the mean operative time was 170 minutes (range 105 to 320 minutes) and mean blood loss was 226 ml (range 50 to 800 ml). The mean hospital stay was 2.3 days, excluding a case converted to laparotomy for presacral hemorrhage. The cure rate for apical prolapse was 100% at 3 to 40 months. Lyons (1995) reported 4 laparoscopic sacrospinous fixations and 10 laparoscopic sacral colpopexies with operative times comparable to vaginal and abdominal approaches. He reported less intraoperative and postoperative morbidity with the laparoscopic route; this was attributed to a superior anatomic approach and visualization of anatomic structures. Nezhat et al. (1994) and Lyons (1995) used mesh and suture and at times they stapled the mesh into the longitudinal ligament of the anterior sacrum.

Ross (1997b) evaluated 19 patients with posthysterectomy vaginal apex prolapse prospectively with extensive preoperative and postoperative testing, including multichannel urodynamics and transperineal ultrasound. All patients underwent sacral colpopexy, Burch colposuspension, and modified culdeplasty. Paravaginal defect repair and posterior colporrhaphy were added as indicated. The author reported seven complications: three cystotomies, two urinary tract infections, one seroma, and one inferior epigastric vessel laceration. Five patients had recurrent defects that were all less than grade 2 (two paravaginal defects and three rectoceles). Vaginal length ranged from 10.8 to 12.1 cm and all sexually active patients reported no sexual dysfunction. All patients but four voided spontaneously and none required more than 4 days of catheterization. All were discharged within 24 hours. The cure rate at 1 year was 100% for vaginal apex prolapse and 93% for GSI, although two patients were lost to follow-up.

## Discussion

Laparoscopy is a means of surgical access, not a unique procedure, and its use is expanding rapidly in all surgical specialties. Despite recent introduction and lack of long-term outcomes, the laparoscopic Burch colposuspension has become popular. We believe that the laparoscopic and open Burch procedures should be identical in operative techniques. Bladder injury is probably more common with laparoscopy, but the risk of cystotomy decreases with surgical experience. Complications associated with open Burch bladder neck suspension, such as wound infection, are rare with the laparoscopic route.

The benefits of improved visualization of anatomic structures and small incisions associated with the laparoscopic approach are desirable, particularly in obese patients. The advantages of less postoperative pain, shorter hospitalization, shortened recovery period, and earlier return to work are partially offset by increased operative time and possibly increased cost. The operative time and cost are likely to decrease as surgeons gain experience with the advanced laparoscopic techniques of suturing and knot-tying. The steep learning curve in development of laparoscopic suturing skills may deter many gynecologic surgeons from performing retropubic procedures by this approach; nevertheless, patient desire will continue to promote laparoscopic access.

Although several case series and cohort studies show comparable cure rates between laparoscopic and open Burch colposuspension, the two prospective trials show lower cure rates associated with laparoscopic Burch colposuspension. The main criticisms of Burton's trial (1993, 1997) are that he had not gained sufficient experience with laparoscopic surgery before embarking on the study and that the suture used was absorbable with a small needle, which may have caused insufficient thickness of sutured tissue. Similarly, Su et al. (1997) used three absorbable sutures in the open Burch colposuspension, compared with a single nonabsorbable suture in the laparoscopic procedure. More prospective clinical trials with identical technique of laparoscopic and open colposuspension and follow-up of 3 or more years are warranted.

The principles of laparoscopic reparative procedures for enterocele, rectocele, and vaginal apex prolapse are not new; it is the route by which they are performed that differs. Adequate laparoscopic suturing skills are essential in performing these procedures. The increase in operating time may increase the cost of the procedure, especially early in a surgeon's experience. Prospective clinical trials with long-term follow-up are warranted.

## BIBLIOGRAPHY
### Laparoscopic Retropubic Surgical Procedures

Adams JB, Schulam PG, Moore RG, et al: New laparoscopic suturing device: initial clinical experience, *Urology* 46:242, 1995.

Albala DM, Schuessler WE, Vancaillie TG: Laparoscopic bladder suspension for the treatment of stress incontinence, *Semin Urol* 10:222, 1992.

Aslan P, Woo HH: Ureteric injury following laparoscopic colposuspension, *Br J Obstet Gynaecol* 104:266, 1997.

Birken RA, Leggett PL: Laparoscopic colposuspension using mesh reinforcement, *Surg Endosc* 11:1111, 1997.

Burton G: A randomised comparison of laparoscopic and open colposuspension, *Neurourol Urodyn* 13:497, 1993 (abstract).

Burton G: A three year prospective randomised urodynamic study comparing open and laparoscopic colposuspension, *Neurourol Urodyn* 16:353, 1997 (abstract).

Carter JE: Laparoscopic bladder neck suspension, *Endosc Surg* 3:81, 1995.

Classi R, Sloan PA: Intraoperative detection of laparoscopic bladder injury, *Can J Anaesth* 42:415, 1995.

Cooper MJ, Cario G, Lam A, et al: A review of results in a series of 113 laparoscopic colposuspensions, *Aust N Z J Obstet Gynaecol* 36:44, 1996.

Das S, Palmer JK: Laparoscopic colpo-suspension, *J Urol* 154:1119, 1995.

Dorsey JH, Cundiff G: Laparoscopic procedures for incontinence and prolapse, *Curr Opin Obstet Gynecol* 6:223, 1994.

Dorsey JH, Sharp HT, Chovan JD, et al: Laparoscopic knot strength: a comparison with conventional knots, *Obstet Gynecol* 86:536, 1995.

Flax S: The gasless laparoscopic Burch bladder neck suspension: early experience, *J Urol* 156:1105, 1996.

Frankel G, Kantpong M: Sixteen-month experience with video-assisted extraperitoneal laparoscopic bladder neck suspension, *J Endourol* 9:259, 1993.

Grossmann T, Darai E, Deval B, et al: Place de l'endoscopie dans la chirurgie de l'incontinence urinaire, *Ann Chir* 50:896, 1996.

Gunn GC, Cooper RP, Gordon NS, et al: Use of a new device for endoscopic suturing in the laparoscopic Burch procedure, *J Am Assoc Gynecol Laparosc* 2:64, 1994.

Hannah SL, Chin AL: Laparoscopic retropubic urethropexy, *J Am Assoc Gynecol Laparosc* 4:47, 1996.

Henley C: The Henley staple-suture technique for laparoscopic Burch colposuspension, *J Am Assoc Gynecol Laparosc* 2:441, 1995.

Kiilholma P, Haarala M, Polvi H, et al: Sutureless colposuspension with fibrin sealant, *Tech Urol* 1:81, 1995.

Kohli N, Jacobs PA, Sze EH, et al: Open compared with laparoscopic approach to Burch colposuspension: a cost analysis, *Obstet Gynecol* 90:411, 1997.

Kung RC, Lie K, Lee P, et al: The cost-effectiveness of laparoscopic versus abdominal Burch procedures in women with urinary stress incontinence, *J Am Assoc Gynecol Laparosc* 3:537, 1996.

Lam AM, Jenkins GJ, Hyslop RS: Laparoscopic Burch colposuspension for stress incontinence: preliminary results, *Med J Aust* 162:18, 1995.

Lam AM, Rosen DMB: Laparoscopic Burch colposuspension for urinary stress incontinence: results from 109 consecutive cases, *Gynaecol Endosc* 6:109, 1997.

Langebrekke A, Dahlstrom B, Eraker R, et al: The laparoscopic Burch procedure: a preliminary report, *Acta Obstet Gynecol Scand* 74:153, 1995.

Liu CY: Laparoscopic retropubic colposuspension (Burch procedure): a review of 58 cases, *J Reprod Med* 38:526, 1993.

Liu CY: Laparoscopic treatment of genuine urinary stress incontinence, *Clin Obstet Gynecol* 8:789, 1994.

Lobel RW, Davis GD: Long-term results of laparoscopic Burch urethropexy, *J Am Assoc Gynecol Laparosc* 4:341, 1997.

Loveridge K, Malouf A, Kennedy C, et al: Laparoscopic colposuspension. Is it cost-effective? *Surg Endosc* 11:762, 1997.

Lyons TL: Minimally invasive retropubic urethropexy: the Nolan-Lyons modification to the Burch procedure, *Gynecol Endocrinol* 3:40, 1994.

McDougall EM, Lutke CG, Cornell T: Comparison of transvaginal versus laparoscopic bladder neck suspension for stress urinary incontinence, *Adult Urol* 45:641, 1995.

Miannay E, Cosson M, Querleu D, et al: Compariaison entre la colposuspension par coelioscopie et laparotomie dans le traitement de l'incontinence urinaire d'effort. Etude comparative a partir de 72 cas apparies, *Contracept Fertil Sex* 26:376, 1998.

Nezhat CH, Nezhat F, Nezhat CR, et al: Laparoscopic cystourethropexy, *J Am Assoc Gynecol Laparosc* 14:339, 1994.

Ostrzenski A: Genuine stress urinary incontinence in women: new laparoscopic paravaginal reconstruction, *J Repro Med* 43:477, 1998.

Ou CS, Presthus J, Beadle E: Laparoscopic bladder neck suspension using hernia mesh and surgical staples, *J Laparoendosc Surg* 3:563, 1993.

Papasakelariou C, Papasakelariou B: Laparoscopic bladder neck suspension, *J Am Assoc Gynecol Laparosc* 4:185, 1997.

Polascik TJ, Moore RG, Rosenberg MT, et al: Comparison of laparoscopic and open retropubic urethropexy for treatment of stress incontinence, *Urology* 45:647, 1995.

Raboy A, Hakim LS, Ferzli G, et al: Extraperitoneal endoscopic vesicourethral suspension, *J Laparoendosc Surg* 3:505, 1995.

Radomski SB, Herschorn S: Laparoscopic Burch bladder neck suspension: early results, *J Urol* 155:515, 1996.

Ross JW: Laparoscopic Burch repair compared to laparotomy Burch for cure of urinary stress incontinence, *Int Urogynecol J* 6:323, 1995.

Ross JW: Two techniques of laparoscopic Burch repair for stress incontinence: a prospective randomized study, *J Am Assoc Gynecol Laparosc* 3:351, 1996.

Ross JW: Multichannel urodynamic evaluation of laparoscopic Burch colposuspension for genuine stress incontinence, *Obstet Gynecol* 91:55, 1998.

Saidi MH, Gallagher MS, Skop IP, et al: Extraperitoneal laparoscopic colposuspension: short-term cure rate, complications, and duration of hospital stay in comparison with Burch colposuspension, *Obstet Gynecol* 92:619, 1998.

Smith ARB, Stanton SL: Laparoscopic colposuspension, *Br J Obstet Gynaecol* 105:383, 1998.

Su TH, Wang KG, Hsu CY, et al: Prospective comparison of laparoscopic and traditional colposuspensions in the treatment of genuine stress incontinence, *Acta Obstet Gynecol Scand* 76:576, 1997.

Tanagho EA: Colpocystourethropexy: the way we do it, *J Urol* 116:751, 1976.

Vancaillie TG, Schuessler W: Laparoscopic bladder neck suspension, *J Laparoendosc Surg* 1:169, 1991.

Von Theobald P, Guillaumin D, Levy G: Laparoscopic preperitoneal colposuspension for stress incontinence in women: technique and results of 37 procedures, *Surg Endosc* 9:1189, 1995.

Wallweiner D, Grischke EM, Maleika RA, et al: Endoscopic retropubic colposuspension: "Retziusscopy" versus laparoscopy: a reasonable enlargement of the operative spectrum in the management of recurrent stress incontinence? *Endosc Surg* 3:115, 1995.

Wattiez A, Boughizane S, Alexandre F, et al: Laparoscopic procedures for stress incontinence and prolapse, *Curr Opin Obstet Gynecol* 7:317, 1995.

## Laparoscopic Surgery for Enterocele, Vaginal Apex Prolapse, and Rectocele

Cadeddu JA, Micali S, Moore RG, et al: Laparoscopic repair of enterocele, *J Endourol* 4:367, 1996.

DeLancey JO: Anatomic aspects of vaginal eversion after hysterectomy, *Am J Obstet Gynecol* 166:1717, 1992.

Dorsey JH, Sharp HT: Laparoscopic sacral colpopexy and other procedures for prolapse, *Baillieres Clin Obstet Gynecol* 9:749, 1995.

Koninckx PR, Poppe W, Deprest J: Carbon dioxide laser for laparoscopic enterocele repair, *J Am Assoc Gynecol Laparosc* 2:181, 1995.

Lyons TL: Minimally invasive treatment of urinary stress incontinence and laparoscopically directed repair of pelvic floor defects, *Clin Obstet Gynecol* 38:380, 1995.

Lyons TL, Winer WK: Vaginal vault suspension, *Endosc Surg* 3:88, 1995.

Lyons TL, Winer WK: Laparoscopic rectocele repair using polyglactin mesh, *J Am Assoc Gynecol Laparosc* 4:381, 1997.

Nezhat CH, Nezhat F, Nezhat C: Laparoscopic sacral colpopexy for vaginal vault prolapse, *Obstet Gynecol* 84:885, 1994.

Richardson AC: The rectovaginal septum revisited: its relationship to rectocele and its importance in rectocele repair, *Clin Obstet Gynecol* 35:976, 1993.

Richardson AC: The anatomic defects in rectocele and enterocele, *J Pelvic Surg* 1:214, 1995.

Ross JW: Apical vault repair, the cornerstone of pelvic floor reconstruction, *Int Urogynecol J* 8:146, 1997a.

Ross JW: Techniques of laparoscopic repair of total vault eversion after hysterectomy, *J Am Assoc Gynecol Laparosc* 4:173, 1997b.

Vancaillie TG: The role of laparoscopy in the management of pelvic floor relaxation, *J Am Assoc Gynecol Laparosc* 4:147, 1997.

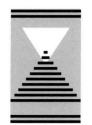

CHAPTER **17**

*Surgical Correction of Anterior Vaginal Wall Prolapse*

Anne M. Weber

Anterior vaginal prolapse occurs commonly and may coexist with disorders of micturition. Mild anterior vaginal prolapse often occurs in parous women but usually presents few problems. As prolapse progresses, symptoms may develop and worsen, and treatment becomes indicated. This chapter reviews the anatomy and pathology of anterior vaginal prolapse and describes methods of surgical repair.

## ANATOMY AND PATHOLOGY

Anterior vaginal prolapse (cystocele) is defined as pathologic descent of the anterior vaginal wall and overlying bladder base. According to the International Continence Society (ICS) standardized terminology for prolapse grading, the term *anterior vaginal prolapse* is preferred over *cystocele* because information obtained at the physical examination does not allow the exact identification of structures behind the vaginal wall. The ICS grading system for prolapse is discussed fully in Chapter 4.

The cause of anterior vaginal prolapse is not completely understood, but it is probably multifactorial, with different factors implicated in prolapse in individual patients. Normal support for the vagina and adjacent pelvic organs is provided by the interaction of the pelvic muscles and connective tissue, as discussed in Chapter 1. The upper vagina rests on the levator plate and is stabilized by superior and lateral connective tissue attachments; the midvagina is attached to the arcus tendineus fasciae pelvis (white line) on

each side. Pathologic loss of that support may occur with damage to the pelvic muscles, connective tissue attachments, or both.

Nichols and Randall (1996) described two types of anterior vaginal prolapse: distention and displacement. Distention was thought to result from overstretching and attenuation of the anterior vaginal wall, caused by overdistention of the vagina associated with vaginal delivery or atrophic changes associated with aging and menopause. The distinguishing physical feature of this type was described as diminished or absent rugal folds of the anterior vaginal epithelium caused by thinning or loss of midline vaginal fascia. The other type of anterior vaginal prolapse, displacement, was attributed to pathologic detachment or elongation of the anterolateral vaginal supports to the arcus tendineus fasciae pelvis. It may occur unilaterally or bilaterally and often coexists with some degree of distention cystocele and with urethral hypermobility. Rugal folds may or may not be preserved.

Another theory ascribes most cases of anterior vaginal prolapse to disruption or detachment of the lateral connective tissue attachments at the arcus tendineus fasciae pelvis or white line, resulting in a paravaginal defect and corresponding to the displacement type discussed earlier. This was first described by White in 1909, but disregarded until reported by Richardson in 1976. Richardson also described transverse defects, midline defects, and defects involving isolated loss of integrity of pubourethral ligaments. Transverse defects were said to occur when the pubocervical fascia separated from its insertion around the cervix, whereas midline defects represented an anteroposterior separation of the fascia between the bladder and vagina.

There has never been a systematic or comprehensive description of anterior vaginal prolapse based on physical findings and correlated with findings at surgery to provide objective evidence for any of these theories of pathologic anatomy. However, recent improvements in pelvic imaging may lead to a greater understanding of normal pelvic anatomy and the abnormalities associated with prolapse. Magnetic resonance imaging (MRI) holds great promise, with its excellent ability to differentiate soft tissues and its capacity for multiplanar imaging. Further work is needed to correlate the different images with anatomy and histology under normal conditions and under conditions of pelvic organ prolapse. The main limitation for imaging related to prolapse has been the inability to image patients in the standing position to evaluate for the effects of gravity and increased intraabdominal pressure; eventually, this limitation will be overcome.

The pelvic organs, pelvic muscles, and connective tissues can be identified easily with MRI. Various measurements can be made that may be associated with anterior vaginal prolapse or urinary incontinence, such as the urethrovesical angle, descent of the bladder base, and the relationship between the vagina and its lateral connective tissue attachments. Aronson et al. (1995) used an endoluminal surface coil placed in the vagina to image pelvic anatomy with MRI, and compared four continent nulliparous women with four incontinent women with anterior vaginal prolapse. Lateral vaginal attachments were identified in all continent women. In Fig. 17-1, the "posterior pubourethral ligaments" (bilateral attachment of arcus tendineus fasciae pelvis to posterior aspect of the pubic symphyses) are clearly seen. In the two subjects with clinically apparent paravaginal defects, lateral

detachments were evident (Fig. 17-2). Although this study involved only a small number of subjects, it provides the basis for further work in describing the anatomic abnormalities that accompany anterior vaginal prolapse and other abnormalities of pelvic support. This may ultimately guide the choice of surgical repair.

## EVALUATION
### History

When evaluating women with pelvic organ prolapse or urinary or fecal incontinence, attention should be paid to all aspects of pelvic support. The reconstructive surgeon must determine the specific sites of damage for each patient, with the ultimate goal of restoring both anatomy and function.

Patients with anterior vaginal prolapse complain of symptoms directly related to vaginal protrusion or of associated symptoms such as urinary incontinence or voiding difficulty. Symptoms related to prolapse may include the sensation of a vaginal mass or bulge, pelvic pressure, low back pain, and sexual difficulty. Stress urinary incontinence commonly occurs in association with anterior vaginal prolapse.

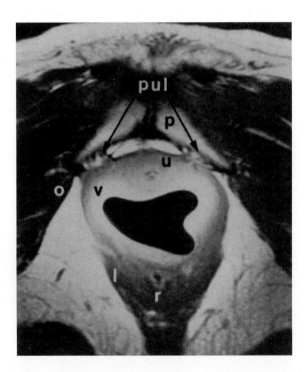

**Fig. 17-1**   Axial T1-weighted image from a continent 38-year-old nulliparous woman, showing the connection of the anterior vaginal wall *(v)* to the posterior pubic symphysis *(p)* by the pubourethral ligaments *(pul)*. The anterior vaginal wall and endopelvic fascia function as a sling or hammock for support of the urethra *(u)*. *o,* Obturator internus muscle; *c,* endovaginal coil; *r,* rectum; *l,* levator ani musculature.

From Aronson MP, Bates SM, Jacoby AF, et al: Periurethral and paravaginal anatomy: an endovaginal magnetic resonance imaging study, *Am J Obstet Gynecol* 173:1702, 1995.

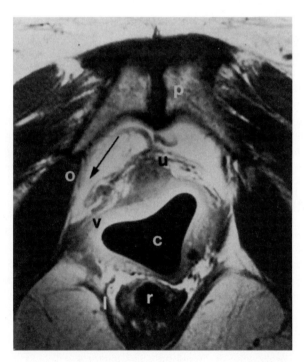

**Fig. 17-2**   Axial T1-weighted image from a 57-year-old woman, para 5, with genuine stress urinary incontinence. The paravaginal detachment *(arrow)* is seen at the level of the urethrovesical junction. *v,* Anterior vaginal wall; *p,* posterior pubic symphysis; *pul,* pubourethral ligaments; *u,* urethra; *o,* obturator internus muscle; *c,* endovaginal coil; *r,* rectum; *l,* levator ani musculature.

From Aronson MP, Bates SM, Jacoby AF, et al: Periurethral and paravaginal anatomy: an endovaginal magnetic resonance imaging study, *Am J Obstet Gynecol* 173:1702, 1995.

Voiding difficulty may result from advanced prolapse. Women may require vaginal pressure or manual replacement of the prolapse in order to accomplish voiding. Women may relate a history of urinary incontinence that has since resolved with worsening of their prolapse. This can occur with urethral kinking and obstruction to urinary flow; women in this situation are at risk for incomplete bladder emptying and recurrent or persistent urinary tract infections.

## Physical Examination

The physical examination should be conducted with the patient in lithotomy position, as for a routine pelvic examination. The examination is first performed with the patient supine. If physical findings do not correspond to symptoms or if the maximum extent of the prolapse cannot be confirmed, the woman is reexamined in the standing position.

The genitalia are inspected, and if no displacement is apparent, the labia are gently spread to expose the vestibule and hymen. The integrity of the perineal body is evaluated, and the approximate size of all prolapsed parts is assessed. A retractor or Sims speculum can be used to depress the posterior vagina to aid in visualizing the anterior vagina. After the resting examination, the patient is instructed to strain down forcefully or to cough vigorously. During this maneuver, the order of descent of the pelvic organs is noted, as is the relationship of the pelvic organs at the peak of straining. It may be possible to differentiate lateral defects, identified as detachment or effacement of the lateral vaginal sulci, from central defects, seen as midline protrusion but with preservation of the lateral sulci. Anterior vaginal wall descent usually represents bladder descent with or without concomitant urethral hypermobility. Less commonly, an anterior enterocele can mimic a cystocele on physical examination. The grading systems for prolapse and measurement of urethral hypermobility are described in Chapters 4 and 5.

## Diagnostic Tests

After a careful history and physical examination, few diagnostic tests are needed to evaluate patients with anterior vaginal prolapse. A urinalysis should be performed to evaluate for urinary tract infection if the patient complains of any lower urinary tract dysfunction. If the patient's estrogen status is unclear, a vaginal cytologic smear can be obtained to assess maturation index. Hydronephrosis occurs in a small proportion of women with prolapse; however, even if identified, it does not change management in women for whom surgical repair is planned. Therefore, routine imaging of the kidneys and ureters is not necessary.

If urinary incontinence is present, further diagnostic testing is indicated to determine the cause of the incontinence. Urodynamic (simple or complex), endoscopic, or radiologic assessments of filling and voiding function are generally indicated only when symptoms of incontinence or

voiding dysfunction are present. Even if no urologic symptoms are noted, voiding function should be assessed to evaluate for completeness of bladder emptying. This procedure usually involves a timed, measured void, followed by urethral catheterization to measure residual urine volume.

In women with severe prolapse, it is important to check urethral function after the prolapse is repositioned. As demonstrated by Bump et al. (1988), women with severe prolapse may be continent because of urethral kinking; when the prolapse is reduced, urethral dysfunction may be unmasked with occurrence of incontinence. A pessary or vaginal packing can be used to reduce the prolapse before office bladder filling or electronic urodynamic testing. If urinary leaking occurs with coughing or Valsalva maneuvers after reduction of the prolapse, the urethral sphincter is probably incompetent, even if the patient is normally continent. In this situation, the surgeon can choose an antiincontinence procedure in conjunction with anterior vaginal prolapse repair. If sphincteric incompetence is not present even after reduction with a pessary, an antiincontinence procedure is not indicated.

## SURGICAL REPAIR TECHNIQUES
### Anterior Colporrhaphy

The objective of anterior colporrhaphy is to plicate the layers of vaginal muscularis and adventitia overlying the bladder (pubocervical fascia) or to plicate the paravaginal tissue in such a way as to reduce the protrusion of the bladder and vagina. Modifications of the technique depend on how lateral the dissection is carried, where the plicating sutures are placed, and whether additional layers (natural or synthetic) are placed in the anterior vagina for extra support.

The operative procedure begins with the patient supine, with the legs elevated and abducted and the buttocks placed just past the edge of the operating table. The chosen anesthetic has been administered, and one perioperative intravenous dose of an appropriate antibiotic may be given as prophylaxis against infection. The vagina and perineum are sterilely prepped and draped, and a 16-French Foley catheter with a 5-ml balloon is inserted for easy identification of the bladder neck. If indicated, a suprapubic catheter is placed into the bladder.

A weighted speculum is placed into the vagina. If a vaginal hysterectomy has been performed, the incised apex of the anterior vaginal wall is grasped transversely with two Allis clamps and elevated. Otherwise, a transverse incision is made in the vaginal mucosa near the apex. A third Allis clamp is placed about 1 cm below the posterior margin of the urethral meatus and pulled up. Additional Allis clamps may be placed in the midline between the urethra and apex. Hemostatic solutions (such as 0.5% lidocaine with 1:200,000 epinephrine) or saline may be injected submucosally, along the midline of the anterior vaginal wall, to decrease bleeding and to aid in dissection. The points of a pair of curved Mayo scissors are inserted between the vaginal epithelium and the vaginal muscularis, or between layers of the vaginal muscularis, and gently forced upward while being partially opened and closed. Countertraction during this maneuver is important to minimize the likelihood of perforation of the bladder. The vagina is then incised in the midline, and the incision is continued to the level of the midurethra. As the vagina is incised, the edges are grasped with Allis or T-clamps and drawn laterally for further mobilization. Dissection of the vaginal flaps is then accomplished by turning the clamps back across the forefinger and incising the vaginal muscularis with a scalpel or Metzenbaum scissors, as shown in Fig. 17-3. An assistant maintains constant traction medially on the remaining vaginal muscularis and underlying vesicovaginal adventitia. This procedure is performed bilaterally until the entire extent of the anterior vaginal prolapse has been dissected; in general, the dissection should be carried further laterally with more advanced prolapse. The spaces lateral to the urethrovesical junction are sharply dissected toward the inferior pubic rami.

In most cases, regardless of whether the patient suffers from urinary incontinence, plicating sutures at the urethrovesical junction should be placed to augment posterior

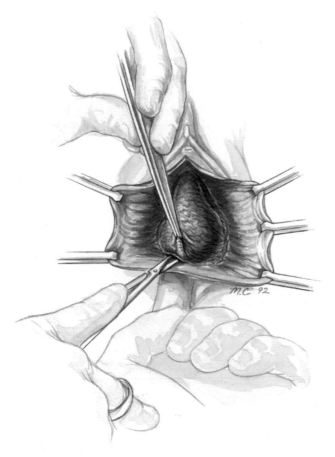

**Fig. 17-3** Sharp dissection is used to mobilize the bladder base from the vaginal apex during anterior colporrhaphy.

urethral support and to ensure that stress incontinence, if not present at the time of operation, does not develop postoperatively. Details on the effectiveness of vesical neck plication for stress incontinence are given in Chapter 15. Once the vaginal flaps have been completely developed, the urethrovesical junction can be identified visually or by pulling the Foley catheter downward until the bulb obstructs the vesical neck. Repair should begin at the urethrovesical junction, using No. 2-0 or 0 delayed absorbable suture. The first plicating stitch is placed into the periurethral endopelvic fascia and tied (Fig. 17-4, A and B). One or two additional stitches are placed to support the length of the urethra and urethrovesical junction.

After the stitches for vesical neck plication have been placed and tied, attention is turned to the anterior vaginal prolapse repair. In a standard anterior colporrhaphy, stitches using No. 2-0 or 0 delayed absorbable sutures are placed in the vaginal tissue (muscularis and adventitia) medial to the vaginal flaps and plicated in the midline without tension. Depending on the severity of the prolapse, one or two rows of plication sutures or a pursestring suture followed by plication sutures are placed (Fig. 17-4, C and D). The vaginal epithelium is then trimmed from the flaps bilaterally, and the remaining anterior vaginal wall is closed with a running No. 3-0 subcuticular or locking suture.

One modification of the standard repair is to extend the dissection and mobilization of the vaginal flaps laterally to the descending pubic rami on each side. After the vesical neck plication has been performed, stitches are then placed laterally in the paravaginal tissue (lateral to the vaginal muscularis and adventitial layers, but not including the epithelium of the vaginal flaps). The paravaginal connective tissue is plicated in the midline under tension using No. 0 delayed absorbable or permanent sutures. This produces a firm bridge of tissue across the anterior vaginal space, but it also results in narrowing of the anterior vagina, which must be considered when planning a concomitant posterior colporrhaphy. The vaginal flaps are trimmed and closed as usual.

Another modification involves the use of an additional layer of support in the anterior vagina. After the plication sutures have been placed and tied, this layer is placed over the stitches and anchored in place at the lateral limit of the previous dissection, using interrupted stitches of No. 3-0 absorbable suture. Natural materials that have been used include resected segments of vaginal wall or rectus fascia. Permanent or absorbable mesh may be used, although permanent material carries a risk of infection or erosion, with need for subsequent removal.

Antiincontinence operations are often performed at the same time as anterior vaginal prolapse repair. Urethral suspension procedures (sling procedures, needle or retropubic urethropexies) may effectively treat mild anterior vaginal prolapse associated with urethral hypermobility. More advanced anterior vaginal prolapse will not be treated adequately, and in these cases, anterior colporrhaphy should be performed as well. Surgical judgment is required to perform the plication tightly enough to sufficiently reduce the anterior vaginal prolapse, yet preserve enough mobility of the anterior vagina to allow adequate urethral suspension. If anterior colporrhaphy is combined with a sling procedure or needle urethropexy, the cystocele should be repaired before the urethropexy sutures are tied.

## Vaginal Paravaginal Repair

The objective of paravaginal defect repair for anterior vaginal prolapse is to reattach the detached lateral vagina to its normal place of attachment at the level of the white line or arcus tendineus fasciae pelvis. This can be accomplished using a vaginal or retropubic approach. Retropubic paravaginal defect repair is discussed in Chapter 14, along with other retropubic procedures such as the Burch colposuspension.

The preparation for vaginal paravaginal repair begins as for an anterior colporrhaphy. Marking sutures are placed on the anterior vaginal wall on each side of the urethrovesical junction, identified by the location of the Foley balloon after gentle traction is placed on the catheter (Fig. 17-5, A). In patients who have had a hysterectomy, marking sutures are also placed at the vaginal apex. If a culdeplasty is being performed, the stitches are placed but not tied until the completion of the paravaginal repair and closure of the anterior vaginal wall. As for anterior colporrhaphy, vaginal flaps are developed by incising the vagina in the midline and dissecting the vaginal muscularis laterally. The dissection is performed bilaterally until the space is developed between the vaginal wall and retropubic space. Blunt dissection using the surgeon's index finger is used to extend the space anteriorly along the inferior pubic rami, medially to the

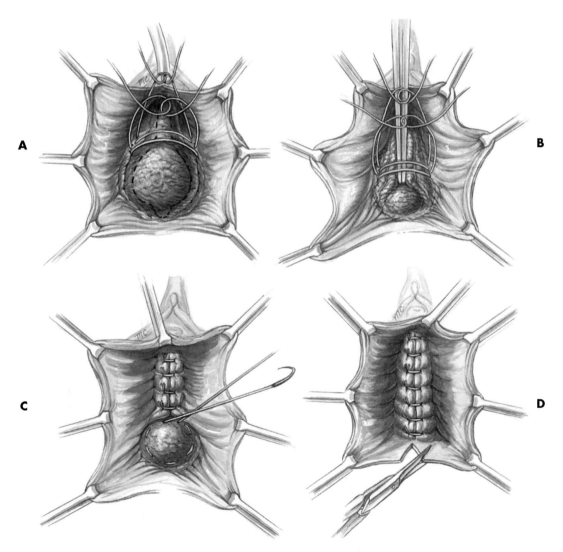

**Fig. 17-4** Technique of anterior colporrhaphy. **A,** After dissection of vaginal wall from the bladder and urethra, one to three plication sutures are placed into the periurethral endopelvic fascia at the urethrovesical junction. **B,** The plication sutures at the vesical neck are tied. **C,** A pursestring suture can be placed in the vaginal muscularis to reduce large cystoceles. **D,** The entire cystocele has been repaired with plication sutures and the vaginal epithelium is trimmed before closure.

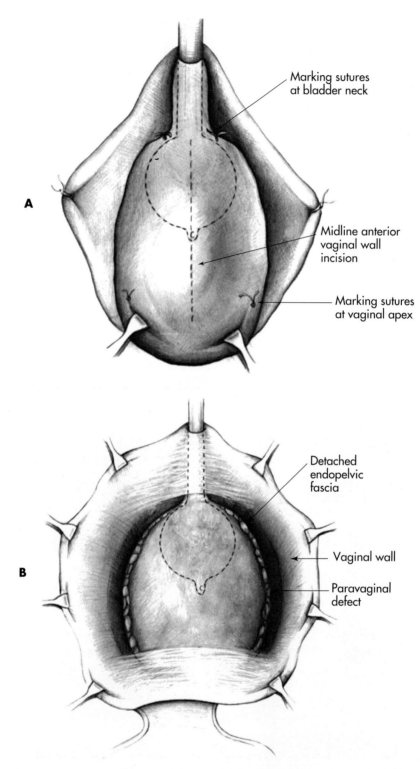

**Fig. 17-5** Technique of vaginal paravaginal repair. **A,** Vagina is opened through a midline incision. Marking sutures are placed at the bladder neck and vaginal apex to ensure proper suture placement on vaginal epithelium. **B,** Opened vagina reveals bilateral paravaginal defects. Note detached endopelvic fascia on lateral edge of bladder.                                                        *Continued*

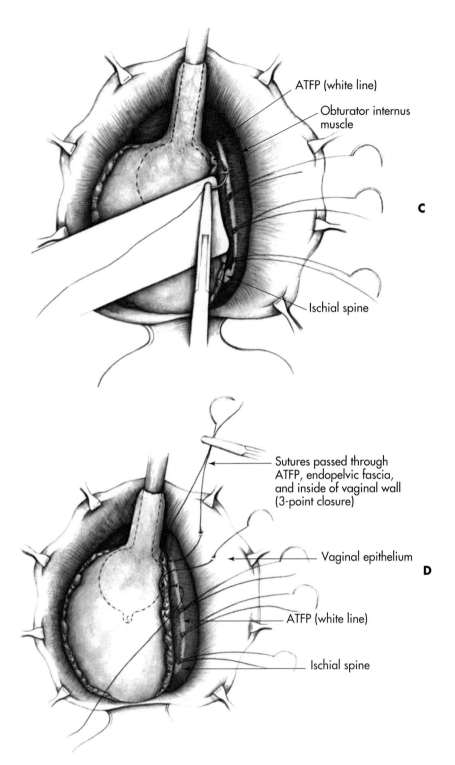

**Fig. 17-5, cont'd** **C,** Access to the arcus tendineus fasciae pelvis *(ATFP)* or white line is obtained by retracting the bladder medially. Permanent sutures are passed through the white line or fascia over the obturator internus muscle. Four or five sutures are placed starting at the ischial spine. Tension on sutures facilitates placement of subsequent sutures. **D,** Each suture is passed through the white line, detached endopelvic fascia, and the inside of the vaginal epithelium, forming the three-point closure. Once sutures have been placed on both sides (if indicated), sutures are individually tied by alternating right and left sides.

pubic symphysis, and laterally toward the ischial spine. If the defect is present and dissection is occurring in the appropriate plane, one should easily enter the retropubic space, visualizing retropubic adipose tissue. The ischial spine can then be palpated on each side. The arcus tendineus fasciae pelvis coming off of the spine can be followed to the back of the symphysis pubis (Fig. 17-5, *B*). After dissection is complete, midline plication of vaginal muscularis can be performed, either at this point or after placement and tying of the paravaginal sutures.

On the lateral pelvic sidewall, the obturator internus muscle and the arcus tendineus fasciae pelvis are identified by palpation and then visualization. Retraction of the bladder and urethra medially is best accomplished with a Briesky-Navratil retractor, and posterior retraction is provided with a lighted right-angle retractor. Using No. 0 nonabsorbable suture, the first stitch is placed around the tissue of the white line just anterior to the ischial spine. If the white line is detached from the pelvic sidewall or clinically not felt to be durable, then the attachment should be to the fascia overlying the obturator internus muscle. The placement of subsequent sutures is facilitated by placing tension on the first suture. A series of four to six stitches are placed and held, working anteriorly along the white line from the ischial spine to the level of the urethrovesical junction (Fig. 17-5, *C*). Starting with the most anterior stitch, the surgeon picks up the edge of the periurethral tissue (vaginal muscularis or pubocervical fascia) at the level of the urethrovesical junction and then tissue from the undersurface of the vaginal flap at the previously marked sites. Subsequent stitches move posteriorly until the last stitch closest to the ischial spine is attached to the vagina nearest the apex, again using the previously placed marking sutures for guidance. Stitches in the vaginal wall must be carefully placed to allow adequate tissue for subsequent midline vaginal closure. After all stitches are placed on one side, the same procedure is carried out on the other side. The stitches are then tied in order from the urethra to the apex, alternating from one side to the other. This repair is a three-point closure involving the vaginal epithelium, vaginal muscularis and endopelvic fascia (pubocervical fascia), and lateral pelvic sidewall at the level of the arcus tendineus fasciae pelvis (Fig. 17-5, *D*). There must be tissue-to-tissue approximation between these structures. Suture bridges must be avoided by careful planning of suture placement. Vaginal tissue should not be trimmed until all the stitches are tied. As previously stated, if not already performed, vaginal muscularis can then be plicated in the midline with several interrupted stitches using No. 0 delayed absorbable suture. The vaginal flaps are trimmed and closed with a running subcuticular or interlocking delayed absorbable suture.

## Abdominal Cystocele Repair

Abdominal repair of mild anterior vaginal prolapse can be accomplished at the time of abdominal hysterectomy. After the cervix has been amputated from the vagina, the bladder is dissected off the anterior vaginal wall, nearly to the level of the ureters. A full-thickness midline wedge of anterior vaginal wall is excised, and the vagina is closed with running delayed absorbable suture. The vaginal cuff then is repaired according to the surgeon's preference. This procedure has no effect on bladder neck or urethral support, and care should be taken not to unmask latent stress incontinence by treating anterior vaginal prolapse without simultaneous urethral suspension.

## COMPLICATIONS

Intraoperative complications are uncommon with anterior vaginal prolapse repair. Excessive blood loss may occur, requiring blood transfusion, or a hematoma may develop in the anterior vagina. The lumen of the bladder or urethra may be entered in the course of dissection. Accidental cystotomy should be repaired in layers at the time of the injury. After repair of cystotomy, the bladder is generally drained for 7 to 14 days to allow adequate healing. Other rare complications include ureteral damage, intravesical or urethral suture placement (and associated urologic problems), and fistula, either urethrovaginal or vesicovaginal. If permanent sutures or mesh material are used in the repair, erosion, draining sinuses, or chronic areas of vaginal granulation tissue can result. The incidence of these complications is unknown. Urinary tract infections occur commonly, but other infections such as pelvic or vaginal abscesses are less common.

Voiding difficulty can occur after anterior vaginal prolapse repair. This problem may occur more often in women with subclinical preoperative voiding dysfunction. Treatment is bladder drainage or intermittent self-catheterization until spontaneous voiding resumes, usually within 6 weeks.

Sexual function may be positively or negatively affected by vaginal operations for anterior vaginal prolapse. Haase and Skibsted (1988) studied 55 sexually active women who underwent a variety of operations for stress incontinence or genital prolapse. Postoperatively, 24% of the patients experienced improvement in their sexual satisfaction, 67% experienced no change, and 9% experienced deterioration. Improvement often resulted from cessation of urinary incontinence. Deterioration was always caused by dyspareunia after posterior colporrhaphy. These authors concluded that the prognosis for an improved sexual life is good after surgery for stress incontinence, but that posterior colpoperineorrhaphy causes dyspareunia in some patients.

## RESULTS

The main indication for surgical repair of anterior vaginal prolapse is to relieve symptoms when they exist, or as part of a comprehensive pelvic reconstructive procedure for multiple sites of pelvic organ prolapse with or without urinary incontinence. Anterior colporrhaphy with vesical neck plication also may be effective for treatment of mild stress incontinence associated with urethral hypermobility.

Few studies have addressed the long-term success of surgical treatments for anterior vaginal prolapse. All published studies are uncontrolled series. Definitions of recurrence vary and sometimes are not stated, and loss to follow-up often is not stated. In our review of surgical techniques for the correction of anterior vaginal prolapse, reported failure rates ranged from 0% to 20% for anterior colporrhaphy and 3% to 14% for paravaginal repair. No controlled studies have compared different procedures performed primarily for anterior vaginal wall prolapse.

Women with advanced anterior vaginal prolapse, with or without stress incontinence, often have other abnormal bladder symptoms such as urgency, urge incontinence, and voiding difficulty. In a study of surgical repair of large cystoceles by Gardy et al. (1991), stress incontinence resolved in 94%, urge incontinence in 87%, and significant residual urine (greater than 80 ml) in 92% of patients 3 months after needle suspension procedures and anterior colporrhaphy. Approximately 5% of patients developed a recurrent anterior vaginal prolapse, and 8% developed a recurrent enterocele after an average of 2 years of follow-up.

Risk factors for failure of anterior vaginal prolapse repair have not been specifically studied. Vaginal prolapse recurs with increasing age, but the actual frequency is unknown. Recurrence may represent a failure to identify and repair all support defects, or weakening, stretching, or breaking of patients' tissues, as occurs with advancing age and after menopause. Sacrospinous ligament suspension of the vaginal apex, with exaggerated retrosuspension of the vagina, may predispose patients to recurrence of anterior vaginal prolapse. Other characteristics that may increase chances of recurrence are genetic predisposition, subsequent pregnancy, heavy lifting, chronic pulmonary disease, smoking, obesity, and absence of estrogen replacement after menopause.

## BIBLIOGRAPHY
### Anatomy and Pathology

Aronson MP, Bates SM, Jacoby AF, et al: Periurethral and paravaginal anatomy: an endovaginal magnetic resonance imaging study, *Am J Obstet Gynecol* 173:1702, 1995.

Nichols DH, Randall CL: *Vaginal surgery,* ed 4, Baltimore, 1996, Williams & Wilkins.

Richardson AC, Lyon JB, Williams NL: A new look at pelvic relaxation, *Am J Obstet Gynecol* 126:568, 1976.

White GR: A radical cure by suturing lateral sulci of vagina to white line of pelvic fascia, *JAMA* 21:1707, 1909.

White GR: An anatomical operation for the cure of cystocele, *Am J Obstet Dis Women Child* 65:286, 1912.

### Evaluation

Beverly CJ, Walters MD, Weber AM, et al: Prevalence of hydronephrosis in women undergoing surgery for pelvic organ prolapse, *Obstet Gynecol* 90:37, 1997.

Bhatia NN, Bergman A: Pessary test in women with urinary incontinence, *Obstet Gynecol* 65:220, 1985.

Bump RC, Fantl JA, Hurt WG: The mechanism of urinary continence in women with severe uterovaginal prolapse: results of barrier studies, *Obstet Gynecol* 72:291, 1988.

deGregorio G, Hillemanns HG: Urethral closure function in women with prolapse, *Int Urogynecol J* 1:143, 1990.

Richardson DA, Bent AE, Ostergard DR: The effect of uterovaginal prolapse on urethrovesical pressure dynamics, *Am J Obstet Gynecol* 146:901, 1983.

### Surgical Repair Techniques and Complications

Beck RP, McCormick S: Treatment of urinary stress incontinence with anterior colporrhaphy, *Obstet Gynecol* 59:269, 1982.

Gardy M, Kozminski M, DeLancey J, et al: Stress incontinence and cystoceles, *J Urol* 145:1211, 1991.

Haase P, Skibsted L: Influence of operations for stress incontinence and/or genital descensus on sexual life, *Acta Obstet Gynecol Scand* 67:659, 1988.

Julian TM: The efficacy of Marlex mesh in the repair of severe, recurrent vaginal prolapse of the anterior midvaginal wall, *Am J Obstet Gynecol* 175:1472, 1996.

Macer GA: Transabdominal repair of cystocele, a 20-year experience, compared with the traditional vaginal approach, *Am J Obstet Gynecol* 131:203, 1978.

Mitchell GW: Vaginal hysterectomy: anterior and posterior colporrhaphy; repair of enterocele; and prolapse of vaginal vault. In Ridley JH, ed: *Gynecologic surgery; errors, safeguards, salvage,* ed 2, Baltimore, 1981, Williams & Wilkins.

Pelusi G, Bacchi P, Demaria F, et al: The use of Kelly plication for the prevention and treatment of genuine stress urinary incontinence in patients undergoing surgery for genital prolapse, *Int Urogynecol J* 1:196, 1990.

Shull BL, Benn SJ, Kuehl TJ: Surgical management of prolapse of the anterior vaginal segment: an analysis of support defects, operative morbidity, and anatomic outcome, *Am J Obstet Gynecol* 171:1429, 1994.

Stanton SL, Norton C, Cardozo L: Clinical and urodynamic effects of anterior colporrhaphy and vaginal hysterectomy for prolapse with and without incontinence, *Br J Obstet Gynaecol* 89:459, 1982.

Symmonds RE, Jordan LT: Iatrogenic stress incontinence of urine, *Am J Obstet Gynecol* 82:1231, 1961.

Weber AM, Walters MD: Anterior vaginal prolapse: review of anatomy and techniques of surgical repair, *Obstet Gynecol* 89:311, 1997.

Zacharin RF: Free full-thickness vaginal epithelium graft in correction of recurrent genital prolapse, *Aust NZ J Obstet Gynaecol* 32:146, 1992.

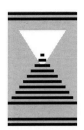

CHAPTER 18

# Enterocele and Rectocele

Bob L. Shull and Claudia G. Bachofen

The management of pelvic organ prolapse is difficult; several support defects often coexist, and simple anatomic correction of the various defects does not always result in normal function of the vagina and surrounding organs. To accomplish the goals of pelvic reconstructive surgery—to restore anatomy, maintain or restore normal bowel and bladder function, and maintain vaginal capacity for sexual intercourse—the surgeon must thoroughly understand normal anatomic support and physiologic function of the vagina, bladder, and rectum.

This chapter discusses the pathophysiology and surgical correction of enterocele and rectocele. Normal anatomy of the pelvic diaphragm is discussed in detail in Chapter 1. The evaluation of patients with pelvic organ prolapse, including their symptoms, physical examination, classification, and diagnostic tests, is discussed in Chapters 4 and 5.

## PATHOPHYSIOLOGY OF PELVIC ORGAN PROLAPSE

Normally the vaginal axis in an erect woman is nearly horizontal in the upper half of the vagina, with the uterus and upper 3 or 4 cm of the vagina lying over the levator plate in the hollow of the sacrum (Fig. 18-1). Funt et al. (1978) found that the vagina is directed toward the S3 and S4 vertebrae and extends approximately 3 cm past the ischial spines in most nulliparous women. Increases in intraabdominal pressure compress the vagina anteriorly to poste-

riorly over the contracted levator muscles in the midline (levator plate). Diminished muscle tone may result in loss of stability of the levator plate, widening of the levator hiatus, and loss of an adequate base to support the upper vagina and uterus in the normal axis.

Pelvic organ prolapse may occur as a result of congenital or acquired factors in the bones, muscles, nerves, or connective tissues that are responsible for normal support and function. Vaginal delivery, chronic increases in intraabdominal pressure, increasing age, and decreased estrogen stimulation are important factors associated with pelvic organ prolapse.

Loss of support of anterior, posterior, and apical vaginal walls results in cystocele, rectocele, enterocele, and vaginal cuff prolapse, respectively. Uterovaginal prolapse occurs secondary to damage of the cardinal-uterosacral ligament complex and endopelvic fascia that normally support the uterus and upper vagina over the pelvic diaphragm.

Connective tissue defects have been found in women with uterine prolapse and stress incontinence. In several studies, Mäkinen et al. (1986, 1987) identified abnormal histologic changes in the pelvic connective tissue in 70% of women with uterine descent, compared to 20% of normal controls. Decreased cellularity (fibroblasts) and an increase in collagen fibers were observed. Ulmsten et al. (1987) reported 40% less total collagen in the skin and round ligaments of women with stress incontinence when compared to that of continent women. These studies suggest that abnormal connective tissue may be associated with pelvic organ prolapse and stress incontinence.

## ENTEROCELE
### Definition and Types

Enterocele is a hernia in which peritoneum is in contact with vaginal mucosa. The normal intervening endopelvic fascia is absent, and small bowel fills the hernia sac.

Generally, enteroceles have been divided into four types: congenital, traction, pulsion, and iatrogenic. Congenital enterocele is rare. Factors that may predispose to the development of congenital enterocele include neurologic disorders, such as spina bifida, and connective tissue disorders. Trac-

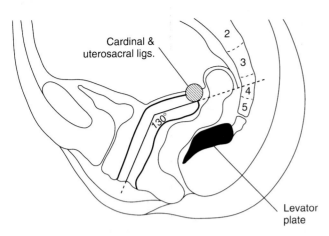

**Fig. 18-1** Normal vaginal axis of nulliparous woman in the standing position. Note that the upper third of the vagina is nearly horizontal and is directed toward the S3 and S4 sacral vertebrae.
From Funt MI, Thompson JD, Birch H: *South Med J* 71:1534, 1978.

tion enterocele occurs secondary to uterovaginal descent, and pulsion enterocele results from prolonged increases in intraabdominal pressure. These two latter types of enterocele may coexist with apical vaginal prolapse, cystocele, or rectocele. Iatrogenic enterocele occurs after surgical procedures that elevate the normally horizontal vaginal axis toward vertical; examples include colposuspension and needle urethropexy operations for stress incontinence, or hysterectomy, with or without repair, when the vaginal cuff and cul-de-sac are not managed effectively.

## Physical Examination

Enteroceles may occur in association with rectocele. When these hernias coexist, rectovaginal examination may demonstrate the rectocele as distinct from the bulging sac that arises from a higher point in the vagina. Visual inspection of the posterior vaginal wall may reveal a transverse furrow between the two hernias.

Initially, the physical examination should be conducted with the patient in lithotomy position, as for a routine pelvic examination. When the physical findings cannot be evaluated adequately in the supine position, the woman is reexamined in the standing position.

Pelvic organ prolapse defects can be identified best by using a Sims speculum or the split blade of a Graves speculum. Following the resting examination, the patient is instructed to strain forcefully or cough vigorously. During this maneuver, descent of the pelvic organs is observed systematically.

Despite the development of many classification systems, researchers have been unable to agree upon a universally accepted set of objective standards until recently. In 1996, the International Continence Society, American Urogynecologic Society, and Society of Gynecologic Surgeons pub-

lished an objective system that is being used by investigators worldwide to determine its clinical utility. This system is described in Chapter 4.

## Surgical Repair Techniques

Surgical repair of enterocele can be performed vaginally or abdominally. No data exist comparing the various types of repairs. The approach and type of procedure performed depend on the surgeon's preference and whether there is concomitant vaginal or abdominal pathology. Vaginal surgical techniques described herein are the traditional vaginal enterocele repair, the McCall culdeplasty, and the specific fascial reconstruction and suspension of the vaginal apex. Torpin (1955) and Waters (1956) each described vaginal procedures involving the excision of a deep cul-de-sac. Abdominal approaches include the Moschcowitz procedure, Halban procedure, and uterosacral ligament plication.

### Vaginal Enterocele Repair

Patients rarely have an isolated enterocele; hence, concurrent vaginal vault suspension and rectocele repair often are necessary. The technique is as follows:

1. The patient is positioned as for posterior colporrhaphy. A midline posterior vaginal wall incision is made over the enterocele sac up to the vaginal apex and extended to the perineum if a rectocele is also present. Dissection of the posterior vaginal wall from the enterocele sac, the anterior rectal wall, and the rectovaginal fascia is accomplished sharply and bluntly. The dissection should extend laterally to the medial margins of the levator ani muscles.
2. The enterocele sac should be mobilized from the vaginal walls and rectum. When the enterocele sac is difficult to distinguish from the rectum, differentiation is aided by a rectal examination with simultaneous dissection of the enterocele sac from the rectal wall. At times, distinguishing the enterocele sac from a large cystocele may prove difficult. In this situation, placement of a probe into the bladder or transillumination with a cystoscope may prove helpful.
3. After the enterocele sac has been dissected from the vagina and rectum, traction is placed on it with two Allis clamps and the sac is entered sharply (Fig. 18-2, *A*). The enterocele sac is explored digitally to ensure that no small bowel or omental adhesions are present; if encountered, they are dissected to the level of its neck.
4. Under direct visualization, two or three circumferential, nonabsorbable, pursestring sutures are used to close the enterocele sac. The cardinal-uterosacral ligaments are incorporated as well (Fig. 18-2, *B*). Once placed, the sutures are tied in sequence. Care should be taken to avoid kinking the ureter.
5. Posterior colporrhaphy and vaginal vault suspension are performed as indicated.

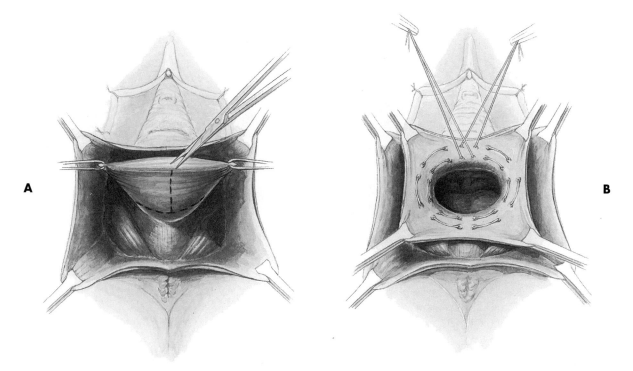

**Fig. 18-2** Vaginal enterocele repair. **A,** Isolation and entry of the enterocele sac in the rectovaginal space. **B,** Pursestring sutures are placed close to the neck of the enterocele sac.

## McCall Culdeplasty

McCall (1957) described the technique of surgical correction of enterocele and deep cul-de-sac at the time of vaginal hysterectomy. The advantage of the McCall culdeplasty is that it not only closes the redundant cul-de-sac and associated enterocele but also provides apical support and lengthening of the vagina. Many authors advocate using this procedure as part of every vaginal hysterectomy, even in the absence of enterocele, to minimize future hernia formation and vaginal vault prolapse.

The technique is as follows (Fig. 18-3):

1. After the vaginal hysterectomy is completed, the surgeon places a finger into the posterior cul-de-sac to evaluate its depth. Lateral traction is placed on the previously tagged uterosacral ligaments.

2. With the patient in Trendelenburg position, a large pack is placed intraperitoneally to prevent descent of omentum or bowel into the field. Using permanent suture, the needle is initially passed through one uterosacral ligament as high as possible. Successive bites are then taken at 1- to 2-cm intervals through the anterior serosa of the sigmoid colon until the opposite uterosacral ligament is reached. This suture is left untied, and one to three more identical sutures are placed caudally, progressing toward the posterior vaginal cuff. The number of internal sutures placed depends on the size and depth of the enterocele or cul-de-sac. The goal is obliteration of the entire dependent portion of the cul-de-sac.

3. After all the internal permanent sutures have been placed and their ends held laterally without tying, one or two sutures of delayed absorbable, No. 0 suture are placed. These are inserted from the vaginal lumen just below the middle of the cut edge of the posterior vaginal cuff, through the peritoneum, and through the right uterosacral ligament. Successive bites are taken across the cul-de-sac as before and into the left uterosacral ligament. This suture is passed through the peritoneum and vaginal epithelium, adjacent to the point of entry.

4. The permanent sutures are tied in sequence. Finally, the delayed absorbable sutures are tied in a manner to bring the posterior vaginal mucosa up to the level of the uterosacral ligaments.

Few studies have reported long-term results after vaginal repair of enterocele. In a study of 48 women who had McCall culdeplasties for large enterocele, complete procidentia, or complete vaginal vault prolapse, only two enteroceles (4%) recurred 2 to 22 years (average, 7 years) postoperatively.

The complications reported after McCall culdeplasty are shown in Table 18-1. Given (1985) reported ureteral injury in 2 of 48 McCall culdeplasty procedures. Stanhope et al. (1991) also found that culdeplasty sutures were implicated in ureteral obstruction after vaginal surgery. Some authors advocate intraoperative cystoscopy after all vaginal reconstructive surgery.

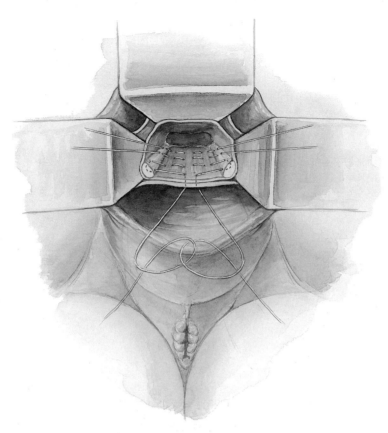

**Fig. 18-3** McCall culdeplasty technique. Note that the lowest suture incorporates the posterior vaginal wall, thus providing additional support.

**Table 18-1**  Complications After McCall Culdeplasty*

| Complication | Percent of patients (N = 48) |
| --- | --- |
| Removal of silk suture | 10 |
| Postoperative cuff infection | 4 |
| High rectocele | 4 |
| Partial prolapse of vaginal vault | 4 |
| Shortened vagina | 4 |
| Introital stenosis | 2 |
| Pulmonary emboli | 2 |
| Nerve palsy | 2 |
| Ureteral obstruction | 2 |

From Given FT: *Am J Obstet Gynecol* 153:135, 1985.
*Follow-up was 2 to 22 (average 7) years.

### Fascial Reconstruction

Another technique for enterocele repair can be performed either transabdominally, laparoscopically, or transvaginally. The approach is not as important as are the concepts involved.

DeLancey (1992) described the anatomy of vaginal vault eversion and divided vaginal support into levels I, II, and III. In level I, the cervix (in a woman who has not had the uterus removed) or the vaginal apex (in a woman who has previously had a hysterectomy) is suspended to the cardinal and uterosacral ligaments. In level II, the area along the base of the bladder anteriorly and along the rectum posteriorly is attached to the arcus tendineus fasciae pelvis or to the fascia over levator muscle. Level III, the area along the base of the urethra or at the distal rectovaginal septum just inside the hymen, is derived from the urogenital sinus and is an area of fusion. Richardson (1995) believes that the connective tissue of the vaginal tube, generally called endopelvic fascia, does not stretch or attenuate but rather breaks at specific definable points. By integrating the concepts of suspension of level I with breaks in pelvic connective tissue, one can conclude that enterocele and vaginal vault prolapse are specific defects that result from failure of the cardinal-uterosacral ligaments to support the most superior or transverse portions of endopelvic fascia at the apex of the vagina. The vaginal epithelium covering the connective tissue is not important in maintaining normal support.

Fig. 18-4 shows a sagittal view of a woman whose uterus has been removed and whose vaginal apex is suspended to the cardinal-uterosacral ligaments. Note the posterior axis of the vagina and the continuity of the endopelvic (pubocervical and rectovaginal) fascia at the vaginal apex. Enteroceles develop as the pubocervical and rectovaginal fasciae separate, allowing a peritoneal sac with its contents to protrude through the fascial defect. The vaginal lining becomes a passive partner in the evolution of the hernia. In a woman

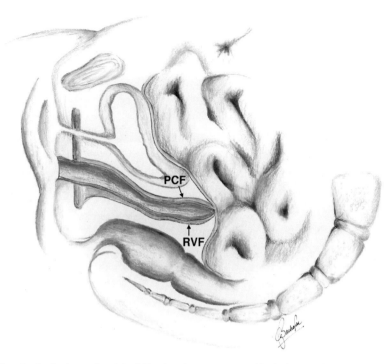

**Fig. 18-4**   Sagittal view of pelvis following hysterectomy. Vaginal apex is suspended via the endopelvic fascia, to the uterosacral ligaments. *PCF,* Pubocervical fascia; *RVF,* rectovaginal fascia. Copyright 1998 by CG Bachofen, MD.

whose uterus remains intact, the hernia predictably occurs posterior to the cervix and anterior to the rectum. These are patients in whom the McCall culdeplasty has been commonly used. Following hysterectomy, enteroceles may occur at the vaginal apex, anterior to the vaginal apex, or posterior to the vaginal apex.

Apical enterocele is perhaps the most common defect seen in women with prior hysterectomy. In this case, both the pubocervical fascia anteriorly and the rectovaginal fascia posteriorly have separated at the apex of the vagina. The enterocele may carry both layers of connective tissue with it as the hernia enlarges (Fig. 18-5, *A*).

An anterior enterocele is a defect in the support of the transverse portion of the pubocervical fascia to the apex of the vagina, and should not be confused with a cystocele. These hernias have a peritoneal sac allowing intraabdominal contents to herniate anterior to the vaginal apex and posterior to the base of the bladder (Fig. 18-5, *B*). The apex and the rectovaginal septum may have normal support in these patients.

A posterior enterocele is a defect at the superior or transverse portion of rectovaginal fascia allowing a peritoneal sac with the intraabdominal contents to herniate anterior to the rectum but posterior to the apex of the vagina (Fig. 18-5, *C*).

When you apply the aforementioned anatomic concepts, the approach to enterocele repair is somewhat different from that described by other gynecologic surgeons. However, it closely follows the principles of hernia surgery used in the management of umbilical, ventral, and inguinal hernias: the identification of a fascial defect, reduction of intraabdominal contents, and closure of the defect. The difference with enterocele is that almost always, not only must the defect be closed but the vagina must also be suspended. In a woman with normal support, the apex is suspended by the cardinal and uterosacral ligaments, the same structures that are used in most operations for enterocele repair.

We prefer the vaginal approach to the management of enterocele and vault prolapse. The patient is placed in dorsal lithotomy position, and the bladder is drained before the first incision. We identify the limits of the hernia by physical examination, looking for the demarcation of rugae along the anterior and posterior walls of the vagina. The absence of rugae implies the absence of connective tissue and, by inference, defines the borders of the hernia itself. The vaginal epithelium is grasped with a series of Allis clamps beginning anterior to the vaginal cuff and continuing vertically until the edge of the hernia sac has been identified along the posterior vagina. The vaginal epithelium is incised with a scalpel, and the edges of the vaginal epithelium are dissected sharply away from the hernia sac until the edges of the pubocervical and rectovaginal fasciae are clearly identified. The hernia sac is opened by sharp dissection and the abdominal cavity inspected for the presence of adhesions or other pathology. A large, moist, soft pack is placed in the posterior cul-de-sac and hollow of the sacrum. A wide

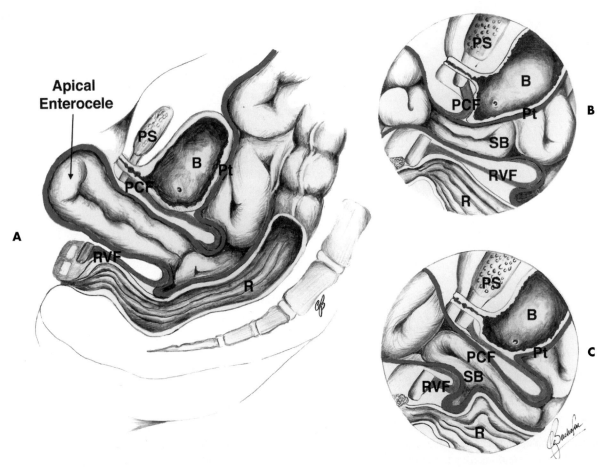

**Fig. 18-5**   Enterocele locations. **A,** Apical enterocele. **B,** Anterior enterocele. **C,** Posterior entero-cele. *PS,* Pubic symphysis; *B,* bladder; *Pt,* peritoneum; *PCF,* pubocervical fascia; *RVF,* rectovaginal fascia; *R,* rectum; *SB,* small bowel.

Copyright 1998 by CG Bachofen, MD.

Deaver retractor is used to elevate the pack and the intestines out of the operative field. The ischial spines are palpated. The remnants of uterosacral ligaments are found posterior and medial to the ischial spine. They can be identified more easily by using an Allis or Babcock clamp at approximately 5 o'clock and 7 o'clock to place tension on structures in the lateral wall of the pelvis. When tension is placed with the clamp, the contralateral index finger can be used to palpate the connective tissue condensations along the side of the pelvis. A series of interrupted nonabsorbable sutures are then placed in each uterosacral ligament beginning at approximately the level of, but posterior and medial to, the ischial spine, and the needle is driven from a lateral to a medial position each time. Care should be taken to avoid the ureter with these sutures. After the first suture has been placed, the second is placed in a more caudal and medial position. The third is placed caudally and medially to the second. We prefer to identify each of these sutures with a numbered clamp, with numbers *1, 2,* and *3* placed sequentially on one side of the pelvis and numbers *4, 5,* and *6* placed on the opposite side (Fig. 18-6).

After the suspensory sutures have been placed, the surgeon must determine whether the connective tissue of the anterior and posterior segments requires midline plication to reconstruct the vaginal connective tissue tube. Once you have established that the connective tissue requires no repair or have done the midline plication, the suspensory sutures are systematically placed into the most superior portions of pubocervical and rectovaginal fasciae. The suspensory suture most proximal to the ischial spine is sewn to the most lateral portion of the pubocervical and rectovaginal fasciae, as shown in Fig. 18-7. The suture caudal to that one is placed more medially into the pubocervical and rectovaginal fasciae. The most caudal suture is then placed most medially into the pubocervical and rectovaginal fasciae. At this point, all packs should have been removed from the operative field. The patient is given intravenous indigo carmine, and the suspensory sutures are tied sequentially, beginning with the most lateral suture on one side followed by the more distal sutures on the same side. The same sequence is followed on the opposite side. Once the suspensory sutures have been tied properly, the apex of the vagina should be in

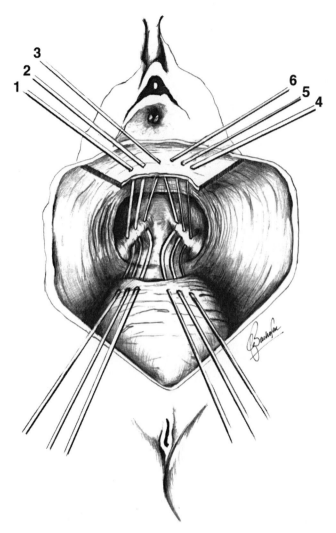

**Fig. 18-6** Suspension of the vaginal apex to the cardinal-uterosacral ligament complex using endopelvic fascia. Note the correct placement of each numbered suture posterior and medial to the ischial spines.

Copyright 1998 by CG Bachofen, MD.

the hollow of the sacrum and the connective tissue tube closed at the vaginal apex (Fig. 18-8).

Cystoscopy is performed to ensure ureteral patency. The vaginal epithelium is assessed and tailored to the contour of the vagina by excising excess tissue. The epithelial incision is closed vertically with an absorbable suture. The same methods for identification of the fascial defect and the use of remnants of uterosacral ligaments can be used endoscopically or transabdominally. Fig. 18-9 shows the approximation of the vaginal cuff to uterosacral ligaments, as seen abdominally. In either situation, there may be a need to perform a perineorrhaphy or a surgical procedure for the management of genuine stress urinary incontinence.

When appropriate, a perineorrhaphy is performed at the completion of the previously described procedure. In the case of a woman who has enterocele and genuine stress

urinary incontinence, our preference would be to perform a retropubic urethropexy at the completion of the reconstructive procedure.

### Abdominal Enterocele Repairs

The apical defect repair of vaginal fascial reconstruction can be done abdominally, as previously illustrated. Three other techniques of abdominal enterocele repair have been described: Moschcowitz and Halban procedures and the uterosacral ligament plication. The Moschcowitz procedure is performed by placing concentric pursestring sutures around the cul-de-sac to include the posterior vaginal wall, the right pelvic side wall, the serosa of the sigmoid, and the left pelvic side wall (Fig. 18-10, *A*). The initial suture is placed at the base of the cul-de-sac. Usually, three or four sutures completely obliterate the cul-de-sac. The pursestring sutures are tied so that no small defects remain that could entrap small bowel or lead to enterocele recurrence. Care should be taken not to include the ureter in the pursestring sutures or to allow the ureter to be kinked medially when tying the sutures.

Halban described a technique to obliterate the cul-de-sac using sutures placed sagittally between the uterosacral ligaments. Four or five sutures are placed in a longitudinal fashion sequentially through the serosa of the sigmoid, into the deep peritoneum of the cul-de-sac, and up the posterior vaginal wall (Fig. 18-10, *B*). The sutures are tied, obliterating the cul-de-sac.

Transverse plication of the uterosacral ligaments can be used to obliterate the cul-de-sac (Fig. 18-10, *C*). Three to five sutures are placed into the medial portion of one uterosacral ligament, into the back wall of the vagina, and into the medial portion of the opposite uterosacral ligament. The lowest suture incorporates the anterior rectal serosa to bring the rectum adjacent to the uterosacral ligaments and vagina. Care must be taken to avoid entrapment or kinking of the ureter. Relaxing incisions can be made in the peritoneum lateral to the uterosacral ligament to release the ureter, if necessary.

## RECTOCELE

Defects of posterior vaginal wall support are common and may be asymptomatic or associated with disorders of defecation. As the pelvic defects become progressively larger and symptoms increase, treatment may be indicated.

### Anatomy and Pathophysiology

Rectocele may be defined as herniation or bulging of the posterior vaginal wall, with the anterior wall of the rectum in direct apposition to the vaginal epithelium. Rectocele is fundamentally a defect of the rectovaginal septum, not the rectum.

Within the rectovaginal septum is a thin, membranous connective tissue called the fascia of Denonvilliers, which is

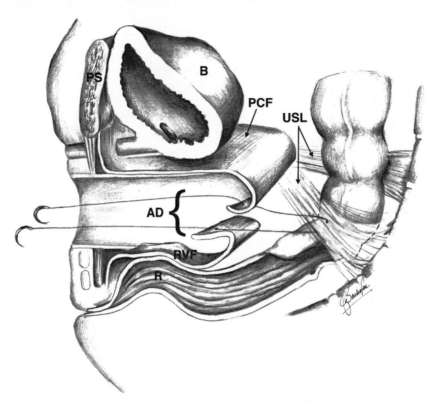

**Fig. 18-7**  Sagittal view of correct suture placement through pubocervical fascia *(PCF)*, left uterosacral ligament *(USL)*, and rectovaginal fascia *(RVF)*. *B,* Bladder; *PS,* pubic symphysis; *AD,* apical defect; *R,* rectum.

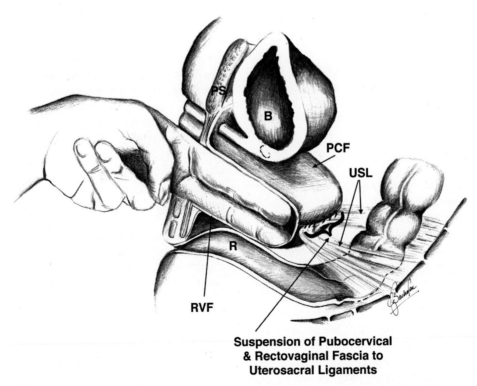

**Suspension of Pubocervical
& Rectovaginal Fascia to
Uterosacral Ligaments**

**Fig. 18-8**  Sagittal view following tying of double-armed sutures. Note restoration of the normal axis. *PS,* Pubic symphysis; *B,* bladder; *PCF,* pubocervical fascia; *USL,* uterosacral ligaments; *RVF,* rectovaginal fascia; *R,* rectum.

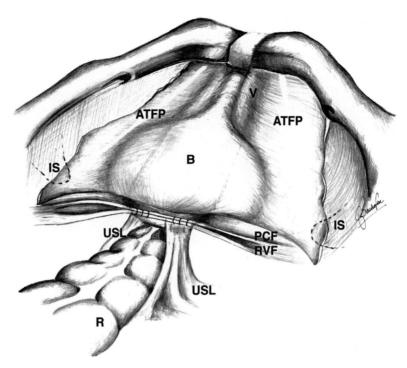

**Fig. 18-9** Intraabdominal view following repair. *ATFP,* Arcus tendineus fasciae pelvis; *B,* bladder; *IS,* ischial spines; *PCF,* pubocervical fascia; *RVF,* rectovaginal fascia; *USL,* uterosacral ligaments; *R,* rectum.

Copyright 1998 by CG Bachofen, MD.

fused to the underside of the posterior vaginal wall. The rectovaginal fascia extends downward from the posterior aspect of the cervix and the cardinal-uterosacral ligaments to its attachment on the upper margin of the perineal body and laterally to the fascia over levator ani muscles. When this caudal attachment is separated, as during childbirth, the perineal body becomes more mobile, leading to rectocele and perineal descent. Rectocele and enterocele appear to be most common in parous women.

## Evaluation

Patients with rectocele may complain of symptoms related directly to the herniated tissue in the vagina or of symptoms of defecation dysfunction, such as the inability to evacuate the distal rectum completely without straining or splinting. Constipation per se is not a symptom of rectocele, although it may coexist. Finally, fecal incontinence often coexists with pelvic prolapse. Symptoms directly related to genital prolapse include the sensation of a mass or bulge in the vagina, pelvic pressure and pain, low back pain, and difficulty with intravaginal intercourse.

Rectocele is suspected on physical examination by observation of posterior vaginal wall bulging, especially during Valsalva maneuver. Anterior displacement of the rectal wall on rectovaginal examination is diagnostic.

## Surgical Repair Techniques
### *Posterior Colporrhaphy and Perineoplasty*

The repairs of a relaxed perineum and rectocele are two distinct operative procedures, although they are usually performed together. Before beginning the repair, the surgeon should estimate the severity of the rectocele and the perineal defect, as well as the desired postoperative caliber of the vagina and introitus. The ultimate size of the vaginal orifice is determined by placing Allis clamps on the inner aspect of the labia minora bilaterally and approximating them in the midline. The final vaginal opening should admit three fingers easily, taking into account that the levator ani and perineal muscles are completely relaxed from the general anesthesia and that the vagina may further constrict postoperatively.

To begin the posterior colporrhaphy, Allis clamps are placed bilaterally on the posterior perineum. A triangular incision is made in the perineal body, and the overlying perineal skin is removed. A subepithelial tunnel is made in the rectovaginal space using Mayo scissors. The dissection is extended to the apex of the vagina and bilaterally in the rectovaginal space using blunt and sharp dissection. The surgeon removes a triangular strip of full-thickness vaginal wall, wide enough to repair the rectocele but leaving an appropriate caliber vagina.

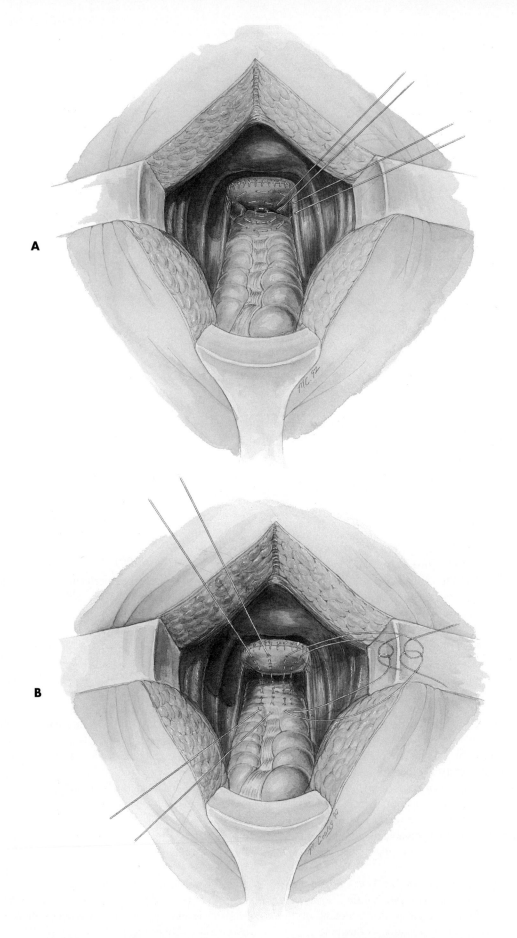

**Fig. 18-10**  Techniques of enterocele repair via the abdominal route. **A,** Moschcowitz procedure.
**B,** Halban procedure.

*Continued*

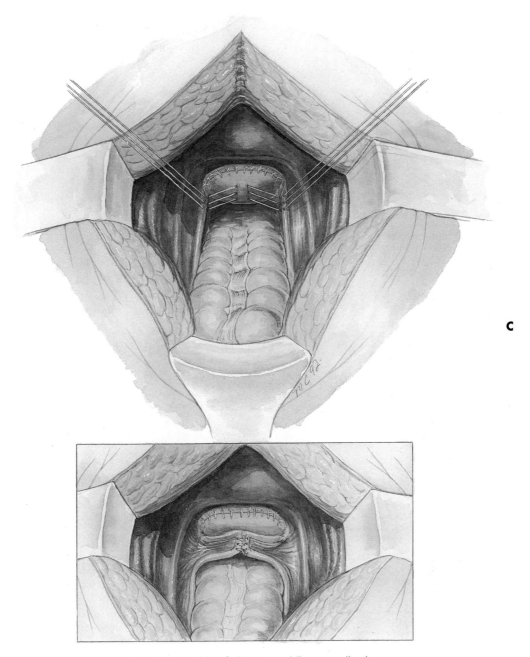

**Fig. 18-10, cont'd    C,** Uterosacral ligament plication.

Alternatively, the posterior vaginal wall is incised in the midline along its entire length. In a manner similar to the anterior colporrhaphy, lateral traction is placed on each vaginal flap and the underlying rectum and rectovaginal fascia are dissected bluntly and sharply from the vaginal epithelium. The dissection should be extended laterally as far as possible to mobilize perirectal fascia and expose the medial margins of the puborectalis muscles. The terminal ends of the bulbocavernosus and transverse perineal muscles are also freed from the adherent epithelium in the lower vagina.

The rectovaginal fascia is identified and any defects or lacerations are repaired with No. 2-0 or 0 delayed absorbable sutures (Fig. 18-11). Identification of rectovaginal de-fects is aided by rectal examination with the surgeon's finger elevated toward the vagina. Vertical mattress sutures then are used to plicate the pararectal and rectovaginal fascia over the rectal wall. Repair and plication of this fascia may be sufficient to treat small rectoceles. However, if the rectocele and levator hiatus are large, additional No. 0 delayed absorbable sutures are placed deeply into the medial portions of the puborectalis muscles, and the muscles are brought together in the rectovaginal space. Although levator plication effectively treats rectocele, it also tends to decrease the caliber of the vaginal lumen and to create a transverse ridge in the posterior vaginal wall, both of which may lead to dyspareunia. After the pararectal fascia and levator

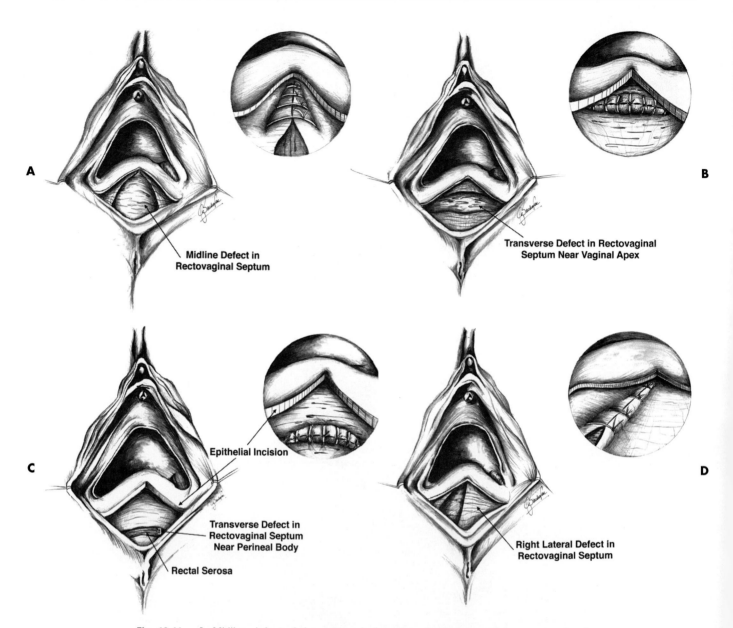

**Fig. 18-11** **A,** Midline defect of the rectovaginal septum. Inset demonstrates reapproximation following repair. **B,** Transverse defect of the rectovaginal fascia in the mid- to upper vagina. Inset depicts reapproximation following repair. **C,** Transverse defect near the junction of the rectovaginal fascia to the perineal body. Inset depicts reapproximation following repair. **D,** Lateral defect in rectovaginal fascia. Inset demonstrates repair with interrupted sutures.

Copyright 1998 by CG Bachofen, MD.

muscles are plicated, as appropriate, redundant vaginal epithelium is trimmed bilaterally, and the posterior vaginal wall and epithelium are closed with No. 3-0 delayed absorbable running suture. A perineoplasty is then performed by placing deep sutures into the perineal muscles and fascia to build up the perineal body. The overlying vulvar skin is closed with No. 3-0 running subcuticular suture.

For anterior and posterior colporrhaphy, a vaginal pack is placed and removed the first postoperative day. Ambulation and diet are advanced rapidly as tolerated by the patient.

## Rectovaginal Fascia Defect Repair

Isolated defects of the rectovaginal fascia can be seen most readily when the vaginal epithelium is dissected sharply from the underlying rectovaginal fascia. The rectovaginal fascia normally is suspended by the cardinal-uterosacral ligaments, and in the case of a woman who has not had a hysterectomy, to the posterior portion of the cervix. In women in whom the uterus has been removed, the most superior portion of rectovaginal fascia should be in direct apposition with the pubocervical fascia. Laterally, the rectovaginal fascia is attached to the fascia over levator muscles and distally is fused with the perineal body.

Transverse defects may occur most superiorly along the posterior wall of the cervix or at the vaginal apex. In these patients with a "high rectocele," an enterocele is present as well. Transverse defects may also occur at midvagina or, more commonly, where the rectovaginal fascia should be connected to the perineal body. The transverse defects may extend laterally and be associated with a tear or separation of the rectovaginal fascia from its normal attachment to the fascia over the levator muscles. Midline defects may occur in association with or separately from the other defects.

The most accurate way to identify fascial defects is in the operating room after the epithelium has been reflected away from the rectovaginal fascia. After obtaining hemostasis, irrigate the field with sterile saline and place the index finger of the nondominant hand into the rectum to elevate the anterior rectal wall. Inspect the entire posterior segment for breaks in the connective tissue. We commonly repair posterior segment defects with delayed absorbable suture using a series of interrupted sutures approximating the broken edges of the connective tissue. Midline repair is shown in Fig. 18-11, *A.* The edges of the fascial defect are generally well defined and are repaired under direct visualization, restoring the integrity of the rectovaginal septum over the rectal mucosa.

Fig. 18-11, *B,* shows a transverse defect of the rectovaginal fascia in the mid- to upper vagina. The defect may be seen more clearly when the examining finger is placed into the rectum and pressure is placed anteriorly. The edges of the defect are closed transversely with a series of interrupted sutures. Fig. 18-11, *C,* shows a transverse defect near the junction of the rectovaginal fascia to the perineal body. This common defect may be associated with prior episiotomy that either was not repaired properly or was repaired but did not heal properly. When repairing these defects, it is important to restore the continuity of the rectovaginal fascia to the perineal body. Fig. 18-11, *D,* demonstrates a lateral defect. The defect is identified, and the fascial edges are reapproximated using a series of interrupted sutures.

Whereas rectocele repair is accomplished by identification of the fascial defect and reapproximation of the connective tissue, evaluation of the levator hiatus is an entirely different issue. In women who have an enlarged levator hiatus, it may be appropriate to place another set of interrupted sutures horizontally to narrow the levator hiatus. That portion of the operation is not necessary in all patients and is independent of the rectocele repair.

Perineorrhaphy is the third part of the posterior segment reconstruction. The perineal body consists of the anal sphincter, the superficial and deep transverse perineus muscles, the bulbocavernosus muscles, and the junction of the rectovaginal fascia to the anal sphincter. Perineorrhaphy implies the identification and reconstruction of these components.

## Results

Few studies have addressed the long-term success of vaginal plastic procedures for treating enterocele and rectocele. Early recurrence is probably caused by failure to identify and individually repair all support defects. Late recurrence is probably caused by the subsequent weakening of the patient's support tissue occurring with advancing age, chronic straining, estrogen deficiency, and other factors.

## Complications

The intraoperative complications of rectocele repair include blood loss requiring a blood transfusion and unintended proctotomy. Proctotomy should be repaired in layers at the time of the injury. Following repair, management of the patient's diet is individualized. Use of a stool softener for 10 to 14 days may be beneficial but is not mandatory.

Sexual function may be affected by vaginal operations for genital prolapse. Francis and Jeffcoate (1961) found that about half of sexually active women had some sexual problems after anterior and posterior colpoperineorrhaphy, with or without hysterectomy. Fifty-five percent of these patients reported loss of sexual desire or impotence (male or female), which often predated the vaginal surgery. The remaining women reported sexual difficulties caused by shortened or stenotic vaginas, dyspareunia, or fear of injury.

Haase and Skibsted (1988) studied 55 sexually active women who underwent a variety of operations for stress incontinence or genital prolapse. Postoperatively, 24% of the patients experienced improvement in their sexual satisfaction, 67% experienced no change, and 9% experienced deterioration. Deterioration was always caused by dyspareunia after posterior colporrhaphy. These authors concluded that the prognosis for an improved sexual life is good after surgery for stress incontinence, but posterior colpoperineorrhaphy causes dyspareunia in some patients.

## BIBLIOGRAPHY
### Anatomy and Pathophysiology

DeLancey JOL: Anatomic aspects of vaginal eversion after hysterectomy, *Am J Obstet Gynecol* 166:1717, 1992.

Funt MI, Thompson JD, Birch H: Normal vaginal axis, *South Med J* 71:1534, 1978.

Harrison JE, McDonagh JE: Hernia of Douglas pouch and high rectocele, *Am J Obstet Gynecol* 60:83, 1950.

Kuhn RJP, Hollyock MD: Observations on the anatomy of the rectovaginal pouch and septum, *Obstet Gynecol* 59:445, 1982.

Mäkinen J, Kähäri V, Söderström K, et al: Collagen synthesis in the vaginal connective tissue of patients with and without uterine prolapse, *Eur J Obstet Gynecol Reprod Biol* 24:319, 1987.

Mäkinen J, Söderström K, Kiilholma P, et al: Histologic changes in the vaginal connective tissue of patients with and without uterine prolapse, *Arch Gynecol* 239:17, 1986.

Milley PS, Nichols DH: A correlative investigation of the human rectovaginal septum, *Anat Rec* 163:443, 1969.

Nichols DH: Posterior colporrhaphy and perineorrhaphy: separate and distinct operations, *Am J Obstet Gynecol* 164:714, 1991.

Nichols DH, Randall CL: *Vaginal surgery,* ed 3, Baltimore, 1989, Williams & Wilkins.

Richardson AC: The anatomic defects in rectocele and enterocele, *J Pelvic Surg* 1:215, 1995.

Richardson AC, Lyon JB, Williams NL: A new look at pelvic relaxation, *Am J Obstet Gynecol* 126:568, 1976.

Ulmsten U, Ekman G, Giertz G, et al: Different biochemical composition of connective tissue in continent and stress incontinent women, *Acta Obstet Gynecol Scand* 66:455, 1987.

### Evaluation

Baden WF, Walker T, Lindsey JH: The vaginal profile, *Tex Med* 64:56, 1968.

Beecham CT: Classification of vaginal relaxation, *Am J Obstet Gynecol* 136:957, 1980.

Bump RC, Mattiasson A, Bo K, et al: The standardization of terminology of female pelvic organ prolapse and pelvic floor dysfunction, *Am J Obstet Gynecol* 175:10, 1996.

Porges RF: A practical system of diagnosis and classification of pelvic relaxations, *Surg Gynecol Obstet* 117:769, 1963.

### Surgical Repair Techniques and Complications

Francis WJA, Jeffcoate TNA: Dyspareunia following vaginal operations, *Br J Obstet Gynaecol* 68:1, 1961.

Given FT: "Posterior culdeplasty": revisited, *Am J Obstet Gynecol* 153:135, 1985.

Haase P, Skibsted L: Influence of operations for stress incontinence and/or genital descensus on sexual life, *Acta Obstet Gynecol Scand* 67:659, 1988.

Harris RL, Cundiff GW, Theofiastous JP, et al: The value of intraoperative cytoscopy in urogynecologic and reconstructive pelvic surgery, *Am J Obstet Gynecol* 177:1367, 1997.

Mattingly RF, Thompson JD: Relaxed vaginal outlet, rectocele, and enterocele. In Thompson JD, Rock JA, eds: *Operative gynecology,* ed 6, Philadelphia, 1985, JB Lippincott.

McCall ML: Posterior culdeplasty, *Obstet Gynecol* 10:595, 1957.

Mitchell GW: Vaginal hysterectomy: anterior and posterior colporrhaphy, repair of enterocele, and prolapse of vaginal vault. In Ridley JH, ed: *Gynecologic surgery: errors, safeguards, salvage,* ed 2, Baltimore, 1981, Williams & Wilkins.

Moschcowitz AV: The pathogenesis, anatomy, and cure of prolapse of the rectum, *Surg Gynecol Obstet* 15:7, 1912.

Stanhope CR, Wilson TO, Utz WJ, et al: Suture entrapment and secondary ureteral obstruction, *Am J Obstet Gynecol* 164:1513, 1991.

Torpin R: Excision of the cul-de-sac of Douglas for the surgical care of hernias through the female caudal wall, including prolapse of the uterus, *J Int Coll Surg* 24:322, 1955.

Waters EG: Vaginal prolapse: technique for correction and prevention at hysterectomy, *Obstet Gynecol* 8:432, 1956.

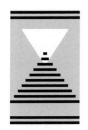

CHAPTER **19**

# Surgical Treatment of Vaginal Vault Prolapse

Mickey M. Karram, Eddie H.M. Sze, and Mark D. Walters

---

In recent years, the problem of pelvic organ prolapse has been given much more attention. Many women are living longer, and there is more interest in maintaining self-image of femininity and the capacity of sexual activity beyond menopause. Although few data on the incidence or prevalence of various forms of pelvic organ prolapse exist, the incidence appears to be rising based on increased longevity of women.

The management of pelvic organ prolapse can be difficult; several support defects often coexist, and simple anatomic correction of the various defects does not always result in normal function of the vagina and surrounding organs. To accomplish the goals of pelvic reconstruction, the surgeon must thoroughly understand normal anatomic support and physiologic function of the vagina, bladder, and rectum. These goals are to restore anatomy, maintain or restore normal bowel and bladder function, and maintain vaginal capacity for sexual intercourse.

This chapter discusses the pathology and surgical correction of uterine prolapse and posthysterectomy apical prolapse. Normal anatomy of the pelvic diaphragm is discussed in detail in Chapter 1. The evaluation of patients with pelvic organ prolapse, especially regarding their symptoms, phys-

ical examination, and diagnostic tests, is discussed in Chapters 4 and 5.

## PATHOLOGY OF PELVIC ORGAN PROLAPSE

Pelvic organ prolapse can result when normal pelvic organ supports are subjected chronically to increases in intraabdominal pressure or when defective genital support responds to normal intraabdominal pressure. Individual organs that pass through the pelvic floor can lose support singly or in combination, resulting in various degrees and combinations of pelvic organ prolapse. This loss of support occurs as a result of damage to any of the pelvic supportive systems. These systems include the bony pelvis, to which the soft tissues ultimately attach; the subperitoneal retinaculum and smooth muscle component of the endopelvic fascia (the cardinal and uterosacral ligament complex); the pelvic diaphragm, with the levator ani muscles and their fibromuscular attachments to the pelvic organs; and the perineal membrane. The perineal body and the walls of the vagina can lose tone and weaken from pathologic stretching from childbirth and attenuating changes of aging and menopause.

Loss of support or integrity of the anterior and posterior vaginal walls results in cystocele and enterorectocele, respectively. Uterovaginal prolapse occurs with damage or attenuation of endopelvic fascia that supports the uterus and upper vagina over the pelvic diaphragm. Furthermore, when the muscles within the pelvic diaphragm weaken as a result of congenital factors, childbirth injury, pelvic neuropathy, or aging, the levator ani lose resting tone and fail to contract quickly and strongly with increases in intraabdominal pressure. Muscle atrophy and a wider levator hiatus result; weaker and less rapid muscle contractions with rises in intraabdominal pressure contribute to related symptoms of urinary and fecal incontinence.

The pathophysiology of pelvic organ prolapse is further discussed in Chapter 18. Fig. 18-1 demonstrates the normal vaginal axis of nulliparous women in the standing position. Distortion of the normal vaginal axis during reconstructive pelvic surgery predisposes women to the development of pelvic organ prolapse at an anatomic site opposite to where

**235**

the repair was performed. Examples of this are the development of posterior vaginal wall prolapse after colposuspension procedures for stress incontinence and the development of anterior vaginal wall prolapse after suspension of the vaginal apex to the sacrospinous ligament.

## GENERAL CONCEPTS

The true incidence and prevalence of vaginal vault prolapse are unknown. Eversion of the vagina probably occurs in about 0.5% of patients who have undergone vaginal or abdominal hysterectomy. Prophylactic measures performed at the time of hysterectomy (vaginal or abdominal) probably decrease the incidence of vaginal vault prolapse. These measures include routine reattachment of endopelvic fascia—cardinal and uterosacral ligaments—to the vaginal vault and routine use of culdeplasty sutures, cul-de-sac obliteration, or enterocele excision after removal of the uterus. This is discussed further in Chapter 18.

When mild forms of isolated uterovaginal prolapse (descent of the cervix not beyond the midportion of the vagina) are present, vaginal hysterectomy and culdeplasty with anterior and posterior colporrhaphy are usually sufficient to relieve the patient's symptoms and restore normal vaginal function.

During the preoperative assessment of these patients, it is important to differentiate true uterine prolapse from cervical elongation. When the vault descends into the lower vagina, simple hysterectomy with repair often does not result in acceptable vaginal depth or prevent vaginal prolapse recurrences. In these cases, one must look to procedures aimed at suspending the apex of the vagina, or in rare circumstances, completely obliterating the vagina. When this has been decided, certain other decisions must be made:

- If the uterus is still present, should hysterectomy be part of the surgical correction? The majority of patients require removal of the uterus. The techniques of vaginal and abdominal hysterectomy are sufficiently discussed in other texts and will not be mentioned further. If hysterectomy is not desired, then pessary use or LeFort partial colpocleisis should be considered. If surgical correction is needed and the patient desires fertility potential, the preferred surgical approach is currently controversial because few data exist. A review of the subject has been published by Nichols (1991). Case 1 in Chapter 34 provides the opinions of two experts regarding the surgical correction of advanced uterovaginal prolapse in a patient who insists on uterine preservation. In the author's opinion, abdominal approaches to such patients via uterosacral ligament plication or modified sacral colopexy provide a more durable repair than commonly performed vaginal procedures such as sacrospinous ligament suspension.

- Is the surgical correction intended to preserve a functional vagina? Most of the operations discussed in this chapter are aimed at preservation of vaginal and coital function. For patients in whom future sexual function is not a goal or operative time and morbidity are best kept at a minimum, colpectomy with partial or complete colpocleisis may be indicated.
- Should the surgical correction be approached via a vaginal or abdominal route? Factors such as the patient's general medical condition and weight, the need for concurrent surgical procedures, and the preference and expertise of the surgeon influence this decision. A prospective randomized trial by Benson et al. (1996) seems to indicate that an abdominal approach to prolapse provides a better anatomic and functional outcome when compared with a vaginal approach.
- Does the patient have occult or potential stress urinary or fecal incontinence? When choosing the route of surgical correction, the surgeon must always consider the correction of lower urinary tract and lower gastrointestinal dysfunction. Preoperative reduction of the prolapse followed by urodynamic or rectal manometric tests will help the physician to answer this question and to determine which operations are required. The clinical utility of reductive maneuvers to predict potential or occult stress incontinence in patients with advanced prolapse has recently been questioned. This topic is nicely discussed by two experts in Case 3 in Chapter 34.

As previously mentioned, any reconstructive surgery should return the upper vagina to the normal near-horizontal axis. Failure to recognize an enterocele or to reconstruct a widened levator hiatus may predispose to postoperative vaginal prolapse. The length of the vagina is also an important factor for surgical success. The upper 3 to 4 cm of the vagina lies horizontally over the levator plate. Operations that shorten the vagina do not allow the upper vagina to lie over the levator plate and may predispose to recurrent vaginal prolapse.

Although many different techniques have been described to suspend or obliterate the vagina, only the most popular vaginal and abdominal techniques will be discussed.

## VAGINAL PROCEDURES THAT SUSPEND THE APEX
### Sacrospinous Ligament Suspension
#### Surgical Anatomy

To perform this procedure correctly and safely, the surgeon must be familiar with pararectal anatomy as well as the anatomy of the sacrospinous ligament and its surrounding structures (Fig. 19-1).

The sacrospinous ligaments extend from the ischial spines on each side to the lower portion of the sacrum and

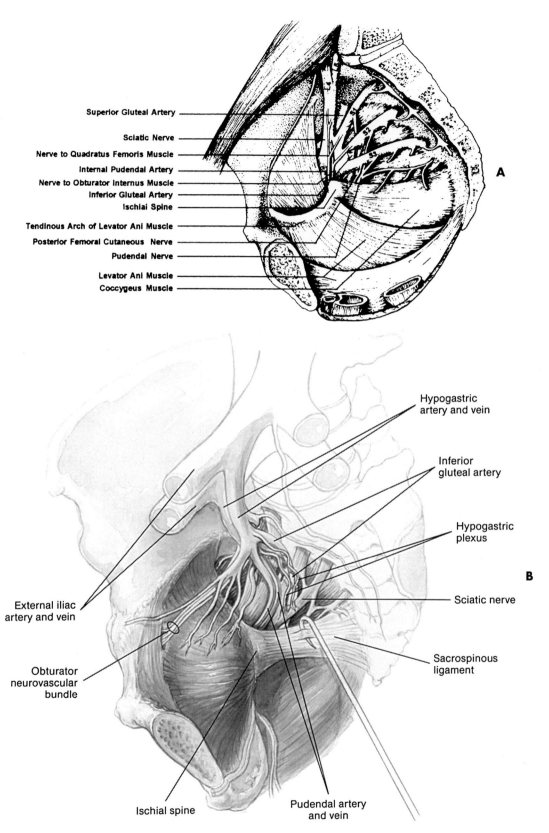

**Fig. 19-1    A,** Anatomy of the coccygeus-sacrospinous ligament (C-SSL) complex. A cross-section of the pelvis, depicting C-SSL and surrounding structures. **B,** Close-up view of C-SSL complex to demonstrate close proximity of various nerves and blood vessels.

**A** from Sze EHM, Karram MM: *Obstet Gynecol* 89:466, 1997.

coccyx. Nichols and Randall (1989) described the sacrospinous ligament as a cordlike structure lying within the substance of the coccygeus muscle. However, the fibromuscular coccygeus muscle and sacrospinous ligament are basically the same structure and are thus called the coccygeus-sacrospinous ligament (C-SSL). The coccygeus muscle has a large fibrous component that is present throughout the body of the muscle and on the anterior surface, where it appears as white ridges. The C-SSL can be identified by palpating the ischial spine and tracing the flat triangular thickening posteriorly to the sacrum. The fibromuscular coccygeus is attached directly to the underlying sacrotuberous ligament.

Posterior to the C-SSL and sacrotuberous ligament are the gluteus maximus muscle and the fat of the ischiorectal fossa. The pudendal nerves and vessels lie directly posterior to the ischial spine. The sciatic nerve lies superior and lateral to the C-SSL. Also superiorly lies an abundant vascular supply that includes inferior gluteal vessels and a hypogastric venous plexus.

### Surgical Technique

Before this operation is initiated, one should have preoperatively recognized the ischial spine and C-SSL on pelvic examination. Preoperative estrogen replacement therapy should be given liberally, if appropriate. We prefer to use a vaginal estrogen cream for 4 to 6 weeks preoperatively.

The performance of this operation almost always requires simultaneous correction of the anterior and posterior vaginal walls and enterocele repair. Displacing the prolapsed vaginal apex to the sacrospinous ligament to see whether the anterior and posterior vaginal wall prolapse disappears with a Valsalva maneuver helps to determine whether cystocele and rectocele repairs are needed. The patient should be routinely consented for these repairs because many times it is difficult to discern the extent of the various defects preoperatively.

The technique of unilateral sacrospinous fixation is as follows:

1. With the patient in dorsal lithotomy position, the vaginal area is prepped and draped. Prophylactic perioperative antibiotics are given routinely.
2. The apex of the vagina is grasped with two Allis clamps, and downward traction is used to determine the extent of the vaginal prolapse and associated pelvic support defects. The vaginal apex is then reduced to the sacrospinous ligament intended to be used. Although bilateral sacrospinous fixations have been described, most surgeons prefer unilateral fixation of the vaginal vault. At times the apex of the vagina is foreshortened and will not reach the intended area of fixation. This is commonly associated with a shortened anterior vaginal wall and a prominent enterocele. The apex should be moved to a portion of the vaginal wall over the enterocele, thus allowing sufficient vaginal

length for suspension to the sacrospinous ligament. The intended apex is tagged with two sutures for its later identification.
3. If the patient has complete eversion of the vagina and requires anterior vaginal wall repair and/or bladder neck suspension, we prefer doing this portion of the operation first. During this procedure, one can separate the bladder base away from the vaginal apex, thus lowering the risk of cystotomy. After these procedures are completed, the anterior vaginal wall is closed with a continuous running suture.
4. The posterior vaginal wall is then incised. After a transverse perineal incision, a midline posterior vaginal wall incision is made just short of the apex of the vagina, leaving a small vaginal bridge approximately 3 or 4 cm wide. In the majority of cases, an enterocele sac is present. This sac should be dissected off the posterior vaginal wall and closed with a high pursestring suture, as described in Chapter 18. Once the enterocele has been incised and ligated, one is ready to begin the sacrospinous fixation.
5. The first step is entry into the perirectal space. The right rectal pillar separates the rectovaginal space from the right perirectal space. The rectal pillar is areolar tissue that extends from the rectum to the arcus tendineus fasciae pelvis and overlies the levator muscle. It has two layers and may contain a few small muscle fibers and blood vessels. In the majority of cases, entry into the perirectal space is best achieved by breaking through the fibroareolar tissue just lateral to the enterocele sac at the level of the ischial spine. This maneuver can usually be accomplished bluntly by mobilizing the rectum medially. At times, however, the use of gauze on the index finger or a tonsil clamp is necessary to break through into this space.
6. Once the perirectal space is entered, the ischial spine is identified and, with dorsal and medial movement of the fingers, the C-SSL is palpated.
7. Blunt dissection is used to further remove tissue from this area. The surgeon should take great care to ensure that the rectum is adequately retracted medially. At this time, we recommend performing a rectal examination to ensure that no inadvertent rectal injury has occurred.
8. Two techniques have been popularized for the actual passage of sutures through the ligament (Fig. 19-2). The first is the technique of Randall and Nichols (1971) using a long-handled Deschamps ligature carrier and nerve hook (Fig. 19-3, A). Long straight retractors are used to expose the coccygeus muscle. Heaney retractors or Briesky-Navratil retractors (Fig. 19-3, B) are preferred. One must take great care not to let the tip of the retractor be pushed across the anterior surface of the sacrum, risking potential damage to vessels and nerves. If the right sacro-

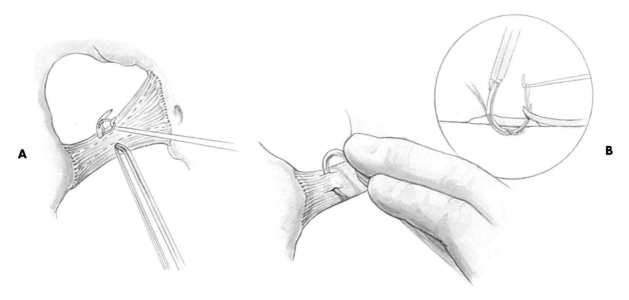

**Fig. 19-2    A,** Passage of Deschamps ligature carrier with suture through C-SSL. Note that needletip is passed in superior direction. Retrieval of suture is with nerve hook. **B,** Passage of Miya hook through C-SSL. Note that needletip is passed inferiorly. Retrieval of suture is facilitated by using notched speculum.

spinous ligament is to be used, the middle and index fingers on the left hand are placed on the medial surface of the ischial spine and, under direct vision, the tip of the ligature carrier penetrates the C-SSL at a point two fingerbreadths medial to the ischial spine. When pushing the ligature carrier through the body of the C-SSL, considerable resistance should be encountered; this must be overcome by forceful yet controlled rotation of the handle of the ligature carrier. If visualization of the C-SSL is difficult, the muscle and ligament can be grasped in the tip of a long Babcock or Allis clamp, which helps to isolate the tissue to be sutured from underlying vessels and nerves. After suture passage, the fingers of the left hand are withdrawn. The retractor is suitably repositioned and the tip of the ligature carrier is visualized. The suture is then grasped with a nerve hook (see Fig. 19-2, *A*). A second suture is similarly placed 1 cm medial to the first. To avoid a second passage of the ligature carrier, the original long suture can be cut in the center and each end of the cut loop paired with its respective free suture. This obtains two sutures through the ligament with only one penetration of the ligature carrier. To ensure that an appropriate bite of tissue has been obtained, one should be able to gently move the patient with traction of the sutures.

A second technique that has been popularized for passing the sutures through the C-SSL is the technique of Miyazaki (1987) using a Miya hook ligature carrier (Fig. 19-4). The proposed advantage of this technique is that it is safer and easier because the ligature carrier enters the C-SSL under direct palpa-

tion of distinct landmarks and is then pulled down into the safe perirectal space below.

To perform this modification, the right middle fingertip is placed on the C-SSL just below its superior margin, approximately two fingerbreadths medial to the ischial spine. The Miya hook, in the left hand in a closed position, is slid along the palmar surface of the right hand. The hook point should come to rest just beneath the previously positioned tip of the right middle finger. The handles are then opened and lowered to a near horizontal position. This points the hook into the C-SSL at about a 45-degree angle. If a high perineum prevents lowering the handle, then an episiotomy should be performed. With the tip of the middle finger, the hook point is placed two fingerbreadths medial to the ischial spine, approximately 0.5 cm below the superior edge. With experience, the hook point can be passed above the superior edge. With the middle and index fingers, apply firm pressure downward just behind the hook hump so the hook point penetrates the C-SSL (see Fig. 19-2, *B*). Downward pressure with two fingers on the top, plus traction with the back of the thumb on the back handle, produces enough force to penetrate the ligament. Close and elevate the handles of the Miya hook, and with the index and middle fingers, push the tissue from the hook point so as to make the suture clearly visible. If too much tissue is in the hook, simply back the hook out a little and take a smaller bite. An assistant should hold the elevated handles in a closed position. A long retractor is then placed to mobilize the rectum medially, and a notched

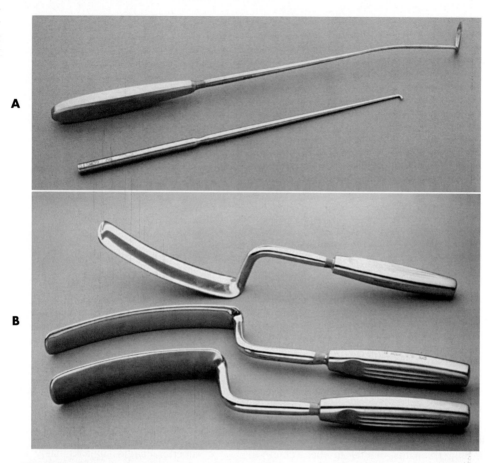

**Fig. 19-3** **A,** Long-handled Deschamps ligature carrier and nerve hook. Note slight bend near the tip to facilitate suture placement into the C-SSL. **B,** Briesky-Navratil retractors, various sizes.

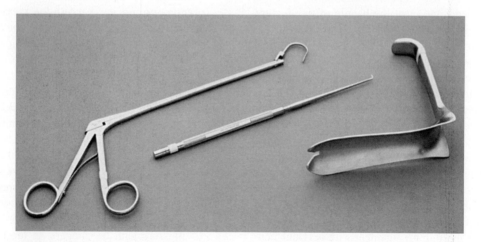

**Fig. 19-4** Miya hook, notched speculum, and suture hook for use during sacrospinous ligament fixation.

speculum is inserted by palpation underneath the hook point. A nerve hook is then used to retrieve the suture.

In addition to these techniques, two new instruments have been designed to facilitate passage of a suture through the ligament. These are shown in Fig. 19-5.

9. Now the surgeon is ready to bring the stitches out to the apex of the vagina. Again, two methods have been popularized for this maneuver (Fig. 19-6). The first involves bringing the vaginal apex to the surface of the C-SSL with the use of a pulley stitch. After the stitch has been placed in the ligament, one end of the suture is rethreaded on a free needle, sewn into

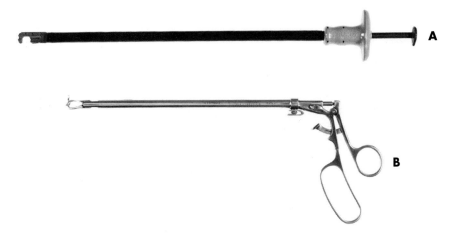

**Fig. 19-5**   Two specially designed instruments to facilitate passage of sutures through the sacrospinous ligament. **A,** Laurus needle driver (Microvasive–Boston Scientific Corp, Watertown, Mass). **B,** Nichols-Veronikis ligature carrier (BEI Medical Systems, Chatsworth, Calif).

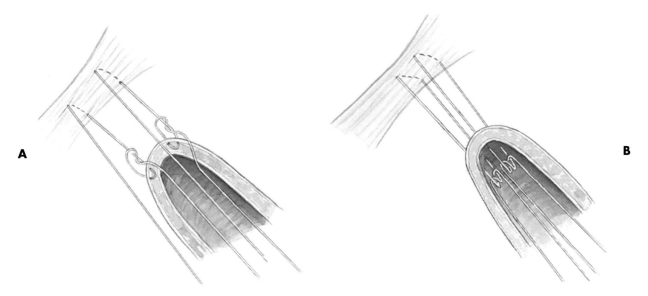

**Fig. 19-6**   Technique of fixing vaginal apex to C-SSL. **A,** Pulley stitch. Permanent sutures should be used. **B,** Stitches are placed through the vaginal epithelium and tied in the vaginal lumen. Delayed absorbable sutures should be used.

the full thickness of the fibromuscular layer of the undersurface of the vaginal apex, and tied by a single half hitch, while the free end of the suture is held long (see Fig. 19-6, *A*). Traction of the free end of the suture pulls the vagina directly onto the muscle and ligament. A square knot then fixes it in place. With this type of fixation, a permanent suture should be used because the suture is not exposed through the epithelium of the vagina.

Some surgeons prefer a second technique, especially if the vaginal wall is thin or if greater vaginal length is desired. This method inserts each end of the suture through the vaginal epithelium (see Fig. 19-6, *B*). When this method is used, a delayed absorbable suture should be used because the knot re-

mains in the vagina. We recommend a No. 2 delayed absorbable suture. After the sutures have been brought out through the vagina, the upper portion of the posterior vaginal wall is closed with interrupted or continuous No. 3-0 sutures. The vaginal vault suspension stitches are then tied, thus elevating the apex of the vagina to the C-SSL (Fig. 19-7). It is important that the vagina comes into contact with the coccygeus muscle and no suture bridge exists, especially if delayed absorbable sutures are being used. While tying these sutures, it may be useful to perform a rectal examination to detect any suture bridges.

10. After these sutures are tied, the posterior colpoperineorrhaphy is completed, as needed, and the vagina is packed with a moist gauze for 24 hours.

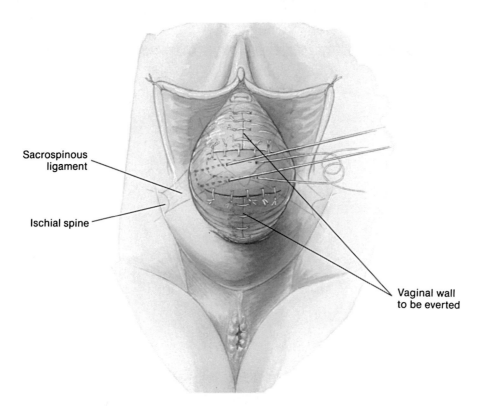

Sacrospinous
ligament

Ischial spine

Vaginal wall
to be everted

**Fig. 19-7** After stitches are passed through C-SSL, a free needle is used to pass through entire thickness of the vaginal wall at the level of the vaginal apex. Tying of suture inverts vagina by fixing vaginal apex to C-SSL.

## Results and Complications

The results of sacrospinous fixation are difficult to evaluate because few studies report long-term follow-up. The largest published series to date is by Nichols (1982), who performed the operation on 163 patients and followed them for at least 2 years. He reported only a 3% incidence of recurrent vaginal eversion and did not specify whether other pelvic support defects recurred. More recently, Morley and DeLancey (1988) reported on 100 patients who underwent sacrospinous fixation with or without anterior and posterior vaginal wall repairs. Subjective 1-year follow-up was available on 71 patients; only three had recurrent vaginal vault prolapse. These authors did note, however, that 22 patients had recurrent or persistent mild to moderate anterior vaginal wall relaxation or symptomatic cystoceles.

Shull et al. (1992) reported the results of sacrospinous ligament fixation, as well as other pelvic reconstructive surgery, in 81 patients. The authors performed site-specific analysis of pelvic support defects preoperatively and at consecutive postoperative visits. The findings at 6 weeks postoperatively and at subsequent visits were noted for each of five sites: urethra, bladder, vaginal cuff, cul-de-sac, and rectum. The most common site for recurrent prolapse was the anterior vaginal wall.

Sze et al. (1997) reported on 75 women who underwent sacrospinous ligament fixation in conjunction with other

reconstructive surgery. Fifty-four of the women were felt to have stress incontinence and also underwent a needle suspension procedure. Patients were objectively followed for an average of 2 years. The rate of recurrence of symptomatic prolapse was 33% in the needle suspension group and 19% in the remainder of the patients. Table 19-1 reviews these and other studies that have reported the long-term follow-up and recurrence of prolapse after sacrospinous ligament suspension.

Miyazaki (1987) reported on 74 cases of sacrospinous fixation using the Miya hook. Results with regard to treatment of the prolapse were not discussed, but the safety of the technique was documented. No patients had injuries to the bladder, rectum, nerves, or blood vessels, and no blood transfusions were performed. Average blood loss was approximately 75 ml.

Although infrequently reported, serious intraoperative complications can occur with sacrospinous fixation. Potential complications of the procedure are as follows:

- **Hemorrhage.** Severe hemorrhage can result from overzealous dissection superior to the coccygeus muscle or lateral to the ischial spine. This can result in hemorrhage from the inferior gluteal vessels, hypogastric venous plexus, or internal pudendal vessels. Hemorrhage from these vessels can be difficult to control. For this reason, we prefer the technique

**Table 19-1**  Long-Term Complications, Follow-Up, and Recurrence of Prolapse After Sacrospinous Ligament Suspension

| Investigator | Duration of follow-up | No. available for follow-up | Surgical repair required/recurrent pelvic relaxation (n) | | | | No. cured (%) | Cure assessment* |
|---|---|---|---|---|---|---|---|---|
| | | | Vault | Anterior wall | Posterior wall | Unspecified/ multiple sites | | |
| Richter and Albright (1981) and Richter (1982) | 1-10 yr | 81 | 2/2 | 0/12 | 0/10 | | 57 (70) | Objective |
| Nichols (1982) | ≥2 yr | 163 | 5/5 | | | | 158 (97)† | |
| Morley and Delancey (1988) | 1 mo-11 yr | 92 | 3/3 | 2/11 | 0/0 | 0/3 | 75 (82) | Subjective/objective |
| Brown et al. (1989) | 8-21 mo | 11 | 1/1 | 0/0 | 0/0 | | 10 (91) | Objective |
| Keetel and Herbertson (1989) | | 31 | 2/6 | | | | 25 (81) | Subjective/objective |
| Cruikshank and Cox (1990) | 8 mo-3.2 yr | 48 | 0/1 | 0/5 | 0/2 | | 40 (83) | Objective‡ |
| Monk et al. (1991) | 1 mo-8.6 yr | 61 | 1/1 | 0/6 | 0/2 | | 52 (85) | Objective |
| Backer (1992) | | 51 | 0/0 | 0/3 | 0/0 | | 48 (94) | Objective |
| Heinonen (1992) | 6 mo-5.6 yr | 22 | 0/0 | 0/1 | 0/2 | | 19 (86) | Objective |
| Imparato et al. (1992) | — | 155 | 0/4 | | | 0/11 | 140 (90) | Objective |
| Shull et al. (1992) | 2-5 yr | 81 | 0/1 | 4/20 | 0/1 | 0/6 | 53 (65) | Objective |
| Kaminski et al. (1993) | — | 23 | 2/2 | 0/1 | 0/0 | | 20 (87) | Objective |
| Carey and Slack (1994) | 2 mo-1 yr | 63§ | 1/1 | 0/16 | 0/0 | | 46 (73) | Objective |
| Porges and Smilen (1994) | — | 76 | | ?/1 | | 0/2 | — | Objective‡ |
| Holley et al. (1995) | 15-79 mo | 36 | | | | 0/33|| | 3 (8) | Objective |
| Sauer and Klutke (1995) | 4-26 mo | 24 | 3/5 | 1/3 | 0/1 | | 15 (63) | Objective‡ |
| Peters and Christenson (1995) | Median = 48 mo | 30 | 0/0 | 0/0 | 4/6 | 0/1 | 23 (77) | Subjective/objective |
| Elkins et al. (1995) | 3-6 mo | 14 | | 0/2 | | | 12 (86) | Objective‡ |
| Sze et al. (1997) | 7-72 mo | 75 | ?/4 | ?/16 | ?/1 | ?/1 | 53 (71) | Objective‡ |
| Total | 1 mo-11 yr | 1137 | 20/36 | 7/96 | 4/25 | 0/57 | | |

From Sze EHM, Karram MM: *Obstet Gynecol* 89:466, 1997.
*Subjective assessment, based on telephone interview or questionnaire; objective assessment, based on findings from pelvic examination.
†Cure rate applies to vaginal vault support only; does not include support defect at other site.
‡Extrapolated from text.
§Includes 11 patients whose uteri were preserved.
||Includes 33 patients with anterior vaginal wall defects, 3 vaginal vault prolapses, and 8 posterior vaginal wall relaxations.

described by Miyazaki in which the needle tip is passed downward into the safe ischiorectal space, rather than the technique using the Deschamps ligature carrier in which the needle tip is passed superiorly toward an abundant vasculature. If severe bleeding occurs in the area around the coccygeus muscle, we recommend initially packing the area. If this does not control the bleeding, then visualization and attempted ligation with clips or sutures should be performed. This area is difficult to approach transabdominally, so bleeding should be controlled vaginally, if possible.

- **Buttock pain.** It has been our experience that approximately 10% to 15% of patients experience moderate to severe buttock pain on the side on which the sacrospinous suspension was performed. This is probably caused by injury of a small nerve that runs through the C-SSL. This nerve injury is always self-limiting and should resolve completely by 6 weeks postoperatively. Reassurance and antiinflammatory agents usually are all that are necessary.

- **Nerve injury.** Because of the close proximity of the sciatic nerve to the C-SSL, the potential for its injury is present. Although it is rarely reported, if this injury occurs, reoperation with removal of suture material may be necessary.

- **Rectal injury.** Rectal examination should be performed frequently during this operation because of the close proximity of the rectum to the C-SSL. Rectal injury can occur during entering of the perirectal space as well as during mobilization of tissue off of the C-SSL. If a rectal injury is identified, it can usually be repaired primarily transvaginally by conventional techniques.

- **Stress urinary incontinence.** This may occur after vaginal vault suspension procedures and is probably secondary to straightening of the vesicourethral junction coincident with restoration of vaginal length and depth. Stress incontinence should be tested for preoperatively by performing a stress test in the standing position with reduction of the vaginal prolapse.

- **Vaginal stenosis.** Stenosis may occur if too much anterior and posterior vaginal wall tissue is trimmed or if too tight a posterior colporrhaphy is performed. We recommend postoperative use of estrogen vaginal cream in these patients in the hope of preventing or decreasing the incidence of this problem.

- **Recurrent anterior vaginal wall prolapse.** As mentioned earlier, the pelvic support defect that recurs with the highest incidence is that of the anterior vaginal wall. Approximately 20% of patients return with a moderate anterior vaginal wall prolapse within a year after surgery. This defect probably results from the alteration of the vaginal axis in an exaggerated posterior direction.

## Endopelvic Fascia Repair (Modified McCall Culdeplasty)

Between 1952 and 1981, two groups of investigators performed a total of 367 surgeries for vaginal eversion by suturing the prolapsed vagina to the endopelvic fascia with few complications (Phaneuf, 1952; Symmonds and Pratt, 1960; Symmonds and Sheldon, 1965; Lee and Symmonds, 1972; Symmonds et al., 1981). More recently, Webb et al. (1998) reported on 660 women who underwent primary endopelvic fascia repair for posthysterectomy vault prolapse between 1976 and 1987.

The technique of this repair is as follows:

1. An elliptical wedge of vaginal mucosa is excised initially from the anterior and posterior walls of the prolapsed vagina to narrow the vault and to allow access to the lateral apical supports of the vagina and rectum. The width and length of the excised wedge are determined by the desired dimensions of the reconstructed vagina.
2. The enterocele sac is isolated and excised, and the ureters are identified by palpation or dissection.
3. Up to three modified McCall stitches are placed (see Chapter 18). Each suture incorporates the full thickness of the posterior vaginal wall, the cul-de-sac peritoneum, the remains of the uterosacral-cardinal complex laterally, and the fascial tissue lateral and posterior to the upper vagina and rectum.
4. Sutures are then tied, resulting in fixation of the prolapsed vaginal vault to the uppermost portion of the endopelvic fascia as well as high closure of the cul-de-sac peritoneum.

The results and complications of this technique were discussed in a review article by Sze and Karram (1997). Of the initial studies reporting 367 patients, 322 (88%) received postoperative follow-up ranging from 1 to 12 years, with a cure rate of 88% to 93%. Thirty-four (11%) patients developed recurrent pelvic relaxation, including 9 with vaginal vault prolapse, 2 with anterior vaginal wall defects, 11 with posterior vaginal wall relaxations, and 12 patients with pelvic support defects at multiple or unspecified sites. The subsequent study by Webb et al. (1998) reported results on 660 women, most of whom were followed up with a

questionnaire. Information about recurrent prolapse was available on 504 women (72.7%). Fifty-eight patients (11.5%) complained of a "bulge" or "protrusion" at the time of questioning. The question about satisfaction with the operation was answered by 385 patients, and 82% indicated that they were satisfied. Forty-two (22%) of 189 sexually active women complained of dyspareunia.

## Iliococcygeus Fascia Suspension

In 1963, Inmon described bilateral fixation of the everted vaginal apex to the iliococcygeal fascia just below the ischial spine in three patients with atrophied uterosacral ligaments.

The technique of this repair is as follows:

1. The posterior vaginal wall is opened in the midline as for a posterior colporrhaphy, and the rectovaginal spaces are dissected widely to the levator muscles bilaterally.
2. The dissection is extended bluntly toward the ischial spines.
3. With the surgeon's nondominant hand depressing the rectum downward and medial, an area 1 to 2 cm caudad and posterior to the ischial spine in the ileococcygeus muscle and fascia is exposed (Fig. 19-8). A single No. 0 delayed absorbable suture is placed deeply into the levator muscle and fascia. Both ends of the suture are then passed through the ipsilateral posterior vaginal apex and held with a hemostat. This is repeated on the opposite side.
4. The posterior colporrhaphy is completed and the vagina closed. Both sutures are tied, elevating the posterior vaginal apices. This repair is often done in conjunction with a culdeplasty or uterosacral suspension.

From 1981 to 1993, Shull et al. (1993) and Meeks et al. (1994) used the Inmon technique to treat 152 patients with posthysterectomy vault prolapse or total uterine procidentia. There were four intraoperative complications, including one rectal and one bladder laceration and two cases of hemorrhage requiring transfusion. Thirteen (8%) patients developed recurrent pelvic support defects at various sites 6 weeks to 5 years after the initial procedure; two had vault prolapse, eight had anterior vaginal wall relaxation, and three had posterior wall defects.

## High Uterosacral Ligament Suspension With Fascial Reconstruction

A new approach to the management of enterocele and vault prolapse is based on the anatomic observations of Richardson (1995), who believes that the connective tissue of the vaginal tube does not stretch or attenuate but rather breaks at specific definable points. This concept and the vaginal approach to enterocele and vault prolapse are discussed in detail by Shull and Bachofen in Chapter 18. The authors believe that this repair may be superior to

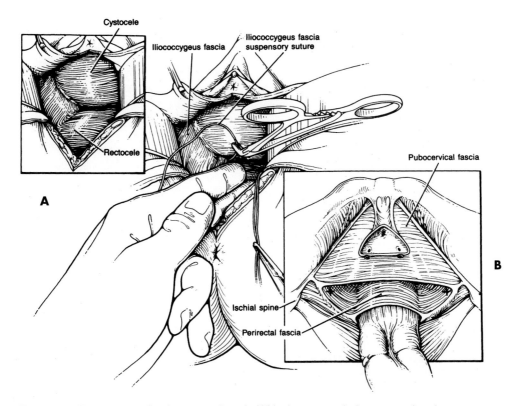

**Fig. 19-8** Iliococcygeus fascia suspension. **A,** With the surgeon's finger pressing the rectum downward, the right iliococcygeus fascia suture is placed. *Inset:* view of the dissected vagina. **B,** Abdominal view of the endopelvic fascia. *Plus marks* show the approximate location of the iliococcygeus fascia sutures.

From Meeks GR, Washburne JF, McGeher RP, et al: *Am J Obstet Gynecol* 171: 1447, 1994.

previously discussed repairs in that it can be performed vaginally, abdominally, or laparoscopically and it suspends the apex of the vagina into the hollow of the sacrum while restoring the continuity of the endopelvic fascia, thus reinforcing the anterior and posterior vaginal walls.

We use a technique similar to the vaginal approach described in Chapter 18 (Fig. 19-9).

1. The vaginal apex is grasped with two Allis clamps (Fig. 19-9, *A*) and incised with a scalpel. The vaginal epithelium is dissected off the enterocele sac up to the neck of the hernia. The enterocele is opened, and the sac of the hernia excised.
2. Numerous moist tail sponges are placed in the posterior cul-de-sac. A wide Deaver retractor is used to elevate the packs and the intestines out of the operative field.
3. The ischial spines are palpated transperitoneally. The remnants of the uterosacral ligaments are found posterior and medial to the ischial spine, and the ureter can usually be palpated along the pelvic side wall anywhere from 2 to 5 cm ventral and lateral to the ischial spine.
4. We prefer to plicate the remnants of the uterosacral ligaments across the midline with two to four

nonabsorbable sutures (Fig. 19-9, *B* and *C*). Tying of these sutures results in a firm ridge of tissue high up in the hollow of the sacrum (Fig. 19-9, *C*).

5. If an anterior colporrhaphy or sling procedure is indicated, it should be performed at this time.
6. Delayed absorbable sutures are then used to suspend the anterior and posterior vaginal walls with their underlying fascia to the plicated uterosacral ligaments (Fig. 19-9, *D*). This results in suspension of the prolapsed apex and establishes continuity of the underlying fascia of the anterior vaginal wall with that of the posterior vaginal wall (Figs. 19-9, *E,* and 19-10).

To date there are no published data reporting the efficacy or complication rate of this type of repair.

## OBLITERATIVE PROCEDURES
### LeFort Partial Colpocleisis

The LeFort partial colpocleisis reduces the uterovaginal prolapse and apposes the anterior and posterior vaginal walls. This operation should be used only as a last resort to cure prolapse because the procedure does not leave a functional vagina. It is useful because it can be performed

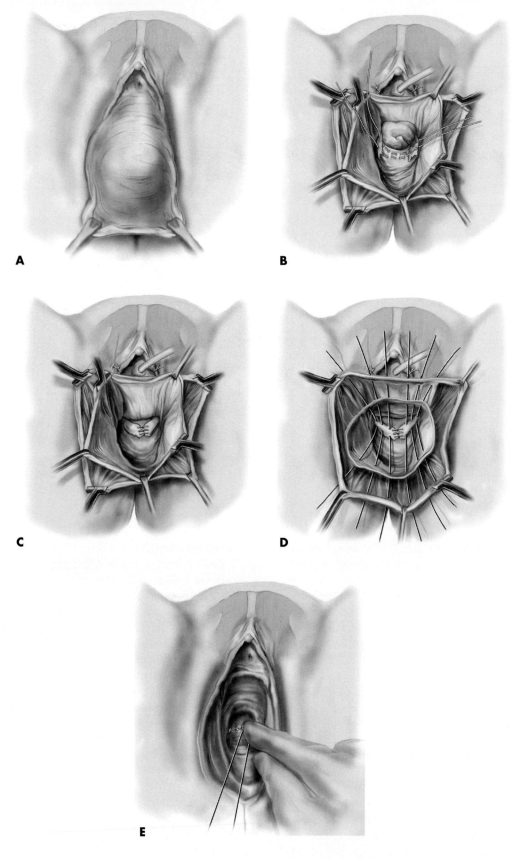

**Fig. 19-9** Uterosacral ligament suspension with fascial reconstruction. **A,** Apex of vagina is grasped with two Allis clamps. **B,** Enterocele has been entered and nonabsorbable sutures have been passed through the uterosacral ligaments at the level of the ischial spines. **C,** Sutures have been tied across midline, creating a firm ridge to which the vagina will be anchored. **D,** Absorbable sutures are used to suspend anterior and posterior vaginal walls with their fascia to uterosacral ligaments. **E,** Tying of these sutures suspends the vagina into the hollow of the sacrum and restores the continuity of the endopelvic fascia of the anterior and posterior vaginal walls.

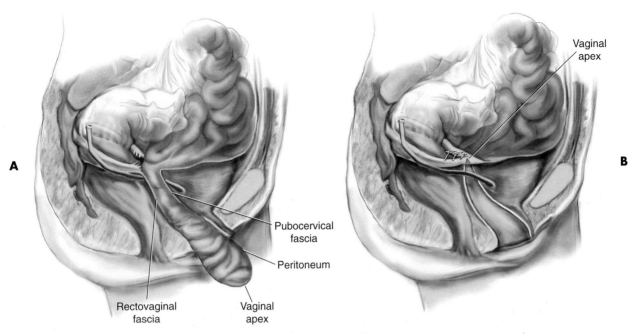

**A**

Pubocervical
fascia

Peritoneum

Rectovaginal
fascia

Vaginal
apex

Vaginal
apex

**B**

**Fig. 19-10    A,** Cross-section of pelvis demonstrating enterocele and vaginal vault prolapse.
**B,** Cross-section of pelvis after excision of enterocele sac and suspension of vaginal apex to
uterosacral ligaments. Note continuity of pubocervical fascia with rectovaginal fascia.

quickly, has minimal risk of blood loss, and can be performed safely under regional or even local anesthesia. The procedure is commonly used in elderly, medically fragile patients who would otherwise have no other treatment options except indefinite pessary use. The patient must understand that the procedure involves complete closure of the vagina and thus will terminate any potential for vaginal intercourse.

Other potential problems are associated with this procedure. A postoperative urinary stress incontinence rate as high as 30% has been reported in some studies. This high rate probably results from the fusion of the anterior rectal wall to the base of the bladder, thus causing descent and flattening of the bladder neck and proximal urethra. Simultaneous bladder neck plication should be performed with the LeFort procedure if stress incontinence or the potential for postoperative stress incontinence exists.

Because the uterus is not removed, any bleeding that the patient has in the future will be difficult to evaluate because the vaginal canal is obstructed. An endometrial biopsy or dilation and curettage and Pap smear with cervical biopsies, if necessary, should always be performed preoperatively to ensure that no cervical or endometrial pathologic condition is present.

The LeFort procedure is as follows:

1. Traction is placed on the cervix to evert the vagina completely. A 0.5% lidocaine in 1:200,000 epinephrine solution is used to inject the vaginal tissue below the epithelium. A pudendal nerve block can be used if the procedure is to be performed under local anesthe-

sia. A Foley catheter with a 30-ml balloon is placed for easy identification of the bladder neck.
2. A dilation and curettage should be performed, if it was not performed preoperatively.
3. The areas to be denuded anteriorly and posteriorly are marked out with a scalpel as indicated in Fig. 19-11, *A* and *B*. The rectangular piece of anterior vaginal wall should extend from 2 cm proximal to the tip of the cervix to approximately 5 cm below the external urethral meatus.
4. Sharp and blunt dissection is used to remove the vaginal epithelium. These flaps should be thin, leaving a maximum amount of underlying fascia on the bladder and rectum. Sufficient vagina should be left bilaterally to form canals for draining cervical secretions or blood. Posteriorly, the cul-de-sac peritoneum may be encountered when vaginal mucosa is excised, but it should not be entered, if possible. Bleeding is controlled with fulguration. Absolute hemostasis is necessary to avoid a postoperative hematoma in the vaginal canal.
5. The cut edge of the anterior vaginal wall is sewn to the cut edge of the posterior vaginal wall with interrupted, delayed absorbable sutures. This is achieved in such a way that the knot is turned into, and remains in, the epithelium-lined tunnels that are created bilaterally. Suturing in this way gradually pushes the uterus and vaginal apex inward (Fig. 19-11, *C*). When the entire vagina has been inverted, the superior and inferior margins of the rectangle can be sutured horizontally.

6. We almost routinely perform a plication of the bladder neck (see Fig. 19-11, *A*) during a LeFort procedure. A perineorrhaphy is usually performed to increase posterior pelvic muscle support and to narrow the introitus.

7. Postoperatively, the patient is mobilized early. Heavy lifting should be avoided for at least 2 months to avoid recurrence of the prolapse secondary to breakdown of repair.

Early complications include hematoma, infection, and nonhealing (with acute herniation) of the prolapse. Urinary urgency and retention can also occur, especially if a bladder neck plication is performed. Because most patients are elderly and may be debilitated, the risk of thromboembolic complications is significant. Pressure stockings and early ambulation should be used.

Late postoperative complications and results of a modified LeFort operation as reported by Goldman et al. (1985) are shown in Table 19-2. In this report, anterior colporrhaphy or other urethropexies were not performed; this may explain the 10.2% rate of postoperative urinary incontinence. In general, total relief of uterine prolapse symptoms with good anatomic results can be expected in more than 90% of patients. Complete breakdown with recurrent prolapse occurs in about 2% to 5% of patients.

## Colpectomy and Colpocleisis

Another operation that can be used for severe posthysterectomy vaginal vault prolapse is colpectomy with colpocleisis. This operation is performed in cases of vault prolapse in which operating time is best kept at a minimum and future

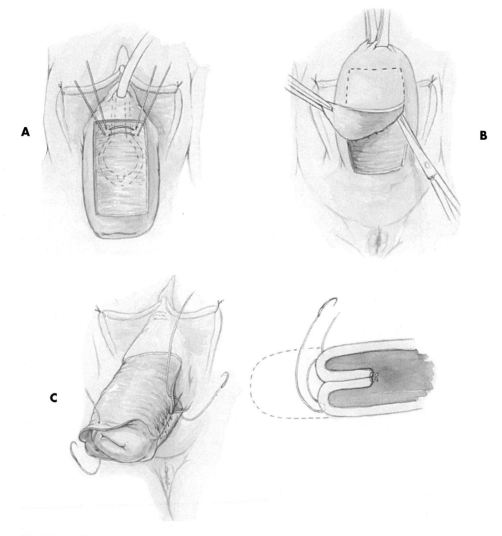

**Fig. 19-11**   Technique of LeFort partial colpocleisis. **A,** Anterior vaginal wall has been removed and plication stitch is placed at the bladder neck. **B,** Posterior vaginal wall is removed. **C,** Cut edge of anterior vaginal wall is sewn to cut edge of posterior vaginal wall in such a way that the uterus and vagina are inverted.

vaginal intercourse is not anticipated by the patient. It can be performed under regional or local anesthesia.

The operation is performed by completely excising the vaginal mucosa from the underlying vaginal or endopelvic fascia. It is not necessary to enter the peritoneum. A series of pursestring, delayed absorbable sutures is placed, slowly inverting the vaginal muscularis and fascia (Fig. 19-12). A posterior colporrhaphy with high levator plication is usually performed, followed by vaginal closure. Like the LeFort procedure, bladder neck plication and perineorrhaphy are often performed with a colpectomy.

Table 19-3 reviews published results of obliterative procedures for vault prolapse.

**Table 19-2** Late Postoperative Complications and Results of Modified LeFort Operation

| Outcome and complications | No. of patients (%) |
| --- | --- |
| Good anatomic results | 107 (90.7) |
| Relief of symptoms | 101 (85.6) |
| Recurrence of prolapse | 3 (2.5) |
| Complete breakdown (1 patient) | |
| Partial recurrence (2 patients) | |
| Urinary tract symptoms, incontinence (minor degrees or worsened by operation) | 12 (10.2) |
| Occurrence of late vaginal bleeding | 2 (1.8) |

From Goldman, J, Ovadia J, Feldberg D: *Eur J Obstet Gynecol Reprod Biol* 12:31, 1985.

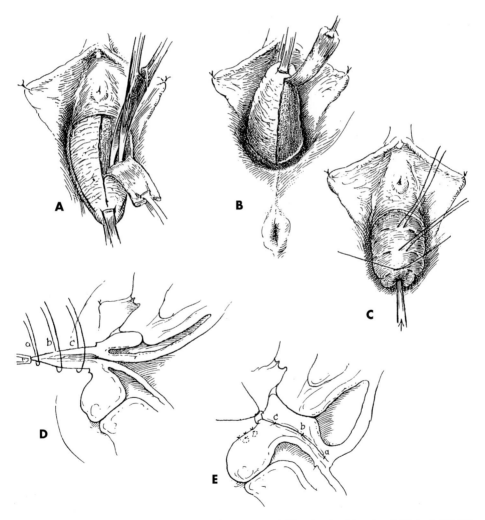

**Fig. 19-12   A** and **B,** Colpectomy. After subcutaneous infiltration by lidocaine 0.5% in 1:200,000 epinephrine solution, the vagina is circumscribed by an incision at the site of the hymen and marked into quadrants. Each quadrant is removed by sharp dissection. **C,** Pursestring sutures using polyglycolic acid–type sutures are placed. The leading edge of the soft tissue is inverted by the tip of a forceps *(arrow).* **D,** Pursestring sutures are tied, *a* before *b* before *c,* with progressive inversion of the soft tissue before the tying of each suture. **E,** Final relationship is shown in sagittal section. An appropriate perineorrhaphy may complete the operation.

From Nichols DH, Randall CL: *Vaginal surgery,* ed 3, Baltimore, 1989, Williams & Wilkins.

**Table 19-3**  Long-Term Follow-Up and Recurrence of Prolapse After LeFort Colpocleisis, Partial Colpectomy, and Total Colpectomy

| Investigator | Duration of follow-up (mo) | No. available for follow-up | Vault* | Anterior wall* | Posterior wall* | Unspecified/ multiple sites* | No. cured/total (%) | Cure assessment |
|---|---|---|---|---|---|---|---|---|
| **LeFort Colpocleisis** | | | | | | | | |
| Phaneuf (1935) | NA | 20 | ?/2 | 0/1 | 0/0 | 0/0 | 17/20 (85) | NA |
| Adair and DaSef (1936) | 3->36 | 38 | 0/0 | 0/2 | 0/0 | 1/1 | 35/38 (92) | Objective† |
| Collins and Lock (1941) | 1-48 | 31 | 0/2 | 0/0 | 0/0 | 0/0 | 29/31 (94) | Objective† |
| Mazer and Israel (1948) | 24-132 | 38 | 1/1 | 0/0 | 0/0 | 0/0 | 37/38 (97) | NA |
| Wolf (1952) | NA | 13 | 0/0 | 0/0 | 0/0 | ?/1 | 12/13 (92) | Objective |
| Falk and Kaufman (1955) | >24 | 100 | 0/0 | 0/2 | 0/2 | 0/0 | 96/100 (96) | Objective |
| Hanson and Keettel (1969) | ≥60 | 216 | 3/3 | 0/1 | 1/1 | 0/8 | 203/216 (94) | Subjective/objective |
| Ridley (1972) | 6-60 | 17 | 2/3 | 0/0 | 0/0 | 0/0 | 14/17 (82) | Subjective/objective |
| Ubachs et al. (1973) | ≥36 | 93 | 2/3 | 0/0 | 0/0 | 0/5 | 85/93 (91) | Objective |
| Denehy et al. (1995) | 4-40 | 20 | 0/0 | 0/0 | 0/0 | 1/1 | 19/20 (95) | Objective |
| **Partial Colpectomy** | | | | | | | | |
| Langmade and Oliver (1986) | 12-144 | 102 | 0/0 | 0/0 | 0/0 | 0/0 | 102/102 (100) | NA |
| **Total Colpectomy** | | | | | | | | |
| Phaneuf (1935) | NA | 5 | 0/0 | 0/0 | 0/0 | 0/0 | 5/5 (100) | NA |
| Adams (1951) | 12-408 | 30 | 0/0 | 0/0 | 0/0 | 0/0 | 30/30 (100) | NA |
| Anderson and Deasy (1960) | 6-12 | 18 | 0/0 | 0/1 | 0/1 | 0/0 | 16/18 (89) | Objective† |
| Ridley (1972) | 6-60 | 41 | 0/0 | 0/0 | 0/0 | 0/0 | 41/41 (100) | Subjective/objective |
| DeLancey and Morley (1997) | Mean = 35 | 33 | 1/1 | 0/0 | 0/0 | 0/0 | 32/33 (97) | Subjective/objective |

*Number of patients with recurrent prolapse who underwent surgical repair/number of patients with recurrent prolapse.
†Extrapolated from text.
*NA*, Not available.

# ABDOMINAL PROCEDURES THAT SUSPEND THE APEX
## Abdominal Sacral Colpopexy

Suspension of the vagina to the sacral promontory via the abdominal approach is an effective treatment for uterovaginal prolapse and vaginal eversion and can offer several advantages over vaginal surgical approaches. It is the procedure of choice for patients who have other indications for abdominal surgery, such as ovarian masses. The laparotomy incision also offers the advantage of performing simultaneous retropubic procedures such as the Burch colposuspension and the paravaginal defect repair.

Many different materials, both autologous and synthetic, have been used for the graft in the sacral colpopexy. Natural materials that have been used include fascia lata, rectus fascia, and dura mater. Synthetic materials include polypropylene mesh, polyester fiber mesh, polytetrafluoroethylene mesh, Dacron mesh, and Silastic silicone rubber. No studies have compared the efficacy of the various graft materials, and individual reports of long-term rates of cure are consistently good.

As was noted earlier, the normal vaginal axis directs toward sacral segments S3 and S4 in the nulliparous woman. Although some authors have advocated connecting the graft material at this level, Sutton et al. (1981) encountered life-threatening hemorrhage from presacral vessels at this low level on the sacrum. As these authors suggest, we recommend fixing the graft to the upper one third of the sacrum, near the sacral promontory, thus improving safety without sacrificing outcome or future vaginal function.

The technique of abdominal sacral colpopexy using graft placement is as follows (Figs. 19-13 and 19-14):

1. The patient should be placed in Allen stirrups or in frogleg position so that the surgeon has digital access to the vagina during the operation. A spongestick or EES sizer can be placed in the vagina for manipulation of the apex, if desired. A Foley catheter is placed into the bladder for drainage. Prophylactic perioperative antibiotics are generally used during this procedure.

2. A laparotomy is performed through a low transverse or midline incision. Small bowel is packed into the upper abdomen, and the sigmoid colon is packed into the left pelvis as much as possible. The ureters are identified bilaterally for their entire course into the bladder. If the uterus is present, a hysterectomy should be performed and the vaginal cuff closed. The depth of the cul-de-sac and the length of the vagina when completely elevated are estimated.

3. While the vagina is elevated cephalad using a spongestick or EES sizer, the peritoneum over the vaginal apex is incised transversely and the bladder

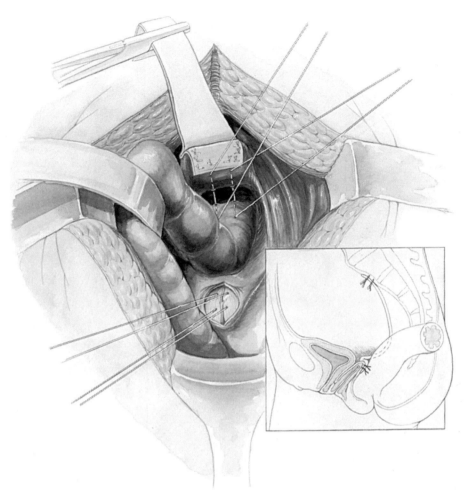

**Fig. 19-13** Abdominal sacral colpopexy. Note that Halban technique is used to obliterate cul-de-sac below graft. *Inset,* Graft connects vagina to sacrum and lies without tension in the deep pelvis.

dissected from the anterior vaginal wall (this may have already been done if the uterus was removed). The peritoneum over the posterior vaginal wall into the cul-de-sac is incised longitudinally and dissected for several centimeters bilaterally. The vaginal apex is elevated bilaterally with clamps or guide sutures.

4. Three to five pairs of nonabsorbable No. 0 sutures are placed in the posterior vaginal wall, transversely, 1 to 2 cm apart. Sutures are placed through the full fibromuscular thickness of the vagina but not into the vaginal epithelium. The spongestick is removed to ensure that no sutures have perforated the sponge. Sutures are then fed through the graft in pairs and tied. The graft should extend approximately halfway down the length of the posterior vaginal wall. We prefer to attach a second smaller piece of mesh to the upper part of the anterior vaginal wall. This piece of mesh is then sewn to the posterior piece of mesh, which will be attached to the sacrum (see Fig. 19-14, *D*). Other potential configurations of mesh attachment are reviewed in Fig. 19-14.

5. A Moschcowitz or Halban procedure is performed to obliterate the lower cul-de-sac. These procedures were described in Chapter 18.

6. A longitudinal incision, approximately 6 cm long, is made in the peritoneum over the sacral promontory. At this point the surgeon should carefully palpate the aortic bifurcation and common and internal iliac vessels and mobilize the sigmoid colon and right ureter so that these structures can be avoided. The left common iliac vein is medial to the left common iliac artery and is particularly vulnerable to damage during this procedure. The middle sacral artery and vein should be identified.

7. Blunt and sharp dissection caudally may be used to create a subperitoneal tunnel into the full depth of the cul-de-sac so that the graft can be extraperitonized. The graft can then be tunneled retroperitoneally or placed above the previous Halban or Moschcowitz cul-de-sac closure. The surgeon can then extraperitonealize the mesh by sewing the serosa of the

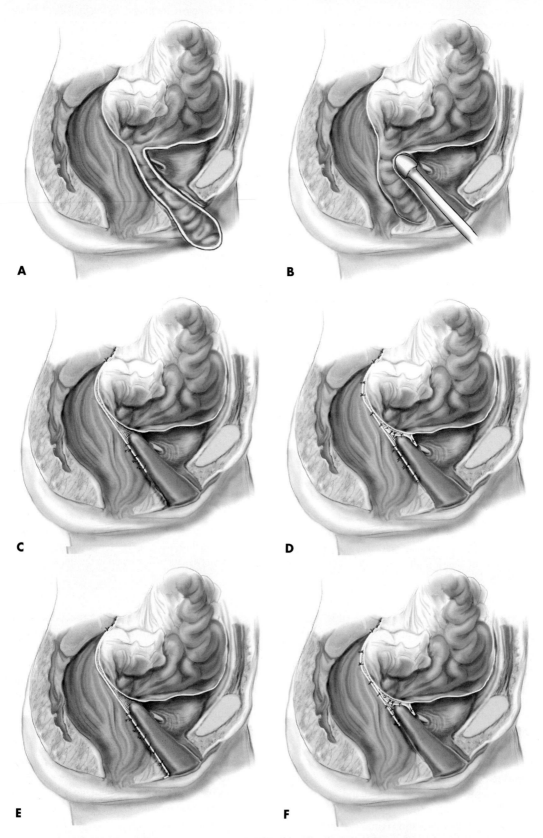

**Fig. 19-14** **A,** Cross-section of the pelvis demonstrating large enterocele and vaginal vault prolapse. **B,** EES sizer placed in vagina to elevate apex. **C** to **F,** Obliteration of cul-de-sac with examples of various configurations for mesh attachment to the vagina. **C,** Mesh attached to upper half of posterior vaginal wall. **D,** Mesh attached as in **C;** second piece of mesh attached to upper part of anterior vaginal wall and sewn to posterior piece of mesh. **E,** Mesh attached along entire length of posterior vaginal wall and fixed to perineum. **F,** Vaginal end of mesh is divided and fixed to upper parts of the anterior and posterior vaginal walls.

**Table 19-4**   Long-Term Follow-Up and Recurrence of Prolapse After Abdominal Sacral Colpopexy

| Investigator | Duration of follow-up (mo) | No. available for follow-up | Vault* | Anterior wall* | Posterior wall* | Unspecified/ multiple sites* | No. cured (%) | Cure assessment |
|---|---|---|---|---|---|---|---|---|
| Rust et al. (1976) | 9-40 | 12 | 0/0 | 0/1 | 0/0 | 0/0 | 12/12 (100) | Objective† |
| Todd (1978) | NA | 93 | 1/2 | 0/0 | 0/1 | 0/1 | 91/93 (98) | Objective† |
| Feldman and Birnbaum (1979) | 1-48 | 21 | 0/1 | 0/2 | 0/1 | 0/1 | 20/21 (95) | Objective† |
| Cowan and Morgan (1980) | ≤60 | 39 | 0/1 | NA | NA | NA | 38/39 (97) | Objective† |
| Addison et al. (1985) | 6-126 | 56 | 2/2 | 0/0 | 0/0 | 0/0 | 54/56 (96) | NA |
| Drutz and Cha (1987) | 3-93 | 15 | 1/1 | 0/0 | 0/2 | 0/0 | 14/15 (93) | Objective† |
| Angulo and Ligman (1989) | 2-36 | 18 | 0/0 | NA | NA | NA | 18/18 (100) | Objective |
| Baker et al. (1990) | 1-45 | 59 | 0/0 | 0/6 | 0/4 | 0/0 | 51/51 (100) | Subjective/objective |
| Maloney et al. (1990) | 12-60 | 10 | 0/1 | 0/0 | 0/0 | 0/0 | 9/10 (90) | NA |
| Creighton and Stanton (1991) | 3-35 | 23 | 2/2 | 0/0 | 0/0 | 0/0 | 21/23 (91) | Objective† |
| Snyder and Krantz (1991) | ≥6 | 116 | ?/8 | NA | NA | ?/24 | 108/116 (93) | Objective |
| Timmons et al. (1992) | 9-216 | 162 | 0/1 | 0/0 | 3/3 | 0/0 | 161/162 (99) | Objective† |
| Imparato et al. (1992) | NA | 63 | ?/4 | 0/0 | 0/0 | ?/10 | 59/63 (94) | Objective† |
| Traiman et al. (1992) | 6-60 | 11 | 0/1 | NA | NA | NA | 10/11 (91) | NA |
| Iosif (1993) | 12-120 | 40 | 1/1 | 0/1 | 0/2 | 0/0 | 39/40 (96) | Objective |
| Grunberger et al. (1994) | 12-240 | 48 | 0/3 | 0/0 | 0/0 | 6/6 | 45/48 (94) | Objective |
| Vitranen et al. (1994) | 12-96 | 27 | 0/1 | 0/1 | 0/0 | 0/1 | 23/27 (85) | Objective |
| Valaitis and Stanton (1994) | 3-91 | 38 | 3/3 | 0/0 | 0/1 | 0/0 | 38/41 (93) | Objective |
| van Lindert et al. (1996) | 15-63 | 61 | 0/0 | 0/0 | 0/0 | 0/2 | 61/61 (100) | Objective† |

*Denotes the number of patients with recurrent prolapse who underwent surgical repair/number of patients with recurrent prolapse.
†Extrapolated from text.
*NA*, Not available.

sigmoid colon to the lateral peritoneum of the cul-de-sac.

8. The bony sacral promontory and anterior longitudinal ligaments are directly visualized for approximately 4 cm by using blunt and sharp dissection through the subperitoneal fat. Special care should be taken to avoid the delicate plexus of presacral veins that is often present, especially as one dissects more caudally.

9. Using a stiff but small half-curved tapered needle with permanent No. 0 suture, two to four sutures are placed through the anterior sacral longitudinal ligament, over the sacral promontory. The graft should be trimmed to the appropriate length. The sutures are then fed through the graft in pairs and tied. The appropriate amount of vaginal elevation should provide gentle tension without undue traction on the vagina.

10. The peritoneum over the presacral space is closed with a running absorbable suture. The bladder-flap peritoneum is also closed transversely over the graft.

11. When appropriate, retropubic urethropexy or paravaginal repair should be accomplished at this time, followed by placement of a suprapubic catheter, if desired, and closure of the abdomen.

12. Posterior colporrhaphy and perineoplasty are generally performed to treat the remaining rectocele and perineal defect.

If attention has been paid to repairing all the support

defects of the vagina at the time of sacral colpopexy, then recurrences of vaginal vault prolapse are uncommon. Addison et al. (1989) reported three cases of recurrent vaginal prolapse after the sacral colpopexy with Mersilene mesh. In two patients, the mesh separated from the vaginal apex. In the remaining patient, the posterior vaginal wall ruptured distal to the attachment of the mesh to the vagina. These authors and others believe that failures of this procedure can be minimized by suturing the suspensory mesh to the posterior vagina and anterior vaginal apex over as extended an area as possible. This is the justification for suturing the graft to the posterior vagina with four to six pairs of permanent sutures.

More recently, some investigators (Cundiff et al., 1997) advocated attaching the mesh along the entire posterior vaginal wall and fixing the mesh to the perineum (see Fig. 19-14, *E*). Table 19-4 reviews published reports on abdominal sacral colpopexy.

Intraoperative complications are uncommon but can be life-threatening. When there is bleeding from presacral vessels, hemostasis can be difficult to achieve because of the complex interlacing of the venous network, both beneath and on the surface of the sacral periosteum. When these veins have been damaged, they can retract beneath the bony surface of the anterior sacrum and recede into the underlying channels of cancellous bone. Communications with adjacent pelvic veins, especially the left common iliac vein, can be particularly troublesome. Packing of the presacral space may control bleeding temporarily, but it often recurs when the pack is removed, and packing may further lacerate delicate veins. Sutures, metallic clips, cautery, and bone wax should be used initially. If these measures are not successful, sterilized stainless steel thumbtacks can be placed on the retracted bleeding presacral vein to treat life-threatening hemorrhage that has not responded to other measures.

Other complications that have been reported after abdominal sacral colpopexy tend to be similar to those of procedures that require laparotomy, retropubic surgery, and extensive pelvic dissection. The complications include enterotomy, ureteral damage, cystotomy, proctotomy, extrafascial wound infections, and persistent granulation tissue in the vaginal vault. Remarkably, graft rejections are exceedingly rare. Lansman (1984) reported a small bowel obstruction after colpopexy that was caused by a loop of ileum adherent to a hole in the posterior peritoneum, near the side wall of the pelvis. This problem underscores the importance of reperitonization over the hollow of the sacrum to prevent small bowel from getting trapped in the cul-de-sac or behind the graft.

The most common long-term complication is erosion of synthetic mesh through the vagina, which has recently been reported to occur in 7% of cases (Kohle et al., 1998). This complication almost always requires partial or complete removal of the mesh. Mesh erosion after sacral colpopexy is further discussed in Case 12 in Chapter 34.

## High Uterosacral Ligament Suspension With Fascial Reconstruction

The vaginal and laparoscopic approaches to this repair are discussed in Chapters 16, 18, and 19. The abdominal repair involves the same concepts.

1. The remnants of the uterosacral ligaments are identified and tagged at the level of ischial spines.
2. The ureters are identified on each side, and the enterocele is addressed by abdominal obliteration of the cul-de-sac.
3. The peritoneum over the apex of the vagina is opened, and the endopelvic fascia of the anterior and posterior vaginal walls are identified and approximated.
4. Nonabsorbable sutures are then used to suspend the prolapsed vagina with its fascia to the uterosacral ligaments (see Fig. 19-10).

## SUMMARY

The prevalence of vaginal prolapse appears to be increasing. This may be because of the increased longevity of women, but also is probably a result of inadequate recognition and repair of pelvic organ support defects when pelvic surgery has been performed. The standard use of cul-de-sac plication at every hysterectomy and urethropexy would probably decrease the likelihood of iatrogenic enterocele. Finally, more education and research in the principles of pelvic and vaginal reconstructive surgery are needed to improve care to all affected women.

## BIBLIOGRAPHY
### Vaginal Procedures

Amreich I: Atiologie und operation des scheiden stump prolapses, *Wien Klin Wochenschr* 65:74, 1951.

Backer MH: Success with sacrospinous suspension of the prolapsed vaginal vault, *Surg Gynecol Obstet* 175:419, 1992.

Brown WE, Hoffman MS, Bouis PJ, et al: Management of vaginal vault prolapse: retrospective comparison of abdominal versus vaginal approach, *J Fla Med Assoc* 76:249, 1989.

Carey MP, Slack MC: Transvaginal sacrospinous colpopexy for vault and marked uterovaginal prolapse, *Br J Obstet Gynaecol* 101:536, 1994.

Cruikshank SH: Sacrospinous fixation: should this be performed at the time of vaginal hysterectomy? *Am J Obstet Gynecol* 164:1072, 1991.

Cruikshank SH, Cox IN: Sacrospinous fixation at the time of vaginal hysterectomy, *Am J Obstet Gynecol* 162:1611, 1990.

DeLancey JO: Anatomic aspects of vaginal eversion after hysterectomy, *Am J Obstet Gynecol* 166:1717, 1992.

Elkins TE, Hopper JB, Goodfellow K, et al: Initial report of anatomic and clinical comparison of the sacrospinous ligament fixation to the high McCall culdeplasty for vaginal cuff fixation at hysterectomy for uterine prolapse, *J Pelvic Surg* 1:12, 1995.

Farrell SA, Scotti RJ, Ostergard DR, et al: Massive evisceration: a complication following sacrospinous vaginal vault fixation, *Obstet Gynecol* 78:560, 1991.

Funt MI, Thompson JD, Birch H: Normal vaginal axis, *South Med J* 71:1534, 1978.

Heinonen PK: Transvaginal sacrospinous colpopexy for vaginal vault and complete genital prolapse in aged women, *Acta Obstet Gynecol Scand* 71:377, 1992.

Holley RJ, Varner RE, Gleason BP, et al: Recurrent pelvic support defects after sacrospinous ligament fixation for vaginal vault prolapse, *J Am Coll Surg* 180:444, 1995.

Imparato E, Aspesi G, Rovetta E, et al: Surgical management and prevention of vaginal vault prolapse, *Surg Gynecol Obstet* 175:233, 1992.

Inmon WB: Pelvic relaxation and repair including prolapse of vagina following hysterectomy, *South Med J* 56:577, 1963.

Kaminski PF, Sorosky JI, Pees RC, et al: Correction of massive vaginal prolapse: an older population, *J Am Geriatr Soc* 41:42, 1993.

Keetel LM, Hebertson RM: An anatomic evaluation of the sacrospinous ligament colpopexy, *Surg Gynecol Obstet* 168:318, 1989.

Kovac SR, Cruikshank SH: Successful pregnancies and vaginal deliveries after sacrospinous uterosacral fixation in five of 19 patients, *Am J Obstet Gynecol* 168:1778, 1993.

Lee RA, Symmonds RE: Surgical repair of posthysterectomy vault prolapse, *Am J Obstet Gynecol* 112:953, 1972.

Mäkinen J, Söderström K, Kiilholma P, et al: Histologic changes in the vaginal connective tissue of patients with and without uterine prolapse, *Arch Gynecol* 239:17, 1986.

McCall ML: Posterior culdeplasty, *Obstet Gynecol* 10:595, 1957.

Meeks GR, Washburne JF, McGeher RP, et al: Repair of vaginal vault prolapse by suspension of the vagina to iliococcygeus (prespinous) fascia, *Am J Obstet Gynecol* 171:1444, 1994.

Miyazaki FS: Miya hook ligature carrier for sacrospinous ligament suspension, *Obstet Gynecol* 70:286, 1987.

Monk BJ, Ramp JF, Montz FJ, et al: Sacrospinous fixation for vaginal vault prolapse. Complications and results, *J Gynecol Surg* 7:87, 1991.

Morley G, DeLancey JO: Sacrospinous ligament fixation for eversion of the vagina, *Am J Obstet Gynecol* 158:872, 1988.

Nagata I, Kato K: Sacrospinous ligament fixation of vaginal apex for repair operation of uterine prolapse: operative procedure and postoperative outcome evaluated with score system and x-ray subtraction colpography, *Acta Obstet Gynaecol Jpn* 38:29, 1986.

Nichols DH: Sacrospinous fixation for massive eversion of the vagina, *Am J Obstet Gynecol* 142:901, 1982.

Nichols D: Massive eversion of the vagina. In *Gynecologic and obstetric surgery,* St. Louis, 1993, Mosby.

Nichols DH, Randall CL: *Vaginal surgery,* ed 3, Baltimore, 1989, Williams & Wilkins.

Peters WA, Christenson ML: Fixation of the vaginal apex to the coccygeus fascia during repair of vaginal vault eversion with enterocele, *Am J Obstet Gynecol* 172:1894, 1995.

Phaneuf TE: Inversion of the vagina and prolapse of the cervix following suprapubic hysterectomy and inversion of the vagina following total hysterectomy, *Am J Obstet Gynecol* 64:739, 1952.

Porges RF, Smilen SW: Long-term analysis of the surgical management of pelvic support defects, *Am J Obstet Gynecol* 171:1518, 1994.

Randall C, Nichols D: Surgical treatment of vaginal inversion, *Obstet Gynecol* 38:327, 1971.

Richardson AL: The anatomic defects in rectocele and enterocele, *J Pelvic Surg* 1:214, 1995.

Richardson DA, Scotti RJ, Ostergard DR: Surgical management of uterine prolapse in young women, *J Reprod Med* 34:388, 1989.

Richter K: Massive eversion of the vagina: pathogenesis, diagnosis, and therapy of the "true" prolapse of the vaginal stump, *Clin Obstet Gynecol* 25:897, 1982.

Richter K, Albright W: Long-term results following fixation of the vagina on the sacrospinal ligament by the vaginal route, *Am J Obstet Gynecol* 151:811, 1981.

Ridley JH: A composite vaginal vault suspension using fascia lata, *Am J Obstet Gynecol* 126:590, 1976.

Sauer HA, Klutke CG: Transvaginal sacrospinous ligament fixation for treatment of vaginal prolapse, *J Urol* 154:1008, 1995.

Seigworth GR: Vaginal vault prolapse with eversion, *Obstet Gynecol* 54:255, 1979.

Sharp TR: Sacrospinous suspension made easy, *Obstet Gynecol* 82:873, 1993.

Shull BL, Capen CV, Riggs MW, et al: Preoperative analysis of site-specific pelvic support defects in 81 women treated with sacrospinous ligament suspension and pelvic reconstruction, *Am J Obstet Gynecol* 166:1764, 1992.

Shull BT, Capen CV, Riggs MW, et al: Bilateral attachment of the vaginal cuff to iliococcygeus fascia: an effective method of cuff suspension, *Am J Obstet Gynecol* 168:1669, 1993.

Stanhope CR, Wilson TO, Utz WJ, et al: Suture entrapment and secondary ureteral obstruction, *Am J Obstet Gynecol* 164:1513, 1991.

Symmonds RE, Pratt JH: Vaginal prolapse following hysterectomy, *Am J Obstet Gynecol* 79:899, 1960.

Symmonds RE, Sheldon RS: Vaginal prolapse after hysterectomy, *Obstet Gynecol* 25:61, 1965.

Symmonds RE, Williams TJ, Lee RA, et al: Posthysterectomy enterocele and vaginal vault prolapse, *Am J Obstet Gynecol* 140:852, 1981.

Sze EHM, Karram MM: Transvaginal repair of vault prolapse: a review, *Obstet Gynecol* 89:466, 1997.

Sze EHM et al: Sacrospinous ligament fixation with transvaginal needle suspension for advanced pelvic organ prolapse and stress incontinence, *Obstet Gynecol* 89:94, 1997.

TeLinde RW: Prolapse of the uterus and allied conditions, *Am J Obstet Gynecol* 94:444, 1966.

Thompson JD, Rock JA, eds: *TeLinde's operative gynecology,* ed 7, Philadelphia, 1992, JB Lippincott.

Torpin R: Excision of the cul-de-sac of Douglas for the surgical care of hernias through the female caudal wall, including a prolapse of the uterus, *J Int Coll Surg* 24:322, 1955.

Waters EG: Vaginal prolapse: technique for correction and prevention at hysterectomy, *Obstet Gynecol* 8:432, 1956.

Webb MJ, Aronson MP, Ferguson LK, et al: Posthysterectomy vaginal vault prolapse: primary repair in 693 patients, *Obstet Gynecol* 92:281, 1998.

### Obliterative Procedures

Adair FL, DaSef L: The LeFort colpocleisis, *Am J Obstet Gynecol* 32:334, 1936.

Adams HD: Total colpocleisis for pelvic eventration, *Surg Gynecol Obstet* 92:321, 1951.

Anderson GV, Deasy PP: Hysterocolpectomy, *Obstet Gynecol* 16:344, 1960.

Collins CG, Lock FR: The LeFort colpocleisis, *Am J Surg* 53:202, 1941.

DeLancey JOL, Morley GW: Total colpocleisis for vaginal eversion, *Am J Obstet Gynecol* 176:1228, 1997.

Denehy TR, Choe JY, Gregori CA, et al: Modified LeFort partial colpocleisis with Kelly urethral plication and posterior colpoperine-oplasty in the medically compromised elderly: a comparison with vaginal hysterectomy, anterior colporrhaphy, and posterior colpoperine-oplasty, *Am J Obstet Gynecol* 173:1697, 1995.

Falk HC, Kaufman SA: Partial colpocleisis: the LeFort procedure, *Obstet Gynecol* 5:617, 1955.

Goldman J, Ovadia J, Feldberg D: The Neugebauer-LeFort operation: a review of 118 partial colpocleises, *Eur J Obstet Gynecol Reprod Biol* 12:31, 1985.

Hanson GE, Keettel WC: The Neugebauer-LeFort operation: a review of 288 colpocleisis, *Obstet Gynecol* 34:352, 1969.

Langmade CF, Oliver JA: Partial colpocleisis, *Am J Obstet Gynecol* 154:1200, 1986.

Mazer C, Israel SL: The LeFort colpocleisis: an analysis of 43 operations, *Am J Obstet Gynecol* 56:944, 1948.

Phaneuf LE: The place of colpectomy in the treatment of uterine and vaginal prolapse, *Am J Obstet Gynecol* 30:544, 1935.

Ridley JG: Evaluation of the colpocleisis: a report of fifty-eight cases, *Am J Obstet Gynecol* 113:1114, 1972.

Ubachs JMH, Van Sante TJ, Schellekens LA: Partial colpocleisis by a modification of LeFort's operation, *Obstet Gynecol* 42:415, 1973.

Wolf WA: The LeFort operation, *Am J Obstet Gynecol* 63:1346, 1952.

### Abdominal Procedures

Addison WA, Livengood CH, Parker RT: Posthysterectomy vaginal vault prolapse with emphasis on management by transabdominal sacral colpopexy, *Postgrad Obstet Gynecol* 8:1, 1988.

Addison WA, Livengood CH, Sutton GP, et al: Abdominal sacral colpopexy with Mersilene mesh in the retroperitoneal position in the management of posthysterectomy vaginal vault prolapse and enterocele, *Am J Obstet Gynecol* 153:140, 1985.

Addison WA, Timmons CM, Wall LL, et al: Failed abdominal sacral colpopexy: observations and recommendations, *Obstet Gynecol* 74:480, 1989.

Angulo A, Ligman I: Retroperitoneal sacrocolpopexy for correction of prolapse of vaginal vault, *Surg Gynecol Obstet* 169:319, 1989.

Baker KR, Beresford JM, Campbell C: Colposacropexy with Prolene mesh, *Surg Gynecol Obstet* 171:51, 1990.

Benson JT, Lucente V, McClellan E: Vaginal versus abdominal reconstructive surgery for the treatment of pelvic support defects: a prospective randomized study with long-term outcome evaluation, *Am J Obstet Gynecol* 175:1418, 1996.

Cowan W, Morgan HR: Abdominal sacral colpopexy, *Am J Obstet Gynecol* 138:348, 1980.

Creighton SM, Stanton SL: The surgical management of vaginal vault prolapse, *Br J Obstet Gynecol* 98:1150, 1991.

Cundiff GW, Harris RL, Coates K, et al: Abdominal sacral colpoperi-neopexy: a new approach for correction of posterior compartment defects and perineal descent associated with vaginal vault prolapse, *Am J Obstet Gynecol* 177:1345, 1997.

Drutz HP, Cha LS: Massive genital and vaginal vault prolapse treated with abdominal-vaginal sacropexy with use of marlex mesh: review of the literature, *Am J Obstet Gynecol* 156:387, 1987.

Feldman GB, Birnbaum SJ: Sacral colpopexy for vaginal vault prolapse, *Obstet Gynecol* 53:399, 1979.

Given FY, Muhlendorf TK, Browning GM: Vaginal length and sexual function after colpopexy for complete uterovaginal eversion, *Am J Obstet Gynecol* 169:284, 1993.

Grunberger W, Grunberger V, Wierrani F: Pelvic promontory fixation of the vaginal vault in sixty-two patients with prolapse after hysterectomy, *Surg Gynecol Obstet* 178:69, 1994.

Iosif CS: Abdominal sacral colpopexy with use of synthetic mesh, *Acta Obstet Gynecol Scand* 72:214, 1993.

Kohle N, Walsh P, Roat TW, et al: Mesh erosion following abdominal sacral colpopexy, *Obstet Gynecol* 92:999, 1998.

Lansman HH: Posthysterectomy vault prolapse: sacral colpopexy with dura mater graft, *Obstet Gynecol* 63:577, 1984.

Maloney JC, Dunton CJ, Smith K: Repair of vaginal vault prolapse with abdominal sacropexy, *J Reprod Med* 35:6, 1990.

Nichols DH: Fertility retention in the patient with genital prolapse, *Am J Obstet Gynecol* 164:1155, 1991.

Rust JA, Botte JM, Howlett RJ: Prolapse of the vaginal vault. Improved techniques for management of the abdominal approach or vaginal approach, *Am J Obstet Gynecol* 125:768, 1976.

Snyder TE, Krantz KE: Abdominal-retroperitoneal sacral colpopexy for the correction of vaginal prolapse, *Obstet Gynecol* 77:944, 1991.

Sutton GP, Addison WA, Livengood CH, et al: Life-threatening hemorrhage complicating sacral colpopexy, *Am J Obstet Gynecol* 140:836, 1981.

Tancer ML, Fleischer M, Berkowitz BJ: Simultaneous colpo-recto-sacropexy, *Obstet Gynecol* 70:951, 1987.

Timmons MC, Addison WA, Addison SB, et al: Abdominal sacral colpopexy in 163 women with posthysterectomy vaginal vault prolapse and enterocele, *J Reprod Med* 37:323, 1992.

Timmons MC, Kohler MF, Addison WA: Thumbtack use for control of presacral bleeding, with description of an instrument for thumbtack application, *Obstet Gynecol* 78:313, 1991.

Todd JW: Mesh suspension for vaginal prolapse, *Int Surg* 63:91, 1978.

Traiman P, De Lucia LA, Silva AAF, et al: Abdominal colpopexy for complete prolapse of the vagina, *Int Surg* 77:91, 1992.

Valaitis SR, Stanton SL: Sacrocolpopexy: a retrospective study of a clinician's experience, *Br J Obstet Gynaecol* 101:518, 1994.

van Lindert ACM, Groenendijk AG, Scholten PC, et al: Surgical support and suspension of genital prolapse, including preservation of the uterus, using Gore-tex soft tissue patch, *Eur J Obstet Gynecol Reprod Biol* 50:133, 1996.

Vitranen H, Hirvonen T, Makinen J, et al: Outcome of thirty patients who underwent repair of posthysterectomy prolapse of the vaginal vault with abdominal sacral colpopexy, *J Am Coll Surg* 178:283, 1994.

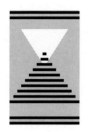

PART IV
*Fecal Incontinence and Defecation Disorders*

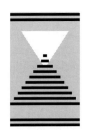

CHAPTER **20**

*Fecal Incontinence*

Tracy L. Hull

## EPIDEMIOLOGY

The inability to control feces is a devastating problem. Many people find this problem socially incapacitating and stay home, thus minimizing social contact to avoid an embarrassing situation. It is difficult to estimate the number of people afflicted with fecal incontinence because many do not mention the problem to their caregivers. In a study by Johanson and Lafferty (1996), only about a third of patients discussed their incontinence with their physicians. Others incorrectly describe their symptoms and may call incontinence diarrhea, making it difficult for the physician to understand the problem without careful questioning. Thus, estimates probably grossly underreport the prevalence, which ranges from 0.1% to 18%. Definitions of fecal incontinence also vary from report to report, making comparisons difficult.

Caring for incontinent patients is a tremendous financial responsibility. Over $400 million is spent annually on adult diapers, and fecal and urinary incontinence are primary reasons for nursing home placement (outnumbering senile dementia). Fecal incontinence probably increases progressively with age, although it can affect all ages, even children. It affects men as well as women, and some studies find men affected more commonly than women.

## ETIOLOGY

Defecation is a complex process that involves an intricate interaction between anal function and sensation, rectal compliance, stool consistency, stool volume, colonic transit, and mental alertness. An alteration in any of these can lead to incontinence. Box 20-1 lists some common causes of fecal incontinence.

Childbirth is increasingly being recognized as commonly injuring the mother's sphincter complex. In an important study by Sultan et al. (1993), women were evaluated before and after childbirth with interviews, anal physiology testing, and anal endosonography. They found that 35% of primiparous women and 44% of multiparous women had sphincter defects after delivery. The internal anal sphincter was injured more often than the external sphincter—sometimes when no breach occurred in the perineal skin. There was a strong correlation between sphincter defects and the development of bowel symptoms, although only about a third of women with sphincter defects developed bowel symptoms. Incontinence may not appear until decades after the obstetric injury, so it remains to be seen how many of these women develop incontinence later in life. In the past these patients, particularly women with delayed symptoms years after childbirth injury, were labeled with idiopathic incontinence. However, with the advent of more sophisticated evaluation techniques, defects in the sphincter complex have been found.

Fecal incontinence also appears to be associated with urinary incontinence and pelvic organ prolapse. In one study by Jackson et al. (1997), a third of women presenting to a urogynecologist for urinary incontinence also had fecal incontinence, and 7% of women with isolated pelvic organ prolapse had fecal incontinence. In another study by Tetzscher et al. (1996), 18% of women who had a previous obstetric anal sphincter disruption had both urinary and fecal incontinence. Besides obstetric injury, other causes thought to possibly contribute to both conditions include

**Box 20-1**

## CAUSES OF FECAL INCONTINENCE

**Anal**

Injury
 Obstetric
 Surgical (fistulotomy, hemorrhoidectomy, sphincterotomy, stretch)
 Irradiation
 Trauma
Congenital (e.g., imperforate anus)

**Intestinal**

Colitis or proctitis
Colon, rectum, or small bowel resection
Tumors
Fecal impaction
Decreased rectal compliance
Rectal prolapse

**Neurologic**

Central nervous system
 Dementia
 Neoplasm
 Stroke
 Trauma
 Multiple sclerosis
Peripheral (e.g., diabetes)

**Other**

Diarrhea
Combinations of anal and rectal causes
Myopathy (e.g., scleroderma)

chronic constipation with straining at stool, aging, and relaxation of pelvic support.

## EVALUATION
### History

Evaluation of a patient with fecal incontinence starts with a comprehensive history. Important questions to ask include duration of the problem, frequency of incontinence, time of day of incontinence, quality of stool lost, ability to control flatus, use of pads, frequency of bowel motions, problems with constipation or diarrhea, and effects of incontinence on daily life. It is important to differentiate incontinence from urgency. Urgency may reflect inability of the rectal reservoir to store stool (as with diarrhea or proctitis) rather than a true sphincter problem. It is also important to differentiate diarrhea from incontinence because many patients incorrectly interchange the two problems. The quality of stool lost gives clues to the severity of the incontinence. Flatus is

more difficult to control than liquid stool, and solid stool is the most easily controlled. Patients with incontinence of solid bowel motions without knowledge of the loss of stool are usually more distressed and reclusive than those with incontinence of flatus only.

Additionally, the physician should obtain a thorough obstetric history: number of vaginal deliveries, duration of second stage of labor, previous episiotomy, use of forceps, perineal tears or infections, weight of babies, and unusual presentations at birth. A sexual history, including the effect of incontinence on sexual behavior, should be obtained. Other medical and surgical conditions must be ascertained, including back injuries, previous anorectal or abdominal surgeries, irradiation history, diabetes, multiple sclerosis, and scleroderma. Medications, food intolerance, and activity restrictions may add information.

## Physical Examination

The physical examination starts with inspection of the anal area, looking for soilage of stool on the skin and evidence of skin irritation. Sometimes the underwear also gives evidence of stool soilage. The anus is inspected, looking for gaping of the muscles and any scarring. The patient is asked to squeeze and simulate holding in a bowel movement to look for uniform circular contraction of muscle. Next, asking the patient to strain may show exaggerated perineal descent or prolapse of hemorrhoids or even the rectum. The anocutaneous reflex can be checked by rubbing the perianal skin gently (a Q-tip works well) and looking for the reflex contraction of the anal sphincter mechanism. Sensation to pinprick can also be checked. Both of these give a crude assessment of sphincter innervation. Palpation of the sphincter is next done with digital examination. The initial tone reflects the internal sphincter and should be noted. Then the patient is asked to squeeze on the index finger in the anus as if she were holding in a bowel movement. Strength, defects in the circle of muscle, and early fatigability are assessed. Scars or masses are appreciated.

A digital rectal examination checks for masses, occult or gross blood, fistula, and the presence of a rectocele. The physical examination is usually completed with a sigmoidoscopy or proctoscopy; this rules out proctitis or neoplasm as a source of the problem.

## Diagnostic Testing

The use of additional testing depends on the severity of the problem and the amount of distress it causes the patient. Further tests may be helpful in establishing the diagnosis and in planning the most appropriate treatment. These tests are discussed individually.

### Enema

To determine whether the patient is truly having incontinence, an enema may help clarify the problem. About 100 ml of tap water is given, and it is noted whether the patient can hold this for more than a few minutes. Because liquid is more difficult to control than solid stool, patients who can hold a tap water enema probably do not have significant incontinence. They may need to be questioned more carefully to fully understand their symptoms.

## Anorectal Physiology Testing

Many methods are available to assess anorectal physiology. Manometry, electromyography (EMG), rectal compliance, and pudendal nerve studies may all be helpful. Manometry provides quantitative information regarding the resting and squeeze pressures of the sphincter muscles. The resting pressures reflect the constant tone of the internal sphincter muscles. The squeeze pressures reflect the pressure generated by the external sphincter muscle. The length of the anal canal can be determined by the measured distance of these pressures. A shortened anal canal length may reflect injury to the muscle. A positive rectoanal inhibitory reflex rules out Hirschsprung's disease (see Chapter 21).

Rectal compliance can be determined by inserting a balloon and determining the minimal volume the rectum can sense, then sequentially inflating the balloon to a volume that cannot be tolerated. Decreased compliance signals a rectal reservoir that does not appropriately store stool and may push the fecal bolus past sphincter muscles, even if the sphincter muscle pressures are adequate. It is important to note that normal manometric findings do not exclude incontinence and normal people without symptoms of fecal incontinence may have abnormal manometry.

EMG is used to study the innervation of the external sphincter complex and to examine for reinnervation seen in pelvic neuropathy. Traditionally, needle EMG has been used with concentric or single-fiber electrodes, although this is quite painful for the patient. An increase in fiber density implies compensatory reinnervation after denervation of the external sphincter. Surface electrodes (attached to the skin overlying the subcutaneous portion of the external anal sphincter) give a less precise EMG but still provide some information.

Pudendal nerve terminal motor latency can be determined using an electrode attached to a glove inserted into the anal canal. A prolonged conduction in the pudendal nerve may signal damage to the innervation of the external sphincter and puborectalis muscle.

## Defecography

Defecography is indicated if rectal prolapse or internal intussusception (occult prolapse) is suspected. See Chapter 23 for a more thorough discussion.

## Colonoscopy and Barium Enema

Proctoscopy, sigmoidoscopy, colonoscopy, and barium enema are appropriate in some patients, particularly if diarrhea and blood are associated or contributing symptoms. Colitis and neoplasms can be ruled out with these tests.

## Endosonography

Endosonography has recently been recognized as a valuable tool in the assessment of fecal incontinence. A probe inserted into the rectum and withdrawn through the anal canal allows for a 360-degree visualization of the internal and external anal sphincters. Particularly in patients with surgical or obstetric injury who did not develop incontinence until many years (even decades) after the insult, endosonography has allowed visualization of defects in the sphincter muscle, which in turn can lead to surgical correction. In the past many of these patients would have been diagnosed with idiopathic incontinence, and surgical repair may have not been considered (Fig. 20-1). Additionally, the pictures obtained from endosonography provide a "road map" for repair of the sphincter. For instance, in some patients who become incontinent after a sphincterotomy for a fissure, it gives visualization of the ends of the internal sphincter muscle and the amount of gap between those ends. This allows planning of the surgical incision. Similarly, in patients with a past obstetric injury, the gap in the internal and external sphincter muscles can be noted and allows planning of the surgical procedure.

## Conclusion

What tests are essential for treating patients with fecal incontinence? A suggested algorithm for the diagnosis and treatment of fecal incontinence is shown in Fig. 20-2. Many excellent caregivers use few of these tests, although recently more testing is being used. To rule out colitis, proctitis, and neoplasia, evaluation of the colon and rectum by endoscopy or barium enema is needed. Defecography may or may not be needed for evaluation of rectal prolapse but may be necessary to diagnose internal intussusception (or occult prolapse). The enema test is easy and inexpensive and helps to determine whether a patient has true fecal incontinence. Many clinicians do not have access to an anorectal physiology laboratory or endosonography machine. Additionally, it takes experienced personnel to perform and interpret the results of these tests. Even for some surgical procedures these tests are not mandatory but may be helpful for planning surgery and predicting success. For complicated surgical repairs or previously failed repairs, anal physiology testing and endosonography have significant value in planning an appropriate repair or determining why a previous repair failed. As caregivers become aware of this previously silent group of patients, more testing will be needed to study these patients in an effort to understand their problem. Then, as incontinence becomes analyzed more accurately, these tests and others yet to be discovered will allow more precise treatment planning.

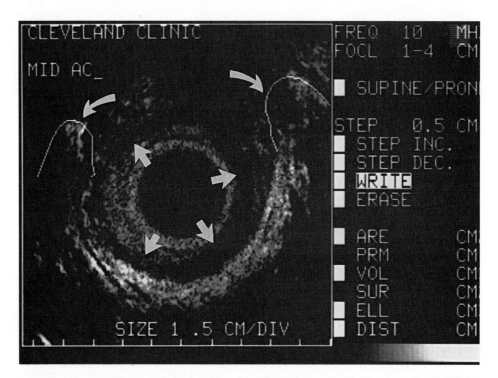

**Fig. 20-1**    Anal endosonography in a woman with "idiopathic incontinence" decades after the birth of her children. The internal anal sphincter is intact *(straight arrows)*. The external anal sphincter has a defect anteriorly *(curved arrows)*. *MID AC,* Midanal canal.

## NONSURGICAL TREATMENT

Treatment begins with correction of underlying medical and surgical problems. Preliminary surgical treatments may include cancer resection, treatment of inflammatory bowel disease, repair of rectal prolapse, and removal of impactions.

### Medical Treatments

In patients with minor incontinence, the use of bulking agents, such as Metamucil, Citracel, or Konsyl, can change the consistency of the stool, making it firmer and more easily controlled. Starting with a teaspoon daily and working up to a tablespoon up to three times daily helps to decrease side effects such as abdominal distention and bloating. If one agent gives these side effects, sometimes switching to another agent produces fewer side effects. Restricting the amount of fluid taken with these products may enhance their ability to increase stool bulk, especially if diarrhea is a problem.

Agents designed to slow down the intestinal tract may also help with stool control. Even in patients without diarrhea, these agents may slightly constipate patients, allowing them to better control their stool. Loperamide hydrochloride (Imodium) is often prescribed in this capacity. It prolongs intestinal transit time, allowing fecal volume to be reduced (secondary to the increased time allowed for removal of fluid from stool) and bulk density to be increased. It also increases rectal compliance, which de-

creases urgency. Side effects are rare, and physical dependence does not occur. The dosage must be individualized for each patient. If patients have particular trouble after meals, 2 to 4 mg may be given before a meal to decrease the chance of stooling. The maximum daily dosage is 16 mg. Some patients with diarrhea require the maximum dosage, but patients with mild incontinence who use it to mildly decrease the intestinal transit may need only two or three, 2-mg doses daily, or as needed. Diphenoxylate hydrochloride (Lomotil) is another agent used in this capacity, especially if diarrhea is a primary contributor to the incontinence. It is less expensive than Imodium, but it is a Schedule V substance (under the Controlled Substances Act). It has minimal potential for physical dependence. Side effects are rare but may include abdominal distention, drowsiness, dizziness, depression, restlessness, nausea, headache, blurred vision, and dry mouth. The dosing is similar to that of Imodium. One or two 2.5-mg tablets are used up to four times daily. As with Imodium, the dosing must be individualized. Other agents that focus on control of diarrhea include tincture of opium, paregoric, and codeine. Side effects and the risk of physical dependence make them less attractive.

### Biofeedback and Pelvic Muscle Exercises

Successful treatment of fecal incontinence has been achieved with biofeedback and pelvic muscle exercises. In addition, Jensen and Lowry (1997) showed that functional

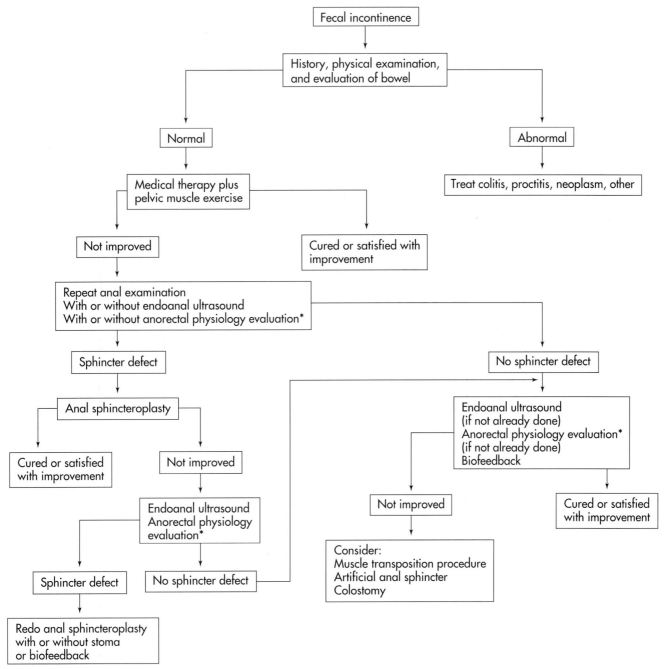

**Fig. 20-2** Algorithm for diagnosis and treatment of fecal incontinence.

*Could include anal manometry, electromyography, rectal compliance studies, and pudendal nerve studies.

outcomes after sphincteroplasty improved in patients who initially did not experience optimal results from surgery. It is indicated for alert, motivated patients as it is labor-intensive and requires a dedicated therapist. Biofeedback involves placement of a balloon in the rectum to simulate stool. Anal sphincter contraction is measured with a different balloon in the anal canal, by an anal plug, or by perianal surface electrodes. When patients sense the balloon in the rectum, contraction of the sphincter muscles is

initiated. Visual feedback is given regarding contraction of the external sphincter, and patients are encouraged when the proper sphincter response is made. Gradually the volume in the balloon is decreased and patients learn to sense smaller volumes with less rectal distention. Finally, the visual feedback is gradually removed. The goal is to increase sphincter strength and to teach patients to respond to smaller volumes of material in the rectum. Improvement has been reported in 63% to 90% of patients. Symptom improvement probably results from heightened rectal sensation. In addition, Rao et al. (1996) found that anal squeeze pressures improved, the duration of squeeze increased, and the capacity to retain liquid increased. These findings correlated with a decrease in the number of episodes of fecal incontinence.

There have been no studies that definitely show that pelvic muscle–strengthening exercises (Kegel exercises) alone benefit patients with fecal incontinence. However, they are safe and cost nothing. Therefore, they should be discussed with most patients afflicted with fecal incontinence. They may particularly benefit patients who have early fatigability of the sphincter muscle on digital examination when asked to squeeze. Sometimes biofeedback is used to assist patients in performing these exercises by giving visual feedback when the correct muscles are contracted. When using biofeedback we attempt to have patients hold the contraction for a full 10 seconds while watching a screen that tells them when the contraction decreases. Consultation with an interested physical therapist may optimize results.

## Bowel Management

Some patients find that daily enemas with approximately 2 pints of tap water, usually at the same time each morning just after eating, induce a bowel motion and empty the rectum. Sometimes a cone-tipped catheter (the same type used for colostomy irrigation) may be needed for incontinent patients to instill an enema so that it does not run out with instillation. Some advocate inserting a glycerine or bisacodyl (Dulcolax) suppository 20 to 30 minutes after eating along with abdominal massage to induce a bowel motion daily. With either method, bulking agents can be used in addition to medications to stop stooling in between desired defecation.

## SURGICAL TREATMENT

For sphincter repairs, the bowel is completely cleansed with an agent such as polyethylene glycol. Prophylactic antibiotics such as intravenous metronidazole and a third-generation cephalosporin are given preoperatively. These antibiotics are continued for variable periods postoperatively at the discretion of the surgeon. For surgery to correct a defect secondary to an injury, the tissue must be soft and pliable, and at least 3 to 6 months should elapse after the injury for the inflammation to subside. A Foley catheter is placed. Patients may be positioned in the lithotomy position or prone jackknife position for procedures directly performed on the sphincter muscle. For muscle wraps or the artificial sphincter, the prone jackknife position is indicated. I prefer the prone jackknife position for almost all anal procedures because it allows the buttock muscles to fall out of the way and gives the surgical assistants optimal viewing of the surgical field. For simple procedures such as

sphincteroplasty or postanal repair, general, epidural, or spinal anesthesia may be used. For complicated sphincter wraps, general anesthesia is needed.

## Sphincteroplasty

When a defect is detected in the sphincter complex, reapproximation of the two ends is attempted. Usually these defects are secondary to obstetric injury, fistula repair, or lateral internal sphincterotomy. Occasionally defects after hemorrhoidectomy can be successfully repaired. An arc type of incision is made over the injury usually about 1 to 1.5 cm beyond the anal verge (Fig. 20-3). For obstetric injuries, this arc spans about 200 degrees anteriorly. It is important to remember that the branches of the pudendal nerves that innervate the external sphincter approach the muscle from the posterolateral position. To avoid nerve injury, the arc of the incision should not extend to the extreme posterolateral position. I prefer to initially dissect down the rectovaginal septum to avoid injury to any remaining muscle and to avoid buttonhole defects into the anal canal or rectum. Sometimes the only remaining perineal body is the vaginal and anal mucosa, so dissection is difficult. The dissection is carried laterally to the ischiorectal fat. Placing a finger in the vagina or rectum and dissecting from lateral to medial may facilitate the dissection. Any tears in the anal mucosa are repaired with No. 4-0 chromic suture. The ends of the sphincter are usually approximated with scar in the midline (or midportion of the injury). This scar is divided in the middle, leaving two ends of sphincter with scar attached. It is important to divide the scar but to not trim it from the ends of the sphincter because it will provide tensile strength when

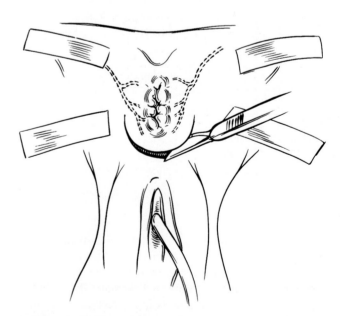

**Fig. 20-3**  Sphincteroplasty repair. The patient is in the prone jackknife position. The buttocks are taped apart. A curved incision is made anteriorly, avoiding the pudendal nerves, which approach the external sphincter from a deep posterolateral position.

the repair is done. If both the internal and external muscles are injured, I prefer to leave them intact and repair them as one unit. If the internal sphincter is not disrupted, I divide and repair only the external sphincter.

The levator ani muscles may be plicated at this point using No. 0 or 2-0 delayed absorbable sutures. This may lengthen the anal canal. The vagina should be checked after the levator plication to ensure that a ridge or narrowing did not occur with levator plication because this may contribute to dyspareunia. If the internal anal sphincter was not injured and hence not divided for the overlapping repair, plication can be done before the sphincteroplasty if there is redundant internal sphincter (Fig. 20-4).

The sphincter ends that have been sufficiently mobilized to allow overlapping of the muscle are grasped. Some advocate merely approximating the muscles, but if possible, I prefer to overlap the muscle ends. I use No. 2-0 polyglactin sutures and place mattress sutures for the sphincteroplasty. Approximately six sutures (three on each side) are used (Fig. 20-5). The repair is performed to tighten the anal canal so that just an index finger is admitted. During the

procedure, irrigation of the wound is carried out with antibiotic solution. The skin edges are closed in a V-Y fashion, starting laterally and leaving the center open for drainage (Fig. 20-6). If there is a significant amount of "dead space," a half-inch Penrose drain can be inserted and then removed on postoperative day 2.

Postoperatively, patients are kept on intravenous antibiotics for 2 to 3 days, and oral intake is withheld. I do not use constipating agents. I also do not use Sitz baths because I feel they macerate the skin edges, but showers are permitted. The Foley catheter is removed on postoperative day 2, and the patient is allowed a high-fiber diet just before discharge. At discharge, patients are placed on Metamucil, Citrucel, or Konsyl daily. Additionally, they take 1 ounce of mineral oil each morning. If they do not move their bowels by postoperative day 7, they take 1 ounce of milk of magnesia twice daily until their bowels move. Because they undergo a complete bowel cleansing before surgery, patients may not move their bowels for several days after surgery.

Diverting stoma is used at the discretion of the surgeon. Preoperatively I discuss the possibility of using a stoma in

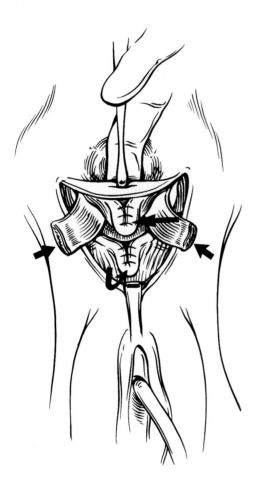

**Fig. 20-4**  If the internal anal sphincter *(long arrow)* is intact, it can be plicated before the external anal sphincter *(short arrows)* is overlapped. The levator muscles can also be plicated *(curved arrow)*.

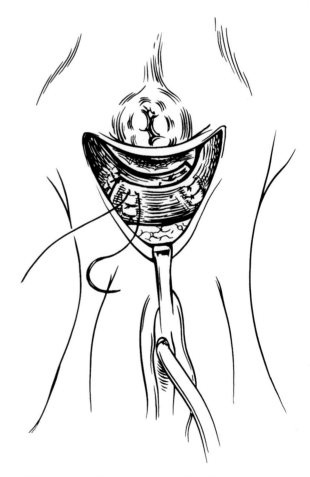

**Fig. 20-5**  The sphincter ends are identified and overlapped. Three mattress sutures are placed on each side to hold the muscle ends in place.

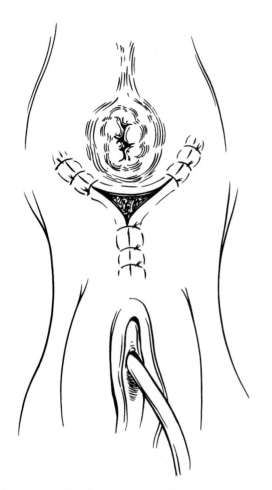

**Fig. 20-6**  The skin edges are closed in a V-Y fashion starting laterally and leaving the center open for drainage.

patients who have had failed repairs previously, have concomitant inflammatory bowel disease or severe diarrhea, or need an extremely complicated repair. A stoma does not ensure success but may aid a successful outcome in such patients.

Functional improvement can be anticipated in 80% to 90% of patients. Pudendal nerve damage is associated with suboptimal results. Age does not seem to significantly affect results, although erratic bowel problems such as urgency and diarrhea may lead to continued incontinence. Wound infection occurs in up to a quarter of patients but does not adversely affect the outcome unless the sphincter repair sutures become disrupted. Complete disruption of the skin sutures usually heals by secondary intention with adequate wound care.

## Postanal Pelvic Floor Repair

The postanal repair has been advocated for patients with incontinence without a sphincter defect or with neuropathic incontinence. This procedure is designed to reestablish the anorectal angle, increase the length of the anal canal, and

tighten the anal canal. Optimal results seem to be in patients with incontinence from anal sphincter stretch or loss of anorectal angulation. Patients with neurogenic incontinence usually do not have significant improvement. Preoperative preparation has been previously described. An inverted V incision is made 5 to 6 cm from the anal verge posteriorly. Flaps are raised and the intersphincteric plane is identified. Dissection is carried in this plane cephalad to Waldeyer's fascia, which is divided to expose the mesorectal fat. Figure-of-eight, No. 2-0 polypropylene sutures are placed to draw the two sides of the ileococcygeus muscle together. The sides will not approximate because of the distance, so the sutures are tied with minimal tension to form a lattice. The pubococcygeus muscle is the next muscle encountered. Sutures are placed and tied to again form a lattice, especially posteriorly, although anteriorly the ends also may be approximated. The last layer plicated is the puborectalis and external sphincter. The skin is closed with absorbable suture in a V-Y fashion. Postoperative care is similar to the sphincteroplasty repair.

Original results by Parks (1975) demonstrated postoperative improvement in incontinence in 80% of patients; however, this degree of success has not been achieved by others. Perhaps 50% of patients experience significant long-term improvement.

## Muscle Transposition Procedures

In some patients, repair of the sphincter does not relieve symptoms. Additionally, some patients have had traumatic loss of sphincter muscle, making approximation of the ends impossible. Transposition of the gracilis or gluteus muscle has been advocated for these patients.

### Gracilis Muscle Transposition

The gracilis muscle is mobilized from the inner thigh, preserving the neurovascular bundle proximally. The tendon of insertion is divided at the knee, preserving as much tendon as possible. The muscle is wrapped around the anus, and the tendon is sewn to the opposite ischial tuberosity. An electrical stimulator is placed at an optimal site on the abdomen. Leads are tunneled from the stimulator and placed onto the proximal portion of the nerve. The entire procedure is done under cover of a stoma and usually in several stages.

Patients appropriate for this procedure include those with incontinence caused by obstetric injury, idiopathic incontinence, traumatic loss of sphincter muscle, and congenital anal sphincter problems. Contraindications include neurologic disease such as multiple sclerosis. This operation carries a high morbidity and has a significant learning curve. Surgeons with considerable experience, such as Baeten et al. (1995), achieve excellent results, especially considering that the only alternative for many of these patients is a permanent stoma. In their study of 1995, about 23% achieved perfect continence for solid and liquid stool and flatus. An additional 50% had continence for solid and liquid stool but not flatus. Others have achieved complete continence in 46% to 65% of patients. As more experience is gained with this procedure, it is hoped that the technical and learning problems will be remedied.

### Gluteus Maximus Muscle Transposition

The gluteus maximus is an accessory muscle of continence even under normal circumstances. It is a powerful muscle able to sustain basal tone. Its inferior aspect has an independent neurovascular pedicle that can be preserved and detached with the muscle's lower portion and wrapped around the anal sphincter. To perform the procedure, a 5-cm strip of muscle is detached from the sacrum and coccyx along with its aponeurotic tissue bilaterally. This strip of muscle is mobilized laterally to the neurovascular bundle. The free ends are split and wrapped around the anal region, securing them to the muscle from the opposite side with sutures. The procedure is done under the cover of a stoma.

Results after gluteus maximus muscle transposition vary. Devesa et al. (1992) reported that 67% of their patients had normal continence or less than one episode of minor soiling per week. Others, in an attempt to improve results, have suggested using an electrical stimulator similar to that used with the gracilis muscle. More experience is needed with this procedure to fully evaluate its place in the treatment of fecal incontinence.

### Artificial Anal Sphincter

As success with the artificial urinary sphincter was attained, efforts turned toward using a modified version of this device for fecal incontinence. This fully implantable device incorporates a balloon that, when fully inflated, occludes the anus. It is indicated for patients in whom conventional management of fecal incontinence has failed. Few centers in the world perform this procedure, and many technical challenges are associated with its implantation. Wong et al. (1996) reported the results from a combined study of the University of Minnesota and The Royal Infirmary in Edinburgh, Scotland. They found infectious or mechanical complications in 33%. Seventy-five percent of patients had improvement in their incontinence, although some of the patients with improvement experienced incontinence of flatus, mucus, or liquid stool at times. As with the muscle transpositions, there is a considerable learning curve with this operation. However, it also holds promise for patients with severe fecal incontinence.

### Colostomy or Ileostomy

Fecal diversion, in the form of an end colostomy or occasionally an ileostomy, sometimes can offer a much better lifestyle for patients with incapacitating incontinence when repairs fail or have no chance of succeeding. They allow patients trapped in their homes from fear of an episode of incontinence the opportunity to leave their "prisons."

## CONCLUSION

Fecal incontinence is a complex problem with many causes. Even though it is not a life-threatening problem, it can be life-devastating. Evaluation is tailored to the patient, and treatment depends on the findings from history, physical examination, and testing. Many patients can obtain improvement or cure from nonsurgical treatment. Others with a demonstrable defect in the sphincter mechanism may be candidates for sphincter repair. New frontiers in muscle transposition techniques and artificial sphincters are emerging for patients who fail sphincter repair or are not suitable candidates. There are still significant disappointments and failures after surgery for incontinence, and fecal diversion still is the appropriate treatment for some.

## BIBLIOGRAPHY

Baeten CG, Geerdes BP, Adang EMM, et al: Anal dynamic graciloplasty in the treatment of intractable fecal incontinence, *N Engl J Med* 332:1600, 1995.

Den KI, Kumar D, Williams JG, et al: The prevalence of anal sphincter defects in faecal incontinence: a prospective endosonic study, *Gut* 34:685, 1993.

Devesa JM, Vicente E, Enriquez JM: Total fecal incontinence—a new method of gluteus maximus transposition: preliminary results and report of previous experience with similar procedures, *Dis Colon Rectum* 35:339, 1992.

Gordon PH. Anal incontinence. In Gordon PH, Nivatvongs S, eds: *Principles and practice of surgery for the colon, rectum, and anus,* St Louis, 1992, Quality Medical Publishing.

Guelinckx PJ, Sinsel NK, Gruwez JA: Anal sphincter reconstruction with the gluteus maximus muscle: anatomic and physiologic considerations concerning conventional and dynamic gluteoplasty, *Plast Reconstr Surg* 98:293, 1996.

Jackson SL, Weber AM, Hull TL, et al: Fecal incontinence in women with urinary incontinence and pelvic organ prolapse, *Obstet Gynecol* 89:423, 1997.

Jensen LL, Lowry AC: Biofeedback improves functional outcome after sphincteroplasty, *Dis Colon Rectum* 40:197, 1997.

Johanson JF, Lafferty J: Epidemiology of fecal incontinence: the silent affliction, *Am J Gastroenterol* 91:33, 1996.

Madoff RD, Williams JG, Caushaj PF: Fecal incontinence, *N Engl J Med* 326:1002, 1992.

Meyenberger C, Bertschinger P, Zala GF, et al: Anal sphincter defects in fecal incontinence: correlation between endosonography and surgery, *Endoscopy* 28:217, 1996.

Oliveira L, Pfeifer J, Wexner SD: Physiological and clinical outcome of anterior sphincteroplasty, *Br J Surg* 83:502, 1996.

Parks AG: Anorectal incontinence, *Proc R Soc Med* 68:681, 1975.

Rao SS, Welcher KD, Happel J: Can biofeedback therapy improve anorectal function in fecal incontinence? *Am J Gastroenterol* 91:2360, 1996.

Sultan AH, Kamm MA, Hudson CN, et al: Anal-sphincter disruption during vaginal delivery, *N Engl J Med* 329:1905, 1993.

Tetzscher T, Sorensen M, Lose G, et al: Anal and urinary incontinence in women with obstetric anal sphincter rupture, *Br J Obstet Gynaecol* 103:1034, 1996.

Wexner SD, Gonzalez-Padron A, Rius J, et al: Stimulated gracilis neosphincter operation: initial experience, pitfalls, and complications, *Dis Colon Rectum* 39:957, 1996.

Wexner SD, Schmitt SL: Fecal incontinence: surgical therapy. In Brubaker LT, Saclarides TJ, eds: *The female pelvic floor,* Philadelphia, 1996, FA Davis.

Wong WD, Jensen LL, Bartolo DCC, et al: Artificial anal sphincter, *Dis Colon Rectum* 39:1345, 1996.

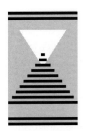

CHAPTER 21
*Constipation*

Tracy L. Hull

## DEFINITION AND ETIOLOGY

Constipation is a commonly encountered problem in most medical practices. It is estimated that 2% of Americans suffer from constipation, and medications are prescribed for 2 to 3 million patients annually. Women are three times more commonly afflicted than men, making this a condition gynecologists and urogynecologists see often.

The term *constipation* means different things to different people. The perception of a normal bowel pattern varies. In fact, in one study normal volunteers had bowel movements from three per day to two or three per week. Additionally, some view infrequent stooling as constipation and others feel that hard or hard-to-pass stool signals constipation. A commonly accepted definition of constipation is straining at stool more than 25% of the time or having two or fewer stools per week. There are many causes of constipation. Box 21-1 lists some common ones.

## EVALUATION

A thorough history and physical examination is the first step toward treatment. Laboratory, radiologic, and other tests are done based on the history and physical examination.

### History

The history begins with clarification of the nature of the defecation problem, such as number of stools per week,

difficulty expelling stool, pain with defecation, consistency of stool, and duration of the problem. Some patients experience rectal pressure or fullness. Others may need to use their fingers to expel stool or stabilize the vagina or surrounding perineum during defecation. They may be embarrassed to admit some of these practices and may need to be encouraged to tell this information. Additional questions that center on the amount of dietary fiber and fluid consumed daily are asked.

It is important to rule out associated medical problems that can lead to constipation. Some of these, as outlined in Box 21-1, are neurologic abnormalities (Parkinson's disease, multiple sclerosis, cerebral vascular accident, immobility, and others), psychiatric disorders, endocrine problems (hypothyroidism, hypercalcemia, hypokalemia, diabetes mellitus, and others), and medications (narcotics, antidepressants, iron, calcium, and others). Past surgeries may also provide clues and should be elicited. Recent changes in routine such as a vacation, smoking cessation, or eliminating caffeine from the diet may contribute to constipation and should be questioned. In patients with severe constipation and no obvious cause, histories of physical and sexual abuse may be helpful.

### Physical Examination

The physical examination is tailored to the patient. The abdominal examination may be normal, but masses, palpable stool in the colon, and surgical scars and hernias should be noted. The perineal examination starts with inspection, looking for fissures or abnormalities. Asking the patient to strain may demonstrate perineal descent or a large rectocele prolapsing into the vagina. Digital examination rules out anal stenosis and pelvic or rectal masses, and a rectocele may be noted anteriorly. The examiner should note the consistency of stool in the rectum.

No physical examination is complete without flexible or rigid proctosigmoidoscopy. This examination rules out neoplasms, a solitary rectal ulcer (erythema or ulceration on the lower anterior rectal wall felt to be from trauma secondary to internal rectal prolapse), or melanosis coli (brown-black discoloration of the mucosa from chronic use of certain laxatives).

## Box 21-1
## CAUSES OF CONSTIPATION

**Personal Habits**

Poor dietary intake of fluids and fiber
Low physical activity
Changes in normal routine

**Obstructive**

*Colon*

Neoplasm
Benign stricture (i.e., diverticula)
Rectal prolapse

*Anal outlet obstruction*

Pain (i.e., fissure)
Stenosis
Rectocele
Pelvic floor dysfunction (i.e., paradoxical puborectalis
   contraction)

**Medications**

Narcotics
Antidepressants
Mineral supplements (i.e., iron, calcium)
Anticholinergics
Beta-blockers, calcium channel blockers

**Endocrine**

Hypothyroidism
Hypercalcemia
Hypokalemia
Diabetes mellitus
Uremia

**Neurologic**

Aganglionosis (congenital: Hirschsprung's disease; acquired:
   Chagas' disease)
Central nervous system or spinal cord trauma or disease
   (Parkinson's disease, multiple sclerosis)

**Pregnancy**

**Psychiatric Causes**

**Other/Unknown**

## Testing

Further testing depends on the severity of symptoms and findings on physical examination. In the majority of patients, at this stage no further testing is needed, and the physician can proceed to medical therapy. However, there is a group of distressed patients who need further evaluation. The tests chosen depend on the patient's characteristics and severity of symptoms.

### Laboratory Testing

Blood work looking at levels of potassium, calcium, renal function, and glucose are performed initially. Thyroid function tests screening for hypothyroidism are also drawn if a problem is suspected.

### Anatomic Studies of the Colon

A barium enema or colonoscopy will diagnose anatomic abnormalities such as stricture or cancer. At times I prefer a barium enema because it defines the borders of the colon and may show a redundant or chronically dilated colon (megacolon) or rectum (megarectum).

Some patients with rectal prolapse may not manifest a protrusion of the rectum through the anal canal but may experience defecation problems such as constipation. If internal prolapse is suspected, a defecating proctogram can establish the diagnosis.

Rectoceles are a common finding in women. A defecating proctogram helps delineate those rectoceles that are displaced anteriorly, not fully emptying, and may require repair (Fig. 21-1). Also, sigmoidoceles can be seen.

Defecating proctograms are performed by placing a paste of contrast material into the rectum to simulate stool. The patients are asked to contract their anal muscles and strain while radiographs are taken. During the examination, they sit on a commode behind a curtain, and fluoroscopy is performed to obtain the pictures. From these pictures, the angle between the anal canal and rectum is measured at rest, strain, and squeeze. During normal defecation the anal canal becomes straighter, which in turn lengthens the angle. If this does not occur, the puborectalis muscle may be inappropriately contracting and may prohibit the expulsion of the contrast (and stool). This is termed *paradoxical puborectalis contraction;* it is a cause of anal outlet obstruction, which is one form of constipation. The amount of descent of the perineum is noted because this may be associated with anal outlet obstruction and constipation. Additionally, infolding of the walls of the rectum with defecation, as is seen with internal prolapse, is evaluated. It is important to remember that this test is embarrassing for the patient and complicated for the radiologist to perform. Therefore, the results may not always demonstrate the abnormality or be totally accurate.

### Functional Studies of the Colon

The colonic transit study is an important test to evaluate the colon for slow transit (colonic inertia). Patients stop all laxatives 48 hours before the study. They also consume a high-fiber diet (30 grams daily) and refrain from using enemas. There have been many variations of this study, but basically patients consume a commercially prepared capsule that contains a certain number of radiopaque markers. Radiographs are then taken daily or every other day and compared. Normally 80% of the markers are passed by the fifth day and all markers should be passed

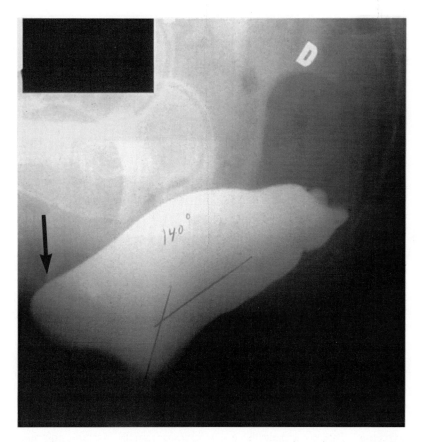

**Fig. 21-1**   Defecating proctogram demonstrating a rectocele *(arrow)* during the defecation.

by the seventh day. Some people divide the colon into right, left, and rectosigmoid to determine the transit time of each segment. This allows distinction between whole gut dysmotility, as seen by evenly distributed markers throughout the colon to the rectum, versus anal outlet obstruction, in which the markers progress quickly through the colon and are held up in the rectal sigmoid region. In another pattern, markers proceed through the colon and accumulate in the left colon and stop. This signals left colonic dysfunction.

Anal physiology testing can be helpful in patients with constipation. Normally, rectal distention, which can be simulated with a fluid-filled balloon in the rectum, leads to reflexive internal sphincter relaxation. This is called the rectal anal inhibitory reflex. In patients with Hirschsprung's disease this does not occur. Compliance of the rectum can be calculated by measuring the sensitivity and maximal volume tolerated in a fluid-filled balloon. An increased compliance can be seen in patients with constipation and signals a megarectum or insensitive rectum. Electromyography (EMG) is done with surface electrodes or needles placed directly in the puborectalis and external sphincter. We prefer to do this test with surface electrodes rather than needles because of the extreme discomfort associated with needles. EMG done during straining (which simulates a bowel movement) should reveal a decrease in electrical activity of these muscles; that is, the muscles should relax to allow passage of stool. If paradoxical contraction is seen in these muscles during straining, this may be a cause of the anal outlet constipation. As mentioned previously, this is called paradoxical puborectalis contraction. The EMG is an important test to distinguish patients with colonic inertia from spastic pelvic floor problems. However, patients may have both disorders.

### Psychiatric Evaluation

The interplay between the emotional being and the colon and anus is not well understood. Some problems with abnormally holding in stool during childhood may be attributed to problems between children and their parents over bowel function. Patients who have experienced sexual trauma or abuse can have defecation problems. Some patients complain of infrequent stools and constipation, but a transit study may be normal; these two findings are not compatible because there must be bowel function to eliminate the markers. Additionally, patients with psychosis, depression, or eating disorders can have severe constipation from a variety of causes. The clinician needs to be alert to possible cues from the patient and, if suspicious, refer him or her for a psychiatric assessment.

**Box 21-2**
## CLASSIFICATION OF LAXATIVES

Bulk laxatives
Hyperosmotic laxatives
Lubricant laxatives
Saline laxatives
Stimulant laxatives
Stool softeners

From the U.S. Food and Drug Administration.

**Box 21-3**
## INSOLUBLE FIBER CONTENT OF SELECTED FOODS

| Food (g Total Fiber) | Insoluble Fiber (g) |
|---|---|
| One pear (4.2) | 2.9 |
| One banana (3.9) | 1.6 |
| One cup strawberries (3.5) | 3.0 |
| One apple with skin (2.9) | 2.8 |
| Half cup frozen boiled peas (10.3) | 3.2 |
| Half cup cooked lima beans (5.5) | 5.5 |
| Half cup frozen broccoli (4.0) | 2.1 |
| Half cup cooked green beans (2.4) | 1.2 |
| Half cup raw tomatoes (1.9) | 1.0 |
| One cup chopped lettuce (0.9) | 0.5 |

Data from Dubuc MB, Lahaie LC. *Nutritive value of foods*, Ottawa, 1987, National Library, pp 16-158.

## NONSURGICAL TREATMENT
### Medications

The majority of patients with constipation can be treated nonsurgically. It is important to correct associated medical or gastrointestinal abnormalities if possible. These include problems such as hypothyroidism and hypokalemia. Hyperparathyroidism should be ruled out in patients with elevated calcium levels. Conditions such as Hirschsprung's disease require surgical intervention. Treating fissures and anal or colonic stenosis may resolve associated constipation. Medications that are known to cause constipation sometimes can be modified to relieve the symptoms. Patients without these obvious or correctable problems should be started on medical management.

Dispelling the myth that a daily bowel movement is "normal" initiates medical treatment. Many laxative manufacturers suggest that daily bowel movements are essential for a happy life in an effort to sell their products. However, this simply is not true. Next, a careful dietary history may provide clues to easily correctable problems that do not require specific drug treatment. Encouraging most patients to drink at least six 8-ounce glasses of fluid daily is important. If treatment is needed, Box 21-2 is a guide to the commonly used laxatives. They are grouped according to the U.S. Food and Drug Administration Classification.

### Bulk-Forming Laxatives and Fiber

Detrimental personal habits play a large role in most cases of constipation. The Western diet is highly refined and low in fiber. Fiber is the nondigestible segment of plants. It is estimated that humans should consume 20 to 35 grams daily for bowel health; however, the average American consumes only 11 grams daily. These agents promote evacuation of the bowel by increasing bulk volume and water content of feces. This may be done in four proposed ways. First, stool is 30% to 50% bacteria. Fiber provides substrate to increase the growth of bacteria and hence increase stool volume. Second, undigested hydrophilic components of fiber absorb fluid and can increase the fluidity of stool. Third, fermentation of fiber produces short chain fatty acids that decrease transit time in the colon. This allows less time for the colonic mucosa to be in contact with the luminal contents to reabsorb water, thus increasing the fluidity of stool. Finally, the weight of the stool is increased simply by the nondigested components in fiber. Natural fiber is classified as soluble or insoluble fiber and foods contain a mixture of these types. Stool size increases from the insoluble component of fiber. Foods high in insoluble fiber and their fiber content are listed in Box 21-3.

Bulk laxatives are felt to be among the safest laxatives. These include familiar product names such as Metamucil, Konsyl, Citrucel, and FiberCon. Dosage varies among products. They should be taken with sufficient fluids to avoid esophageal bolus obstruction and bowel obstruction from fecal impaction. The optimum quantity of "sufficient fluids" is unknown, but in adults a full 8-ounce glass of fluid is recommend. For diabetics, sugar-free varieties are manufactured. Side effects of bulk laxatives include increased flatus and bloating. Generally, I instruct patients to start with a teaspoon of Metamucil, Citrucel, or Konsyl daily for a week, then increase to a tablespoon daily. This can be further increased, if needed. These agents take 12 to 72 hours to exert an effect, so patients should be encouraged to try the product for 1 to 2 weeks. Sometimes the problems of increased flatus and bloating decrease with continued use. If these symptoms are too distressing, the patient should switch to another bulk laxative because the side effects may not be as distressing with another product.

### Hyperosmotic Laxatives

Hyperosmotic agents contain poorly absorbed substances that remain in the intestinal lumen, increasing the intraluminal osmotic pressure by drawing water into the lumen. The volume increases as the consistency decreases. The increased volume induces peristalsis. Lactulose is a synthetic disaccharide that is not digested by gastrointestinal enzymes and is not significantly absorbed in the small intestine. It is metabolized by colonic bacteria to short-chain organic acids. The osmotic activity of the nonabsorbable short chain organic acids draws water into the lumen. Lactulose is a syrup and the dosage is 15 to 30 ml daily, increased to 60 ml daily if necessary. It may take up to 2 days to produce stool. Use as an enema in a 25% to 30% solution has been reported. Side effects include diarrhea, and the dosage must be titrated to each patient. Increased flatus and intestinal cramps can occur but usually subside with time. Lactulose contains galactose and lactose in small amounts and may alter serum glucose in diabetics.

Sorbitol, another poorly absorbed carbohydrate, can cause chronic diarrhea in people who consume sugarless candy and gum that contain it. It works similarly to lactulose by reaching the colon as an active osmol. It can be administered orally or as an enema to treat constipation.

Glycerin suppositories promote fecal evacuation 15 to 30 minutes after administration by stimulating rectal evacuation as a hyperosmotic agent drawing fluid into the rectum. Possible side effects are abdominal cramping, rectal discomfort, and irritation of the rectal mucosa.

## Lubricant Laxatives

Mineral oil is the most common lubricant laxative. It is a nondigested hydrocarbon with limited absorption, which decreases the absorption of water from stool and penetrates the stool to lubricate and soften. It can be used orally (15 to 45 ml daily in single or divided doses for adults) or in an enema (120 ml). There are major concerns with long-term use of this product (more than 4 months). Oral use for more than 2 weeks coats the small intestine and may interfere with vitamin absorption, especially of D, E, K, and A (the fat-soluble vitamins). For this reason, it is recommended that mineral oil should not be taken with meals. Additionally, many feel it should not be administered at bedtime to reduce the occurrence of aspiration of the mineral oil, which can produce lipoid pneumonia. Administration with docusate salts may enhance absorption of mineral oil, which can form lipoid granulomas in the reticuloendothelial system; therefore, administration of both together is usually avoided. Other side effects include pruritus ani, anal leakage, and diarrhea.

## Saline Laxatives

Saline laxatives are usually used to prepare patients for diagnostic bowel procedures and testing. They contain a magnesium cation or phosphate anion. Some believe that the nonabsorbed ion produces an osmotic effect, which increases the intraluminal fluid and thus increases the volume of stool. However, recent studies suggest that their method of action may be to stimulate the release of cholecystokinin, which stimulates small bowel motility and inhibits absorption of fluid and electrolytes from the small intestine. Saline laxatives can produce an evacuation within 2 to 6 hours if given orally or 15 minutes if given rectally. Oral administration should be accompanied by sufficient amounts of fluid to decrease holdover in the stomach and limit the possible effect of dehydration. Examples of these agents are magnesium citrate, milk of magnesia (magnesium hydroxide), magnesium sulfate, Phospho-soda (sodium phosphate and biphosphate), and Fleet enema (sodium biphosphate and phosphate). These agents should be used cautiously in patients with impaired renal function because magnesium and phosphate may be partially absorbed. The sodium salts may cause congestive heart failure in susceptible patients. Electrolytes should be monitored in selected patients with use of these products. Additionally, enema preparations can cause rectal irritation.

## Stimulant Laxatives

Stimulant laxatives produce their effect by irritating the intestinal mucosa or by selective action on the enteric nervous system. This reduces the water absorption and increases secretions, probably through prostaglandins. They are extremely potent and should be used only for short-term treatment. Long-term use may lead to cathartic colon syndrome (a dilated and atonic colon following extensive and prolonged use of laxatives), melanosis coli (dark pigmentation of the colonic mucosa), or neuronal degeneration.

Classes of stimulant laxatives include anthraquinones (cascara, senna [Senokot], and aloe), polyphenolic derivatives (phenolphthalein [Feen-a-Mint, Correctol, Ex-Lax] and bisacodyl [Dulcolax, Carter's Little Pills]), and castor oil. Oral and some rectal preparations are available for these medications. The anthraquinones and polyphenolic derivatives work in 6 to 8 hours. Short-term side effects include cramps, nausea, and abdominal pain. Castor oil works in 2 to 6 hours and is used mainly as a preparation for colonic procedures or radiologic studies.

## Stool Softener Laxatives

Stool softeners exert a detergent-type effect through their hydrophilic and hydrophobic properties, which break down surface barriers, allowing water and lipids to enter the stool. This softens the stool and increases the fecal mass. Onset of action may take several days when administered orally because it may take that long for the softened stool to reach the rectum. Rectal administration produces an effect in 2 to 15 minutes. Examples include docusate calcium (Surfak), docusate potassium (Dialose, Kasof), and docusate sodium (Colace, Comfolax, Modane Soft). Preparations of these in combination with stimulant laxatives include Feen-a-Mint, Correctol, Peri-Colace, and Doxidan. It has been suggested that these agents can decrease jejunal absorption and damage villi, resulting in increased absorption of substances such as mineral oil and phenolphthaleins. However, no serious adverse action is usually seen if these agents are taken alone. Side effects include diarrhea and mild abdominal cramping.

### Other Agents

Prokinetic agents enhance normal propulsive action of the bowel. Metoclopramide and domperidone have not been found to have significant colonic effects. However, cisapride is the most promising of these agents. It works as a cholinergic agent by facilitating the release of acetylcholine at the level of the myenteric plexus. In several studies involving constipated patients, it has been shown to significantly increase stooling frequency without affecting fecal water content. The only side effect was mild, occasional crampy abdominal pain. The dosage is 5 to 20 mg two to four times daily, but should be adjusted to the lowest effective dosage.

Patients with intractable constipation may benefit from daily administration of polyethylene glycol solutions such as GoLYTELY or Colyte. These solutions are not absorbed and thus are safe for patients with concerns of fluid overload or renal insufficiency. A daily dosage of 8 to 16 ounces has been shown to improve stool frequency in chronically constipated patients.

Enemas or suppositories used on an intermittent basis may relieve some patients of constipation. Some patients find that daily tap water enemas eliminate their need for oral laxatives. There are many suppository and enema preparations. If considering long-term enema use, the tap water variety may be the least irritating to the rectal mucosa. Potential side effects of enemas include electrolyte depletion, water intoxication, and colonic perforation.

### Biofeedback

Patients with rectal evacuation problems manifested only by a hold up of markers in the rectum during the colonic transit study may benefit from biofeedback. Additionally, patients with paradoxical puborectalis contractions may benefit from biofeedback. Neither of these conditions responds to current surgical treatment, and medication therapy often is not effective. Biofeedback allows patients to be more aware and responsive to biological information provided to them. There are many different treatment protocols, making comparison of results difficult. Success rates vary from 18% to 100%. However, because this treatment is painless and harmless and can have a reasonable chance of success in patients otherwise difficult to treat, biofeedback should be considered.

### SURGICAL TREATMENT

Surgical treatment is required for patients with constipation caused by Hirschsprung's disease. It is also considered for patients with idiopathic constipation in whom an adequate course of medical therapy has failed. However, Pemberton et al. (1991) at the Mayo Clinic found that only 15% of constipated patients referred to them fall into the category that may benefit from surgery. Preoperative evaluation is essential in determining which patients will benefit from surgery and which surgical procedure to perform.

### Colonic Inertia
#### Normal Size Colon and Rectum

Severely constipated patients with colonic inertia demonstrated on colonic transit studies, a normal caliber colon and rectum, and a normal defecography may benefit from colectomy. When properly selected, this group of patients experienced a 70% improvement with surgery. Operative choices include colectomy with ileosigmoid, ileorectal, or cecorectal anastomosis. Cecorectal anastomosis, preserving the ileocecal valve, seems preferable. However, persistent constipation may be slightly more common with cecorectal and ileosigmoid anastomoses than with ileorectal anastomosis. Despite the entire colon being removed, a subset of patients still have constipation and require enemas. In addition, diarrhea can be a new problem after surgery (seen in 30%) along with fecal incontinence (seen in 0% to 38%).

Colonic inertia coexisting with paradoxical puborectalis muscle contractions creates a dilemma. Which problem should be treated first? Many favor biofeedback to treat the nonrelaxing puborectalis because the colonic inertia can be a result of the abnormal pelvic muscle problem. If patients respond and demonstrate relaxation of the puborectalis with straining, colectomy may be offered. Some surgeons would offer colectomy to those without demonstrated relaxation of the puborectalis, contending that the liquid stool resulting after colectomy is easier to pass and not as problematic for the patient.

Our approach for patients with colonic inertia is to perform a colectomy with ileorectal anastomosis. If a paradoxical puborectalis contraction is seen preoperatively, biofeedback treatment is tried initially. Patients are counseled that this operation might not improve their constipation and will probably produce diarrhea. For patients with marginal sphincters detected on preoperative evaluation, an ileostomy may be a better option because of the diarrhea that can result from the colectomy. Even those with normal anal sphincters are warned about the possible postoperative problem of fecal incontinence. If abdominal pain and bloating are part of their preoperative constellation of symptoms, patients are warned that these may not improve after a colectomy.

#### Megacolon and Megarectum

In some patients with constipation, preoperative studies may demonstrate a megacolon and/or megarectum. Hirschsprung's disease is initially ruled out. In patients with a megacolon and normal-sized rectum, colectomy with ileorectal anastomosis is the preferred treatment. In patients with a rectum more than 6.5 cm in diameter at the pelvic brim and a normal transit time, the Duhamel operation may be an option. (In the Duhamel operation, the colon is removed and the rectal stump is closed. After presacral dissection, the posterior wall of the rectum is anastomosed to the end of the proximal bowel.) However, if the transit time is prolonged, a proctocolectomy and pelvic pouch is reasonable. Some advocate anorectal myomectomy to treat megarectum not associated with Hirschsprung's disease.

This procedure has been used successfully in the pediatric population, but more positive data are needed before this approach can be recommended in adults.

### Left Colonic Dysfunction

In the select group of patients who exhibit delayed passage of markers in the left colon (i.e., distal to the splenic flexure), a left colectomy and proctectomy with low colorectal or coloanal anastomosis has been done. The proximal colon was preserved in an attempt to decrease diarrhea. Conflicting results regarding success have been reported in the literature and reflect only small numbers of patients studied. Additionally, it is unclear whether the patients had segmental or diffusely abnormal colonic transit studies. More data are needed to judge whether this is a viable option for patients with segmental colonic dysfunction.

## Anorectal Outlet Obstruction
### Paradoxical Puborectalis Contraction

Surgical division of the pelvic floor or sphincter muscles has been tried for nonrelaxing or paradoxical puborectalis contraction. However, long-term improvement is seen in few patients, and biofeedback has become the mainstay of treatment for this problem.

### Rectal Prolapse

Rectal prolapse or intussusception can be entirely internal (occult) or external and protrude through the anal sphincter complex. Patients with rectal prolapse and constipation should undergo a complete evaluation before surgery. If diffuse, slow transit constipation (colonic inertia) is found, a colectomy with ileorectal anastomosis and rectopexy may be the procedure of choice. Patients with a normal transit and mild constipation may benefit from a sigmoid resection with a colorectal anastomosis and rectopexy. Chapter 23 more fully discusses this condition.

### Rectocele

Rectoceles are commonly seen in women. Some produce significant symptoms by sequestering stool in the pocket formed by the herniation into the vagina. Initially, nonsurgical treatment is attempted by increasing fiber and fluids in the diet. In patients who have symptoms attributed to the rectocele, such as needing to insert their finger into the vagina to defecate, repair either transvaginally or transanally can be performed. Gynecologic issues related to rectocele are fully discussed in Chapter 18.

## CONCLUSION

Constipation is a complex constellation of known and unknown problems that can produce mild or incapacitating symptoms. History and physical examination initiate therapy. Further laboratory, anatomic, and functional testing depend on the history and physical examination. The majority of patients can be helped with dietary improve-

ments and increased fluid consumption. Some patients not helped by simple dietary measures require laxatives. There are many types of laxatives. The bulk-forming laxatives (and dietary fiber) are probably safest for long-term use. For patients with continued constipation, in addition to fiber and bulk laxative supplementation, Sloan (1996) advocates medical therapy with nonstimulant laxatives such as milk of magnesia. If constipation continues to be intolerable, the addition of stimulant laxatives on an intermittent basis may be needed. Chronic use of stimulant laxatives should be tempered because of possible colonic neuronal degeneration (especially with the anthraquinones). Sloan (1996) also recommends combination therapy, such as milk of magnesia at bedtime and a suppository in the morning, repeated every 3 or 4 days to minimize patient discomfort. Cisapride may help some patients.

For patients unresponsive to these measures, behavioral or surgical therapy may be offered. Those with anal outlet constipation caused by paradoxical puborectalis contraction usually do not benefit from surgical therapy and biofeedback is the mainstay of treatment for this group. Surgical intervention is mandated for patients with Hirschsprung's disease and external rectal prolapse. Surgical treatment (after failed medical therapy) is suggested for patients with colonic inertia, internal rectal prolapse, and symptomatic rectocele. A small group of patients with idiopathic constipation benefit from surgical intervention.

## BIBLIOGRAPHY

Andorsky RI, Goldner F: Colonic lavage solution (polyethylene glycol electrolyte lavage solution) as a treatment for chronic constipation: a double-blind placebo-controlled study, *Am J Gastroenterol* 85:261, 1990.

Binder HJ: Use of laxatives in clinical medicine, *Pharmacology* 36(suppl 1):226, 1988.

Cerulli MA, Schuster MM: Medical treatment of constipation and fecal incontinence. In Phillips SF, Pemberton JH, Shorter RG, eds: *The large intestine physiology, pathophysiology, and disease,* New York, 1991, Raven.

Dahl J, Lindquist BL, Tysk C, et al: Behavioral medicine treatment in chronic constipation with paradoxical anal sphincter contraction, *Dis Colon Rectum* 34:769, 1991.

Drossman DA, Sandler RS, McKee DC, et al: Bowel patterns among subjects not seeking health care, *Gastroenterology* 83:529, 1982.

Dubuc MB, Lahaie LC: *Nutritive value of foods,* Ottawa, 1987, National Library.

Hull TL, Milsom JW: Constipation: results of surgical therapy. In Brubaker LT, Saclarides TJ, eds: *The female pelvic floor: disorders of function and support,* Philadelphia, 1996, FA Davis.

Nicholls RJ, Kamm MA: Proctocolectomy with restorative ileo-anal reservoir for severe idiopathic constipation, *Dis Colon Rectum* 31:968, 1988.

Pemberton JH, Rath DM, Ilstrup DM: Evaluation and surgical treatment of severe chronic constipation, *Ann Surg* 214:403, 1991.

Schouten WR, Gordon PH: Constipation. In Gordon PH, Nivatvongs S, eds: *Principles and practice of surgery for the colon, rectum, and anus,* St Louis, 1992, Quality Medical Publishing.

Sloan S: Medical management of constipation, In Brubaker LT, Saclarides TJ, eds: *The female pelvic floor: disorders of function and support,* Philadelphia, 1996, FA Davis.

Sonnenberg A, Koch TR: Epidemiology of constipation in the United States, *Dis Colon Rectum* 32:1, 1989.

Vickery G: Basics of constipation, *Gastroenterol Nurs* 20:125, 1997.

Wexner SD, Cheape JD, Jorge JM, et al: Prospective assessment of biofeedback for the treatment of paradoxical puborectalis contraction, *Dis Colon Rectum* 35:145, 1992.

Wexner SD, Daniel N, Jagelman DG: Colectomy for constipation: physiologic investigation is the key to success, *Dis Colon Rectum* 34:851, 1991.

Young FE, Heckler MM: Laxative drug products for over the counter human use: tentative final monograph, *Fed Reg* 50:2124, 1985.

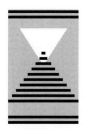

CHAPTER *22*

# *Rectovaginal Fistula*

Janice F. Rafferty

Etiology
   *Trauma*
   *Inflammatory bowel disease*
   *Infection*
   *Radiation*
Surgical Treatment
   *Preoperative preparation*
   *High fistula repair*
   *Midlevel fistula repair*
   *Low fistula repair*
   *Fecal diversion*

Rectovaginal fistula is a congenital or acquired tract between the rectum and the vagina. The communication is lined with epithelium and may occur at any point along the vagina. Rectovaginal fistulas are classified according to their location and size; careful attention to both features allows determination of the approach for surgical repair. In a low rectovaginal fistula, the rectal opening is located close to the dentate line, with the vaginal opening just inside the hymen. In a high rectovaginal fistula, the vaginal opening is near the cervix (or apex of the vagina in a posthysterectomy patient); the communication into the intestinal tract may be located in either the sigmoid colon or rectum. A mid-rectovaginal fistula is found somewhere between the hymen and the cervix. Rectovaginal fistulas range in size from tiny (less than 1 mm in diameter) to large where the rectovaginal defect encompasses the entire posterior vaginal wall.

A patient with a rectovaginal fistula is usually symptomatic. She most often complains of passage of flatus or stool through the vagina. Occasionally the presenting complaint is a recurrent vaginal or bladder infection, the result of fecal soilage. A small fistula may be symptomatic only when loose or liquid stool is passed. It is important to determine the status of the anal sphincter mechanism when the patient's complaints are consistent with fecal seepage.

## ETIOLOGY

There are many different causes of an abnormal epithelialized tract between the rectum and the vagina (Box 22-1); the cause varies with the location of the fistula. Congenital rectovaginal fistulas are rare and are not discussed here.

## Trauma
### *Obstetric*

Episiotomy is commonly performed in the practice of obstetrics. Kozok (1989) reported that approximately 62% of vaginal deliveries in the United States required episiotomy (80% of nulliparous patients and 20% of multiparous patients). A rectal tear or anal sphincter disruption complicates up to one fourth of episiotomies. Although the majority of perineal injuries are successfully repaired at the time of the delivery, dehiscence of an episiotomy repair can occur and is associated with infection, abscess, fistula, or sphincter disruption. It is usually evident by day 3 or 4 after delivery. Up to 1.5% of women who undergo an episioproctotomy develop a rectovaginal fistula. Midline episiotomy with resulting third- or fourth-degree laceration appears to be the greatest risk factor for development of a rectovaginal fistula. Mediolateral episiotomy, more common in British obstetric practice, causes fewer tears into the rectum when compared to midline incision. Rectovaginal fistula following infection and dehiscence of an episiotomy most commonly occurs low in the rectovaginal septum but may extend much higher, especially in the case of a traumatic cloaca.

### *Iatrogenic*

Rectovaginal fistula can follow any surgical procedure that involves the posterior wall of the vagina or the anterior wall of the rectum, such as rectocele repair or transanal excision of tumor. The fistula may result from a direct or unrecognized rectal injury, cautery, anastomotic leak, or infection.

## Inflammatory Bowel Disease

Proctitis from inflammatory bowel disease (IBD), either ulcerative colitis or Crohn's disease, occurs in up to 10% of patients with IBD. Most commonly, a rectovaginal fistula from Crohn's disease is located in the mid-rectovaginal septum. However, in patients with anorectal Crohn's disease, a fistula can extend into the most distal aspect of the vagina or perineum. An anovaginal or rectovaginal fistula in Crohn's disease is more likely to result in proctectomy or

**277**

defunctioning stoma than anal Crohn's disease without rectovaginal fistula.

## Infection

The most common nonobstetric infection causing a rectovaginal fistula is a cryptoglandular abscess located in the anterior aspect of the anal canal. Extension of such an abscess into the vaginal wall can result in fistula formation. Other infectious processes that may fistulize into the vagina include lymphogranuloma venereum, tuberculosis, and Bartholin's abscess. Acquired rectovaginal fistula may be an early manifestation of human immunodeficiency virus infection in girls. Some authors implicate human papilloma virus in poor healing of episiotomy wounds, which may contribute to the development of a postpartum rectovaginal fistula, although this is controversial.

## Radiation

Rectovaginal fistulas develop in up to 6% of women following pelvic irradiation and are dependent on the radiation dosage. Rectovaginal fistulas are most commonly associated with radiation therapy for endometrial, cervical, and vaginal cancer. Fistulas that present early during radiation therapy are more likely to be caused by destruction of the carcinoma, whereas fistulas caused by radiation injury may occur as late as 2 years after therapy. Late fistulas are commonly associated with a rectal stricture. It is critical to determine whether the rectovaginal fistula is caused by recurrent cancer in a patient with a history of genital carcinoma. This often requires examination under anesthesia, with biopsies of the margins of the fistula. Rectovaginal fistulas caused by radiation injury are usually located in the midvagina or proximal vagina; the exact location of the connection with the intestinal tract must be determined before commencing surgical treatment.

**Box 22-1**
### CAUSES OF RECTOVAGINAL FISTULA

Congenital
Trauma
    Obstetric
    Postsurgical
Inflammatory bowel disease
Infection
Radiation
Carcinoma
Lymphoproliferative malignancy
Endometriosis

## SURGICAL TREATMENT
### Preoperative Preparation

Treatment of a rectovaginal fistula depends on the cause, location, and size of the fistula, as well as the condition of the involved tissues. The majority of rectovaginal fistulas following obstetric trauma spontaneously heal, whereas those associated with Crohn's disease or radiation injury have little chance of healing without surgical intervention. The tissues involved in a rectovaginal fistula should be given adequate time to heal following the acute injury. This allows maximum resolution of inflammation as well as a decrease in size of the fistula tract. Most authors recommend a waiting period of 8 to 12 weeks after the injury before attempting surgical repair, although immediate operative repair of a fourth-degree episiotomy dehiscence is recommended by some. Fistulas associated with IBD are unlikely to heal if severe proctitis is present. Inflammation must be controlled by medical treatment, especially if the rectovaginal fistula is low. A reparative procedure is more likely to be successful if the proctitis has been controlled.

For most rectovaginal fistulas, especially postobstetric low fistulas, preoperative evaluation of the anal sphincter with transrectal ultrasound should be considered. This allows clear visualization of the sphincter mechanism, which may be very useful in preoperative surgical planning. Proctoscopy may also be necessary to evaluate for coexisting anorectal disease.

Preoperative bowel preparation should be done for all patients. This reduces the fecal and bacterial load, reducing the risk of postoperative infection and dehiscence of repair. Perioperative antibiotics, both oral and intravenous, should be administered. Consideration should be given to the placement of intraoperative ureteral catheters when using a transabdominal approach to repair a rectovaginal fistula in a previously radiated pelvis.

Several surgical techniques, alone or in combination, are used for the repair of rectovaginal fistulas. Approaches include transanal, transvaginal, perineal, abdominal, and transsacral; most postpartum rectovaginal fistulas are repaired transanally or transvaginally.

### High Fistula Repair

Most surgeons use a transabdominal approach for the repair of a high rectovaginal, or colovaginal, fistula. The cause of high fistulas is usually inflammatory, including diverticulitis and Crohn's disease. Radiation injury, traumatic injury, and carcinoma also must be considered. Bowel resection with primary reanastomosis using nondiseased tissue is the most successful approach.

### Midlevel Fistula Repair

A midlevel rectovaginal fistula caused by trauma can be successfully repaired transrectally or transvaginally once local tissue inflammation has resolved. For the patient with an intact perineum, an intact external anal sphincter, and a fistula in the lower third of the vagina, an endorectal advancement flap repair is usually straightforward (Figs. 22-1 through 22-4). Alternatively, a transvaginal fistula excision and layered closure can be done.

In the endorectal advancement flap procedure, the patient is prone with the hips elevated (Fig. 22-1). The fistula is identified through the anus, and a small probe may be used to follow the tract into the vagina (Fig. 22-2). A hemostatic solution of 0.5% lidocaine with 1:200,000 epinephrine may be injected submucosally. The rectal ostium is circumscribed by an incision placed 0.5 to 1 cm from the margins of the tract. A broad-based flap of mucosa, submucosa, and circular muscle is developed and advanced distally. Before suturing the flap over the fistula site, the epithelium-lined tract is excised and the muscular wall of the rectum is reapproximated with absorbable suture (Fig. 22-3). The flap is then secured with interrupted absorbable sutures (Fig. 22-4). The vaginal side is left open to provide drainage of the surgical site. Several authors report a high rate of success with this approach, even when used for the treatment of rectovaginal fistula in the setting of Crohn's disease. Care must be taken to ensure that the rectal mucosa is not advanced too far, creating a mucosal ectropion and "wet anus."

If the rectovaginal fistula is caused by radiation, local repair is not likely to be successful; healing is impaired by radiation-induced vasculitis. Proctectomy may be required, and if the anal sphincter mechanism is competent, a coloanal pull-through procedure or coloanal anastomosis can be performed. Proximal diversion of the fecal stream should accompany this technically demanding procedure. A more complex repair has been described by Bricker et al. (1986) but is not commonly used. It involves an onlay patch of well-vascularized intestine and has the advantage of requiring only anterior mobilization of the rectum. Bricker's success rate has been difficult to duplicate.

## Low Fistula Repair

Simple fistulotomy is the treatment of choice for very low fistulas lying distal to the anal sphincter mechanism. Extreme caution must be taken when considering a fistulotomy near the anterior anal sphincter mechanism because even a normal sphincter mechanism is attenuated in this region.

For rectovaginal fistulas in the lower third of the vagina, especially those that have followed obstetric trauma and have resulted in a damaged perineal body and anal sphincter mechanism, most gynecologists favor conversion of the fistula to an episioproctotomy followed by layered closure. This is done with the patient in supine position via a perineal approach and has been described by Nichols (1993). Episioproctotomy permits excision of the entire fistulous tract followed by repair similar to that of a fresh fourth-degree perineal laceration (Fig. 22-5). The technique requires transection and reunification of the external anal sphincter and the lower part of the internal sphincter. There

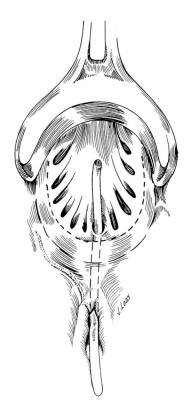

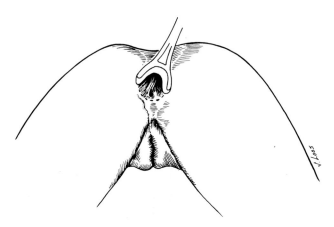

**Fig. 22-1**  The patient is placed in prone position with the hips elevated in preparation for a low or midlevel rectovaginal fistula repair.

**Fig. 22-2**  With the patient in prone position, the anal speculum is placed posteriorly. The rectovaginal fistula is identified by placing a small probe from the anus into the vagina. The dotted line outlines the incision in the rectal mucosa used to develop the advancement flap.

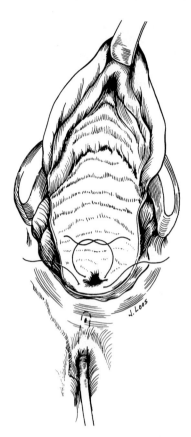

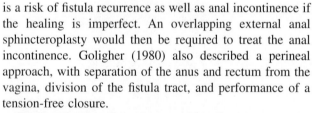

**Fig. 22-3** The epithelium-lined fistula tract is excised, and the muscular wall of the rectum is reapproximated with absorbable suture. The rectal advancement flap has been mobilized and is ready to be placed over the site of the fistula repair.

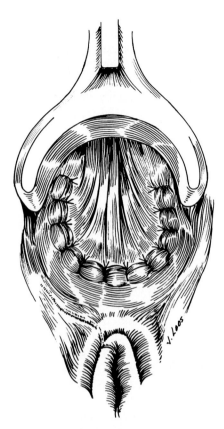

**Fig. 22-4** The flap is secured with interrupted absorbable sutures.

is a risk of fistula recurrence as well as anal incontinence if the healing is imperfect. An overlapping external anal sphincteroplasty would then be required to treat the anal incontinence. Goligher (1980) also described a perineal approach, with separation of the anus and rectum from the vagina, division of the fistula tract, and performance of a tension-free closure.

For low fistulas above the external anal sphincter, as for lower midlevel fistulas, the approach favored by many colorectal surgeons is transanal repair using an endorectal advancement flap (see Figs. 22-1 through 22-4). Repair from the rectal side has the advantage of correction of the defect from the high-pressure side, perhaps resulting in less frequent failure of repair. Endorectal advancement flap also has the benefit of the interposition of healthy tissue, which is beneficial in the repair of both complex and recurrent fistulas. Interpositions of bulbocavernosus muscle, gracilis muscle, and labial fat have been reported.

### Fecal Diversion

Diversion of the fecal stream is sometimes required to allow adequate healing of the rectovaginal septum. Construction

of a stoma is rarely necessary before attempt at primary repair. However, if perineal sepsis is severe, early diversion of the fecal stream may be necessary. Diversion of the fecal stream by construction of a proximal stoma should be considered following a complex repair of rectovaginal fistula, such as a coloanal anastomosis, a Bricker onlay-type repair, or myofascial grafting. In addition, if previous attempts at repair of a rectovaginal fistula have failed, consideration should be given to construction of a stoma before an additional attempt at surgical reconstruction.

### SUMMARY

Rectovaginal fistula can be congenital or the result of trauma, IBD, carcinoma, radiation, or infection. The cause, location, and size of the fistula, as well as the competence of the anal sphincter mechanism, must be determined before repair. Repair of fistula resulting from obstetric trauma has a high rate of success, but those from other causes are more difficult to cure. Several different approaches to surgical repair have been described; the best approach is determined by the location and cause of the fistula.

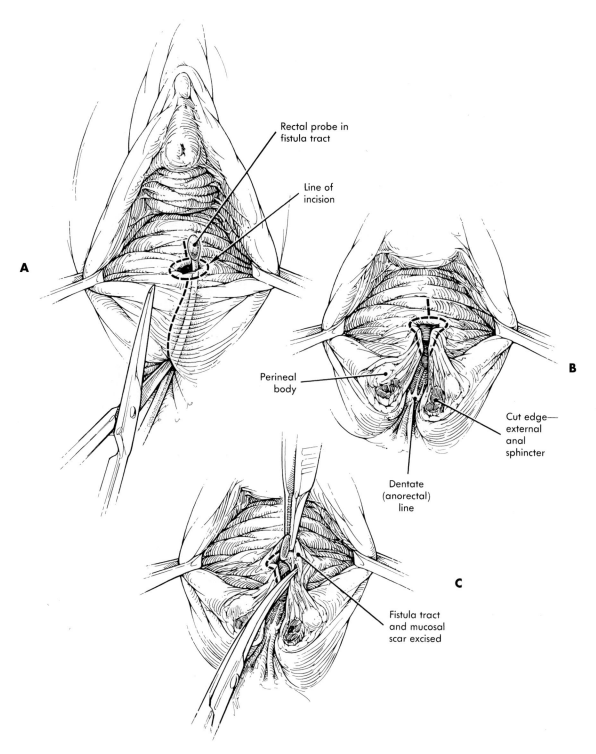

Rectal probe in
fistula tract

Line of
incision

**A**

Perineal
body

**B**

Cut edge—
external
anal
sphincter

Dentate
(anorectal)
line

**C**

Fistula tract
and mucosal
scar excised

**Fig. 22-5**   Repair of a fourth-degree perineal laceration with coexistent low rectovaginal fistula. A malleable probe is inserted through the fistula tract, as shown in **A,** and an incision along this probe exposes the tissue, as shown in **B.** The fistula tract is excised along the site of the dashed line, as shown in **B** and **C.**

From Nichols DH: Repair of rectal fistula and of old complete perineal laceration. In Nichols DH, ed: *Gynecologic and obstetric surgery,* St Louis, 1993, Mosby.                    *Continued*

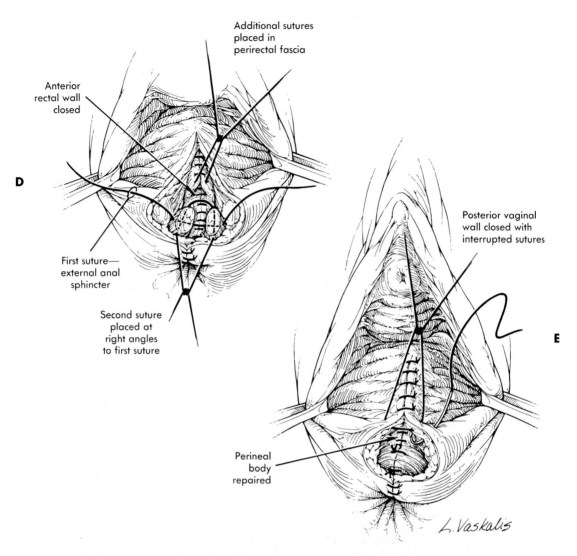

**Fig. 22-5, cont'd** The submucosa and muscularis of the anterior rectal wall are closed with interrupted sutures, as shown in **D,** and this is inverted by an additional layer of sutures placed in the perirectal fascia. The edges of the external anal sphincter are dissected out, and the scar tissue around their severed ends is reapproximated with two interrupted sutures placed at right angles to one another. As shown in **E,** the full thickness of the posterior vaginal wall is closed with interrupted sutures and the perineal body restored with a few interrupted stitches.

From Nichols DH: Repair of rectal fistula and of old complete perineal laceration. In Nichols DH, ed: *Gynecologic and obstetric surgery,* St Louis, 1993, Mosby.

## BIBLIOGRAPHY

Allen-Mersh TC, Wilson EJ, Hope-Stone HF: The management of late radiation-induced rectal injury after treatment of carcinoma of the uterus, *Surg Gynecol Obstet* 164:521, 1987.

Barber HR, Graser EA: *Surgical disease in pregnancy,* Philadelphia, 1976, WB Saunders.

Borgstein ES, Broadhead RL: Acquired rectovaginal fistula, *Arch Dis Child* 71:165, 1994.

Bricker EM, Kraybill WG, Lopez MJ: Functional results after postirradiation rectal reconstruction, *World J Surg* 10:249, 1986.

Coats PM, Chan KK, Wilkins M, et al: A comparison between midline and mediolateral episiotomies, *Br J Obstet Gynaecol* 87:408, 1980.

Froines EJ, Palmer DL: Surgical therapy for rectovaginal fistulas in ulcerative colitis, *Dis Colon Rectum* 34:925, 1991.

Fry RD, Kodner IJ: Rectovaginal fistula, *Surg Ann* 27:113, 1995.

Goligher JC: Rectovaginal fistula. In Goligher JC, ed: *Surgery of the anus, rectum and colon,* ed 4, London, 1980, Spottiswoode Ballantyne.

Homsi R, Daikoku NH, Littlejohn J, et al: Episiotomy: risks of dehiscence and rectovaginal fistula, *Obstet Gynecol Surv* 49:803, 1994.

Kimose H, Fischer L, Spjeldnaes N, et al: Late radiation injury of the colon and rectum: surgical management and outcome, *Dis Colon Rectum* 32:684, 1989.

Kodner IJ, Mazor A, Shemesh EI, et al: Endorectal advancement flap repair of rectal, vaginal, and other complicated anorectal fistulas, *Surgery* 114:682, 1993.

Kozok LJ: Surgical and non-surgical procedures associated with hospital delivery in the United States: 1980-1987, *Birth* 16:209, 1989.

Legino LJ, Woods MP, Rayburn WF, et al: Third and fourth degree perineal tears. Fifty years' experience at a university hospital, *J Reprod Med* 33:323, 1988.

Lowry AC, Thorsen AG, Rothenberger DA: Repair of simple rectovaginal fistulas: influence of previous repairs, *Dis Colon Rectum* 31:676, 1988.

Mattingly RF: Anal incontinence and rectovaginal fistulas. In Mattingly RF, ed: *TeLinde's operative gynecology,* ed 5, Philadelphia, 1977, JB Lippincott.

Nichols DH: Repair of rectal fistula and of old complete perineal laceration. In Nichols DH, ed: *Gynecologic and obstetric surgery,* St Louis, 1993, Mosby.

Nowacki MP: Ten years of experience with Park's coloanal sleeve anastomosis for the treatment of post-irradiation rectovaginal fistula, *Eur J Surg Oncol* 17:563, 1991.

Radcliffe AG, Ritchie JK, Hawley PR, et al: Anovaginal and rectovaginal fistulas in Crohn's disease, *Dis Colon Rectum* 31:94, 1988.

Scott NA, Nair A, Hughes LF: Anovaginal and rectovaginal fistula in patients with Crohn's disease, *Br J Surg* 79:1379, 1992.

Snyder RR, Hammond TL, Hankins GDV: Human papilloma virus associated with poor healing of episiotomy repairs, *Obstet Gynecol* 76:664, 1990.

Thacker SB, Banta HD: Benefits and risks of episiotomy: an interpretive review of the English language literature, 1860-1980, *Obstet Gynecol Surv* 38:322, 1983.

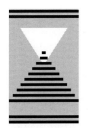

CHAPTER 23
# Rectal Prolapse

Feza H. Remzi and Tracy L. Hull

Rectal prolapse is full-thickness intussusception of the rectum toward and sometimes through the anal canal (Fig. 23-1). It can be entirely internal (occult) or external to the anal sphincters. It has been known for centuries and described in the medical literature. Although its cause is still unclear, it is much more common in adult parous women, and thus occasionally presents to gynecologists. Various operations have been described in the surgical literature, but the types of treatment and the surgical approach still vary significantly from one institution to another. In this chapter we discuss the etiology, epidemiology, clinical features, and evaluation of rectal prolapse. Common surgical techniques, published results, and our experience with this disorder are described.

## ETIOLOGY

There are two accepted theories regarding the etiology of rectal prolapse. In 1912, Moschcowitz proposed that rectal prolapse is a sliding hernia that protrudes through a defect in the pelvic fascia at the anterior rectal wall level. In 1968, a second theory was proposed by Broden and Snellman. These authors demonstrated with cine-defecography full-thickness prolapse starting as an internal intussusception of the rectum with a lead point proximal to the anal verge. Currently, rectal intussusception is the accepted mechanism of rectal prolapse. This theory was reinforced by Theuerkauf et al. (1970), who used radio-opaque markers applied to the rectal mucosa to demonstrate prolapse secondary to intussusception.

Various anatomic disorders are related to prolapse. These include a deep peritoneal cul-de-sac or pouch of Douglas,

loss of posterior rectal fixation, patulous anal sphincter, diastasis of the levator ani, redundant rectum and sigmoid colon, and loss of a horizontal position of the rectum with attenuation of its sacral and pelvic attachments. In women, uterine and vaginal support abnormalities often coexist with rectal prolapse. The ideal rectal prolapse repair should correct as many of these abnormalities as possible and a multidisciplinary approach may be advisable. For rectal prolapse, the best repair is achieved not by addressing each abnormality individually, but by addressing them in unity while repairing the intussusception itself.

## EPIDEMIOLOGY

The true incidence of rectal prolapse is unknown. It occurs at the extremes of age and can even be seen in children less than 3 years old. Malnutrition and cystic fibrosis appear to be predisposing factors in this young age group. There is equal gender distribution and conservative management is usually successful for children with rectal prolapse. In adults, rectal prolapse is more common in women. Peak incidence is after the fifth decade and there is a 6:1 female-to-male ratio. Men are equally distributed throughout age groups. Rectal prolapse can be seen in nulliparous women, but is more common in multiparous women.

## CLINICAL FEATURES

Patients afflicted with rectal prolapse usually present to their physicians because of social embarrassment from soilage. The typical symptoms are prolapse of tissue through the anal sphincter complex, mucus discharge, and bleeding. The prolapse is covered with mucosa, which can secrete a significant amount of mucus. This may lead to perianal excoriation and itching. Bleeding is caused by trauma or venous mucosal congestion. Patients with internal (occult) prolapse experience incomplete evacuation of rectal contents, tenesmus, and rectal pain.

Association of rectal prolapse with a history of senile dementia, neurologic disorders, and infectious disorders has been reported. Rectal prolapse is also associated with straining, constipation, previous gynecologic surgery, and

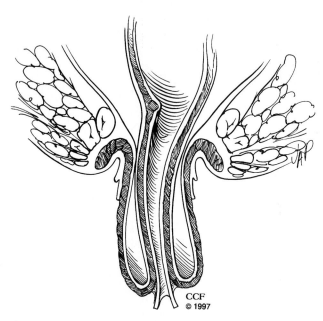

**Fig. 23-1** Full-thickness rectal prolapse protruding through the anal canal.

incontinence. Straining (or other unknown anatomic abnormalities) in men and younger women may push the anterior wall of the upper rectum against the anal canal and cause trauma leading to ulceration, irritation, and bleeding. This is known as a solitary rectal ulcer. At our institution, 18% of patients with prolapse reported straining. Constipation is also associated with rectal prolapse. At our institution, 42% of 169 patients had associated constipation. This rate varies between 15% and 65% in the literature. Previous gynecologic surgery is reported to be associated with rectal prolapse; 35% of our patients had undergone a previous hysterectomy. In addition, uterine and/or vaginal support abnormalities and their associated symptoms may coexist with rectal prolapse. Fecal incontinence varies from 28% to 88% in the literature; 38% of our patients experience this symptom. Thus, complete assessment of patients with prolapse should include evaluation for constipation, incontinence, and other pelvic floor disorders such as rectocele, cystocele, and enterocele. Staged or combined surgical correction of pelvic floor disorders may be needed for resolution of the patient's symptoms.

## EVALUATION

Evaluation of the patient with rectal prolapse starts with a thorough history and physical examination. The evaluation is important in confirming the diagnosis and in decision-making for the surgical alternatives. Age, level of activity, comorbid conditions, and living conditions are important issues in determining the type of surgical therapy for individual patients. A careful neurologic history and examination are done. An obstetric history as well as a gynecologic and surgical history, specifically for hysterectomy and vaginal prolapse repairs, should be taken in all women. Symptoms related to fecal and urinary incontinence and constipation should be sought.

Occasionally prolapse is not externally visible in the office. A Fleet enema along with straining on the commode may be needed to reproduce the prolapse. It is important to differentiate full-thickness rectal prolapse from hemorrhoidal prolapse. The position of the prolapse on the commode is helpful.

A thorough anorectal examination starts with inspection of the perianal skin, where signs of excoriation secondary to itching or mucus soiling may be noted. The anocutaneous reflex can then be tested. Digital examination includes checking for sphincter defects, along with squeeze and resting pressures. Occasionally, the prolapsing segment can be felt on digital examination. An associated rectocele, cystocele, or enterocele should be sought. Proctoscopy or flexible sigmoidoscopy is needed to exclude the possibility of a neoplasm and allows the opportunity to biopsy ulcers or other localized inflammation.

Because a significant portion of patients with prolapse have associated constipation, incontinence, or pelvic floor disorders, it is worthwhile to include certain investigational tools in the workup of these patients. These must be individualized, however, with tests obtained based on the patient's symptoms and level of disability. A colonic transit marker study may be important in patients with severe constipation. This test measures the amount of time it takes for markers to traverse the colon. Patients swallow a set number of radio-opaque markers and serial abdominal radiographs are obtained to evaluate passage of these markers. Patients with a prolonged time of transit through the colon may benefit from resection of their colon with preservation of the rectum and a rectopexy. When additional pelvic outlet obstruction or pelvic support disorders are suspected, defecography can be obtained. It may show a sigmoid colon that prolapses into the anal canal with straining or internal intussusception (occult) that does not go through the anal canal.

Anal manometry is used to address associated incontinence. Matheson and Keighley (1981) found normal anal pressures in continent patients; however, incontinent patients had decreased resting and squeeze anal pressures. Many patients with prolapse associated with incontinence have nerve damage that is believed to be due to traction injury of the pudendal nerves caused by prior obstetric injury or the rectal prolapse. Continent prolapse patients may not show manometric or electromyographic signs of denervation. Anal manometry may help to determine which patients will regain continence after their prolapse repair. Studies from Yoshioka et al. (1989) and Williams et al. (1991) showed that patients who remained incontinent had significantly lower resting and squeeze pressures preoperatively than those whose incontinence improved postoperatively. Thus, anal manometry gives preoperative information that distinguishes patients who may have a more optimal outcome. However, it often does not change the clinical or surgical approach to the patient.

## COMMON SURGICAL REPAIRS FOR PROLAPSE

The type of surgical procedure is determined by many of the patient's characteristics such as age, comorbid conditions, degree of the prolapse, and associated pelvic disorders. The goals of the surgical procedure are to repair the prolapse and to attempt to improve associated constipation or incontinence. Over 50 procedures have been described for rectal prolapse. These procedures can be classified into two main categories: perineal and transabdominal repairs. Perineal repairs are felt to be less invasive and hence viewed as causing less morbidity for patients. They are generally favored for frail elderly patients but some institutions also favor this approach for their younger patients. The perineal approach carries the risk of infection and possible suture line or wound breakdown. Alternatively, abdominal operations are favored by some surgeons because it is felt that prolapse recurrence is less common with transabdominal than perineal procedures. This approach can have complications such as anastomotic leak, abdominal sepsis, stricture, and adhesions and generally requires a general anesthetic. Therefore, abdominal operations are reserved for patients who can tolerate the rigors of a laparotomy. The introduction of laparoscopy in the last decade has added a new dimension to prolapse surgery. If shown to be feasible and equally efficacious, it will reduce the postoperative recovery time of transabdominal repairs.

Our preference for all repairs is to have the patient undergo a full mechanical bowel preparation. We give perioperative antibiotics such as 500 mg metronidazole and a second-generation cephalosporin intravenously (for patients allergic to these medications, alternative broad-spectrum medications are used for prophylaxis against enteric organisms). All patients have a Foley catheter and pneumatic compression stockings during prolapse surgery.

## Perineal Repairs
### Delorme Procedure

The Delorme procedure was first described in 1900. It was not used commonly until Uhlig and Sullivan reported their experience in 1979. The technique is simple and can be done under regional or local anesthesia, so it is an option for the severely debilitated patient. We prefer to perform the operation in the prone jackknife position, but it can also be done in the lithotomy position. After the patient is positioned, the perineum and vagina are prepped. We use No. 1 sutures applied in four places around the perianal skin to evert the anus. Others prefer retractors such as the Lone Star. The operation is begun by injecting 1:100,000 epinephrine solution circumferentially into the submucosal plane just proximal to the dentate line (some surgeons prefer a Pratt

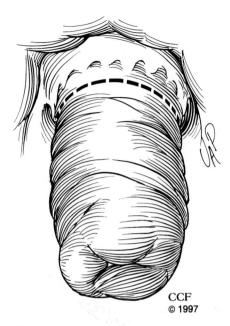

**Fig. 23-2** Incision for a Delorme procedure 1 to 1.5 cm above the dentate line. The incision goes through the mucosa and submucosa initially, stripping this tube from the underlying internal anal sphincter and, more proximally, from the rectal muscular cuff.

bivalve speculum or a Hill Fergeson retractor to enhance visualization). This injection delineates the dissecting plane and diminishes blood loss. Using electrocoagulation, the dissection is started in a circumferential manner 1 to 1.5 cm above the dentate line (Fig. 23-2), creating a plane between the submucosa and the internal sphincter muscle. Once this plane is started, the free edge of mucosa and submucosa is tagged with sutures for ease in handling and for creating traction to ease dissection. Continuing in a circumferential direction and using liberal amounts of injectable saline in the plane between the submucosa and the muscular cuff, scissors (we prefer fistula scissors) are used to divide the attachments and deliver the submucosa and mucosal cuff out of the rectum and anus. Penetrating blood vessels encountered during the dissection can be treated with coagulation. It is important to maintain strict hemostasis during the dissection to avoid hematoma after completion of the procedure. The dissection continues until the rectal mucosa cannot be pulled down any further; usually 10 to 15 cm can be mobilized.

During this phase of the operation we use copious amounts of antibiotic solution such as tetracycline to irrigate the surgical field. After the dissection is completed, the rectal muscle is plicated with sutures such as No. 2-0 Polyglactin 910 suture on a UR-6 needle (Vicryl; Ethicon, Inc., Somerville, New Jersey). A total of eight sutures spaced circumferentially are used for this plication. The dissected mucosa is excised and the proximal line of resection is approximated to the distal line of the incision using delayed absorbable suture (Fig. 23-3).

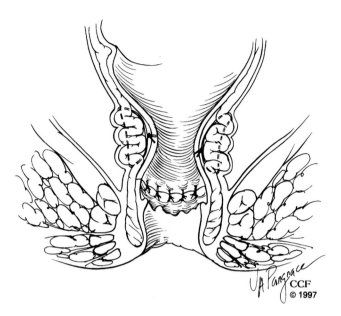

**Fig. 23-3**  Completed Delorme procedure. Notice that the rectal wall is plicated with sutures in an accordion-type fashion and is situated above the anal sphincters. The anastomosis is just above the dentate line.

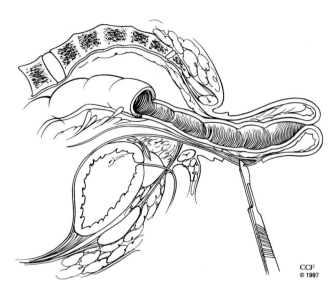

**Fig. 23-4**  Altmeier procedure (perineal proctosigmoidectomy). An incision is made with the bovie or knife (as shown here) 1 to 1.5 cm above the dentate line. Note that the patient is depicted in the prone jackknife position.

The recurrence rate after this procedure ranges from 7% to 22% in different series and is tolerated well in high-risk patients. Incontinence usually improves after this repair and is felt to be secondary to the rectal muscle wall plication, which creates a bulky, donutlike circumferential mass around the upper anal canal. Improvement in incontinence is reported in 44% to 83% of patients. Constipation has not been reported to worsen after this repair.

### Altmeier Procedure (Perineal Rectosigmoidectomy)

Perineal rectosigmoidectomy was first described by Mikulicz in 1889. Altmeier et al. (1971) first reported its safe use in elderly and debilitated patients, describing excellent results. Many prefer this procedure for incarcerated or gangrenous prolapse. This procedure removes the rectum by the perineal approach and a potential disadvantage is the loss of the rectal reservoir. Additionally, in patients who have undergone previous rectal or sigmoid resections, care must be exercised in doing this operation because the inferior mesenteric vessels may have been previously ligated and the blood supply to this area may have been altered.

This procedure can be done in the lithotomy position or prone jackknife position under general or regional anesthesia. We prefer the prone jackknife position because it allows all assistants to see the field and illumination of the pelvis is superior in this position. First the prolapse is reproduced by gentle traction with clamps such as Allis or Babcock. The submucosa is injected with 1:100,000 epinephrine solution. A circumferential incision is made 1.5 to 2.0 cm above the dentate line (Fig. 23-4) with the bovie or a scalpel. The

incision is deepened through the muscular layer until extrarectal fat is encountered (Fig. 23-5). Mesorectal vessels are ligated (Fig. 23-6), proceeding in a circumferential manner. As the cephalad dissection continues, a hernia sac may be encountered anteriorly and opened, and the abdominal cavity may be entered. When no additional bowel can be delivered without tension, the bowel is marked; this will become the line of transection. At this stage, particularly in incontinent patients, a levatorplasty can be performed by placing nonabsorbable sutures such as No. 2-0 polypropylene suture (Prolene; Ethicon, Inc., Somerville, New Jersey) anteriorly, loosely approximating the levators (Fig. 23-7). Some surgeons prefer to place sutures posteriorly also. The prolapsed segment is transected (Fig. 23-8) and an anastomosis is created with circumferential, full-thickness interrupted No. 2-0 delayed absorbable sutures (Fig. 23-9).

An alternative to the hand-sewn technique is to use a circular stapler. After transection of the bowel, pursestring sutures are placed using No. 0 polypropylene suture on an SH needle at the proximal and distal lines of resection. This stapling technique is shown in Fig. 23-10, A through D.

The major advantage of this procedure is that it can be done without a formal laparotomy. Postoperative constipation is also low. This procedure can be complicated by anastomotic leak, infection, and stricture. The postoperative incontinence rate is less dramatically improved than with abdominal procedures and incontinence can be worsened by resection of the rectal reservoir. However, eliminating the prolapse may allow the sphincters to regain strength and improve continence. Adding a levator repair can dramatically improve continence postoperatively. Williams et al.

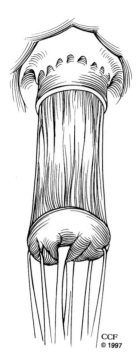

**Fig. 23-5** The incision for the perineal proctosigmoidectomy divides all layers of the rectal wall until the extrarectal fat is encountered.

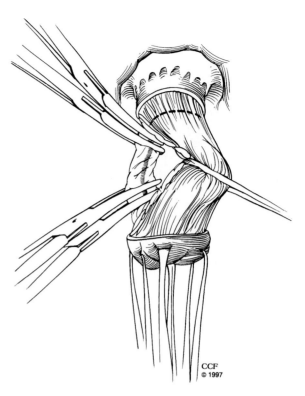

**Fig. 23-6** The mesorectal vessels are divided and ligated.

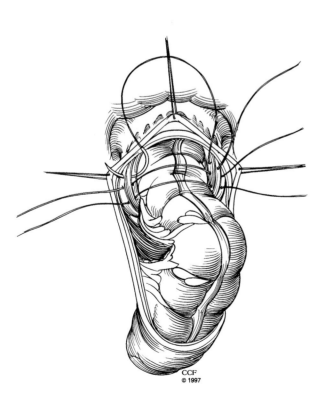

**Fig. 23-7** Levatorplasty may be performed posteriorly and/or anteriorly.

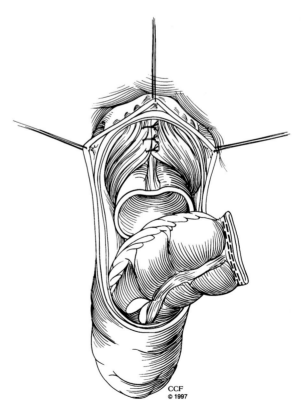

**Fig. 23-8** The prolapsed segment is transected. Note the completed levatorplasty.

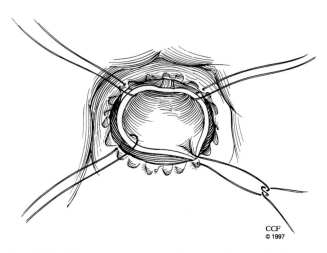

CCF
© 1997

**Fig. 23-9** The anastomosis can be sewn by hand with full-thickness circumferential interrupted sutures.

(1991) from the University of Minnesota demonstrated a 91% rate of improved incontinence with addition of a levator repair, compared to 46% improvement without the levatorplasty. Additionally, others have reported improved incontinence with a levator repair. This approach should be considered for patients with severe full-thickness rectal prolapse and incontinence who otherwise may not tolerate an abdominal procedure. Additionally, some surgeons use this approach as the preferred treatment for healthy or young patients with prolapse. Reported recurrence rates vary between 0% and 39% and complication rates are low.

### Anal Encirclement

Perineal procedures that narrow the anal orifice by encircling them with an artificial material, such as the Thiersch procedure, are associated with a high incidence of complications and do not address the underlying problem. They have a limited place in the current management of rectal prolapse.

## Transabdominal Repairs

Transabdominal repairs provide the best outcome and functional results for the treatment of rectal prolapse. They allow restoration of the normal anatomy and repair of associated abnormalities. They can be classified as rectal mobilization with rectopexy alone, rectal mobilization with rectopexy and resection, or resection alone. In the last decade, the laparoscopic approach has been successfully used to perform each of the abdominal repairs. It has brought a new dimension to the management of this problem in colorectal surgery.

Types of transabdominal repair vary greatly from one country to another, from one institution to another, and even from one surgeon to another in the same institution.

### Rectal Mobilization with Rectopexy

Rectal mobilization is performed posteriorly in the presacral space and carried to the coccyx or levators. Some surgeons preserve the lateral stalks; others divide all or part of these. Anteriorly the mobilization is carried to the upper third of the vagina. All rectopexies require this degree of rectal mobilization. There are many variations of the rectopexy; however, the basic principle is to suspend the rectum to the sacrum either with a suture material or with the assistance of a foreign material such as Teflon mesh (CR Bard, Inc., Billerica, Massachusetts) or polyvinyl alcohol (Ivalon) sponge. Each of these types of rectopexy is individually discussed.

### Ripstein Procedure

Ripstein and Lanter (1963) described an anterior rectopexy that is commonly performed in the United States. After mobilization of the rectum, the rectopexy is performed by placing a 5-cm by about 20-cm strip of mesh around the rectum and suturing the free ends of the mesh to the presacral fascia with nonabsorbable sutures. The mesh is also secured to the antimesenteric border of the rectum and the rectum is pulled straight out of the pelvis while the sutures are being placed. The mesh is wrapped loosely enough to allow a thumb or two fingers between the rectum and the sacrum. Alternatively, some secure the mesh to the fascia at its midportion and wrap each free end of mesh around the rectum, securing it to the antimesenteric border of the rectum. This leaves about a third of the antimesenteric surface uncovered with mesh. This modification has been done to decrease the rate of impaction seen when the mesh completely encircles the rectum. Ripstein himself now uses the posterior rectal sling rather than an anterior sling to decrease the problem with constipation.

This procedure has been praised for the low recurrence rate and criticized for the postoperative obstructive complications. Gordon and Hoexter (1978) polled members of the American Society of Colon and Rectal Surgeons, obtaining information on 1111 Ripstein procedures. This revealed a recurrence rate of 2.3%, sling-related complication rate of 16.5%, and a reoperation rate of 4.1%. Postoperative constipation should be interpreted carefully because many patients who undergo prolapse surgery suffer from constipation preoperatively. One of the largest series using the Ripstein repair was reported from the Cleveland Clinic Foundation. Tjandra et al. (1993) reported the outcomes of 129 patients, of whom 42 (33%) had constipation after the Ripstein procedure. Of these 42, 27 (64%) had constipation before the procedure. The recurrence rate of prolapse was 7%. Additionally, 35% of patients were dissatisfied after the Ripstein procedure, based on a personal interview using a standard questionnaire. Because of these results, we prefer not to perform a Ripstein procedure in patients with preoperative obstructive symptoms or significant bowel dysfunction.

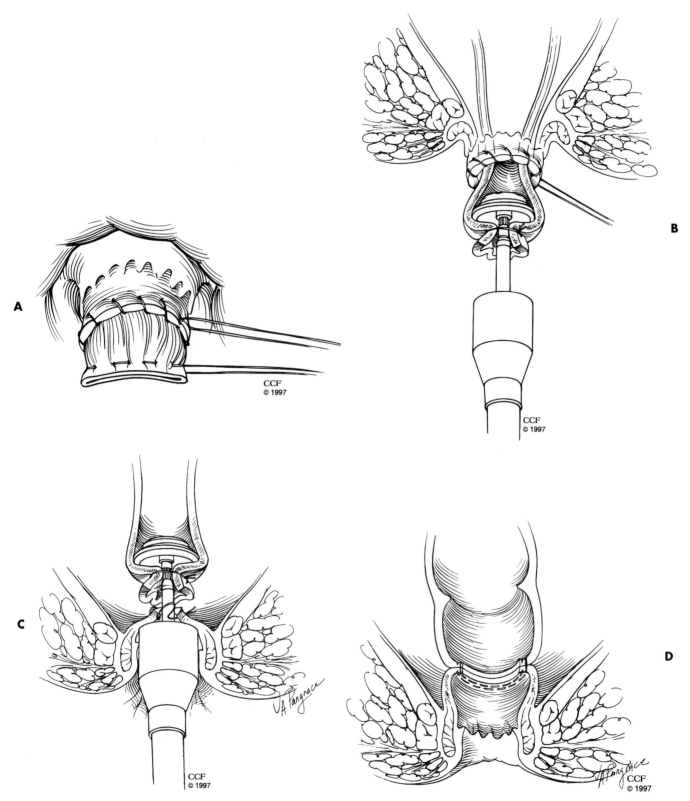

**Fig. 23-10**    Altmeier procedure using circular stapler. **A,** Pursestring sutures are placed on the proximal and distal lines of transected bowel. **B,** The anvil is extruded from the gun and the proximal pursestring is tied. Note that the anvil and gun remain intact for this anastomosis. **C,** The proximal resection line is pushed into the pelvis and the distal pursestring is tied. **D,** The completed anastomosis.

### Wells Procedure (Ivalon Sponge)

Historically, British surgeons have preferred the posterior rectopexy wrap described by Wells (1959) over the Ripstein procedure. In the Wells procedure, an Ivalon sponge made of polyvinyl alcohol is used instead of the mesh. It is placed posteriorly and wrapped partially around the bowel. This repair was believed to prevent the constipation associated with the traditional anterior Ripstein repair. Nonetheless, it is important to note that the constipation rate following the Wells procedure is 44% to 48%.

### Sutured Rectopexy

Some surgeons have argued that the use of foreign material to perform a rectopexy is not only unnecessary but also risky in the event of postoperative complications such as an abscess. Additionally, in patients with preoperative constipation or extremely redundant sigmoid, resection of this redundant colon may be contemplated. It is controversial to use synthetic material in the setting of bowel resection because it may increase the risk of infection. For this reason, sutured rectopexy has been advocated. In fact, excellent results have been obtained in a number of series by suturing the lateral stalks to presacral fascia. These results are similar or even superior to those reported with rectopexy procedures using foreign material. However, 31% to 87% of patients are severely constipated after this procedure.

### Resection and Rectopexy

Rectopexy along with resection was initially described by Frykman in 1955. As originally described, this operation includes mobilization of the rectum via the abdominal route, elevation of the rectum as high as possible out of the pelvis, suturing the rectum to the periosteum of the sacrum, suturing the endopelvic fascia anteriorly to the rectum to obliterate the cul-de-sac, and segmental resection of excessive sigmoid colon with an end-to-end anastomosis. Most surgeons performing this procedure no longer repair the pelvic floor.

We perform this operation by mobilizing the sigmoid colon and dividing the mesentery. The rectum is mobilized as previously described. We prefer to resect the sigmoid colon and then perform the anastomosis either by handsewing or with the circular stapler. The splenic flexure is mobilized if needed. The rectopexy is performed by straightening the rectum (pulling out of the pelvis) and placing two or three nonabsorbable sutures from the lateral stalks to the flat portion of the sacrum at the level of S2 or S3 (Fig. 23-11). We prefer No. 0 braided polyester (Ethibond; Ethicon, Inc., Somerville, New Jersey) suture; others at our institution use No. 0 or 1 polypropylene suture. Before tying the rectopexy sutures, we place a rigid proctoscope through the anus and above the anastomosis to ensure that the sutures are not tied too tightly, contributing to defecation problems.

Excellent results have been reported with this technique. Watts et al. (1985) reported on 102 patients with only a

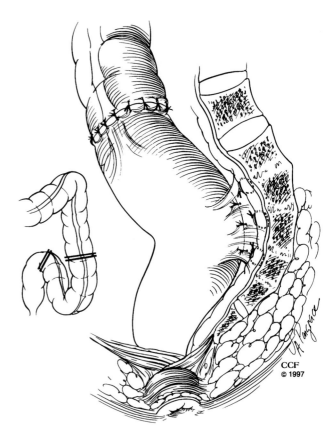

**Fig. 23-11**  Rectopexy with sigmoid resection. A sigmoid resection with a colorectal anastomosis has been performed. The rectum has been pulled out of the pelvis and straightened. The lateral rectal stalks have been sutured to the sacrum.

1.9% recurrence rate. Anastomotic complications occurred in 4% of these patients, with half requiring surgical intervention. Other authors have also reported low recurrence rates (0% to 9%). We obtained improved functional outcome in 18 patients who went through this type of repair. Incontinence rates decreased from 28% to 17% and constipation decreased from 37% to 19% postoperatively.

### Resection

Resection alone has been advocated with an anastomosis in the mid- to low- rectum. The Mayo Clinic (Schlinkert et al.) reported in 1985 on 92 patients who underwent this technique. The recurrence rate was 9%; however, there was significant morbidity with this low anastomosis and increased incontinence was observed postoperatively.

## OUTCOME AND CHOICE OF PROCEDURE

In this review, different types of procedures for the treatment of rectal prolapse have been discussed. There is no one "best" procedure for patients with rectal prolapse. To determine which operation is appropriate for each individual patient, the entire patient must be considered. Perineal repairs are associated with higher recurrence rates, but the morbidity is lower than with an abdominal approach. Therefore, the perineal approach may be the procedure of choice in frail patients with extensive comorbid conditions. If the prolapse is extensive, perineal proctosigmoidectomy is considered. Levatorplasty (posterior and/or anterior) may be added, particularly if the patient is incontinent. In debilitated patients with previous left colon resections or minimal prolapse, the Delorme procedure may be optimal.

Overall, the abdominal approach is favored when comparing recurrence rates and the improvement in functional outcome (in regard to incontinence and constipation). However, the abdominal approach is associated with higher morbidity and mortality. In healthy patients without significant risk factors, this may be the preferred approach. If the patient has no preoperative incontinence but constipation is a contributing symptom, the resection and rectopexy is favored. Also, if the sigmoid is redundant or kinks after the rectum is pulled out of the pelvis to perform the rectopexy, a resection should be entertained. In patients with preoperative incontinence, resection may add to the incontinence. At our institution, the Ripstein procedure is rarely used because of problems with postoperative constipation. Many patients with rectal prolapse have functional defecation problems. Correcting the prolapse may not alleviate the defecation problems, so the patient must be appraised of this preoperatively.

Regarding laproscopic surgery, recently Eu et al. (1995) presented our experience with this approach and the results were encouraging. In patients without associated constipation, rectal mobilization and suture rectopexy was performed. If constipation was an associated symptom, sigmoid resection was added to the procedure. The procedures performed are the same as are done during an open laparotomy. Over 20 patients were treated using a laparoscopic approach. There have been no recurrences and the postoperative recovery time appears to be faster.

In conclusion, the choice of surgical procedures are tailored to each individual person with rectal prolapse. Associated conditions and problems are considered to provide optimal results with the lowest morbidity and mortality.

## BIBLIOGRAPHY

Abou-Enein A: Prolapse of the rectum in young men: treatment with a modified Roscoe Graham operation, *Dis Colon Rectum* 22:117, 1978.

Altmeier WA, Culbertson WR, Schowengerdt C, et al: Nineteen years' experience with the one-stage perineal repair of rectal prolapse, *Ann Surg* 173:993, 1971.

Altmeier WA, Giusefi J, Hoxworth P: Treatment of extensive prolapse of the rectum in aged or debilitated patients, *Arch Surg* 65:72, 1952.

Blatchford GJ, Perry RE, Thorson AG, et al: Rectopexy without resection for rectal prolapse, *Am J Surg* 158:574, 1989.

Broden B, Snellman B: Procidentia of the rectum studied with cine radiography: a contribution to the discussion of causative mechanism, *Dis Colon Rectum* 11:330, 1968.

Deen KI, Grant E, Billingham C, et al: Abdominal resection rectopexy with pelvic floor repair versus perineal rectosigmoidectomy and pelvic floor repair for full-thickness rectal prolapse, *Br J Surg* 81:302, 1994.

Delorme E: On the treatment of total prolapse of the rectum by excision of the rectal mucous membranes, *Bull Mem Soc Chir Paris* 26:499, 1900.

Eu KW, Milsom JW, Hull T, et al: Laparoscopic suture rectopexy for rectal prolapse without constipation (abstract 69). In *Program and Abstracts of the Annual Meeting of the American Society of Colon and Rectal Surgeons,* Montreal, Quebec, 1995, p. 24.

Finlay IG, Aitchison M: Perineal excision of the rectum for prolapse in the elderly, *Br J Surg* 78:687, 1991.

Frykman HM: Abdominal proctopexy and primary sigmoid resection for rectal procidentia, *Am J Surg* 90:780, 1955.

Gordon PH, Hoexter B: Complications of Ripstein procedure, *Dis Colon Rectum* 21:277, 1978.

Gordon SM, Gordon PH, Nivatvongs S: *Essentials of anorectal surgery,* Philadelphia, 1980, JB Lippincott.

Houry S, Lechaux JP, Huguier M, et al: Treatment of rectal prolapse by Delorme's operation, *Int J Colorectal Dis* 2:149, 1987.

Husa A, Sainio P, von Smitten K: Abdominal rectopexy and sigmoid resection for rectal prolapse, *Acta Chir Scand* 154:221, 1988.

Jacobs LK, Lin YJ, Orkin BA: The best operation for rectal prolapse, *Surg Clin North Am* 77:49, 1997.

Johansen OB, Wexner SD, Daniel N, et al: Perineal rectosigmoidectomy in the elderly, *Dis Colon Rectum* 36:767, 1993.

Kling KM, Rongione AJ, Evans B, et al: The Delorme procedure: a useful operation for complicated rectal prolapse in the elderly, *Am Surg* 62:857, 1996.

Kupfer CA, Goligher JC: One hundred consecutive cases of complete rectal prolapse of the rectum treated by operation, *Br J Surg* 57:481, 1970.

Lechaux JP, Lechhaux D, Perez M: Results of Delorme's procedure for rectal prolapse: advantages of a modified technique, *Dis Colon Rectum* 38:301, 1995.

Matheson DM, Keighley MRB: Manometric evaluation of rectal prolapse and fecal incontinence, *Gut* 22:126, 1981.

McKee RF, Lauder JC, Poon FW, et al: A prospective randomized study of abdominal rectopexy with and without sigmoidectomy in rectal prolapse, *Surg Gynecol Obstet* 174:145, 1992.

McMahan JD, Ripstein CB: Rectal prolapse. An update on the rectal sling procedure, *Am Surg* 53:37, 1987.

Mikulicz J: Zur operativen Behandlung des Prolapsus recti et Coli invaginati, *Arch Klin Chir* 38:74, 1889.

Monson JR, Jones AN, Vowden P, et al: Delorme's operation: the first choice in complete rectal prolapse? *Ann R Coll Surg Engl* 68:143, 1986.

Moschcowitz AV: The pathogenesis, anatomy and cure of prolapse of the rectum, *Surg Gynecol Obstet* 15:7, 1912.

Novell JR, Osborne MJ, Winslet MC, et al: Prospective randomized trial of Ivalon sponge versus sutured rectopexy for full-thickness rectal prolapse, *Br J Surg* 81:904, 1994.

Oliver GC, Vachon D, Eisenstat TE, et al: Delorme's procedure for complete rectal prolapse in severely debilitated patients: an analysis of 41 cases, *Dis Colon Rectum* 37:461, 1994.

Ramanjam PS, Venkatesh KS, Fietz MJ: Perineal excision of rectal procidentia in elderly high risk patients: a ten year experience, *Dis Colon Rectum* 37:1027, 1994.

Ripstein CB, Lanter B: Etiology and surgical therapy of massive prolapse of the rectum, *Ann Surg* 157:259, 1963.

Sayfan J, Pinho M, Williams JA, et al: Sutured posterior abdominal rectopexy with sigmoidectomy compared with Marlex rectopexy for rectal prolapse, *Br J Surg* 77:143, 1990.

Schlinkert RT, Beart RW, Wolf BG, et al: Anterior resection for complete rectal prolapse, *Dis Colon Rectum* 28:409, 1985.

Stern RC, Izant RJ, Boat TF, et al: Treatment and prognosis of rectal prolapse in cystic fibrosis, *Gastroenterology* 82:707, 1982.

Theuerkauf FJ, Beahrs OH, Hill JR: Rectal prolapse: causation and surgical treatment, *Ann Surg* 171:819, 1970.

Tjandra JJ, Fazio VW, Church JM, et al: Ripstein procedure is an effective treatment for rectal prolapse without constipation, *Dis Colon Rectum* 36:501, 1993.

Tobin SA, Scott IHK: Delorme operation for rectal prolapse, *Br J Surg* 81:1681, 1994.

Uhlig BE, Sullivan ES: The modified Delorme operation: its place in surgical treatment for massive rectal prolapse, *Dis Colon Rectum* 22:513, 1979.

Vongsangnak V, Varma JS, Watters D, et al: Clinical, manometric and surgical aspects of complete prolapse of rectum, *J R Coll Surg Edinb* 30:251, 1985.

Watts JD, Rothenberger DA, Buls JG, et al: The management of procidentia: 30 years' experience, *Dis Colon Rectum* 28:96, 1985.

Wells C: New operation for rectal prolapse, *Proc R Soc Med* 52:602, 1959.

Williams JG: Perineal approaches to repair of rectal prolapse, *Semin Colon Rectal Surg* 2:198, 1991.

Williams JG, Wong WD, Jenson L, et al: Incontinence and rectal prolapse: a prospective manometric study, *Dis Colon Rectum* 34:209, 1991.

Yoshioka K, Hyland G, Keighley MR: Anorectal function after abdominal rectopexy: parameters of predictive value in identifying return of continence, *Br J Surg* 76:64, 1989.

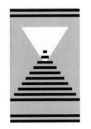

PART V
*Specific Conditions*

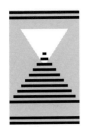

CHAPTER **24**
# Detrusor Instability and Hyperreflexia

Mickey M. Karram

The unstable bladder is one that contracts involuntarily or can be made to contract involuntarily. Urinary incontinence secondary to this condition occurs in many patients without any other recognizable abnormalities. Bladder instability is the second most common cause of incontinence in women, after genuine stress incontinence.

Bladder instability was described initially by Hodgkinson et al. in 1963, when they observed this condition in approximately 8% of their patients with urinary incontinence. Over the years, many terms have been used to describe involuntary detrusor contractions: *unstable bladder, detrusor instability, motor urge incontinence, spastic bladder, hyperreflexic bladder, detrusor dyssynergia, hypertonic bladder, automatic bladder, systolic bladder,* and *uninhibited bladder.* Standardization of definitions and diagnostic criteria has allowed more specific categorization

and terminology. Currently, two terms are accepted by the International Continence Society (ICS) for use in describing an overactive detrusor. The first, *unstable bladder* or *detrusor instability,* is a condition in which the bladder is objectively shown to contract, either spontaneously or with provocation, during the filling phase of a cystometrogram in a neurologically intact female patient while she is attempting to inhibit micturition. Unstable detrusor contractions may be asymptomatic or they may cause abnormal symptoms, most commonly urgency, frequency, and urge incontinence. Patients who present with symptoms suggestive of bladder hyperactivity, who do not demonstrate involuntary bladder contraction on provocative cystometry but have a reduced bladder capacity, are described as having sensory rather than motor urgency.

*Detrusor hyperreflexia* is defined as detrusor overactivity caused by disturbances of the nervous control mechanisms. This term should be used only when the bladder dysfunction can be explained by objective evidence of a relevant neurologic disorder. This chapter reviews the characteristics, clinical presentation, diagnosis, and management of detrusor instability and hyperreflexia in women.

## PREVALENCE AND INCIDENCE

Recent epidemiologic data suggest that the prevalence of urinary incontinence is higher in the general population than has been previously appreciated. The true prevalence, incidence, and spontaneous regression rates of detrusor instability are still unknown because the condition cannot be diagnosed clinically. Turner-Warwick (1979) reported that the lowest prevalence of instability is found in women between the ages of 10 and 30, with an overall prevalence in the general population of approximately 10%. He noted that after age 30, the prevalence increases with age, partly because of cerebrovascular deterioration in older patients.

Currently, the best data available are by Diokno et al. (1988), who performed cystometrograms on 169 randomly selected, community-dwelling women and found 7.9% to have detrusor instability. This represented 4.9% of continent women and 12.2% of incontinent women.

The prevalence is much higher in elderly hospitalized or nursing home patients. Ouslander et al. (1988) found detrusor instability or hyperreflexia in 46% of 135 elderly incontinent women. A review by Abrams (1985) of urodynamic findings in 2124 women found detrusor instability in 38% of women over 65 years of age and in only 27% of those under 65 years.

The prevalence of detrusor instability in women who present for evaluation of incontinence ranges from 10% to 55%. Webster et al. (1984) noted detrusor instability to be a contributing factor in incontinence in 73 of 133 (55%) women referred for evaluation. Forty-five percent of patients with prior failed surgery for stress incontinence were noted to have detrusor instability. Walters and Shields (1988) found detrusor overactivity in 31% of incontinent women referred for urodynamic testing. Twenty-two percent had isolated detrusor instability, 14% had mixed detrusor instability and stress incontinence, and 2% had detrusor hyperreflexia.

The term *de novo detrusor instability* has been used to describe the instability that can arise after antiincontinence operations. This occurs in 7% to 27% of cases.

## ETIOLOGY

The two factors known to produce involuntary contraction of the detrusor muscle are outflow obstruction and neurologic dysfunction. Because outflow obstruction is very rare in women and the majority of women with detrusor overactivity are neurologically intact, detrusor instability is felt to be an idiopathic condition. The following is a discussion of detrusor instability, hyperreflexia, and a variety of other factors that have been associated with involuntary detrusor contractions (Box 24-1).

### Idiopathic Detrusor Instability

With our current diagnostic capabilities, more than 90% of women with this condition appear to have no other recognizable disorder. Kinder and Mundy (1987) studied detrusor muscle strips in vitro from patients with detrusor instability and from normal, continent subjects. The unstable muscle strips showed an increased response to direct electrical stimulation and an increase in sensitivity to stimulation with acetylcholine. In vivo, this response would correspond to a higher sensitivity of efferent neurologic activity or to a lower level of acetylcholine release necessary to initiate a detrusor contraction. However, it is not clear whether this supersensitivity of the detrusor smooth muscle cell membrane is caused by a relative cholinergic denervation or by reduced inhibitory or modulatory neurologic activity, possibly mediated by vasoactive intestinal polypeptide (VIP). VIP is a 28-amino-acid neuropeptide with powerful relaxant effects on smooth muscle. It is abundant in normal human bladders and markedly decreased in the bladders of patients with detrusor instability. It has been hypothesized that deficiency of this substance or a similar

**Box 24-1**

### CONDITIONS ASSOCIATED WITH INVOLUNTARY DETRUSOR CONTRACTIONS

Idiopathic detrusor instability
  Congenital
  Aging
Detrusor hyperreflexia
  Multiple sclerosis
  Cerebrovascular disease
  Parkinson's disease
  Dementia
  Neoplasia
  Spinal cord injury
Bladder outlet obstruction
  Antiincontinence surgery
  Advanced pelvic organ prolapse
Psychosomatic disease
Urine in proximal urethra
Inflammation
Previous pelvic surgery
Orgasm
Detrusor hyperreflexia with impaired contractility
Mixed incontinence

neuroregulatory peptide is the key to development of unstable bladder activity.

It has also been shown that spinal infiltration with a local anesthetic, which blocks the micturition reflex, abolishes detrusor instability, suggesting that a hyperexcitable micturition reflex may exist in these patients.

In the infant, because of absence of inhibition of the spinal reflex, bladder instability is initially a physiologic event. Between 1 and 2 years of age, cortical lobes mature and conscious awareness of bladder activity is perceived. Persistence of spontaneous involuntary detrusor contractions and the child's response to them play a key role in the origin of many pediatric urologic conditions, including enuresis, recurrent cystitis, vesicoureteral reflux, and nonneurogenic neurogenic bladder.

In a study of cerebral perfusion by positron emission tomography (PET) scanning in elderly patients with detrusor instability, reduced perfusion was shown in the frontal lobes, suggesting that a subclinical neuropathic origin may exist in these patients.

### Neurologic Disease

Detrusor hyperreflexia is associated with neurologic lesions of the suprasacral cord and higher centers. These lesions block the sacral reflex arc from the cerebral cortex and other higher centers that are crucial to both voluntary and involuntary inhibition of the bladder. In this group of patients, involuntary detrusor contractions usually are associated with appropriate relaxation of the urethral sphincter

**Table 24-1** Summary of Urodynamic Findings in Patients With MS

| Authors | Patients | Hyperreflexia detrusor (%) | Underactive or areflexic detrusor (%) | Detrusor-sphincter dyssynergia (%) |
|---|---|---|---|---|
| Andersen and Bradley (1976) | 51 | 63 | 33 | 30 |
| Ketelaer et al. (1977) | 100 | 49 | | 86 |
| Bradley et al. (1973) | 301 | 62 | 34 | 72 |
| Schoenberg et al. (1979) | 39 | 74 | | 50 |
| Blaivas et al. (1979) | 41 | 56 | 40 | 27 |
| Piazza and Diokno (1979) | 27 | 85 | 13 | 50 |
| Beck et al. (1981) | 46 | 87 | | |
| Philp et al. (1981) | 52 | 99 | 0 | 88 |
| Goldstein et al. (1982) | 84 | 76 | | 50 |
| Van Poppel et al. (1983) | 160 | 66 | 24 | 33 |
| Awad et al. (1984) | 39 | 67 | | 51 |
| Petersen and Pederson (1984) | 88 | 82 | 16 | 41 |
| Hassouna et al. (1984) | 70 | 70 | 18 | 75 |
| Gonor et al. (1985) | 64 | 78 | 20 | 12 |

From Fowler CJ, Betts CD, Fowler CG: Bladder dysfunction in neurologic disease. In Asbury AK, McKhann GM, McDonald WI, eds: *Diseases of the nervous system: clinical neurobiology,* vol 1, Philadelphia, 1992, WB Saunders.

because there is preservation of long tracts from the pontine region. Neurologic conditions resulting in detrusor hyperreflexia include multiple sclerosis, dementia, cerebrovascular disorders, and Parkinson's disease.

### Multiple Sclerosis

Multiple sclerosis (MS) is a disease of unknown etiology characterized by varying neurologic signs and symptoms; it usually affects patients between 20 and 40 years of age. Demyelinating plaques in the white matter of the cerebral cortex, cerebellum, brain stem, spinal cord, and optic nerve may produce varied neurologic dysfunction and symptoms. MS is characterized by evidence of multiple lesions and usually a progressive course of bladder dysfunction. Plaques in the frontal lobe or in the lateral columns usually produce lower urinary tract dysfunction.

The incidence of bladder dysfunction as an initial symptom is 5%; however, up to 90% of patients with MS show evidence of bladder dysfunction during the course of their disease. Approximately 60% of patients with lower urinary tract dysfunction show detrusor hyperreflexia on cystometry. Up to half of these patients demonstrate detrusor sphincter dyssynergia and the others demonstrate adequate and appropriate sphincter relaxation. Approximately 30% of patients are noted to have an underactive or areflexic detrusor. Table 24-1 summarizes the urodynamic findings in patients with MS.

Management is aimed at reducing the high intravesical pressures associated with hyperreflexia and dyssynergia to prevent vesicoureteric reflux and subsequent renal damage.

### Cerebrovascular Disease

Cerebrovascular disease affects 300,000 people per year in the United States. The disease is associated with varying degrees of chronic disability, including bladder dysfunction. Atherosclerosis, arteritis, intracranial hemorrhage, and arterial malformations may be etiologic factors. Infarction of discrete areas of the frontal lobe, internal capsule, brain stem, or cerebellum can result in bladder dysfunction. During the initial phase of a cerebrovascular accident, urinary retention secondary to detrusor areflexia is common. During recovery, detrusor hyperreflexia with an appropriate sphincteric response usually occurs. Very rarely, detrusor-sphincter dyssynergia results.

### Parkinson's Disease

Parkinson's disease occurs in 100 to 150 per 100,000 persons. Onset usually occurs after age 50, and the course of the disease is progressive. The incidence of bladder dysfunction ranges from 40% to 70%. The extrapyramidal system is believed to have an inhibitory effect on the micturition center, so loss of dopaminergic activity in the substantia nigra, caudate, putamen, and globus pallidus results in loss of detrusor inhibition. This theory was recently challenged by Malone-Lee et al. (1993). They performed urodynamic studies on 2526 patients of whom 76 had Parkinson's disease. They found no evidence of a disease-specific parkinsonian bladder, suggesting that changes seen in such patients are simply age-related phenomena. Obstructive symptoms occasionally can result from therapy with antiparkinsonian agents.

### Dementia

Dementia is a diffuse deterioration in intellectual function manifested primarily by memory deficits and secondarily by changes in conduct. The causes of dementia include aging, severe head injury, encephalitis, presenile dementias (including Alzheimer's disease, Pick's disease, and

Jakob-Creutzfeldt disease), hydrocephalus, and syphilis. The mechanism of bladder dysfunction can be direct involvement of the cerebrocortical areas concerned with bladder control. It is sometimes also related to inattention to personal hygiene. Detrusor hyperreflexia or areflexia may occur, depending on the cause and severity of the dementia.

### Neoplasia

Brain tumors in the superior medial frontal lobe can result in bladder dysfunction. Cystometry generally shows some degree of detrusor hyperreflexia, as well as irritative voiding symptoms. Spinal cord tumors above the level of the conus medullaris and cervical spondylosis also can produce detrusor hyperreflexia.

### Spinal Cord Injury

Spinal cord injury is a common cause of detrusor hyperreflexia. All cord injuries that are complete and spare S2, S3, and S4 segments eventually produce upper motor neuron lesions with resultant detrusor hyperreflexia. However, during the initial phase of spinal shock following suprasacral spinal cord injury, the bladder is areflexic, resulting in urinary retention and overflow incontinence.

## Bladder Outlet Obstruction

Bladder outlet obstruction is rare in women. When abnormal voiding patterns occur, they are usually caused by poor detrusor function rather than physical obstruction. However, obstructive voiding may contribute to detrusor instability that sometimes occurs with advanced pelvic organ prolapse and after operations for stress incontinence, most commonly suburethral sling procedures.

Although not directly relevant to the gynecologist, bladder outflow obstruction often occurs in men. Relief of the obstruction, whether caused by bladder neck dysfunction, prostatic enlargement, or distal urethral stricture, usually leads to relief of the instability.

## Psychosomatic Causes

The psychologic status of women with detrusor instability has been investigated by several authors with conflicting results. Norton et al. (1990) performed psychiatric evaluation on 117 women attending the urodynamic clinic before urodynamic investigation. There was no more psychiatric morbidity in women with detrusor instability than in women with stress incontinence. Interestingly, women in whom no urodynamic abnormality could be detected had the highest scores for anxiety and neuroticism. Moore and Sutherst (1990) analyzed the response to treatment of idiopathic detrusor instability relative to the "psychoneurotic" status in 53 women. Poor responders had a higher mean psychoneurotic score than responders, although one third of poor responders were normal. Patients who responded well to therapy had scores similar to those of normal urban females. These studies emphasize the need for future research in this area.

## Urine in the Proximal Urethra

Some authors believe that urine in the proximal urethra may elicit a urethral reflex resulting in urgency to void and an involuntary bladder contraction. However, studies of bladder pressure while saline is injected into the proximal urethra have not provoked bladder contractions.

## Inflammation

Inflammation of the bladder mucosa, with or without associated bacteriuria, has been suggested as a cause of bladder instability. Bhatia and Bergman (1986) performed urodynamic studies on women with acute urinary tract infections before treatment. Half of those with urodynamic evidence of detrusor instability before treatment had stable cystometrograms after the infection was treated.

However, Bates et al. (1970) reported on more than 2000 patients examined by video-cystography on whom culture and sensitivity studies of midstream urine specimens were performed. They found that of 35 patients infected at the time of the study, only 3 had nonneuropathic detrusor instability.

## Instability After Pelvic Surgery

The correlation between detrusor instability and pelvic surgery is confusing and at times unexplainable. Studies on patients operated on for stress incontinence who had stable cystometrograms preoperatively note that 7% to 27% develop detrusor instability postoperatively. Postoperative detrusor instability is more common in patients with previous bladder neck surgery and in those with coexistent detrusor instability and sphincteric incompetence preoperatively.

Radical pelvic surgery, hysterectomy, and pelvic prolapse surgery can result in an unstable bladder. Partial denervation of the bladder during the operative process with subsequent development of detrusor dysfunction is currently the most accepted theory.

## Orgasm

Orgasm may be a cause of detrusor instability. The exact pathogenesis is unknown, but patients sometimes experience urgency or urge incontinence associated with a gush of urine during climax. Treatment is the same as for idiopathic detrusor instability; sexual counseling and education often are helpful.

## Detrusor Hyperactivity With Impaired Contractility

Resnick and Yalla (1987) noted that there is a subgroup of elderly women with detrusor instability resulting in incontinence, but these patients cannot effectively empty their bladders when attempting to void. Detailed urodynamic testing revealed that impaired contractility caused impaired emptying and may represent the last stage of detrusor instability, in which there is a deterioration of detrusor function.

## Mixed Incontinence

Detrusor instability can coexist with genuine stress incontinence in up to 30% of patients. Whether this is a coincidental finding or whether there is some underlying relationship between these two conditions is unknown. Interestingly, after antiincontinence surgery the detrusor instability may disappear, remain the same, or worsen.

Karram and Bhatia (1989) treated 52 women with coexistent genuine stress incontinence and detrusor instability. Of these, 27 underwent colposuspension and 25 were given oxybutynin hydrochloride together with imipramine or estrogen. Of those who were surgically treated, 59% were cured and 22% improved; of those who were given medical treatment, 32% were cured and 28% improved. This study suggests that medical management reduces the need for surgical intervention.

In a matched control study, Colombo et al. (1996) noted that 95% of their patients were cured of their stress incontinence after a Burch urethropexy was performed if they had a stable preoperative cystometrogram. On the other hand, only 75% were cured if they had a low compliance or unstable bladder preoperatively.

If patients fail medical management and bladder neck surgery is recommended, the patient should understand that the postoperative course of detrusor instability is unpredictable.

## CLINICAL FEATURES

The fundamental feature of an unstable bladder is that it contracts involuntarily. This contraction causes the sensation of impending voiding or urgency. If urgency regularly occurs before the bladder is full, frequency results. If frequency occurs at night, nocturia occurs. If the patient is unable to resist the involuntary contraction, urge incontinence results. Thus, the typical clinical presentation involves urgency, frequency, nocturia, and urge incontinence, with urgency being the cardinal symptom.

Frequency is related to fluid intake and should always be verified with a voided volume diary. Nocturia is a symptom only if the desire to void wakes the patient from sleep. Patients who awake for other reasons and decide to urinate are not categorized as having nocturia.

These symptoms are not exclusive to bladder instability. A variety of conditions that may present with similar symptoms are listed in Box 24-2.

Less common symptoms of detrusor instability include bedwetting, which occurs in about one third of patients, and voiding difficulty. Patients may feel urgency and then rush to relieve themselves, only to find that they have difficulty voiding. This difficulty may occur because the detrusor contraction that gave the patient urgency has subsided, and the patient now has difficulty initiating another contraction to void adequately.

Pain is not a common symptom of women with detrusor instability. Pain with a full bladder in conjunction with

**Box 24-2**

### CONDITIONS THAT PRODUCE SYMPTOMS OF URINARY FREQUENCY AND URGENCY

Urogynecologic
  Detrusor instability
  Genuine stress incontinence
  Sensory urgency
  Interstitial cystitis
  Urinary tract infection
  Radiation cystitis
  Urogenital atrophy
  Urethral syndrome
  Pelvic organ prolapse
  Urethral diverticulum
  Pregnancy
  Pelvic mass
  Intravesical lesion
Medical
  Detrusor hyperreflexia
  Congestive heart failure
  Diabetes mellitus
  Diabetes insipidus
  Diuretics
Psychologic
  Habit
  Anxiety
  Excessive fluid intake

urgency and frequency suggests a hypersensitive bladder condition, such as interstitial cystitis.

When obtaining the urologic history, it is important to inquire into the patient's personal, family, social, sexual, and environmental history. Frewen (1978) emphasized that the stimulus for bladder activity is not a local one, but is central in origin and influenced by psychologic, social, and environmental factors. Great care must be exercised in obtaining a psychiatric history. The suggestion of a psychiatric basis for the problem may be extremely harmful to the doctor-patient relationship, making subsequent trust and compliance difficult.

Numerous studies have evaluated the accuracy of diagnosing detrusor instability based on symptoms alone. Farrar et al. (1975) noted that patients who complained only of stress incontinence with no other symptoms usually were found to have stable bladders. If they complained of urgency, frequency, or nocturia in addition to the stress incontinence, the incidence of detrusor instability increased. If urgency and urge incontinence accompanied stress incontinence, the bladder was unstable 80% of the time. Patients who complained of frequency, nocturia, urgency, and urge incontinence without any stress incontinence were all noted to have an unstable bladder. Eighty percent of patients who complained of incontinence upon getting out of a chair or of constant wetness regardless of any provoking factor were noted to have detrusor instability.

Walters and Shields (1988) studied clinical symptoms in 106 incontinent women. The urologic symptom frequencies showed marked overlap among answers to individual questions and urologic diagnoses. Of the 10 questions studied, only 2—sensory urgency and enuresis—were associated with overactive detrusor function. Sensory urgency was often found in both groups, including 71% of women with genuine stress incontinence; however, only 9% of women in the detrusor instability group had no sensory urgency, making genuine stress incontinence more likely in incontinent women with no symptom of urgency. A recent history of enuresis was strongly associated with overactive detrusor function and uncommon (8%) in the genuine stress incontinence group.

Cardozo and Stanton (1980) also presented a clinical and urodynamic review comparing the symptoms of 100 women shown objectively to have genuine stress incontinence and 100 women shown to have an unstable bladder. Their results confirm that a definite diagnosis cannot be made by history alone.

## PHYSICAL EXAMINATION

General physical and neurologic examinations should be performed, as in all incontinent patients. Anal sphincter tone and perineal sensation, as well as anal cutaneous and bulbocavernosus reflex tests, are the most important aspects of the neurologic examination. However, it is unusual for a neurologic examination to reveal unsuspected neuropathy. Pelvic and vaginal speculum examination are performed to identify pelvic organ prolapse, pelvic masses, and local irritative factors, including mucosal atrophy.

Characteristically, idiopathic detrusor instability produces no physical signs that are pathognomonic for the disease. An examination should be conducted to identify the presence or absence of the sign of urinary incontinence. The examination is best accomplished if the patient has a full bladder. If incontinence occurs simultaneous with a rise in intraabdominal pressure, as with coughing, it is most likely caused by sphincteric weakness (genuine stress incontinence). On the other hand, if it occurs shortly after the cough and is more prolonged, it is probably caused by an uninhibited bladder contraction precipitated by the cough. If incontinence cannot be demonstrated in the supine position, the patient should be asked to stand and again undergo various provocative maneuvers.

## INVESTIGATIONS
### Urinalysis and Culture

Because the symptoms of urinary infection and other irritative bladder conditions commonly mimic detrusor instability, urinalysis should be performed before further investigation is initiated. As previously mentioned, bacteriuria may cause bladder instability and sometimes resolves after the infection has been treated. Urine cytology should be performed to rule out neoplasia in patients with chronic bladder irritative symptoms, particularly elderly patients and those with microscopic hematuria.

### Voided Volume Chart

A chart of the timing and volume of intake and output is indispensable for corroborating the patient's history and symptoms. Typically, a patient with an unstable bladder voids different volumes of urine at different intervals, whereas patients with sensory urgency tend to void consistently small volumes at fairly regular intervals. We usually ask patients to keep a 48-hour chart, usually over a weekend so as to avoid the possible interference of the pressures of work. Follow-up charts are also useful to provide evidence to both patient and physician of a response to treatment. This procedure is particularly important when bladder retraining is used for treatment.

### Urodynamic Tests
#### Cystometry

Cystometry is the mainstay of investigation for bladder storage function and is the only method of objectively diagnosing detrusor instability or hyperreflexia. The first ICS report on standardization of terminology of the lower urinary tract in 1976 stated that for a diagnosis of unstable bladder, contractions must be noted to exceed 15 cm $H_2O$ on filling cystometry. Since then, many studies have noted that contractions less than 15 cm $H_2O$ also can produce symptoms. The ICS has subsequently changed the definition to state that any rise in true detrusor pressure that is not felt to be due to bladder compliance can be called an overactive detrusor. If detrusor overactivity occurs in the absence of a neurologic lesion, it is called an unstable bladder. These conditions may be symptomatic or asymptomatic.

Coolsaet et al. (1985) investigated 334 women with either isolated detrusor instability or coexistent detrusor instability and genuine stress incontinence and noted that 87 of the 334 (26%) women had contractions of less than 15 cm $H_2O$ during cystometry. In this group, 7% were asymptomatic, 10% had subthreshold detrusor instability leading to urinary incontinence, and 85% had symptoms of urgency and frequency. This study clearly showed that contractions of a magnitude less than 15 cm $H_2O$ are clinically significant.

The rise in pressure that occurs on cystometry may be phasic (i.e., a pressure rise followed by a pressure fall) or constant. Many investigators believe that the latter situation should be called a low-compliance bladder because it is sometimes secondary to conditions resulting in changes in the passive elastic properties of the bladder wall, such as interstitial or radiation cystitis. Fig. 24-1 reviews the various cystometric patterns that can be seen in patients with detrusor instability.

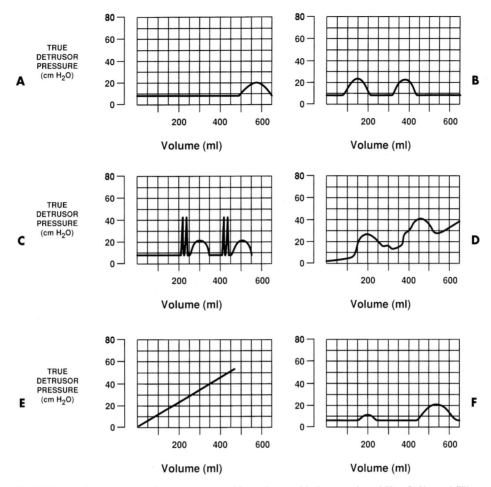

**Fig. 24-1** Various cystometric patterns noted in patients with detrusor instability. **A,** Normal filling cystometry with voluntary terminal contraction. **B,** Phasic involuntary detrusor contractions that return to baseline. **C,** Cough-provoked detrusor instability (intravesical instead of true detrusor pressure is depicted here). **D,** Phasic contractions with steady rise in detrusor pressure. **E,** Steady rise in detrusor pressure (low-compliance bladder). **F,** Subthreshold detrusor instability with voluntary terminal contraction.

During the cystometric evaluation of patients with suspected detrusor instability, one must use provoking stimuli if detrusor instability is not elicited during filling. Sometimes the provocation needed to reproduce a detrusor contraction cannot be performed in a laboratory setting. This problem has been demonstrated in numerous ambulatory monitoring studies in which symptomatic patients were noted in the urodynamic laboratory to have normal bladder filling, but, when monitored on a continuous basis, uninhibited contractions were elicited.

Testing should always be performed with the patient in a sitting or erect position because supine filling cystometry alone fails to uncover a significant proportion of unstable bladders. Other provoking factors are coughing, straining, heel-bouncing, jogging in place, listening to running water, and placing the patient's hands under running water.

The terminal bladder contraction completes the cystometrogram. In a patient without neurologic or urologic disease, this contraction requires voluntary facilitation by the patient. If the patient can suppress the terminal contraction, the controlling central nervous system reflexes are intact.

### Urethral Pressure Studies

These studies add little to the diagnosis of detrusor instability or to the differentiation of patients with stress incontinence from those with urgency incontinence. If simultaneous urethrocystometry is performed during filling, the diagnosis of urethral instability or uninhibited urethral relaxation can be made.

Detrusor contractions are almost always preceded by a drop in urethral pressure (Fig. 24-2). Bergman et al. (1989) studied urethral pressure tracings in 72 women with detrusor instability to learn whether urethral pressure changes may be the cause, rather than the effect, of bladder contractions. Patients who had urethral relaxation before the detrusor

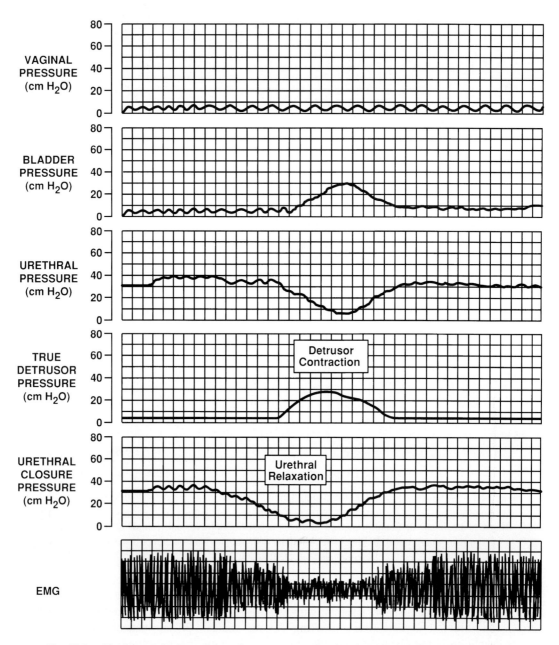

**Fig. 24-2** Multichannel subtracted urethrocystometry showing detrusor instability. Note urethral relaxation and quieting of EMG activity.

contractions responded better to alpha-sympathomimetic drugs, whereas patients without urethral pressure changes responded more favorably to anticholinergic drugs.

In another study, urethral instability (defined as a spontaneous fall in maximum urethral pressure exceeding one third of the resting maximum urethral pressure in the absence of detrusor activity) occurred in 42% of patients with detrusor instability and was strongly associated with the sequence of urethral relaxation before an unprovoked contraction. This study also concluded that, based on a urethral response, there may be two subgroups of detrusor instability.

## Electromyography

Electromyography (EMG) gives information only on activity of the external striated urethral sphincter muscles. Its potential value in patients with detrusor instability is to document voluntary control of this sphincter, as well as demonstrate that the external sphincter and detrusor muscle function in a coordinated fashion (Figs. 24-2 and 24-3). Mayo (1978) found that 48% of patients with idiopathic detrusor instability exhibited reflex relaxation of the sphincter at the time of a detrusor contraction. This observation is important because these patients are probably unable to voluntarily contract the external sphincter at the moment of the

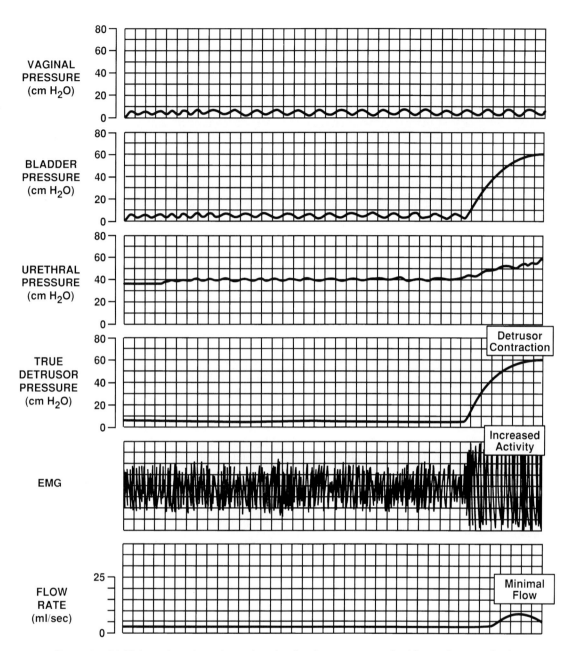

**Fig. 24-3** Multichannel urodynamic tracing showing detrusor–external sphincter dyssynergia. As patient tries to void, an increase in EMG activity is associated with a strong bladder contraction, rise in urethral pressure, and minimal urine flow.

detrusor contraction, thus inhibiting urine loss. Spontaneous sphincter relaxation can also be detected during EMG studies, leading to the diagnosis of uninhibited urethral relaxation. External sphincter EMG studies are used for the diagnosis of detrusor–external sphincter dyssynergia, which is a rare condition and occurs only in patients with neurologic disease (see Fig. 24-3). EMG adds little to the evaluation and management of neurologically intact female patients.

## Bethanechol Supersensitivity Test

Ordinarily, one should attempt to perform all urodynamic studies in the absence of pharmacologic interference.

Medications often must be discontinued 24 to 48 hours before any urodynamic tests are performed. However, pretest administration of some pharmacologic agents may improve the interpretability of cystometric studies. Bethanechol chloride, which has acetylcholine-like activity and acts on the postganglionic parasympathetic effector cells to enhance contractility of the bladder, has been used for this purpose. Although it has minimal effect on a normal bladder, an unstable bladder, whether idiopathic or neurogenic in origin, demonstrates detrusor contractions after the administration of this compound. It has been used to identify patients who are suspected of having detrusor instability that cannot be elicited on provocative cystometry. To perform the test, 2.5 mg of bethanechol chloride is administered subcutaneously and the cystometrogram is repeated approximately 30 minutes later.

## Endoscopy

The role of cystourethroscopy in the patient with urgency and urge incontinence is questionable. Definitive indications include microscopic hematuria and abnormal urine cytology. Cystoscopy should also be considered if the diagnosis is in doubt, if interstitial cystitis must be ruled out, or if the patient shows no response to appropriate behavioral and pharmacologic therapy.

## MANAGEMENT

Incomplete understanding of the causes of detrusor instability has led to several treatment plans. Comparison of various methods is difficult because of differences in patient population, methods of diagnosis, cystometric techniques, and follow-up protocols. The following is a discussion of a variety of treatment modalities that have been advocated (Box 24-3).

---

**Box 24-3**

**TREATMENT OPTIONS FOR DETRUSOR INSTABILITY AND HYPERREFLEXIA**

Treatment of associated conditions
    Stress incontinence
    Outlet obstruction
Treatment of instability
    Behavioral treatment
        Bladder drill
        Biofeedback
    Pharmacologic treatment
        Anticholinergics
        Smooth muscle relaxants
        Tricyclic antidepressants
        Antidiuretic drugs
        Estrogen replacement
    Psychotherapy
    Acupuncture
    Electrical stimulation
    Surgical treatment
        Phenol injections
        Sacral blockade
        Sacral neurectomy
        Sacral electrical stimulation
        Transvaginal denervation
        Bladder transection
        Augmentation cystoplasty
        Detrusor myomectomy
        Urinary diversion

---

## Nonsurgical Management
### Bladder Retraining Drills

This method of therapy institutes a program of scheduled voiding with progressive increases in the interval between each void. Therapy is based on the assumption that conscious efforts to suppress sensory stimuli will reestablish cortical control over an uninhibited bladder, thus reestablishing a normal voiding pattern. This mode of therapy has been studied most thoroughly by Frewen (1982) and by Fantl et al. (1981). In several studies, Frewen reported success rates of approximately 80%. However, his protocol included primarily in-hospital behavioral management and concurrent pharmacologic therapy. Fantl et al. reported on 92 patients with objective evidence of detrusor instability treated by bladder drill, with or without anticholinergic therapy. Cure rates were the same in both groups: 83% in patients treated with bladder drill and drugs and 79% in patients treated with bladder drill alone. These high cure rates with bladder retraining drills have been substantiated by other authors.

The technique used for bladder retraining involves giving the patient insight into the nature of her dysfunction. Drawings demonstrating cerebral cortical inhibitory effect over bladder reflexes can be shown to the patient to assist in explaining the lower urinary tract dysfunction. The patient's own cystometric tracing also can be shown to her to illustrate the dysfunction. The patient then is taught scheduled voidings at timed intervals, which can vary from 15 minutes to 1 hour, according to the patient's own frequency or incontinence intervals. We usually start patients at voiding intervals of 30 to 60 minutes. They are given preprinted cards, which they maintain daily. Voiding events (daily and nightly), involuntary leaking episodes, and occurrences that precipitate incontinence should be checked. The patients are instructed to make an earnest effort to follow the schedule. They should try to suppress urgency and void only at the scheduled times. At these times, the patient is asked to attempt to void regardless of the presence or absence of urinary urgency. Schedules are not followed during sleeping hours. Follow-up visits are scheduled every 1 to 2 weeks, at which time the cards are reviewed with the patient. Micturition intervals are increased periodically by 15 to 60 minutes, according to the response. A 6- to 12-week treatment program is anticipated in most cases.

Enthusiastic patient contact, reassurance, good long-term support, and follow-up are important. The degree of patient compliance determines success. Because the success rate is so good and this mode of therapy involves low cost, bladder retraining drills should be the first line of therapy in patients with detrusor instability.

### Biofeedback

Biofeedback is a form of patient reeducation in which a closed feedback loop is created so that one or more of her normally unconscious physiologic processes are made accessible to her by auditory, visual, or tactile signals. An attempt is made to modify the physiologic process by manipulating the signal presented to the patient. This method has been used with some success in the treatment of autonomic dysfunctions, hypertension, and cardiac dysrhythmias. Cystometry is explained to the patient, the test is begun, and an audible signal is used to let the patient know that her bladder pressure is rising. The tone of the signal varies according to the amount of bladder pressure rise. The patient also visualizes the urodynamic tracing throughout the test. The bladder is repeatedly filled while the patient attempts to inhibit detrusor contractions. Individual treatment sessions are approximately 1 hour and are repeated weekly for up to 8 weeks.

Cardozo et al. (1978) have reported 81% subjective and objective improvement with biofeedback. They noted that biofeedback was not as successful in patients with severe detrusor instability, particularly in women with large detrusor contraction occurring at small volumes. Burgio et al. (1985) reduced incontinence episodes by 85% in patients with biofeedback and by 94% in patients with both sensory and motor urge incontinence. Patients must be highly motivated to improve with this form of therapy. Many investigators also use biofeedback techniques aimed at identifying and strengthening pelvic floor muscles. Also, appropriate control of the external sphincter mechanism may enhance the urethrovesical inhibitory reflex.

### Psychotherapy

The possible psychosomatic origin of this condition has been discussed. Hafner et al. (1972) studied psychotherapy as a method of treatment in 26 patients with urgency, frequency, and urge incontinence. Patients were treated with six 1-hour sessions of group psychotherapy. Approximately one third of the patients benefitted considerably, one third refused treatment or ceased treatment prematurely, and one third improved slightly or not at all. MacCaulay et al. (1987) randomized 50 patients with detrusor instability or sensory urgency to receive bladder retraining drills, propantheline bromide, or psychotherapy. Patients who received psychotherapy showed significant improvement, and no patient had more than minor incontinence at follow-up; however, urinary frequency was unaffected.

### Acupuncture

Acupuncture is thought to act by increasing levels of endorphins and enkephalins in the cerebrospinal fluid. The original work was carried out by Philip et al. (1988), who treated 20 patients with detrusor instability using Chinese acupuncture. Seventy-seven percent of patients improved, but only one was converted to a stable bladder on cystometry.

### Functional Electrical Stimulation

Functional electrical stimulation (FES) works by stimulating the afferent limb of the pudendal reflex arc, resulting in an increase in pelvic floor and urethral striated muscle contractility. In addition, stimulation of the afferent portion of the pudendal nerve can result in the reflex inhibition of detrusor contractility. Clinical studies have supported this finding for patients with hyperreflexic bladders, as well as those with idiopathic detrusor instability. Some patients with detrusor instability respond to FES after having been refractory to behavioral and pharmacologic therapies. The main difficulty with FES is patient acceptance of intravaginal or transrectal stimulation. Patients must wear these devices for several hours each day, and many patients reject this for psychologic or aesthetic reasons. The dismal results of Leach and Bavendam (1989) in using the Incontan transrectal stimulating device—a 94% dropout rate in a study of 36 patients—clearly points out these limitations.

More recently, investigators have studied the efficacy of intermittent maximal electrical stimulation in treating incontinence. With this form of therapy, a short period of stimulation (for example, 30 minutes) is given to the patient at maximum tolerable intensity and the treatment continued over several weeks. Eriksen et al. (1989) reported a trial involving acute short-term maximal pelvic floor electrical stimulation of 48 patients with idiopathic detrusor instability. Each received 20 minutes of simultaneous vaginal and anal electrical stimulation for an average of seven treatments. Initial clinical and urodynamic cures were observed in 50% of patients, and significant improvement occurred in an additional 33%. At 1-year follow-up, persistent positive therapeutic effects were found in 77% of patients. In another study, Plevnik et al. (1986) treated 30 patients with detrusor instability with maximal electrical stimulation at home for 20 minutes per day for 30 days. A cure was noted in 29%; an additional 22% reported improvement. Bent et al. (1989) noted a significant subjective improvement in 69% of patients with detrusor instability, using a regimen of 15 minutes of maximal stimulation twice daily for 6 weeks. Wise et al. (1992) compared maximum electrical stimulation with oxybutynin therapy. Both treatments were associated with a significant reduction in reporting of symptoms on visual analog scales and reduction in diurnal frequency as measured in a voiding diary.

The role of FES as therapy for detrusor instability is still evolving. Although currently not a first-line therapy, it may benefit certain groups of patients who have failed multiple treatment regimens.

### Drug Therapy

Although behavior modification improves or cures most patients with detrusor instability, pharmacologic therapy remains the most popular mode of treatment. A number of pharmacologic agents are effective. Because the cause of detrusor instability is unknown, however, the response to treatment is often unpredictable and side effects are common with effective doses.

**Table 24-2**  Pharmacologic Therapy for Detrusor Instability

| Mechanism of action | Name of drug | Minimum and maximum dosage | Potential side effects | Contraindications |
|---|---|---|---|---|
| Anticholinergic | Propantheline bromide | 15 mg BID to 30 mg QID | Anticholinergic effects (dry mouth, blurred vision, drowsiness, tachycardia, constipation) | Glaucoma, intestinal obstruction, cardiac dysrhythmia, myasthenia gravis |
| Smooth muscle relaxant, anticholinergic, local anesthetic | Oxybutynin chloride | 2.5 mg BID to 5 mg QID | Anticholinergic effects | As above |
| | Flavoxate hydrochloride | 100 mg BID to 200 mg QID | Anticholinergic effects | As above |
| Smooth muscle relaxant (antispasmodic) | Dicyclomine hydrochloride | 10 mg BID to 40 mg QID | Anticholinergic effects | As above |
| Smooth muscle relaxant | Tolterodine | 1 mg BID to 2 mg BID | Anticholinergic effects | As above |
| Tricyclic antidepressant, anticholinergic, alpha-adrenergic agonist, antihistaminic | Imipramine hydrochloride | 25 mg QD to 75 mg BID | Anticholinergic effects, orthostatic hypotension, hepatic dysfunction, mania, cardiovascular effects (especially in the elderly) | Glaucoma, intestinal obstruction, cardiac dysrhythmia, myasthenia gravis, monoamine oxidase inhibitors prohibited |
| Antidiuretic drugs | DDAVP (synthetic vasopressin) | 20 to 40 μg intranasally at bedtime | Higher doses have produced transient headache, nausea, nasal congestion, rhinitis, flushing, and mild abdominal cramps | Coronary artery disease, hypertension, heart failure or epilepsy |

In general, drugs improve detrusor instability by inhibiting the contractile activity of the bladder. These agents can be broadly classified into anticholinergic drugs, calcium channel blockers, tricyclic antidepressants, musculotropic drugs, and a variety of less commonly used drugs (Table 24-2).

**Anticholinergic Agents.** A variety of anticholinergic drugs are effective in the management of detrusor instability, although certain agents have more specific activity on the detrusor muscle than on other cholinergically innervated organs. One of the earliest anticholinergic agents used for detrusor instability was methantheline bromide. Use of this drug for peptic ulcer disease led to acute urinary retention in some patients. This reaction prompted urologists to use it for refractory cases of urgency and frequency, with good preliminary results. Propanthaline bromide, a related but more potent compound, was later found to be as efficacious as methantheline bromide in controlling this condition, but with fewer side effects.

For many years, propantheline bromide was the treatment of choice for detrusor instability and the drug to which most other new compounds were compared. Numerous trials have shown this drug to inhibit involuntary detrusor contractions and increase bladder capacity. The dosage is 15 to 30 mg orally three to four times a day. Side effects are those of parasympathetic blockade: dry mouth caused by suppression of the salivary or pharyngeal secretions, constipation caused by decreased gastrointestinal motility, tachycardia caused by vagal blockade, and transient blurring of vision from blockade of the sphincters of the iris and ciliary muscles of the eye. Dry mouth is the most common side effect; others are likely to occur with higher drug dosages. In general, the maximum dose is usually determined by patient tolerance to side effects rather than by other forms of toxicity. These drugs should be used with caution in patients with narrow-angle glaucoma and in patients with significant cardiac dysrhythmias.

Emepronium bromide is an anticholinergic agent whose potentially dangerous side effects have prevented it from becoming a popular medication. However, Massey and Abrams (1986) studied a new formulation, emepronium carrageenate, in a dose titration trial. They noted that symptoms improved with increasing total daily doses without serious side effects. This improvement was confirmed by urodynamic data. Therefore, this drug may hold some promise for treatment of detrusor instability.

**Musculotropic Agents.** Smooth muscle relaxant drugs used for detrusor instability include oxybutynin chloride (Ditropan, Marion Laboratories, Inc., Kansas City, Missouri), tolterodine (Detrol, Pharmacia and Upjohn,

Bridgewater, New Jersey), dicyclomine hydrochloride (Bentyl, Lakeside Pharmaceuticals, Cincinnati, Ohio), and flavoxate hydrochloride (Urispas, SmithKline Beecham Consumer Products, Pittsburgh, Pennsylvania).

Oxybutynin chloride is currently the most used drug available for the treatment of detrusor instability. It is a tertiary amine compound that has strong musculotropic, antispasmodic, and local anesthetic effects in addition to moderate anticholinergic and antihistaminic properties. This drug is marketed specifically for urologic indications and is prescribed in a dosage of 2.5 to 10 mg one to four times daily. It is also available in a liquid suspension, which is suitable for use in children and elderly patients. Diokno and Lapides (1977) have demonstrated the effectiveness of this drug in reducing the amplitude and frequency of detrusor contractions and in increasing cystometric bladder capacity in patients with detrusor hyperreflexia. In a placebo-controlled trial, 30 unselected patients with detrusor instability underwent treatment. Symptomatic improvement was achieved in 69% of those receiving oxybutynin chloride and only 8% receiving placebo. Urodynamic improvement occurred in one half of the patients on oxybutynin chloride. Seventeen (57%) of the patients suffered side effects; in five, side effects were so severe that the drug was discontinued.

Numerous clinical trials have confirmed that symptoms of urgency, frequency, and urge incontinence are significantly improved or eradicated in a large proportion of patients using oxybutynin chloride. It is effective for both neuropathic and idiopathic detrusor instability. However, some patients are unable to tolerate its anticholinergic side effects.

Tolterodine is a new, potent, competitive muscarinic receptor antagonist developed specifically for the treatment of the overactive bladder. Appell (1997) recently reported that in four double-blind, randomized 12-week trials conducted in nine countries, tolterodine significantly reduced the number of micturitions in 24 hours and the number of incontinence episodes in 24 hours with an efficiency equivalent to that of oxybutynin. Unlike oxybutynin, however, tolterodine is far more selective for muscarinic receptors in the bladder as opposed to the parotid gland, thus avoiding the side effects (particularly dry mouth) that often cause patients to discontinue oxybutynin treatment. Tolterodine is available in 1-mg and 2-mg tablets and is given twice per day.

Dicyclomine hydrochloride is an alternative to oxybutynin chloride and tolterodine when side effects are intolerable. Dicyclomine is usually used to treat gastrointestinal disorders. It has few side effects, but is considerably less effective.

Flavoxate hydrochloride inhibits phosphatide esterase activity and increases intracellular cyclic adenosine diphosphate, a mediator of smooth muscle relaxation. Published data on this drug do not support its effectiveness in the treatment of detrusor instability, even though it is still commonly used in clinical practice.

**Imipramine Hydrochloride.** The tricyclic antidepressant imipramine hydrochloride (Tofranil, Geigy Pharmaceuticals, Ardsley, New York) improves bladder storage significantly. This medication appears to improve bladder hypertonicity or compliance rather than uninhibited contractions. It has been prescribed for treatment of enuresis in children for many years. The drug is given in a dosage of 25 mg, one to three times a day for adults and 5 to 10 mg, four times a day for children. Single nightly doses can be given in patients for the treatment of nocturnal enuresis. As compared to placebo, the drug causes a statistically significant improvement in frequency of bedwetting. It has a complex pharmacologic action, with anticholinergic, antihistaminic, and local anesthetic properties. It also increases bladder outlet resistance through a peripheral blockade of noradrenaline uptake. Because of this dual action, the drug also may be effective for patients with combined stress incontinence and detrusor instability. The side effects are anticholinergic, as well as tremor and fatigue. One must also be aware of the cardiovascular side effects that can occur in elderly patients, the most common of which is orthostatic hypotension.

**Calcium Channel Blockers.** Bodner et al. (1989) used verapamil alone and in combination with oxybutynin in 14 patients with detrusor hyperreflexia. No improvement was noted in patients using verapamil alone; however, when it was used in combination with oxybutynin, 13 patients showed greater improvement than with oxybutynin alone. Until 1991, terodoline (micturin) was the most commonly prescribed drug in Europe for the treatment of detrusor instability. It was voluntarily withdrawn from the market by its manufacturer following cardiac adverse events mainly in elderly patients taking the drug.

**Other Agents.** Other drugs that have been shown to possibly inhibit bladder contractility include beta-adrenergic agonists, such as clenbuterol and terbutaline. These drugs have been shown in animal studies to increase bladder capacity; however, their role in the management of detrusor instability in humans is uncertain. In addition, alpha-adrenergic antagonists and prostaglandin synthetase inhibitors reduce bladder capacity in animals; however, no significant benefit has been reported in humans.

Synthetic vasopressin, DDAVP (1-desamino-8-D-arginine vasopressin), decreases urine production. It is given in doses of 20 to 40 μg intranasally as a spray or snuff at bedtime. This dosage has been shown to decrease urine production by up to 50%. Ramsden et al. (1982) showed that DDAVP was superior to placebo in reducing the number of bedwetting episodes in 21 severely enuretic patients. Hilton and Stanton (1981) found that the drug produced fewer nighttime voids, as compared to placebo, in 25 women with nocturia.

DDAVP is helpful in patients with troublesome nocturnal urinary symptoms, but is contraindicated in patients with hypertension, ischemic heart disease, or congestive heart failure.

Although abundant literature exists regarding estrogen therapy and lower urinary tract dysfunction, there have been very few placebo-controlled trials using standard outcome measures. No studies have shown that estrogen therapy improved incontinence caused by detrusor instability. However, sensory urgency is improved by estrogen therapy, which is thought to raise the sensory threshold of the bladder.

Certain considerations should always be kept in mind regarding drug therapy for detrusor instability: each drug should be given for at least 6 weeks before it is deemed a failure, as the onset of benefit may, at times, be delayed; drug doses must be titrated, based on subjective response and the presence or absence of side effects; if one drug is not beneficial, it is worth trying other drugs with different modes of action or combining drugs; placebo effects are high and may be present in as many as 50% of patients; and detrusor instability is a relapsing and remitting condition, and treatment may need to be adjusted accordingly.

## Surgical Management

Surgery is reserved for the treatment of associated urologic conditions and in the uncommon case in which intractable symptoms of detrusor overactivity persist despite exhausting all conservative measures previously discussed. Historically, many different surgical procedures have been used, but only a few have stood the test of time.

Transvaginal infiltration of the pelvic plexus with phenol was described by Ewing et al. (1982) as a less traumatic alternative to bladder transection. Initial studies reported success rates around 60% for refractory detrusor instability and detrusor hyperreflexia. A more recent study by Wall and Stanton (1989) reported on a series of 28 patients with refractory urge incontinence who underwent a total of 40 transvesical phenol injections. Only eight patients (29%) achieved a significant response, and all relapsed during the 22-month follow-up period.

A similar denervation procedure is selective blockade of the sacral pelvic nerves, which involves the injection of a local anesthetic into the foramina of sacral segment S3. Permanent neurolysis can be obtained by the injection of 6% aqueous phenol. The few studies on this procedure have reported variable results. Awad et al. (1987) developed a similar technique using a cryoprobe instead of phenol injections. They reported good or excellent results in 16 of 17 patients with idiopathic detrusor instability. Mean duration of follow-up was 4.8 months. The technique was safe; temporary sensory disturbances were the only side effects.

A more recent therapy involving the electrical stimulation of the sacral nerve is the Interstim Continence Control System (Medtronic, Minneapolis, Minnesota). Similar to the way a pacemaker delivers electrical stimulation, an implanted neurostimulation system delivers small electrical impulses to the appropriate sacral nerve that controls bladder function (Fig. 24-4). One advantage of this system is that a trial stimulation performed over several days allows the patient and physician to assess the effects of treatment before permanent implantation.

Selective sacral neurectomy is a neurosurgical procedure that involves identification of the sacral roots through a limited sacral laminectomy. Electrical stimulation is used to determine which of the roots should be sectioned, as judged by the effect of stimulation on intravesical pressure. Usually the S3 root is divided bilaterally. Studies on this procedure have reported good results on small numbers of patients.

The Ingelman-Sundberg procedure is a transvaginal partial denervation of the bladder originally described in 1959. In this procedure the inferior hypogastric pelvic nerve plexus is resected after a preliminary local anesthetic block has indicated the likelihood of a successful outcome. Successful outcomes have been reported in 50% to 80% of patients.

Bladder transection was initially described by Turner-Warwick and Ashken in 1967. This operation involved complete transection of the bladder above the trigone and ureteric orifices and division of all inferior lateral communications. The largest series was reported by Mundy (1983), who noted a 74% subjective cure rate at 1-year follow-up.

Augmentation cystoplasty also has been used for resistant cases of detrusor instability. The bladder is bisected almost completely and a patch of gut, usually ileum, equal in length to the circumference of the bisected bladder (almost 25 cm), is sewn in place. The operation often cures the symptoms of detrusor instability but results in inefficient voiding. Patients may have to learn to strain to void or resort to clean intermittent self-catheterization. Mundy and Stephenson (1985) reported on a series of 40 patients treated by "clam" ileocystoplasty. Thirty-six (90%) were cured of their symptoms and 30 were able to void spontaneously and efficiently.

Recent concerns regarding the possible long-term untoward sequelae of enterocystoplasty have led to a search for an alternative. Detrusor myomectomy may achieve the same improvement in bladder compliance and is currently under study in a variety of clinical situations.

For women with severe detrusor instability or hyperreflexia in whom all other methods of treatment have failed, urinary diversion via an ileal conduit may be considered as a last resort. This mode of therapy is particularly useful in young disabled patients with severe neurologic dysfunction.

## SUMMARY

Detrusor instability is a common condition characterized by multiple symptoms, some of which are embarrassing and

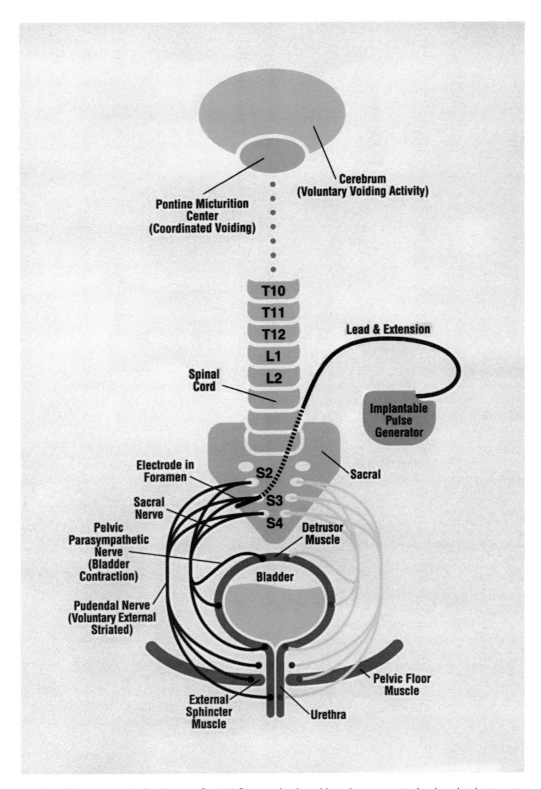

**Fig. 24-4** Interstim Continence Control System. Implantable pulse generator is placed subcutaneously and connected to a lead, which is passed through the sacral foramen usually at the S3 level. Small electrical pulses are delivered to the sacral nerve that controls bladder function.

Courtesy Medtronic, Minneapolis, Minnesota.

may cause an increasingly restricted lifestyle. A lack of understanding of the pathophysiology of this condition is reflected in the numerous methods of currently available treatments. It is important to elicit the patient's main complaints and aim treatment accordingly. Although complete, indefinite cure is rare, the majority of patients can achieve significant reduction of their symptoms. As the pathophysiology of detrusor instability becomes better understood, it is hoped that there will be significant advances in management.

## BIBLIOGRAPHY
### Prevalence and Incidence

Abrams P: Detrusor instability and bladder outlet obstruction, *Neurourol Urodyn* 4:317, 1985.

Arnold EP, Webster JR, Loose H, et al: Urodynamics of female incontinence: factors influence the results of surgery, *Am J Obstet Gynecol* 117:805, 1973.

Couillard DR, Webster GD: Detrusor instability, *Urol Clin North Am* 22:593, 1995.

Diokno AC, Brown MB, Brock BM, et al: Clinical and cystometric characteristics of continent and incontinent noninstitutionalized elderly, *J Urol* 140:567, 1988.

Hodgkinson CP, Ayers MA, Drukker BH: Dyssynergic detrusor dysfunction in the apparently normal female, *Am J Obstet Gynecol* 87:717, 1963.

Sand PK, Hill RC, Ostergard DO: Supine urethroscopic and standing cystometrogram as screening methods for the detection of detrusor instability, *Obstet Gynecol* 70:57, 1987.

Turner-Warwick RT: Observations on the function and dysfunction of the sphincter and detrusor mechanism, *Urol Clin North Am* 6:13, 1979.

Walters MD, Shields LE: The diagnostic value of history, physical examination, and the Q-tip cotton swab test in women with urinary incontinence, *Am J Obstet Gynecol* 159:145, 1988.

Webster GD, Sihelnik SA, Stone AR: Female urinary incontinence: the incidence, identification and characteristics of detrusor instability, *Neurourol Urodyn* 3:235, 1984.

### Etiology

Anderson JT, Bradley WE: Bladder and urethral innervation in multiple sclerosis, *Br J Urol* 48:193, 1976.

Awad SA, Gajewski JB, Sogbein SK, et al: Relationship between neurological and urological status in patients with multiple sclerosis, *J Urol* 132:499, 1984.

Barrington FJ: The component reflexes of micturition in the cat, *Brain* 54:177, 1931.

Bauer SB, Retic AB, Colodny AH, et al: The unstable bladder of childhood, *Urol Clin North Am* 7:321, 1980.

Beck RP, Armsch D, King C: Results in treating 210 patients with detrusor overactivity incontinence of urine, *Am J Obstet Gynecol* 125:593, 1976.

Beck RP, Warren KG, Whitman P: Urodynamic studies in female patients with multiple sclerosis, *Am J Obstet Gynecol* 139:273, 1981.

Bhatia NN, Bergman A: Cystometry: unstable bladder and urinary tract infection, *Br J Urol* 58:134, 1986.

Blaivas JG, Bhimani G, Labib KB: Vesicourethral dysfunction in multiple sclerosis, *J Urol* 122:342, 1979.

Bradley WE, Logothetis JL, Timm GW: Cystometric and sphincter abnormalities in multiple sclerosis, *Neurology* 23:1131, 1973.

Cardozo LD, Stanton SL, Williams JE: Detrusor instability following surgery for genuine stress incontinence, *Br J Urol* 51:204, 1979.

Cucchi A: Detrusor instability and bladder outflow obstruction. Evidence for a correlation between the severity of obstruction and the presence of instability, *Br J Urol* 61:420, 1988.

Frewen WK: An objective assessment of the unstable bladder of psychosomatic origin, *Br J Urol* 50:246, 1978.

Goldstein I, Siroky MB, Sax DS, et al: Neurourologic abnormalities in multiple sclerosis, *J Urol* 128:541, 1982.

Gonor SE, Carroll DJ, Metcalfe JB: Vesical dysfunction in multiple sclerosis, *Urology* 25:429, 1985.

Gu J, Restorick JM, Blank MA, et al: Vasoactive intestinal polypeptide in the normal and unstable bladder, *Br J Urol* 55:645, 1983.

Hassouna M, Lebel M, Elhilali M: Neurologic correlation in multiple sclerosis, *Neurourol Urodyn* 3:73, 1984.

Hilton P: Urinary incontinence during sexual intercourse: a common, but rarely volunteered, symptom, *Br J Obstet Gynaecol* 95:377, 1988.

Hodgkinson CP, Ayers MA, Drukker BH: Dyssynergic detrusor dysfunction in the apparently normal female, *Am J Obstet Gynecol* 87:717, 1963.

Ketelaer P, Leruitte A, Vereecker RL: Striated sphincter urethral and anal sphincter electromyography during cystometry in multiple sclerosis, *Electromyogr Clin Neurophysiol* 17:427, 1977.

Khan Z, Bhola A, Starer P: Urinary incontinence during orgasm, *Urology* 21:279, 1988.

Kinder RB, Mundy AR: Inhibition of spontaneous contractile activity in isolated human detrusor muscle strips by vasoactive intestinal peptide, *Br J Urol* 57:20, 1985.

Kinder RB, Mundy AR: Pathophysiology of idiopathic detrusor instability and detrusor hyper-reflexia: in vitro study of human detrusor muscle, *Br J Urol* 60:509, 1987.

Kinder RB, Restorick JM, Mundy AR: Vasoactive intestinal polypeptide in the hyper-reflexic neuropathic bladder, *Br J Urol* 57:289, 1985.

Petersen T, Pederson E: Neurourodynamic evaluation of voiding dysfunction in multiple sclerosis, *Acta Neurol Scand* 69:402, 1984.

Philp T, Read DJ, Higson RH: The urodynamic characteristics of multiple sclerosis, *Br J Urol* 53:672, 1981.

Piazza DH, Diokno AC: Review of neurogenic bladder in multiple sclerosis, *Urology* 14:33, 1979.

Rees DLP, Whickham JEA, Whitfield HN: Bladder instability in women with recurrent cystitis, *Br J Urol* 50:524, 1978.

Resnick NM, Yalla SV: Detrusor hyperactivity with impaired contractile function, *JAMA* 257:3076, 1987.

Resnick NM, Yalla SV, Laurino E: The psychophysiology of urinary incontinence among institutionalized elderly persons, *N Engl J Med* 320:1, 1989.

Schoenberg HW, Gutrich J, Banno J: Urodynamic patterns in multiple sclerosis, *J Urol* 122:648, 1979.

Sutherst JR, Brown M: The effect on the bladder pressure of sudden entry of fluid into the posterior urethra, *Br J Urol* 50:406, 1978.

Van Poppel H, Vereecken RL, Leruitte A: Neuro-muscular dysfunction of the lower urinary tract in multiple sclerosis, *Paraplegia* 21:374, 1983.

Wise BG, Cardozo LD, Cutner A, et al: Prevalence and significance of urethral instability in women with detrusor instability, *Br J Urol* 72:26, 1993.

### Mixed Incontinence

Colombo M, Zanetta G, Vitobello D, et al: The Burch colposuspension for women with and without detrusor over activity, *Br J Obstet Gynaecol* 103:255, 1996.

Karram MM, Bhatia NN: Management of coexistent stress and urge urinary incontinence, *Obstet Gynecol* 73:4, 1989.

Lockhart JL, Vorstman B, Politano VA: Anti-incontinence surgery in females with detrusor instability, *Neurourol Urodyn* 3:201, 1984.

McGuire EJ, Savastano JA: Stress incontinence and detrusor instability/urge incontinence, *Neurourol Urodyn* 4:313, 1985.

McGuire EJ: Bladder instability and stress incontinence, *Neurourol Urodyn* 7:563, 1988.

### Diagnosis

Awad SA, McGinnis RH: Factors that influence the incidence of detrusor instability in women, *J Urol* 130:114, 1983.

Bates CP, Whiteside CG, Turner-Warwick RT: Synchronous cine/pressure/ flow cystourethrography with special reference to stress and urge incontinence, *Br J Urol* 42:714, 1970.

Bent AE, Richardson DA, Ostegard DR: Diagnosis of lower urinary tract disorders in postmenopausal patients, *Am J Obstet Gynecol* 145:218, 1983.

Bergman A, Koonings PP, Ballard CA: Detrusor instability. Is the bladder the cause or the effect? *J Reprod Med* 34:834, 1989.

Bhatia NN, Bradley WE, Haldeman S: Urodynamics: continuous monitoring, *J Urol* 128:963, 1982.

Bradley WE, Timm GE: Cystometry VI. Interpretation, *Urology* 2:231, 1976.

Cantor TJ, Bates CP: A comparative study of symptoms and objective urodynamic findings in 214 incontinent women, *Br J Obstet Gynaecol* 87:889, 1980.

Cardozo LD, Stanton SL: Genuine stress incontinence and detrusor instability: a review of 200 cases, *Br J Obstet Gynaecol* 87:184, 1980.

Coolsaet BLRA: Bladder compliance and detrusor activity during the collection phase, *Neurourol Urodyn* 4:263, 1985.

Coolsaet BLRA, Blok C, van Venrouij GEFM, et al: Subthreshold detrusor instability, *Neurourol Urodyn* 4:309, 1985.

Diokno AC, Wells TJ, Brock BM, et al: Urinary incontinence in elderly women: urodynamic evaluation, *J Am Geriatr Soc* 35:940, 1987.

Eastwood HDH, Warrell R: Urinary incontinence in the elderly female: prediction in diagnosis and outcome of management, *Age Aging* 13:230, 1984.

Farrar DJ, Whiteside CG, Osborne JL, et al: A urodynamic analysis of micturition symptoms in the female, *Surg Gynecol Obstet* 141:875, 1975.

Griffiths CJ, Assi MS, Styles RA, et al: Ambulatory monitoring of bladder and detrusor pressure during natural filling, *J Urol* 142:780, 1989.

Haylen BT, Sutherst JR, Frazer MI: Is the investigation of most stress incontinence really necessary? *Br J Urol* 61:147, 1989.

Hilton P, Stanton SL: Algorithmic method for assessing urinary incontinence in elderly women, *BMJ* 282:940, 1981.

Jeffcoate TNA, Francis WJA: Urgency incontinence in the female, *Am J Obstet Gynecol* 94:604, 1966.

Korda A, Krieger M, Hunter P, et al: The value of clinical symptoms in the diagnosis of urinary incontinence in the female, *Aust NZ J Obstet Gynaecol* 27:149, 1987.

Kulseng-Hanssen S, Klevmark B: Ambulatory urethro-cysto-rectometry: a new technique, *Neurourol Urodyn* 7:119, 1988.

Lockhart JL, Sherrel F, Weinstein D, et al: Urodynamics in women with stress and urge incontinence, *Urology* 20:333, 1982.

Low JA, Mauger GM, Drajovic J: Diagnosis of the unstable detrusor: comparison of an incremental and continuous infusion technique, *Obstet Gynecol* 65:99, 1985.

Malone-Lee JG, Saadu A, Lieu PK: Evidence against the existence of a specific Parkinsonian bladder, *Neurourol Urodyn* 12(4):341, 1993.

Mayo ME: Detrusor hyperreflexia: the effect of posture and pelvic floor activity, *J Urol* 119:635, 1978.

Ouslander J, Leach G, Abelson S, et al: Simple versus multichannel cystometry in the evaluation of bladder function in an incontinent geriatric population, *J Urol* 140:1482, 1988.

Sutherst JR, Brown MC: Comparison of single and multichannel cystometry in diagnosing bladder instability, *BMJ* 288:1720, 1984.

Turner-Warwick RT: Some clinical aspects of detrusor dysfunction, *J Urol* 113:539, 1975.

Webster GE, Older RA: The value of subtracted bladder pressure measurements in routine urodynamic studies, *Urology* 16:656, 1980.

## Treatment: Behavioral, Psychotherapy, and Acupuncture

Burgio KL, Whitehead WE, Engel BT: Urinary incontinence in the elderly: bladder-sphincter biofeedback and toileting skills training, *Ann Intern Med* 103:507, 1985.

Cardozo LD, Abrams PD, Stanton SL, et al: Idiopathic bladder instability treated by biofeedback, *Br J Urol* 50:512, 1978.

Cardozo LD, Stanton SL: Biofeedback: a 5-year review, *Br J Urol* 56:220, 1984.

Cardozo LD, Stanton SL, Hafner J, et al: Biofeedback in the treatment of detrusor instability, *Br J Urol* 50:250, 1978.

Fantl JA, Hurt WG, Dunn LJ: Detrusor instability syndrome: the use of bladder retraining drills with and without anticholinergics, *Am J Obstet Gynecol* 140:885, 1981.

Ferrie BG, Smith JS, Logan D, et al: Experience with bladder training in 65 patients, *Br J Urol* 56:482, 1984.

Frewen WK: A reassessment of bladder training in detrusor dysfunction in the female, *Br J Urol* 54:372, 1982.

Hadley EC: Bladder training and related therapies for urinary incontinence in older people, *JAMA* 256:372, 1986.

Hafner RJ, Stanton SL, Guy J: A psychiatric study of women with urgency and urgency incontinence, *Br J Urol* 49:211, 1977.

Jarvis GJ: A controlled trial of bladder drill and drug therapy in the management of detrusor instability, *Br J Urol* 53:565, 1981.

MacCaulay AJ, Stern RS, Holmes DM, et al: Micturition and the mind: psychological factors in the aetiology and treatment of urinary symptoms in women, *BMJ* 294:540, 1987.

Millard RJ, Oldenburg BF: The symptomatic, urodynamic, and psychodynamic results of bladder re-education programs, *J Urol* 130:715, 1983.

Moore KH, Sutherst JR: Response to treatment of detrusor instability in relation to psychoneurotic status, *Br J Urol* 66:486, 1990.

Norton KRW, Bnat AV, Stanton SL: Psychiatric aspects of urinary incontinence in women attending an outpatient clinic, *BMJ* 301:271, 1990.

Pengelly AW, Booth CM: A prospective trial of bladder training as treatment of detrusor instability, *Br J Urol* 52:463, 1980.

Philip T, Shah PJR, Worth PHL: Acupuncture in the treatment of bladder instability, *Br J Urol* 1:490, 1988.

## Treatment: Functional Electrical Stimulation

Bent AE, Sand PK, Ostergard DR: Transvaginal electrical stimulation in the treatment of genuine stress incontinence and detrusor instability, *Neurourol Urodyn* 8:363, 1989.

Eriksen BC, Bergmann S, Eik-Nes SH: Maximal electrostimulation of the pelvic floor in female idiopathic detrusor instability and urge incontinence, *Neurourol Urodyn* 8:219, 1989.

Fall M: Does electrostimulation cure urinary incontinence? *J Urol* 131:664, 1984.

Fall M, Ahlstrom K, Carlsson C, et al: Contelle: pelvic floor stimulation for female stress-urge incontinence: a multicenter study, *Urology* 27:282, 1986.

Fossberg E: Urge incontinence treated with maximal electrical stimulation, *Neurourol Urodyn* 7:270, 1988.

Leach GE, Bavendam TG: Prospective evaluation of the Incontan transrectal stimulator in women with urinary incontinence, *Neurourol Urodyn* 8:231, 1989.

McGuire EJ, Shi-Chun Z, Horwinski R, et al: Treatment of motor and sensory detrusor instability by electrical stimulation, *J Urol* 129:78, 1983.

Merrill D: The treatment of detrusor incontinence by electrical stimulation, *J Urol* 122:515, 1979.

Plevnik S, Janez J: Maximal electrical stimulation for urinary incontinence. Report of 98 cases, *Urology* 14:638, 1979.

Plevnik S, Janez J, Vrtenik P, et al: Short-term electrical stimulation: home treatment for urinary incontinence, *World J Urol* 4:24, 1986.

Wise BG, Cardozo LD, Cutner A, et al: Maximal electrical stimulation: an acceptable alternative to anticholinergic therapy, *Int Urogynecol J* 3(3):270, 1992.

## Treatment: Drug Therapy

Abrams P, Freeman R, Anderstrom C, et al: Tolterodine, a new antimuscarinic agent: as effective but better tolerated than oxybutynin in patients with an overactive bladder, *Br J Urol* 81:801, 1998.

Appell RA: Clinical efficacy and safety of tolterodine in the treatment of overactive bladder: a pooled analysis, *Urology* 50(suppl 6A):90, 1997.

Barker G, Clenning PP: Treatment of the unstable bladder with propantheline and imipramine, *Aust NZ J Obstet Gynaecol* 27:152, 1987.

Blaivas JG, Labib KB, Michalik SJ, et al: Cystometric response to propantheline in detrusor hyperreflexia: therapeutic implications, *J Urol* 124:259, 1980.

Bodner DR, Lindan R, Leffler E, et al: The effect of verapamil on the treatment of detrusor hyperreflexia in the spinal cord injured population, *Paraplegia* 27:364, 1989.

Briggs RS, Castleden CM, Asher MJ: The effect of flavoxate on uninhibited detrusor contractions and urinary incontinence in the elderly, *J Urol* 123:665, 1980.

Brooks ME, Braf ZF: Oxybutynin chloride (Ditropan): clinical uses and limitations, *Paraplegia* 18:64, 1980.

Cardozo LD, Stanton SL: An objective comparison of the effects of parenterally administered drugs in patients suffering from detrusor instability, *J Urol* 122:58, 1979.

Cardozo LD, Stanton SL: A comparison between bromocriptine and indomethacin in the treatment of detrusor instability, *J Urol* 123:399, 1980.

Cardozo LD, Stanton SL, Robinson H, et al: Evaluation of flurbiprofen in detrusor instability, *Br Med J* 280:281, 1980.

Castleden CM, Duffen CM, Gulati RS: Double-blind study of imipramine and placebo for incontinence due to bladder instability, *Age Aging* 15:299, 1986.

Diokno AC, Lapides J: Oxybutynin: a new drug with analgesic and anticholinergic properties, *J Urol* 108:307, 1977.

Fantl JA, Wyman JF, Anderson RL, et al: Postmenopausal urinary incontinence: comparison between nonestrogen supplemented and estrogen supplemented women, *Obstet Gynecol* 71:823, 1988.

Farrar DJ, Osborne JL: The use of bromocriptine in the treatment of the unstable bladder, *Br J Urol* 48:235, 1976.

Finkbeiner AE, Bissada NK, Welch LT: Uropharmacology: part VI. Parasympathetic depressants, *Urology* 10:503, 1977.

Fischer-Rasmussen W, Korhonon M, Bossberg E, et al: Evaluation of long-term safety and clinical benefit of terodiline in women with urgency/urge incontinence: a multicentre study, *Scand J Urol Nephrol Suppl* 87:35, 1984.

Gajweski JB, Awad SA: Oxybutynin versus propantheline in patients with multiple sclerosis and detrusor hyperreflexia, *J Urol* 135:966, 1986.

Gruneberger A: Treatment of motor urge incontinence with clenbuterol and flavoxate hydrochloride, *Br J Obstet Gynaecol* 91:275, 1984.

Holmes DM, Montz FJ, Stanton SL: Oxybutynin versus propantheline in the management of detrusor instability. A patient-regulated variable dose trial, *Br J Obstet Gynaecol* 96:607, 1989.

Kohler FP, Morales P: Cystometric evaluation of flavoxate hydrochloride in normal and neurogenic bladders, *J Urol* 100:729, 1968.

Levin RM, Staskin DR, Wein AJ: The muscarinic cholinergic binding kinetics of the human urinary bladder, *Neurourol Urodyn* 1:221, 1982.

Macfarlane JR, Tolley D: The effect of terodiline on patients with detrusor instability, *Scand J Urol Nephrol* 87(suppl):51, 1984.

Massey JA, Abrams P: Dose titration in clinical trials. An example using emepronium carrageenate in detrusor instability, *Br J Urol* 58:125, 1986.

Molsey CV, Stephenson TP, Brendler CB: The urodynamic and subjective results of treatment of detrusor instability with oxybutynin chloride, *Br J Urol* 52:472, 1980.

Ramsden PD, Hindmarsh JR, Price DA, et al: DDAVP for adult enuresis—a preliminary report, *Br J Urol* 54:256, 1982.

Stanton SL: A comparison of emepronium bromide and flavoxate hydrochloride in the treatment of urinary incontinence, *J Urol* 110:529, 1973.

Tapp A, Fall M, Norgaard J, et al: Terodiline: a dose-titrated, multicenter study of the treatment of idiopathic detrusor instability in women, *J Urol* 142:1027, 1989.

Thompson IM, Lauvetz R: Oxybutynin in bladder spasm, neurogenic bladder, and enuresis, *Urology* 8:452, 1976.

Ulmsten U, Ekman G, Andersson KE: The effect of terodiline treatment in women with motor urge incontinence. Results from a double-blind study and long-term treatment, *Am J Obstet Gynecol* 153:619, 1985.

Wein AJ: Drug therapy for detrusor instability: where are we? *Neurourol Urodyn* 4:337, 1985.

**Treatment: Surgery**

Awad SA, Flood HD, Acker KL, et al: Selective sacral cryoneurolysis in the treatment of patients with detrusor instability/hyperreflexia and hypersensitive bladder, *Neurourol Urodyn* 6:307, 1987.

Blackford HN, Murray K, Stephenson TP, et al: Results of transvesical infiltration of the pelvic plexuses with phenol in 116 patients, *Br J Urol* 56:647, 1984.

Clarke SJ, Forster DM, Thomas DG: Selective sacral neurectomy in the management of urinary incontinence due to detrusor instability, *Br J Urol* 51:510, 1979.

Ewing R, Bultitude MI, Shuttleworth KED: Subtrigonal phenol injection for urge incontinence secondary to detrusor instability in females, *Br J Urol* 54:689, 1982.

Ingelman-Sundberg A: Partial bladder denervation for detrusor dyssynergia, *Clin Obstet Gynecol* 21:797, 1978.

Lucas MG, Thomas DG, Clarke S, et al: Long-term follow-up of selective sacral neurectomy, *Br J Urol* 61:218, 1988.

McGuire EJ, Savastano JA: Urodynamic findings and clinical status following vesical denervation procedures for control of incontinence, *J Urol* 132:87, 1981.

Mundy AR: The surgical treatment of urge incontinence of urine, *J Urol* 128:481, 1982.

Mundy AR: Long-term results of bladder transection for urge incontinence, *Br J Urol* 55:642, 1983.

Mundy AR: The surgical treatment of detrusor instability, *Neurourol Urodyn* 4:352, 1985.

Mundy AR, Stephenson TP: "Clam" ileocystoplasty for the treatment of refractory urge incontinence, *Br J Urol* 57:641, 1985.

Opsomer RJ, Klarskov P, Holm-Bentzen M, et al: Long-term results of superselective sacral nerve resection for motor urge incontinence, *Scand J Urol Nephrol* 18:101, 1984.

Rosenbaum TP, Shah PJR, Worth PHL: Trans-trigonal phenol: the end of an era? *Neurourol Urodyn* 7:294, 1988.

Torrens MJ: The role of denervation in the treatment of detrusor instability, *Neurourol Urodyn* 4:353, 1985.

Turner-Warwick RT, Ashken MH: The functional results of partial, subtotal and total cystoplasty with special reference to ureterocaecocystoplasty, selective sphincterotomy, and cystocystoplasty, *Br J Urol* 39:3, 1967.

Wall LL, Stanton SL: Transvesical phenol injection of pelvic nerve plexuses in females with refractory urge incontinence, *Br J Urol* 63:465, 1989.

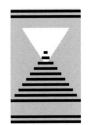

CHAPTER 25

# Hypersensitivity Disorders of the Lower Urinary Tract

Raymond A. Bologna, Le Mai Tu, and Kristene E. Whitmore

Interstitial Cystitis
    *Etiology*
    *Diagnosis*
Urethral Syndrome
Management of Hypersensitivity Disorders
    *Hydrodistention of the bladder*
    *Pharmacologic therapy*
    *Bladder instillations*
    *Refractory symptoms*
Future Directions

Hypersensitivity or sensory disorders of the lower urinary tract in women have been poorly elucidated, and management has been mandated by anecdotal evidence. Reliable and standardized testing to make an accurate diagnosis remains elusive. These disorders represent a spectrum of symptoms and conditions that include chronic bacterial cystitis, urgency and frequency syndrome, sensory urgency, and urethral syndrome. This may be one disease process in different phases or degrees of severity (Fig. 25-1). This chapter focuses on what may be the ultimate expression of this disease process: interstitial cystitis (IC).

Anatomically, the short female urethra lends itself to infectious invasion. Childbirth and sexual activity cause displacement and trauma to the bladder neck. The postmenopausal state subjects the female lower urinary tract to the effects of chronic estrogen deprivation. This leads to ischemia, with a decrease in the urethral mucosal cushion and increased susceptibility of the bladder to bacterial adherence. The result is potential exposure of the neurovascular elements of the bladder wall to urinary toxins and infectious agents. The physiologic ramifications of chronic overstimulation of the sensory nerve components of the lower urinary tract are under investigation.

Hypersensitivity disorders affect most physicians' practices. It is estimated that 15% of the 5 million women who experience a urinary tract infection (UTI) annually will have recurrences (>2 episodes in 6 months or >3 in 1 year). Of the 8.5 million women with urinary incontinence, about 40% have detrusor instability and/or sensory urgency. More than 500,000 women have IC, and their quality of life is often

lower than that of age-matched patients on renal dialysis. Significant clinical depression is present in 68% of these patients. In the absence of infection, patients with frequency, urgency, and pain are often classified as having one or more of the following: a painful bladder syndrome, urethral syndrome, frequency and urgency syndrome, urethral instability, sensory urgency, or IC. Appropriate classification is forthcoming, with current research efforts working toward defining etiology.

## INTERSTITIAL CYSTITIS

IC is the most challenging and encompassing hypersensitivity disorder. Tremendous efforts have been made to gain an understanding of this disease, but the etiology remains unclear. This section presents the current understanding of the pathogenesis and diagnostic approach to IC.

### Etiology

Skene first suggested the term *interstitial cystitis* in 1887. In 1907 Nitze described a painful bladder condition associated with urinary frequency and bladder ulcerations. In 1915, Guy Hunner reported the classic ulcer associated with a contracted fibrotic bladder, mucosal congestion adjacent to the ulcers, and hemorrhage following bladder hydrodistention. Although IC was described early in this century, it was not until the 1970s that epidemiologic studies were done to evaluate and characterize this disease.

The reported prevalence of IC varies greatly. Population prevalence estimates of IC have ranged from 30 in 100,000 to 501 in 100,000 of the total population (as many as 1 million Americans). Many of these studies were self-reported questionnaires and were not confirmed by medical record review. It is also important to note that diagnostic criteria were not established until 1987.

In 1987, for research purposes, the National Institutes of Health (NIH) established standardized diagnostic criteria for IC (Box 25-1). The Interstitial Cystitis Data Base (ICDB), a cooperative multicenter longitudinal observation study group established in 1991, was sponsored to study the natural history of the disease and was based on a large population with symptoms consistent with IC.

**315**

Severity of symptoms

Recurrent UTI diagnosis · Urethral syndrome · Mild interstitial cystitis · NIH cases · Advanced interstitial cystitis

**Fig. 25-1** Spectrum of interstitial cystitis. *NIH,* National Institutes of Health; *UTI,* urinary tract infection.

The etiology of IC is currently unknown. Most authors believe it is multifactorial. Currently proposed causes include infectious agents, quantitative glycosaminoglycan (GAG) layer deficiency, ultrastructural abnormality of the lamina propria or interstitium of the bladder, mast cells, and neurogenic inflammation.

### Infectious Agents

Extensive efforts have been made, with limited success, to establish an infectious agent as the cause of IC. Hunner (1915) first suggested a hematogenously disseminated bacterial cystitis as the cause. Most patients with IC report a history of UTI and have received several courses of antibiotics based on their symptoms, not on positive urine cultures. To date, no single bacterium, virus, fungus, or fastidious microorganism has been isolated as an etiologic factor in IC.

Some authors believe that a low bacterial count, bacterial antigens, or by-products such as endotoxins or P-fimbriae may be involved. These substances can activate an autoimmune response or cause sensory nerve stimulation, thus activating the neurogenic inflammation model of IC. DNA sequencing of bladder biopsies searching for bacteria or their by-products has demonstrated controversial results.

### GAG Layer Deficiency

The concept of a defective urothelium resulting from a quantitative deficiency of its surface coat of GAGs and thereby allowing access of a toxic urothelial substance into the interstitium of the bladder was once the leading theory of the pathogenesis of IC. Current research is focusing on biochemical and ultrastructural studies of the surface layer of urothelium. This may provide a more comprehensive understanding of the pathogenesis of IC.

### Ultrastructural Abnormalities

Ultrastructural studies of bladder biopsy specimens following hydrodistention have revealed a number of distinct features. Abnormalities are observed in all tissue components of the bladder wall, including tissue cells, interstitial tissue, blood vessels, and intrinsic nerves. These features include urothelium with disrupted permeability barrier and accelerated turnover, abnormal profiles of detrusor muscle cells, and damage of intrinsic nerves and blood vessel walls.

**Box 25-1**
## NIH-NIDDK DIAGNOSTIC CRITERIA OF INTERSTITIAL CYSTITIS

Category A: At least one of the following findings on cystoscopy:
- Diffuse glomerulations (at least 10 per quadrant) in at least three quadrants of the bladder
- A classic Hunner's ulcer

Category B: At least one of the following symptoms:
- Pain associated with the bladder
- Urinary urgency

Exclusion criteria:
- Age <18 years*
- Urinary frequency while awake <8 times per day
- Nocturia fewer than two times per night
- Maximal bladder capacity >350 ml while patient is awake
- Absence of an intense urge to void with bladder filled to 150 ml of water with medium filling rate (30-100 ml/min) during cystometry
- Involuntary bladder contractions on cystometry using medium filling rate
- Duration of symptoms <9 months*
- Symptoms relieved by antimicrobial agents (antibiotics, urinary antiseptics), anticholinergics, or antispasmodics*
- Urinary tract or prostatic infection in the past 3 months*
- Active genital herpes
- Vaginitis*
- Uterine, cervical, vaginal, or urethral cancer within the past 5 years*
- Bladder or ureteral calculi*
- Urethral diverticulum*
- History of cyclophosphamide or chemical cystitis or tuberculous or radiation cystitis
- Benign or malignant bladder tumors

NOTE: These are the original criteria and are changing.
*Relative exclusion criteria.
*NIH-NIDDK,* National Institutes of Health–National Institute of Diabetes and Digestive and Kidney Diseases.

Significant fluid engorgement, with diffuse or loculated edema of tissue cells and extracellular tissue, is also seen. Lymphocytes are the predominant component, distributed unevenly throughout the tissue. Activated mast cells are readily identified adjacent to intrinsic nerves, but they are less commonly seen near blood vessels and in the suburothelium. These distinctive features are most prominent and extensive in biopsies from areas of glomerulations (submucosal hemorrhages) following diagnostic hydrodistention. These features, although recognizable, are less dramatic in severity and extent of distribution in biopsies from cystoscopically normal-appearing areas of the bladder lining. This transitional dysfunction or abnormality in epithelial permeability has led to the development of the potassium sensitivity test.

### Mast Cells

Mast cells examined ultrastructurally in IC are intimately associated with nerve fibers and terminals in the suburothelium and are found in the interstitium of the detrusor, often next to nerves and blood vessels. Mast cells are essential for the development of allergic hypersensitivity reactions. Their activation and subsequent degranulation trigger the secretion of many biologically active chemicals. These substances include histamine, serotonin, cytokines, neuropeptides (substance P), and vasoactive intestinal peptide. These mediators, especially histamine, may play a role in stimulating reactions such as vasodilation, leukocyte infiltration, and angiogenesis.

An elevated mast cell count in the bladder muscularis has been promoted as a diagnostic histopathologic feature of IC, and *detrusor mastocytosis* has been advocated as a more appropriate name for IC. Different values for mast cell counts in the detrusor layer have been proposed as a diagnostic marker. These values and their validity are debated. Detrusor mastocytosis has been found in 20% to 65% of patients with IC; patients with classic ulcer-type or late-stage IC have demonstrated an even higher percentage. Recently, investigators have attempted to compare the ratio of detrusor to mucosal mast cells and the relationship of nerve fibers to mast cells. The ultrastructure of the mast cell, demonstrated by electron microscopy, has shown the proximity of nerves and activated mast cells. Researchers are investigating mast cell activation and the subsequent mediator release as an origin of some of the symptoms and cystoscopic findings seen with IC. Current research involving the role of mast cells in IC has brought forth three findings: the intimate association and interaction of mast cells with intrinsic nerves in the bladder wall; the unlikeliness, if not incompatibility, of an immunologic pathogenetic mechanism of immunoglobulin E–mediated immediate hypersensitivity; and the relationship of stress and female hormones to IC.

### Neurogenic Inflammation

Neurogenic inflammation may provide the nidus for induction, establishment, and chronicity of the various tissue changes seen in IC. Other conditions in which neurogenic inflammation may be implicated include irritable bowel syndrome, vulvodynia, migraines, fibromyalgia, and multiple sclerosis. It has been shown that mast cells are located in close proximity to the peripheral and central nervous systems. In addition, an intimate association between mast cells and sensory nerve fibers has been demonstrated in the integumentary, pulmonary, and gastrointestinal systems.

Excitation of sensory nerves, especially small pain C-fibers, triggers an inflammatory process through release of neuropeptides (substance P) and calcitonin gene-related peptide. Substance P causes vasodilation and increased vasopermeability and activates mast cells, causing injury with increased permeability of epithelial surfaces. Multiple

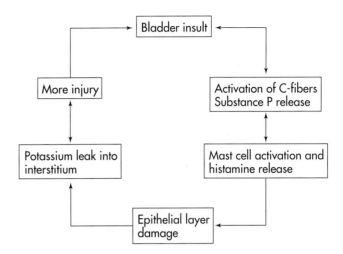

**Fig. 25-2** Pathogenesis of interstitial cystitis.

events or factors trigger neurogenic inflammation. These include bacterial cystitis or the antigen from the organism; an increased level of estrogen; toxins of endogenous and exogenous origin including drugs, their metabolites, and certain foods; and a potent mediator such as the histamine released by activated mast cells. As our understanding of neurogenic inflammation and the role of mast cell activation progresses (Fig. 25-2), the diagnosis and treatment of IC will evolve.

### Diagnosis

Hypersensitivity disorders of the lower urinary tract are diagnosed by exclusion (see Box 25-1). Patients cannot have evidence of cystitis caused by infection, use of cyclophosphamide or other chemical agents, radiation, or tuberculosis. Other infections such as vaginitis, urethritis, or genital herpes cannot be present. Also, urethral diverticulum, bladder carcinoma, and carcinoma in situ must be excluded. However, patients with hypersensitivity disorder may have concomitant lower urinary tract or pelvic floor disorders.

### History

Frequency (>8 voids during waking hours), nocturia (>2 voids during sleeping hours), urgency, suprapubic pressure on bladder filling, and bladder pain are the most common symptoms. Secondary symptoms include burning during or after urination; a feeling of decreased bladder emptying; hesitancy; interruption of urinary stream; double voiding; referred pain to the abdomen, lower back, or medial thighs; abdominal bloating; postvoid urethral pain; incontinence without sensation; or detrusor instability. The severity and duration of each flare over the previous year should be recorded. The physician should also inquire about previous UTI, types of incontinence, parity, previous pelvic surgery, radiation therapy, chemotherapy, previous treatments, menstrual history, history of endometriosis, and dyspareunia. All patients should be asked to do a voiding diary (see Fig. 13-1) and fill out the O'Leary-Sant symptom and problem index (Fig. 25-3). A medical history should include associated diseases such as migraines, fibromyalgia, sinusitis, drug hypersensitivity, sicca syndrome (dry eyes/ dry mouth), Sjögren's syndrome, vulvodynia, and irritable bowel syndrome.

### Physical Examination

The abdominal examination detects the presence of costovertebral tenderness and abdominal tenderness or mass. The external genitalia are examined for signs of infection and vulvodynia/vestibulitis (tenderness over the vulvar vestibular glands or Bartholin's glands). The pelvic examination includes a vaginal and urethral culture if appropriate, evaluation for signs of atrophic vaginitis or a urethral caruncle, and a Pap smear if indicated. Perineometry may help evaluate the pelvic floor muscles to rule out pelvic floor dysfunction (the inability to optimally contract and relax the pelvic floor muscles). Evaluation of bladder and pelvic organ support is done in both the dorsal lithotomy and standing positions to determine and grade bladder neck hypermobility, cystocele, enterocele or uterine prolapse, and rectocele. The posterior bladder wall and urethra should be palpated to check for tenderness and masses, and a bimanual examination should be performed to detect pelvic or adnexal masses and tender nodules. A rectovaginal examination is performed to evaluate tenderness along the uterosacral ligaments. Finally, a neurourologic examination ascertains the presence of the bulbocavernosus reflex and grades perineal sensation and anal sphincter strength.

### Laboratory and Radiographic Evaluation

Initial laboratory examination should include urinalysis, urine culture and sensitivity, and measurement of postvoid residual urine volume (catheterized or with bladder ultrasound). Urine cytology is indicated in the presence of microscopic hematuria and persistent urgency. A 24-hour voiding diary measures input and output, number and quantity of voids, and number and severity of leakage episodes in a 24-hour period. A renal ultrasound or intravenous pyelogram (IVP) is indicated in the presence of hematuria, history of recurrent UTI, or history of pelvic surgery. An IVP is obtained if the renal ultrasound shows obstruction or calculi or if an anatomic defect is suspected (fistula or urethral diverticulum). A voiding cystourethrogram (VCUG) is useful in ruling out vesicoureteral reflux and evaluating the bladder neck in patients with concomitant incontinence or suburethral diverticulum. An awake cystoscopy is indicated in the presence of hematuria, persistent or recurrent UTI, or suspected fistula or urethral diverticulum.

### Potassium Sensitivity Test

Parsons (1996) designed the potassium sensitivity test to measure epithelial permeability. Instilling a solution of potassium chloride (KCl) into a normal bladder will not promote urgency or pain (Box 25-2). If a patient's bladder has an leaky epithelium, the KCl mixture readily diffuses across the transitional cells and stimulates sensory nerves, causing urgency and pain. A recent study demonstrated that 70% of patients with IC had provocation of symptoms, whereas only 4% of normal subjects responded with pain.

### Cystoscopy

Cystoscopy is both diagnostic and therapeutic. Cystoscopy with hydrodistention of the bladder has traditionally been performed under general or regional anesthesia. Our experience has been that intravenous sedation, bupivacaine hydrochloride (Marcaine) bladder instillation, and pudendal nerve block are effective diagnostic and therapeutic alternatives with minimal morbidity and increased postoperative patient satisfaction. Cystoscopy is performed to eliminate other causes of persistent patient symptoms and hematuria and to detect findings consistent with early- or late-stage IC (Table 25-1). The classic Hunner's ulcer (late stage), an area of erythema with small vessels radiating to a central, pale scar after bladder filling, is found in only 8% of patients with IC. Previous biopsy sites and carcinoma in situ can be confused with ulcers. Before hydrodistention, an inclusive evaluation of the entire bladder is performed, and the degree of hypervascularity and linear scarring (mild, moderate, severe) is assessed. Hydrodistention is performed by filling the bladder under gravity at 80 cm $H_2O$ with urethral compression for 2 to 7 minutes. The bladder is then drained, looking for a terminal bloody effluent, and the capacity is measured (>350 ml is defined as early-stage IC and ≤350 ml as late-stage IC). The average bladder capacity for patients with IC has been reported as 575 ml, and as 1115 ml for patients without persistent irritative voiding symptoms. On redistention of the bladder, the presence and severity of glomerulations, strawberry-like petechial hemorrhages, are determined. Not all patients with significant symptoms have glomerulations or a reduced bladder capacity. Bladder biopsy is performed after hydrodistention to reduce the risk of perforation. The biopsy eliminates the presence of carcinoma in situ and infection, and it can quantitate the number of mast cells in the lamina propria and detrusor muscle. The diagnosis of IC cannot be ruled out based on normal cystoscopic findings; the findings of glomerulations and a terminal bloody effluent suggest the diagnosis of IC. A capacity below 350 ml or the presence of a Hunner's ulcer confirms the diagnosis of late IC. Concomitant laparoscopy may be performed when there is tenderness in the adnexa, a history of previous pelvic surgery, an abnormal pelvic ultrasound, suspected endometriosis, dysmenorrhea, or dyspareunia in the absence of vulvodynia.

### Urodynamic Tests

Urodynamic evaluations are performed on patients with hypersensitivity symptoms to evaluate the following features: volume at first sensation of filling, volume at first

Check the one best answer for each question.

1. <u>During the past month,</u> how often have you felt the strong need to urinate with little or no warning?

|  | Score |  | Score |
|---|---|---|---|
| [ ] Not at all | [0] | [ ] About half the time | [3] |
| [ ] Less than 1 time in 5 | [1] | [ ] More than half the time | [4] |
| [ ] Less than half the time | [2] | [ ] Almost always | [5] |

2. <u>During the past month,</u> have you had to urinate less than 2 hours after you finished urinating?

|  | Score |  | Score |
|---|---|---|---|
| [ ] Not at all | [0] | [ ] About half the time | [3] |
| [ ] Less than 1 time in 5 | [1] | [ ] More than half the time | [4] |
| [ ] Less than half the time | [2] | [ ] Almost always | [5] |

3. <u>During the past month,</u> how often each night did you most typically get up at night to urinate?

|  | Score |  | Score |
|---|---|---|---|
| [ ] None | [0] | [ ] 3 times per night | [3] |
| [ ] Once per night | [1] | [ ] 4 times per night | [4] |
| [ ] 2 times per night | [2] | [ ] 5 or more times per night | [5] |

4. <u>During the past month,</u> have you experienced pain or burning in your bladder?

|  | Score |  | Score |
|---|---|---|---|
| [ ] Not at all | [0] | [ ] Usually | [3] |
| [ ] A few times | [1] | [ ] Almost always | [4] |
| [ ] Fairly often | [2] |  |  |

### Interstitial Cystitis Problem Index (ICPI)

<u>During the past month,</u> how much has each of the following been a problem for you?

1. Frequent urination during the day?

|  | Score |  | Score |
|---|---|---|---|
| [ ] No problem | [0] | [ ] Medium problem | [3] |
| [ ] Very small problem | [1] | [ ] Big problem | [4] |
| [ ] Small problem | [2] |  |  |

2. Getting up at night to urinate?

|  | Score |  | Score |
|---|---|---|---|
| [ ] No problem | [0] | [ ] Medium problem | [3] |
| [ ] Very small problem | [1] | [ ] Big problem | [4] |
| [ ] Small problem | [2] |  |  |

3. Need to urinate with little warning?

|  | Score |  | Score |
|---|---|---|---|
| [ ] No problem | [0] | [ ] Medium problem | [3] |
| [ ] Very small problem | [1] | [ ] Big problem | [4] |
| [ ] Small problem | [2] |  |  |

4. Burning, pain, discomfort, or pressure in your bladder?

|  | Score |  | Score |
|---|---|---|---|
| [ ] No problem | [0] | [ ] Medium problem | [3] |
| [ ] Very small problem | [1] | [ ] Big problem | [4] |
| [ ] Small problem | [2] |  |  |

(Patients without IC will score less than 6 on either index.)

**Fig. 25-3**  O'Leary-Sant Interstitial Cystitis Symptom Index.

**Box 25-2**
**POTASSIUM SENSITIVITY TEST**

Measure of epithelial permeability: KCl solution (40 ml; 400 mEq/L)

Normal bladder/intact epithelium: KCl provokes no symptoms

Epithelial dysfunction: $K^+$ diffuses across transitional cells and stimulates sensory nerves, causing urgency or pain

Positive response: No response to $H_2O$; ≥2 response to KCl (scale 0-5)

**Table 25-1** Most Common Cystoscopic Findings in Interstitial Cystitis

| Early | Late |
|---|---|
| Glomerulations (petechial submucosal hemorrhages) | Bladder capacity <300 ml |
| Hypervascularity and linear scarring | Hunner's ulcers |
| Bloody terminal effluent after hydrodistention | |

sensation to void, maximum cystometric capacity, detrusor compliance, the presence or absence of detrusor instability, and reproduction of bladder pain and/or patients' symptoms. Patients with interstitial cystitis often have symptoms suggestive of an overactive bladder, specifically sensory urgency. The International Continence Society (ICS) refers to the term *overactive bladder* as a storage phase disease diagnosed by urodynamics. An overactive bladder is characterized by involuntary detrusor contractions that may occur spontaneously or may be provoked. The overactive bladder is referred to as unstable when the cause is nonneurogenic and hyperreflexic when the cause is neurogenic. Patients with interstitial cystitis typically have severe urgency and frequency. Urgency is divided into two categories: motor urgency and sensory urgency. Motor urgency describes those patients who demonstrate a strong desire to void and have urodynamic findings consistent with an overactive bladder. Sensory urgency defines a subset of patients who present with urinary frequency and urgency without the cystometric evidence of uninhibited bladder contractions or an overactive bladder.

Jarvis (1982) defined sensory urgency as an abnormal first sensation on bladder filling less than 75 ml and a bladder capacity less than 400 ml in the absence of involuntary bladder contractions. Normal first sensation of filling occurs between 50 to 150 ml, with a first urge to void between 200 and 500 ml, and a maximum capacity between 400 and 700 ml. Kirkemo et al. (1997) found that patients enrolled in the National Interstitial Cystitis Data Base (NICDB) had a correlation between reported daytime, nighttime, and 24-hour frequency and both volume at first sensation to void (VFSV) and volume at maximum cystometric capacity (VMCC). VFSV decreased as awake frequency increased. Patients who voided ≤5 times during awake hours had a mean VFSV of $114 \pm 81$ ml versus $74 \pm 61$ ml for those voiding >15 times. Similarly, this was seen with VMCC with mean volumes of $244 \pm 149$ ml versus $184 \pm 114$ ml, respectively for those voiding ≤5 times and those >15 times. This same trend was seen with nocturia and 24-hour voiding frequency. Patients with a 24-hour voiding frequency of >15 times/day had a mean VFSV of $70 \pm 59$ ml and a VMCC of $190 \pm 112$ ml.

In addition to comparing a patient's symptoms to urodynamic findings, a correlation has been made between urodynamic findings, cystoscopic findings, and a patient's severity of disease. Most authors have noted a decrease in volume at first sensation to void and maximum cystometric capacity. Nigro et al. (1997) compared the findings of 150 women involved in the NICDB who underwent cystoscopy, bladder overdistention, and urodynamics. The mean volume at first sensation to void was $81 \pm 64$ ml and a mean volume at maximum capacity was $198 \pm 107$ ml. Many authors feel that patients with a Hunner's ulcer have a more severe form of interstitial cystitis. The NICDB noted that patients with a Hunner's ulcer had a mean volume at first sensation of $34.7 \pm 20.5$ ml. This was statistically lower than the volume at first sensation of patients without a Hunner's ulcer. None of the urodynamic criteria were statistically significant when related to the presence or absence of bloody effluent, presence and degree of glomerulations, presence of involuntary bladder contractions, or end-filling pressures. Twenty-six patients (17.5%) in this study had involuntary bladder contractions. Other studies have found that 5% to 26% of patients with the symptom complex of interstitial cystitis had involuntary bladder contractions. The original exclusion criteria for interstitial cystitis included involuntary bladder contractions; this is now a debatable issue. However, there does appear to be a relationship between the severity of a patient's symptoms and the urodynamic findings.

Currently, there are no specific urodynamic values that diagnose interstitial cystitis or predict the characteristic cystoscopic findings of the disease. Patients with the symptom complex of a hypersensitive lower urinary tract tend to have an early first sensation of bladder filling, a decreased volume at first sensation to void, and a decreased maximum capacity during urodynamic studies.

## URETHRAL SYNDROME

Urethral syndrome, part of the spectrum of lower urinary tract hypersensitivity disorders, was once considered a separate diagnosis. Now it appears to be a mild or early stage of IC (see Fig. 25-1). Urethral syndrome is characterized by symptoms similar to those of IC: frequency, urgency, nocturia, dysuria, urethral pain, and a feeling of decreased bladder emptying. A certain subgroup of patients specifically isolate urethral pain from bladder pain. As with other hypersensitivity disorders, all other diagnoses must be excluded. Of particular importance with urethral pain is the exclusion of cystitis, including bacterial and tuberculosis, as well as various sexually transmitted diseases including chlamydia, *Trichomonas, Gardnerella,* genital herpes, and human papilloma virus. A hypoestrogenic state can produce symptoms of urethral syndrome. Symptoms of urethral syndrome can also be caused by allergic hypersensitivity reactions related to personal hygiene products and other external chemical exposure, including chlorine and spermicides. A urethral stricture, diverticulum, or other anatomic abnormality can be found at the time of cystoscopy. Finally, many patients with early IC or urethral syndrome have pelvic floor dysfunction or pelvic muscle spasticity that may respond to biofeedback or physical therapy.

Diagnosis and treatments are similar to those for IC. Historically, urethral dilation was felt to help by relieving infected urethral glands. There are no controlled studies in the literature to establish the benefit of urethral dilation. Typically these patients respond to treatment of the underlying disorder. Once all other disorders are excluded, patients benefit from conservative measures similar to those for early-stage IC.

## MANAGEMENT OF HYPERSENSITIVITY DISORDERS

After all other diagnoses are excluded, hypersensitivity disorders of the lower urinary tract can be managed successfully in over 85% of patients by using a combination of anecdotal and conventional modalities. A multidisciplinary approach and patient self-care regimens are most successful.

Initial management should promote bladder retraining, relieve irritative voiding symptoms, enhance healing of potential bladder lining defects, and correct pelvic floor dysfunction. Learning how to keep a voiding diary, with emphasis on the time and amount of fluid intake, amount and time between voids, and comments about exacerbation of symptoms with food and fluid intake and activity, will aid in formulating intake and voiding schedules in a 24-hour period. Adequate hydration with frequent sips of water during waking hours aids in urinary dilution. Voiding on a regular schedule can significantly decrease leakage and pain. For example, voiding every 2 hours is recommended if pain or leakage occurs at intervals greater than every 2 hours on the voiding diary. On the other hand, if the patient is a frequent voider, bladder holding to increase the voiding interval by 10 to 15 minutes per week over a 3-month period can significantly decrease frequency, especially if pain is controlled. A low-potassium, low-acid diet (Box 25-3) and urinary alkalinization with potassium citrate may decrease symptoms in 40% to 65% of patients (Table 25-2). The addition of bladder analgesics or antispasmodics may

## Box 25-3
## ANTIINFLAMMATORY DIET

*Alcoholic beverages
Apples
Apple juice
Cantaloupe
*Carbonated beverages
Chili and other spicy foods
*Citrus fruits, including lemons, limes, oranges, and grapefruit
*Coffee (may use decaf or Kava)
Cranberries
Grapes
Peaches
*Pineapple
Plums
*Berries
*Tea
Herbal tea
*Tomatoes
*Vinegar and other condiments
Avocado
Bananas
*Cheeses, particularly hard and soft brie-type cheeses
*Chocolate (may use white chocolate)
Corned beef
Beans
Nuts
Prunes and raisins
Rye bread
Yogurt and sour cream
*Aspartame and saccharin
*Onions
*Pepper
Vitamins buffered with aspartame

---

*Foods to be avoided by patients with IC and vulvodynia.
Non-asterisk entries may be ingested in moderation only. Asterisk entries should be avoided altogether whenever possible.
The acid-restricted diet is most effective when 64 ounces of water is ingested daily and urine is alkalinized.

further decrease hypersensitivity symptoms. Anticholinergic medications such as tolterodine tartrate may also help to decrease symptoms and are currently under investigation. Anecdotally, baking soda and hydrogen peroxide baths have helped patients with pelvic floor dysfunction and urethral syndrome. If these conservative measures fail, the patients proceed to diagnosis with cystoscopy, bladder hydrodistention, bladder biopsy, and video or office urodynamics, depending on the symptoms and history (Fig. 25-4).

## Hydrodistention of the Bladder

Hydrodistention of the bladder under anesthesia improves symptoms in 30% to 54% of patients. Patients who have significant improvement for 6 months or more are candidates for a repeat hydrodistention. The physiology of how

**Table 25-2**   Food Sensitivity in Interstitial Cystitis Patients*

| Diet | Exacerbation N (%) | Worst symptoms (hours) | Dietary quantity |
|---|---|---|---|
| Pizza | 91 (45.5) | 0-4 | 1-2 Slices |
| Tomato | 125 (62.5) | 0-2 | 1 Serving |
| Spicy foods | 111 (55.5) | 0-2 | 1 Serving |
| Coffee | 119 (59.5) | 0-2 | 1 Cup |
| Acidic juice or fruit | 125 (62.5) | 0-2 | 1 Serving or glass |
| Carbonated drink | 114 (57.0) | 0-2 | 1 Glass |
| Alcohol | 106 (53.0) | 0-2 | 1 Glass |
| Chocolate | 82 (41.0) | 0-2 | 1 Piece |

*This table reflects the results of a survey of 200 patients with the symptom complex of IC. Patients were asked a series of questions regarding foods and events that exacerbate their symptoms. This table demonstrates the type of foods that most commonly exacerbated the patients' symptoms, the time to exacerbation, and the amount of food required for exacerbation.

this improves symptoms is not known. In patients with a capacity of less than 600 ml under anesthesia, the therapeutic result was excellent in 26% and fair in 29%, compared with 12% with an excellent and 43% with a fair response in patients whose capacity was greater than 600 ml. Patients for whom hydrodistention fails are begun on oral medications. Oral therapy includes antidepressants (amitriptyline), antihistamines (hydroxyzine), alpha-blockers, pentosanpolysulfate (Elmiron), antianxiety agents, narcotics, and anticonvulsants (Fig. 25-5).

## Pharmacologic Therapy
### Antidepressants

Most patients with IC suffer from anger, anxiety, depression or fatigue caused by the lack of sleep, and chronic pain. Tricyclic antidepressants work as central and peripheral anticholinergic agents, blocking the reuptake of serotonin

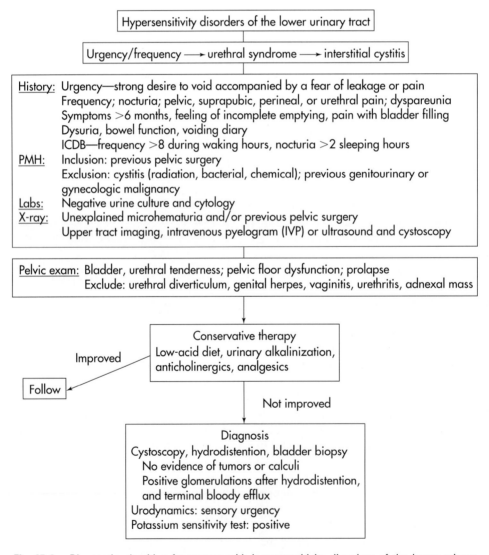

**Fig. 25-4**   Diagnostic algorithm for women with hypersensitivity disorders of the lower urinary tract. *ICDB,* Interstitial Cystitis Data Base; *PMH,* past medical history.

and norepinephrine, and they have antihistaminic properties. Amitriptyline is usually started at a low dosage, 10 to 25 mg before bedtime and titrated up to 75 mg taken 1 hour before bedtime (patients should be advised that they will feel tired for 12 hours after taking the medication). Substitutes may be given if side effects are unacceptable. These include doxepin hydrochloride 10 to 75 mg 1 hour before bedtime, paroxetine hydrochloride (Paxil) 10 to 20 mg before bedtime, or fluoxetine hydrochloride (Prozac) 20 mg a day.

### Antihistamines

Hydroxyzine has been shown to provide symptomatic relief, especially in patients with a history of allergies or biopsy-proven mast cell activation. In a study of 90 patients, 40% were noted to have a reduction in symptom scores using hydroxyzine up to 75 mg/day. The reason hydroxyzine is effective is not completely understood; theories include stabilization of mast cells, anticholinergic properties, and a sedative effect.

### Pentosanpolysulfate

Pentosanpolysulfate (Elmiron) is a synthetic sulfated polysaccharide with properties of sulfated GAGs and an affinity for mucosal membranes. Its use is based on the concept of stabilizing urothelial permeability (the GAG layer) to prevent irritating solutes in the urine from reaching the bladder interstitium. Elmiron is excreted in the urine and attempts to correct the permeability defect in the GAG layer. A randomized clinical trial noted a 38% improvement in symptoms (predominately pain) compared with an 18% response in the placebo group during a 3-month treatment period. A subsequent review of the long-term therapy (up to

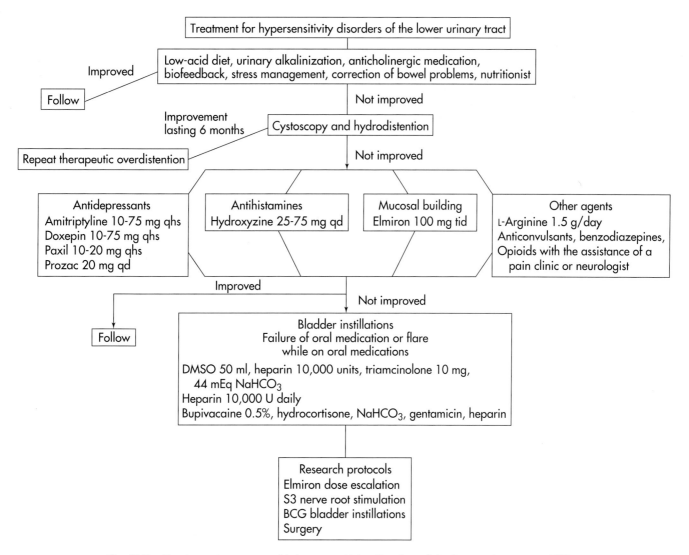

**Fig. 25-5**   Treatment for women with hypersensitivity disorders of the lower urinary tract. *BCG,* Bacillus Calmette–Guérin.

3 years) with Elmiron showed that patients had a 42% to 62% improvement in their overall symptoms (pain and urgency). This study also demonstrated that the medication is safe and effective for 3 years. A dosage escalation study using Elmiron is currently in progress. Side effects occur in less than 5% of patients and include alopecia, diarrhea, nausea, and headache. Elmiron should be taken for 6 months or longer to achieve effectiveness.

### Other Oral Agents

Between 10% to 15% of patients with IC have severe, unrelenting pain. L-Arginine, a nitric oxide synthetase inhibitor and dietary supplement, significantly decreased pain when taken daily for 6 months at 1.5 g/day. After appropriate functional assessment, opioids, anticonvulsants, or benzodiazepines may be administered and titrated often in coordination with a pain specialist.

## Bladder Instillations

Bladder instillations are reserved for patients who are not responding to oral therapy and for those who are doing well on oral therapy and have a flare in their symptoms. A common instillation mixture includes 50 ml dimethyl sulfoxide (DMSO), 10,000 units heparin, 10 mg triamcinolone, and 44 mEq $NaHCO_3$ instilled once a week for 6 weeks. The pharmacologic properties of DMSO include antiinflammatory and analgesic effects, collagen dissolution, muscle relaxation, and mast cell histamine release. Heparin is a GAG that is thought to mimic the activity of the bladder's mucopolysaccharide lining. An improvement in symptoms for up to 6 months has been achieved using the DMSO cocktail in 78% of patients receiving six weekly treatments. Intravesical heparin (20,000 units in 10 ml of sterile water) self-administered daily for 4 to 12 months has resulted in a 60% or better response rate. A combination of 0.5% bupivacaine, heparin, hydrocortisone, $NaHCO_3$, and gentamicin (pH 6.5) given to patients with IC and a history of recurrent UTI resulted in an improvement in 78% of patients that lasted up to 6 months.

Clorpactin, a derivative of hypochlorous acid in a buffered base, has also been used as an instillation agent. Messing and Stamey (1987) described using a 0.4% solution administered at 10 cm $H_2O$ under anesthesia. They reported a success rate of 72% with a duration of improvement of 6 months. Vesicoureteral reflux is a contraindication for usage due to a case of ureteral fibrosis following clorpactin usage; therefore, a pretherapy cystogram is recommended. Intravesical hyaluronic acid, a GAG, showed a 71% response rate that was sustained for up to 6 months. Bacillus Calmette–Guérin (BCG), an immunogenic agent used to treat superficial transitional cell carcinoma of the bladder, is under investigation as an alternative for instillation therapy. Preliminary studies in patients with IC showed a response rate of 60% (compared with a 27% placebo response rate) that lasted for at least 6 months.

## Refractory Symptoms

Patients with intractable pain despite an adequate trial of conservative interventions, such as physical therapy, biofeedback, and oral and intravesical therapies, may benefit from evaluation at a pain clinic. Pain diversion with the use of transcutaneous electrical stimulation may be helpful. Studies report a 26% improvement in pain symptoms for patients with nonulcer (early) IC and a 54% improvement for ulcer (late) IC patients. Epidural nerve blocks have been used in the management of chronic pain. Continued neurogenic inflammation of the bladder may lead to fibrosis and neurologic ischemia or reflex sympathetic dystrophy. Refractory IC pain may respond to a series of epidural nerve blocks.

Peripheral denervation (cystolysis) and central denervation (presacral neurectomy or rhizotomy) techniques were popular in the 1970s and 1980s. Unfortunately, the duration of results was short, and complication rates were high. Currently, an implantable sacral nerve root (S3) electrical stimulator is under investigation.

Surgery is considered a last resort for patients with IC. Less than 10% of patients are unresponsive to all other therapeutic modalities and undergo surgery. Augmentation cystoplasty using ileum, cecum, or colon with a supratrigonal cystectomy was popularized in the early 1980s. The fate of the augmented bowel remains undetermined. These patients can experience recurrent symptoms or pain, and self-catheterization (necessary in up to 80% of the patients) of the patient's inflamed bladder and urethra may be painful. The bowel segment may develop mast cell infiltration and contraction. Therefore, the use of augmentation cystoplasty should be reserved for the rare IC patient with a small-capacity bladder and no pain.

The currently accepted modality of surgical therapy is urinary diversion (ileal loop or conduit, continent diversion or pouch), with or without cystectomy. Before urinary diversion is chosen as therapy for intractable pain, a psychologic evaluation is recommended. A differential epidural block may help distinguish between psychogenic, sympathetic, and somatic pain. Reported success rates of urinary diversion have been approximately 70%. The physician and patient choose between a continent diversion (pouch) or ileal loop (conduit). Several reports of recurrent symptoms (pouchitis) have led surgeons to recommend an ileal loop.

Urinary diversion without cystectomy is particularly attractive in younger patients with the hope of finding a cure and possible undiversion. Morbidity from the in situ bladder has been reported in up to 80% of patients. These complications include pyocystis (67%), hemorrhage (23%), severe pain (13%), and intractable spasm (17%). Many of these patients will require cystectomy. Our own experience has shown that patients with continent diversions experience significant pouch spasms. Total cystourethrectomy is indicated in patients with urethral pain to avoid persistent pain from the urethral remnant. Patients must be informed that their pelvic pain may persist with urinary diversion with or without cystectomy.

## FUTURE DIRECTIONS

A multidisciplinary approach to treating patients with hypersensitivity disorders of the lower urinary tract is comprehensive and cost-effective (Box 25-4). A pelvic floor team provides a detailed history, physical examination, and management based on input from several specialties. The urologist, urogynecologist, or pelvic floor specialist evaluates the patient initially. A gastroenterologist or colorectal surgeon is helpful because many patients have irritable bowel syndrome or constipation. A rheumatologist or internist should evaluate the patient's general medical and autoimmune status because many patients are chronically debilitated or have the systemic features of IC (fibromyalgia, migraines, sinusitis, drug hypersensitivity). Up to 70% of patients with severe symptoms have pelvic floor dysfunction, which is conservatively treated with physical therapy (exercise, myofascial massage, and manual therapy) or biofeedback with or without electrical stimulation. A psychologist is invaluable in providing stress reduction techniques such as self-visualization, self-hypnosis, baths, deep breathing, and meditation. Behavioral therapy, including the development of coping mechanisms, problem solving, and sex therapy are also very useful. Nutritional counseling is beneficial to any patient with a painful or chronic illness. A chemical pain manager (neuropsychiatrist) and invasive pain manager (anesthesiologist) make intractable pain tolerable for most patients.

Complementary medicine has been effective in the treatment of IC. Acupuncture reduced pain by at least 50% in more than 60% of patients after an average of 12 treatments. Anecdotally, herbal therapy may be useful in up to 75% of patients. Nutritional supplements may be useful in boosting the immune system in patients with long-standing disease.

A multidisciplinary approach to research will improve our ability to study the epidemiology, diagnosis, and management of IC. Procurement of increased funding for clinical and basic science research will aid in defining the hypersensitivity pelvic floor disorder population, finding markers for etiology and treatment efficacy, determining the effect of hormones on these disorders, and defining outcome measures for treatment protocols. Unbiased randomized controlled trials for the prevention of IC by treating lower urinary tract hypersensitivity disorders appropriately and in a timely fashion will improve the quality of women's pelvic health. Increased funding for public education, medical student and resident education, and education of primary care providers will allow access to treatment at an earlier point in the hypersensitivity spectrum.

## BIBLIOGRAPHY
### History and Prevalence

Christmas TJ: Historical aspects of interstitial cystitis. In Sant GR, ed: *Interstitial cystitis,* Philadelphia, 1997, Lippincott.

Gillenwater JY, Wein AJ: Summary of the National Institute of Arthritis, Diabetes, Digestive and Kidney Diseases Workshop on Interstitial Cystitis, National Institutes of Health, Bethesda, MD, August 28-29, 1987, *J Urol* 140:203, 1988.

Hanash KA, Pool TL: Interstitial and hemorrhagic cystitis: viral, bacterial, and fungal studies, *J Urol* 104:705, 1970.

Hunner GL: A rare type of bladder ulcer in women: report of cases, *Boston Med Soc J* 172:660, 1915.

Jones CA, Nyberg L: Epidemiology of interstitial cystitis, *Urology* 49S(5A):2, 1997.

Nitze M: *Lehrbuch de cystoscopie: ihre technik und kinsche bedeutung,* Berlin, 1907, JE Bergman.

O'Leary MP, Sant GR, Fowler FJ, et al: The interstitial cystitis symptom index and problem index, *Urology* 49S(5A):58, 1997.

Skene AJ: *Diseases of bladder and urethra in women,* New York, 1887, William Wood.

### Etiology

Alagiri M, Chottiner S, Ratner V, et al: Interstitial cystitis: unexplained associations with other chronic disease and pain syndromes, *Urology* 49S(5A):52, 1997.

Aldenborg F, Fall M, Enerback L: Proliferation and transepithelium migration of mucosal mast cells in interstitial cystitis, *Immunology* 58:411, 1986.

Boucher W, El-Mansoury M, Pang X, et al: Elevated mast cell tryptase in the urine of patients with interstitial cystitis, *Br J Urol* 76:94, 1995.

Buffington CT, Wolfe SA: High affinity binding sites for [$^3$H] substance P in urinary bladders of cats with interstitial cystitis, *J Urol* 160:605, 1998.

Christmas TJ, Rode J, Chapple CR, et al: Nerve fiber proliferation in interstitial cystitis, *Virchow Arch Pathol Anat* 416:447, 1990.

Collan Y, Alfthan O, Kivilaakso E, et al: Electron microscopic and histologic findings on urinary bladder epithelium in interstitial cystitis, *Eur Urol* 2:242, 1976.

Domingue GJ, Ghoniem GM, Bost KL, et al: Dormant microbes in interstitial cystitis, *J Urol* 153:1321, 1995.

Domingue GJ, Ghoniem GM, Human L, et al: Bacteriology of urinary bladder tissue and urine in interstitial cystitis, *J Urol* 155S(5A):432, 1996.

### Box 25-4
### MEMBERS OF A MULTIDISCIPLINARY IC TEAM

Urologist
Urogynecologist
Gastroenterologist
Colorectal surgeon
Rheumatologist or internist
Nutritionist
Psychologist (stress, behavioral, and sex therapy)
Physical therapist (biofeedback)
Neuropsychiatrist
Chemical and invasive pain management specialist
Acupuncture or herbal therapy specialist

Elbadawi A: Interstitial cystitis: a critique of current concepts with a new proposal for pathologic diagnosis and pathogenesis, *Urology* 48S(5A): 14, 1997.

Elbadawi A, Light JK: Distinctive ultrastructural pathology of nonulcerative interstitial cystitis: new observations and their potential significance in pathogenesis, *Urol Int* 56:137, 1996.

Elliott TS, Slack RC, Bishop MC: Scanning electron microscopy of the human bladder mucosa in acute and chronic urinary tract infection, *Br J Urol* 56:38, 1984.

El-Mansoury M, Boucher W, Sant GR, et al: Increased histamine and methylhistamine in interstitial cystitis, *J Urol* 152:350, 1994.

Erickson DR: Inflammatory cell types and other clinical features of interstitial cystitis, *J Urol* 155S(5):440A, 1995.

Fall M, Johasson SL, Vahlne A: A clinicopathological and virological study of interstitial cystitis, *J Urol* 133:771, 1985.

Haarla M, Jalava J, Laato M, et al: Absence of bacterial DNA in the bladder of patients with interstitial cystitis, *J Urol* 156:1843, 1996.

Hampson S, Christmas T, Moss M: Search for mycobacteria in interstitial cystitis using mycobacteria-specific DNA probes with signal amplification by polymerase chain reaction, *Br J Urol* 72:303, 1993.

Hanno PM, Levin RM, Monson FC, et al: Diagnosis of interstitial cystitis, *J Urol* 143:278, 1990.

Hedelin HH, Mardh PA, Brorson JE, et al: Mycoplasma hominis and interstitial cystitis, *Sex Trans Dis* 10S:327, 1980.

Hofmeister MA, He F, Ratliff TL, et al: Mast cells and nerve fibers in interstitial cystitis: an algorithm for histologic diagnosis via quantitative image analysis and morphometry, *Urology* 49:41, 1997.

Hohenfellner M, Nunes L, Schmidt RA, et al: Interstitial cystitis: increased sympathetic innervation and related neuropeptide synthesis, *J Urol* 147:587, 1992.

Holm-Bentzen M, Sondergaard I, Hald T: Urinary excretion of a metabolite of histamine (1,4 methyl-imidazole, acetic-acid) in painful bladder disease, *Br J Urol* 59:230, 1987.

Johansson SL: Interstitial cystitis, *Mod Pathol* 6:738, 1993.

Kastrup J, Hald T, Larsen S, et al: Histamine content and mast cell count of detrusor muscle in patients with interstitial cystitis and other types of chronic cystitis, *Br J Urol* 55:495, 1983.

Keay S, Schwalbe RS, Warren JW, et al: A prospective study of microorganisms in urine and bladder biopsies from interstitial cystitis patients and controls, *Urology* 45:223, 1995.

Larsen S, Thompson SA, Hald T, et al: Mast cells in interstitial cystitis, *Br J Urol* 54:283, 1982.

Leon A, Buriani A, Dal Toso R, et al: Mast cells synthesize, store, and release nerve growth factor, *Proc Natl Acad Sci USA* 91:3739, 1994.

Letourneau R, Pang X, Sant GR, et al: Intragranular activation of bladder mast cells and their association with nerve processes in interstitial cystitis, *Br J Urol* 77:41, 1996.

Lundenberg T, Lieberg H, Nordling L, et al: Interstitial cystitis: correlation with nerve fibers, mast cells and histamine, *Br J Urol* 71:427, 1993.

Lynes WL, Flynn SD, Shortliffe LD, et al: The histology of interstitial cystitis, *Am J Surg Pathol* 14:969, 1990.

Marshall JS, Wasserman S: Mast cells and the nerves: potential interactions in the context of chronic disease, *Clin Exp Allergy* 25:102, 1995.

Messing EM, Stamey TA: Interstitial cystitis. Early diagnosis, pathology and treatment, *Urology* 12:381, 1987.

Miller CH, MacDermott JP, Quattrocchi GA, et al: Lymphocyte function in patients with interstitial cystitis, *J Urol* 157:592, 1992.

Myers G, Donlon M, Kaliner M: Measurement of urinary histamine: development of methodology and normal values, *Allerg Clin Immunol* 67:305, 1981.

Newson B, Dahlstrom A, Enerback L, et al: Suggestive evidence for a direct innervation of mucosal mast cells, *Neuroscience* 10:565, 1983.

Ochs RL, Stein TW, Peebles CL, et al: Autoantibodies in interstitial cystitis, *J Urol* 151:587, 1994.

Pang X, Boucher W, Triadafilopoulos G, et al: Mast cell and substance P-positive nerve involvement in a patient with both irritable bowel syndrome and interstitial cystitis, *Urology* 47:436, 1996.

Pang X, Marchand J, Sant GR, et al: Increased number of substance P positive nerve fibers in interstitial cystitis, *Br J Urol* 75:744, 1995.

Parsons CL: Potassium sensitivity test, *Tech Urol* 2:171, 1996.

Purcell WM, Aterwill CK: Mast cells in neuroimmune function: neurotoxicological and neuropharmacological perspectives, *Biochem Res* 20:521, 1995.

Saban R, Keith IM, Bjorling DE: Neuropeptide-mast cell interaction in interstitial cystitis. In Sant GR, ed: *Interstitial cystitis,* Philadelphia, 1997, Lippincott.

Sant GR, Theoharides TC: The role of the mast cell in interstitial cystitis, *Urol Clin North Am* 21:41, 1994.

Stead RH, Dixon MF, Bramwell NH, et al: Mast cells are closely apposed to nerves in the human gastrointestinal mucosa, *Gastroenterology* 97:575, 1989.

Steers W, Tuttle JB: Neurogenic inflammation and nerve growth factor: possible roles in interstitial cystitis. In Sant GR, ed: *Interstitial cystitis,* Philadelphia, 1997, Lippincott.

Theoharides TC, Sant GR: Bladder mast cell activation in interstitial cystitis, *Semin Urol* 9:74, 1991.

Theoharides TC, Sant GR, El-Mansoury M, et al: Activation of bladder mast cells in interstitial cystitis: a light and electron microscopic study, *J Urol* 153:629, 1995.

Warren JW: Interstitial cystitis as an infectious disease, *Urol Clin North Am* 21:31, 1994.

Yun SK, Laub DJ, Weese DL, et al: Stimulated release of urine histamine in interstitial cystitis, *J Urol* 148:1145, 1992.

## Diagnosis

Abrams P, Blavis JG, Stanton SL, et al: The standardization of terminology of lower urinary tract function recommended by the International Continence Society, *Int Urogynecol J* 1:45, 1990.

Alagiri M, Chottiner S, Ratner V, et al: Interstitial cystitis: unexplained associations with other chronic disease and pain syndromes, *Urology* 49S(5A):52, 1997.

Goldwasser B: Urodynamics. In Wein AJ, Barrett DM, eds: *Voiding function and dysfunction: a logical and practical approach.* Chicago, 1988, Year Book Medical Publishers.

Jarvis GJ: The management of urinary incontinence due to primary vesical sensory urgency by bladder drill, *Br J Urol* 54:374, 1982.

Kirkemo A, Peabody M, Diokno AC, et al: Associations among urodynamic findings and symptoms in women enrolled in the interstitial cystitis data base (ICDB) study, *Urology* 49S(5A):76, 1997.

Koziol JA, Clark DC, Gittes RF, et al: The natural history of interstitial cystitis: a survey of 374 patients, *J Urol* 149:465, 1993.

Messing EM, Pauk D, Schaeffer A, et al: Associations among cystoscopic findings and symptoms and physical examination findings in women enrolled in the interstitial cystitis data base (ICDB) study, *Urology* 49S(5A):81, 1997.

Nigro DA, Wein AJ, Foy M, et al: Associations among cystoscopic and urodynamic findings from women enrolled in the interstitial cystitis data base (ICDB) study, *Urology* 49S(5A):86, 1997.

Parsons CL: Interstitial cystitis: clinical manifestations and diagnostic criteria in over 200 cases, *Neurourol Urodyn* 9:241, 1990.

Parsons CL, Stein PC, Bidair M, et al: Abnormal sensitivity to intravesical potassium in interstitial cystitis and radiation cystitis, *Neurourol Urodyn* 13:515, 1994.

Ratner V, Salde D, Whitmore KE: Interstitial cystitis: a bladder disease finds legitimacy, *J Women's Health* 1:63, 1992.

Simmon LJ, Landis JR, Erickson DR, et al: The interstitial cystitis data base (ICDB) study: concepts and preliminary baseline descriptive statistics, *Urology* 49S(5A):64, 1997.

Whitmore KE: Self-care regimens for patients with interstitial cystitis, *Urol Clin North Am* 21:121, 1994.

## Urethral Syndrome

Allen PM, Davis GD, Bowen LW, et al: The female urethral syndrome is rarely associated with human papilloma virus infection types 6/11, 16, 18, 31, 33, *Int Urogynecol J* 6:195, 1995.

Bodner DR: The urethral syndrome, *Urol Clin North Am* 15:699, 1988.

Bump RC, Copeland WE: Urethral isolation of genital mycoplasmas and chlamydia trachomatis in women with chronic urologic complaints, *Am J Obstet Gynecol* 152:38, 1985.

Hamilton-Miller JT: The urethral syndrome and its management, *J Antimicrob Chemother* 33S:63, 1994.

Ishigooka MH: Effect of hormonal replacement therapy in postmenopausal women with chronic irritative voiding symptoms, *Int Urogynecol J* 5:211, 1994.

Wilkens EG, Payne SR, Pead PJ, et al: Interstitial cystitis and the urethral syndrome: a possible answer, *Br J Urol* 64:39, 1989.

## Management of Hypersensitivity Disorders

Bade JJ, Peeters JM, Mensink HJ: Is the diet of patients with interstitial cystitis related to their disease? *Eur Urol* 32:179, 1997.

Bardot SF, Weigel JW, Krueker DC: Treatment of intractable interstitial cystitis with cystourethrectomy and continent urinary diversion, *J Urol* 143:375A, 1990.

Baskin LS, Tanagho EA: Pelvic pain without pelvic organs, *J Urol* 147:683, 1992.

Brookoff D: The causes and treatment of pain in interstitial cystitis. In Sant GR, ed: *Interstitial cystitis,* Philadelphia, 1997, Lippincott.

Chaiken DC, Blaivas JG, Blaivas ST: Behavioral therapy for the treatment of refractory interstitial cystitis, *J Urol* 149:1445, 1993.

Eigner EB, Freiha FS: The fate of the remaining bladder following supravesical diversion, *J Urol* 144:31, 1990.

Fall M: Transcutaneous electrical nerve stimulation in interstitial cystitis, *Urology* 29:40, 1987.

Fall M, Lindstrom S: Transcutaneous electrical nerve stimulation in classic and nonulcer interstitial cystitis, *Urol Clin North Am* 21:131, 1994.

Galloway NT, Gabale DR, Irwin PP: Interstitial cystitis or reflex sympathetic dystrophy of the bladder? *Semin Urol* 9:148, 1991.

Hanno PM: Amitriptyline in the treatment of interstitial cystitis, *Urol Clin North Am* 21:21, 1994.

Hanno PM: Analysis of long-term Elmiron therapy for interstitial cystitis, *Urology* 49S(5A):99, 1997.

Hanno PM, Fritz R, Wein AJ, et al: Heparin as an antibacterial agent in rabbit bladder, *Urology* 12:411, 1978.

Hanno PM, Wein AJ: Conservative therapy of interstitial cystitis, *Semin Urol* 9:143, 1991.

Hohenfellner M, Lin JF, Hampel C, et al: Surgical treatment of interstitial cystitis. In Sant GR, ed: *Interstitial cystitis,* Philadelphia, 1997, Lippincott.

Irwin P, Galloway NT: Letter to the editor: pelvic pain without pelvic organs, *J Urol* 148:1265, 1992.

Irwin P, Galloway NT: Surgical management of interstitial cystitis, *Urol Clin North Am* 21:145, 1994.

Keselman I, Austin P, Anderson J, et al: Cystectomy and urethrectomy for disabling interstitial cystitis: a long term followup, *J Urol* 153:290A, 1995.

Kirkemo AK, Miles BJ, Peters JM: Use of amitriptyline in the treatment of interstitial cystitis, *J Urol* 143:279A, 1990.

Kisman OK, Lycklama AB, Nijeholt A, et al: Mast cell infiltration in intestine used for bladder augmentation in interstitial cystitis, *J Urol* 146:1113, 1991.

Lotenfoe RR, Christie J, Parsons A, et al: Absence of neuropathic pelvic pain and favorable psychological profile in the surgical selection of patients with disabling interstitial cystitis, *J Urol* 154:2039, 1995.

MacDermitt JP, Charpied GL, Tesluk H: Recurrent interstitial cystitis following cystoplasty: fact or fiction? *J Urol* 144:37, 1990.

Messing EM, Freiha FL: Complications of Clorpactin WCS90 therapy for interstitial cystitis, *Urology* 13:389, 1979.

Morales A, Emerson L, Nickel JC: Intravesical hyaluronic acid in the treatment of refractory interstitial cystitis, *Urology* 49S(5A):111, 1997.

Nielsen KK, Kromann-Andersen B, Steven K, et al: Failure of combined supratrigonal cystectomy and Mainz ileocecocystoplasty in intractable interstitial cystitis: is histology and mast cell count a reliable predictor for the outcome of surgery? *J Urol* 144:255, 1990.

Nurse DE, Parry JW, Mundy AR: Problems in the surgical treatment of interstitial cystitis, *Br J Urol* 68:153, 1991.

Parsons CL: A quantitatively controlled method to prospectively study interstitial cystitis and demonstrate the efficacy of pentosanpolysulfate, *J Urol* 150:845, 1993.

Parsons CL: Epithelial coating techniques in the treatment of interstitial cystitis, *Urology* 49S(5A):100, 1997.

Parsons CL, Housley T, Schmidt JD, et al: Treatment of interstitial cystitis with intravesical heparin, *Br J Urol* 73:504, 1994.

Peters K, Diokno A, Steinert B, et al: The efficacy of intravesical Tice strain bacillus Calmette-Guérin in the treatment of interstitial cystitis: a double-blind, prospective, placebo controlled trial, *J Urol* 157:2290, 1997.

Pontari MA, Hanno PM, Wein AJ: Logical and systematic approach to the evaluation and management of patients suspected of having interstitial cystitis, *Urology* 49S(5A):114, 1997.

Sant GR: Intravesical 50% dimethylsulfoxide (DMSO-50) in treatment of interstitial cystitis, *Urology* 29:17, 1987.

Sant GR: Interstitial cystitis, *Monographs Urol* 12:37, 1991.

Schwartzmann R, Mclellan R: Reflex sympathetic dystrophy: a review, *Arch Neurol* 44:555, 1987.

Smith SD: Improvement in interstitial cystitis syndrome scores during treatment with oral L-arginine, *J Urol* 158:703, 1997.

Theoharides TC: Hydroxyzine for interstitial cystitis, *J Allergy Clin Immunol* 91:686, 1993.

Theoharides TC, Sant GR: Hydroxyzine therapy for interstitial cystitis, *Urology* 49S(5A):108, 1997.

Torens M, Hald T: Bladder denervation procedures, *Urol Clin North Am* 6:283, 1978.

Webster GD, MacDiarmid SA, Timmons SL, et al: Impact of urinary diversion procedures in the treatment of interstitial cystitis and chronic bladder pain, *Neurourol Urodyn* 11:417, 1992.

Whitmore KE, Tu LM, Gordon DA, et al: Self-care and interstitial cystitis: identification of the food-sensitive IC patient, Inter Research Symposium on IC, Washington, DC, October 1997.

Worth PL: The treatment of interstitial cystitis by cystolysis with observation on cystoplasty. A review after 7 years, *Br J Urol* 52:232, 1980.

Worth PL, Turner-Warwick R: The treatment of interstitial cystitis by cystolysis with observation on cystoplasty, *Br J Urol* 45:65, 1973.

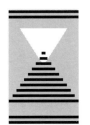

CHAPTER **26**
# Voiding Dysfunction and Retention

Linda M. Partoll

Voiding dysfunction can be defined as difficulty emptying the bladder in a controlled, efficient, and comfortable manner. The lower urinary tract functions as a storage and eliminatory unit. Storage and voiding are both possible because pressure gradients in the bladder and urethra reflexedly change as needed. Voiding dysfunction occurs when the balance of pressure shifts more toward the storage function than the voiding function. In the end stage, voiding dysfunction can progress to urinary retention. In this chapter, we discuss normal and abnormal voiding, urinary retention, evaluation of voiding dysfunction, and treatment modalities.

## NORMAL VOIDING

Bladder control is learned during childhood and usually taken for granted thereafter. However, the control and mechanics of normal voiding involve an intricate neurophysiologic network, and an abnormality at any level can lead to voiding dysfunction. Required components include normal function of the central and peripheral nervous systems; a normal bladder wall and detrusor muscle; and normal anatomy and function of the bladder neck, urethra, and pelvic floor.

A brief review of the neurophysiology of micturition will help clarify how voiding occurs. A more detailed discussion is found in Chapter 2.

Voiding is controlled by the summation of input from four different areas: cerebral cortex, brain stem, sacral spinal cord, and peripheral innervation. Of these areas, the brain stem, primarily the pons, is the most important coordination center because detrusor and sphincter activity are coordinated here in the pontine micturition center.

The cerebral cortex provides both conscious and unconscious control of the micturition reflex. Cortical control allows humans to dampen the micturition reflex until it is socially acceptable. The cortical input required to achieve this is complex, as evidenced by the variety of symptoms noted in patients with cortical lesions. Depending on where the lesion is, patients may suffer from urgency and urge incontinence or from urethral spasticity and retention. Patients may or may not have social concerns about their incontinence.

The pontine reticular formation accepts input from the peripheral nerves, the sacral spinal cord, and various cortical centers and then coordinates detrusor and sphincter activity so that normal voiding can occur. Suprapontine lesions can result in involuntary voiding via a detrusor contraction with coordinated urethral relaxation.

Sacral spinal cord segments S2, S3, and S4 contain detrusor motor neurons that control micturition. Lesions between the sacral spinal cord and the brain stem tend to produce a simultaneous uncoordinated contraction of the detrusor and external urethral sphincter, described as detrusor-sphincter dyssynergia.

Peripheral innervation is transmitted via both sympathetic and parasympathetic fibers. Sacral parasympathetic fibers are the primary motor supply to the detrusor. Parasympathetic neuron cell bodies are located in the sacral spinal cord; their preganglionic fibers travel via the pelvic nerves to synapse in ganglia in and near the bladder wall. The cell bodies of sympathetic preganglionic neurons are located in the thoracolumbar spinal cord; they synapse in the inferior mesenteric and hypogastric ganglia. Their postganglionic fibers either synapse with parasympathetic fibers in or near the bladder wall, allowing for interaction between sympathetic and parasympathetic systems, or terminate directly in the detrusor or urethral musculature.

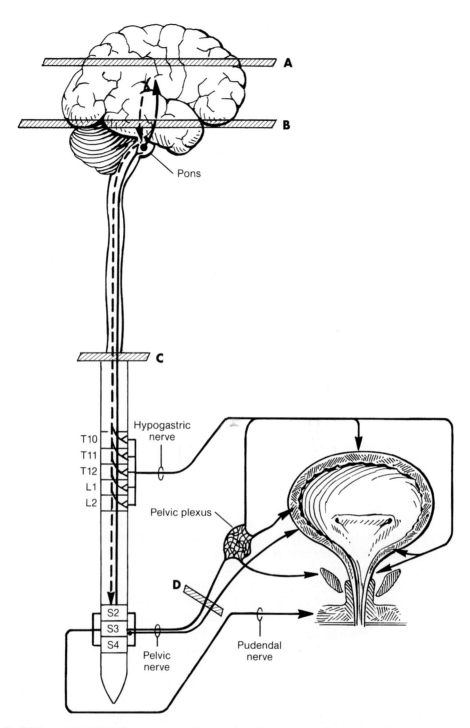

**Fig. 26-1**   Interruption of nervous system at various levels and subsequent voiding dysfunction. *A,* Lesions in higher cortical centers have various effects, including inability to voluntarily postpone voiding, urge incontinence, enuresis, urethral spasm, and loss of social concern about incontinence. *B,* Suprapontine lesions result in involuntary detrusor contractions with coordinated urethral relaxation. *C,* High spinal cord (upper motor neuron) lesions lead to detrusor hyperreflexia without coordinated urethral relaxation (detrusor-sphincter dyssynergia). *D,* Lower motor neuron lesions cause detrusor areflexia.

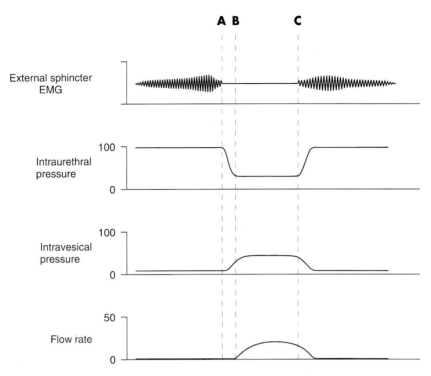

**Fig. 26-2**  Urodynamic representation of normal female micturition. *A,* Voluntary initiation of voiding with relaxation of external urethral sphincter and pelvic floor muscles and associated decrease in urethral pressure. *B,* Detrusor contraction occurs with increase in intravesical pressure; intraurethral pressure equals intravesical pressure, and urine flow is initiated. *C,* Voluntary termination of voiding.

From Walters MD: *Obstet Gynecol Clin North Am* 16:773, 1989.

A simplified schematic diagram of bladder and urethral innervation and the effects of lesions at various levels is found in Fig. 26-1.

Normal voiding is accomplished by relaxation of the urethra, followed by a sustained contraction of the detrusor so that the bladder empties completely. This process begins when bladder distention causes stimulation of bladder wall pressure sensors. After cortical inhibition of the reflex is released, the micturition reflex is activated. The reflex is carried out in two steps: relaxation of the periurethral striated musculature and pelvic floor muscles, resulting in a decrease in intraurethral pressure and funneling and descent of the bladder neck, and a coordinated contraction of the detrusor, increasing intravesical pressure to surpass urethral pressure. Urine flow results, reaching a peak flow rate of 25 to 30 ml/sec. Brain stem modulation of the arc instructs the bladder how long to contract so that the bladder empties completely. When voiding is complete, the detrusor muscle is reflexively inhibited and intravesical and intraurethral pressures return to prevoiding levels. Normal voiding, therefore, is characterized by a sharp start, a smooth sustained flow, and a sharp conclusion. The urodynamic features of normal voiding are seen in Fig. 26-2.

## VOIDING DYSFUNCTION

Voiding dysfunction and urinary retention are points in a spectrum of incomplete voiding. Voiding difficulty may present acutely (e.g., following surgery or with a urinary tract or herpes infection) and is usually transient. Sometimes voiding difficulty progresses slowly over time and is not detected until it becomes symptomatic. Thus, urinary retention, especially when associated with a neurologic or other disease process, is more likely to become a chronic disorder. When urinary retention or voiding dysfunction is detected, a thorough evaluation to determine the cause is needed. Treatment should be initiated, even while the evaluation is ongoing, to help prevent infection, ureteral reflux, and subsequent deterioration of renal function. One can often determine whether the problem is likely to be transient or chronic after a probable cause is identified and treatment is refined appropriately.

### Prevalence

The prevalence of voiding dysfunction in women is difficult to estimate because only those referred to specialty clinics are fully evaluated. Stanton et al. (1983) reported on 600 women referred to a clinic for various urologic symptoms. Thirty-three percent of the patients who presented with

**Box 26-1**

**INTERNATIONAL CONTINENCE SOCIETY CLASSIFICATION OF VOIDING PHASE DYSFUNCTION**

**Detrusor Function During Voiding**

Normal
Underactive
Acontractile

**Urethral Function During Voiding**

Normal
Obstructive
 Overactive
 Mechanical

**Box 26-2**

**CAUSES OF VOIDING DYSFUNCTION AND RETENTION**

Neurologic (see Box 26-3)
 Lesions of the brain
 Lesions of the spinal cord
 Autonomic and peripheral lesions
 Local pain reflex
Pharmacologic (see Table 26-1)
Inflammatory
 Acute urethritis or cystitis
 Acute vulvovaginitis
 Herpes simplex or zoster infection
Obstructive
 Extramural
 Pelvic or vaginal mass
 Uterovaginal and posterior vaginal wall prolapse
 Retroverted impacted gravid uterus
 Hematocolpos
 Fecal impaction
 Intramural
 Intraluminal
 Detrusor-sphincter dyssynergia
Medical disorders
 Diabetes mellitus
 Hypothyroidism
 Porphyria
 Scleroderma
Overdistention
 Postoperative, postpartum
 Associated with acute or chronic disease
Psychogenic
 Nonneurogenic neurogenic bladder
 Psychiatric disorder
 Hysteria
 Schizophrenia
 Depression
Postoperative voiding dysfunction
 Operations that elevate or obstruct bladder neck
 Procedures that denervate the bladder
 Procedures that cause localized edema and pain

urinary problems complained of symptoms suggestive of voiding dysfunction, but the diagnosis was confirmed by urodynamic testing in only one third of those patients. Voiding difficulty was confirmed in 25.5% of patients over 65 years old, 13.6% of patients less than 65 years old, and 16.5% of patients overall. An additional 12 patients (out of 600) had no symptoms of abnormal voiding but were found to have voiding dysfunction on urodynamic testing. Symptoms were generally unreliable in predicting voiding function.

## Classification

The International Continence Society (ICS) established a classification of lower urinary tract dysfunction (see Chapter 4 and Appendix A). This classification divides abnormalities into those of the storage and voiding phases. In the voiding phase, detrusor and urethral function are examined separately, as shown in Box 26-1. An underactive detrusor denotes a detrusor contraction that is of inadequate strength or duration to empty the bladder efficiently. Detrusor areflexia is defined as acontractility caused by an abnormality of nervous control and denotes the complete absence of a centrally coordinated contraction.

## Etiology

The various causes of voiding dysfunction and retention can be grouped based on the underlying causes into neurologic, pharmacologic, inflammatory, obstructive, endocrine, overdistention, and psychogenic (Box 26-2).

### Neurologic Causes

Neurologic lesions cause voiding dysfunction in multiple ways and depend on the level of central nervous system disruption (see Fig. 26-1). Although one cannot predict with complete accuracy the symptoms that a particular lesion will cause, certain patterns of dysfunction are observed after certain insults. Lesions in higher cortical centers have

various effects, including inability to voluntarily postpone voiding, urge incontinence, enuresis, and loss of social concern about incontinence. It is sometimes difficult to ascertain whether the resulting incontinence is caused by detrusor hyperreflexia or reflects a situation in which the patient has lost social concern about voluntary urinary control. Lesions above the brain stem that affect micturition generally result in detrusor hyperreflexia with smooth and striated muscle synergy. Sensation and voluntary striated sphincter function are usually preserved. High spinal cord lesions lead to detrusor hyperreflexia without coordinated urethral relaxation (detrusor-sphincter dyssynergia). The

**Box 26-3**

**NEUROLOGIC DISORDERS CAUSING VOIDING DYSFUNCTION AND RETENTION**

**Lesions of the Brain**

Cerebrovascular disease
Parkinsonism
Multiple sclerosis
Concussion
Brain tumor
Shy-Drager syndrome
Normal pressure hydrocephalus

**Lesions of the Spinal Cord**

Multiple sclerosis
Spinovascular disease
Conus medullaris or cauda equina tumors
Prolapsed intervertebral disk
Spinal stenosis
Spinal arachnoiditis
Tabes dorsalis
Spinal cord injury
Dysraphic lesions

**Lesions of Autonomic and Peripheral Innervation**

Autonomic neuropathy
Sacral agenesis
Spinal cord injury
Diabetes mellitus
Tabes dorsalis
Pernicious anemia
Herpes zoster
Radical pelvic surgery

**Table 26-1** Drugs That Can Cause Voiding Dysfunction and Retention

| Drug | Decreases bladder contractility | Increases outlet resistance |
|---|---|---|
| Atropine-like agents | + | |
| Ganglionic blockers | + | |
| Musculotropic relaxants (antispasmodics) | + | |
| Calcium antagonists | + | |
| Antihistamines | + | |
| Theophylline | + | |
| Phenothiazines | + | |
| Tricyclic antidepressants | + | + |
| Alpha-adrenergic agonists | | + |
| L-dopa | | + |
| Amphetamines | | + |

dysfunctions that occur with interruption of the peripheral reflex usually involve detrusor areflexia; low bladder compliance may result. A list of neurologic disorders that cause voiding difficulty and retention is shown in Box 26-3.

Voiding dysfunction is common after cerebrovascular accidents. Urodynamic evaluation of 33 patients after cerebrovascular accidents revealed involuntary bladder contractions in 26 and poor bladder contractions in 7. Correlation of bladder dysfunction with the anatomic location of the brain injury was inconclusive.

Detrusor hyperactivity with impaired contractility (DHIC) is a condition in which the detrusor is overactive but the bladder does not empty completely, causing incontinence. The impaired emptying is caused by diminished detrusor contractile function. Resnick and Yalla (1987) described associated findings of bladder trabeculation, a slow velocity detrusor contraction, diminished detrusor reserve on isometric (stop flow) testing, and elevated postvoid residual volumes. It is seen most often in elderly patients.

Patients experiencing prolonged voiding dysfunction after pelvic floor surgery can also be classified as having neurologic lesions because the primary lesion is peripheral denervation of the bladder and urethra secondary to surgical dissection. This problem is seen most often in women undergoing abdominoperineal resection of the rectum or radical hysterectomy. Over 50% of patients who have undergone radical hysterectomy report persistent urinary complaints, including voiding dysfunction, incontinence, and decreased sensation. Because of the anatomic location of the pelvic parasympathetic nerves and sympathetic plexi, neurologic damage and subsequent voiding dysfunction occur more commonly after rectal surgery than uterine surgery. The effect of simple abdominal hysterectomy on bladder function and urinary symptoms is unclear; conclusions of the few objective studies are contradictory. Voiding dysfunction after bladder neck surgery is often caused by functional obstruction; this is discussed in greater detail later in this chapter.

### Pharmacologic Causes

Numerous classes of drugs can have detrimental effects on voiding. Any drug that inhibits bladder contractility or increases outlet resistance can result in incomplete emptying (Table 26-1). Clinically obvious voiding difficulty is not seen in most patients using these drugs; symptoms usually appear in patients who already have borderline voiding dysfunction. Any drug that interferes with the action of acetylcholine at vesical cholinergic receptors can result in voiding dysfunction. These drugs include anticholinergic agents, tricyclic antidepressants, and ganglionic blockers (e.g., mecamylamine). Alpha-adrenergic stimulants (e.g., epinephrine) increase urethral tone and can impair voiding by increasing outflow resistance.

Epidural anesthetics cause temporary retention primarily by inhibiting afferent neuronal transmission from the bladder, thereby decreasing the sensation of bladder fullness and the urge to void.

### Inflammatory Causes

Acute inflammation or infection of the bladder, urethra, vulva, or vagina can cause voiding dysfunction via localized pain and edema. This reaction is seen in the immediate postoperative period as well as with various inflammatory processes. Primary herpes simplex infection (Elsberg syndrome) can cause radiculitis with subsequent detrusor underactivity.

### Obstruction

Urethral or bladder neck obstruction is the most common cause of voiding dysfunction in men; however, it is rare in women. Massey and Abrams (1988) reported that evaluation of 5948 women referred to a urodynamic unit revealed obstruction in only 163 patients (2.7%), although the classic symptoms of hesitancy, poor stream, and incomplete emptying were present in 40%. Causes of obstruction can be extramural (23.9%), intramural (73.6%), or intraluminal (2.5%). Extramural causes include pelvic or vaginal masses such as a myomata, retroverted impacted gravid uterus, and hematocolpos. Pelvic organ prolapse usually must be beyond the hymen to cause enough urethral distortion so that obstruction occurs. Intramural causes include urethral stenosis, acute urethral edema, and chronic fibrosis secondary to surgery or radiation. Urethral masses such as condyloma and urethral cancer are causes of intraluminal obstruction.

Obstruction can also be caused by urethral sphincter activity or contraction during voiding. A detrusor contraction occurring simultaneously with a sphincteric contraction is called detrusor-sphincter dyssynergia. This occurs only in patients with neurologic lesions, particularly high spinal cord (upper motor neuron) lesions. Functional obstruction occurs despite high detrusor pressures. The degree of dysfunction depends on the contractile strength of the detrusor; as long as the detrusor can overcome urethral resistance, some amount of voiding can occur. An obstructed flow pattern is found on urodynamic testing. Urethrovesical backwash, ureterovesical reflux, and high residual urine volumes all can lead to recurrent infection. Treatment is aimed at inhibiting the detrusor hyperreflexia with medical and behavioral therapy. Drugs that can be used to relax the external striated sphincter include alpha-sympathetic antagonists, such as prazosin and phenoxybenzamine. Centrally acting muscle relaxants, such as baclofen, dantrolene, or diazepam, can be used in an attempt to relax the pelvic floor musculature. Conversely, detrusor contractility can be inhibited with anticholinergic agents, such as oxybutynin or tolterodine. Finally, a schedule of intermittent self-catheterization (ISC) can be instituted.

### Medical Disorders

Endocrine causes of detrusor dysfunction include hypothyroidism and diabetes mellitus, both of which can cause a peripheral neuropathy in poorly controlled patients.

### Overdistention

Overdistention, especially iatrogenic overdistention, is an often preventable cause of voiding dysfunction. Overdistention of the bladder can cause voiding dysfunction from stretch injury to the detrusor. The degree of distention required to incur injury varies depending on individual bladder capacity, but it is rare with volumes under 1000 ml. Overdistention can occur because of poorly managed acute or chronic retention; patients at risk include diabetic patients and stroke victims. Patients are also at risk in the postoperative or postpartum period, especially if epidural or spinal anesthesia was used. All at-risk patients must be monitored carefully for adequate urine output. Voiding dysfunction caused by overdistention should be managed with an indwelling Foley catheter for 24 to 48 hours. Dysfunction is usually transient, but even one episode of overdistention can lead to a large hypotonic bladder.

### Psychogenic Causes

Although psychogenic causes of voiding dysfunction are well known, it should be considered a diagnosis of exclusion. Criteria for the diagnosis are no detectable neurologic or other significant organic disease, positive correlation of psychiatric symptoms and the onset of voiding dysfunction, and clinical response to psychotherapy and pharmacologic treatment. Psychiatric disorders sometimes seen with voiding dysfunction include hysteria, depression, and schizophrenia.

Nonneurogenic neurogenic bladder (psychologic nonneuropathic bladder, or Hinman's syndrome) is a voiding dysfunction with a behavioral cause and is not attributable to a neurologic lesion. The precise psychologic or behavioral cause is unclear and the clinical presentation varied, but the urodynamic findings are fairly precise. External urethral sphincter electromyogram (EMG) studies of patients with a true neurogenic bladder and detrusor-sphincter dyssynergia show an increase in EMG activity before and during the upslope of a detrusor contraction, and EMG activity quiets on the downslope. In contrast, patients with nonneurogenic neurogenic bladder show quieting of the external sphincter EMG before and during the upslope of a detrusor contraction and augmented EMG activity during the downslope of the detrusor contraction. (EMG tracings in normal voiding show a quieting of activity before and during a detrusor contraction.) Patients may have a large-capacity bladder with poor compliance or ineffective detrusor contractions during voiding. The urinary flow rate is often intermittent because of failure of the external sphincter to relax. Medical, behavioral, and psychologic treatments are usually used; ISC may be needed in children or adults who fail to respond.

### Postoperative Voiding Dysfunction

Postoperative voiding dysfunction is often seen in patients undergoing a variety of reconstructive pelvic floor procedures. It is usually transient but can be distressing for the patient and surgeon. Problems with voiding postoperatively can be eased by identifying patients at risk preoperatively and avoiding surgical techniques that may encourage postoperative dysfunction. It is best to educate patients about the potential for voiding dysfunction preoperatively and have in place a well-structured plan of management. A relative degree of risk can be assigned preoperatively by noting the patient's history, the planned procedure, and her urodynamic findings. Women with an elevated postvoid residual urine volume on routine evaluation, a history of voiding difficulty or bladder overdistention, or urinary retention after other operations or postpartum are at risk for voiding dysfunction postoperatively. Patients with underlying neurologic disease such as multiple sclerosis, dementia, and cerebral vascular accident are also at increased risk.

Any type of reconstructive pelvic floor surgery can cause postoperative voiding dysfunction. Anterior colporrhaphy, for example, can cause periurethral tissue edema or partial outlet obstruction leading to transient voiding difficulty. Likewise, posterior colporrhaphy can cause voiding dysfunction by stimulation of the levator ani muscles (from pain, for example), causing inability to relax the pelvic floor muscles to initiate voiding. Voiding dysfunction commonly occurs following various colorectal procedures, radical hysterectomy, and other extensive pelvic surgery because these procedures require dissection of the cardinal ligaments, thereby interfering with autonomic innervation of the bladder.

Antiincontinence surgery often results in voiding dysfunction. The degree of voiding dysfunction specifically relates to the amount of outlet obstruction produced by the operation and the ability of the detrusor muscle to overcome this obstruction. Preoperative urodynamic findings can help identify patients at risk for postoperative voiding dysfunction. Women who void without or with a very weak detrusor contraction may be at increased risk for postoperative voiding dysfunction. Clinically, this manifests as difficulty initiating a stream, a weak stream or prolonged voiding time, or inability to void at all. These symptoms can be objectively confirmed by the following urodynamic parameters: peak flow rate less than 15 ml/sec on uroflowmetry, flow time greater than 30 seconds, maximum detrusor pressure during voiding less than 20 cm $H_2O$, and an increase in detrusor pressure on isometric "stop flow" test less than 10 cm $H_2O$. Individually, each test has pitfalls. Uroflowmetry itself is a poor predictor of postoperative voiding because patients may attain a normal flow rate by straining. Likewise, detrusor pressure during voiding often depends on urethral resistance; women with stress urinary incontinence may void with little or no increase in detrusor pressure preoperatively but may have a detrusor contraction postoperatively. The "stop flow" or isometric detrusor pressure test may help identify these women. These tests are discussed in detail in Chapter 7.

## Evaluation

Patients with voiding dysfunction present with a variety of symptoms, including a weak stream, incomplete emptying, straining to void, urinary frequency, and incontinence. Unfortunately, these symptoms are nonspecific, and there is little correlation between symptoms, postvoid residual volumes, and urodynamic findings.

A thorough evaluation is required in most patients with dysfunctional voiding symptoms. The history includes inquiring about prior voiding dysfunction postoperatively or postpartum, neurologic complaints or conditions, current medications, previous pelvic surgery, and general health problems such as diabetes and hypothyroidism. The physical examination must include pelvic, neurologic, and mental status examinations. Urinalysis should be done to rule out cystitis or urethritis.

Diagnostic studies can be simple or complex, depending on the amount of disability and the need for making an exact (versus general) diagnosis. Basic screening studies include measurement of postvoid residual volume and uroflowmetry. Multichannel urodynamic testing, with simultaneous measurement of bladder, intraabdominal, and urethral pressures, can aid in detecting detrusor and urethral abnormalities during filling and voiding and are necessary, when combined with flow rate, to determine obstructed and nonobstructed voiding patterns. Concomitant sphincter electromyography is helpful in measuring the activity of the pelvic floor musculature during filling and voiding. Pressure-flow voiding studies with fluoroscopy allow visualization of the bladder and urethra during voiding.

Debate continues regarding what constitutes normal and abnormal voiding parameters in women. To establish voiding dysfunction, Massey and Abrams (1988) suggested as diagnostic criteria a maximum flow rate ($Q_{max}$) of less than 15 ml/sec with a residual urine volume greater than 100 ml on two occasions or any two of the following: flow rate less than 12 ml/sec, detrusor peak flow pressure (PFP) greater than 50 cm $H_2O$, urethral resistance ($PFP/Q_{max}^2$) greater than 0.2, and significant residual urine in the presence of elevated PFP or urethral resistance.

It is difficult to assign an absolute volume to "significant" postvoid residual urine. Postvoid residual volume should be evaluated in context with the voided volume, the clinical situation, and the desired outcome. For example, if the voided volume is 500 ml, a postvoid residual volume of 100 ml is insignificant; if the voided volume is 50 ml, the same residual volume is significant. In general, women should be able to void spontaneously at least 80% of their total bladder volume. Residual urine volumes consistently above 100 ml may warrant monitoring for bladder overdistention, infection, and upper tract damage.

## MANAGEMENT OF VOIDING DYSFUNCTION AND RETENTION
### Basic Concepts and Techniques

Prompt treatment of voiding dysfunction and urinary retention is important for three reasons: to provide relief of symptoms, to prevent bladder overdistention and the possible sequelae, and to prevent the development of a high-pressure system causing ureteral reflux, upper tract dilation, and subsequent deterioration of renal function. Acute and chronic retention are usually treated similarly initially because when retention is first diagnosed, it is often unclear whether it will be acute or become a chronic problem. Postoperative retention is a somewhat special situation that is discussed separately.

First, bladder drainage must be established. This is accomplished most easily with a transurethral Foley catheter. If more than 500 ml is drained, continuous drainage should be used for 24 to 48 hours because the overdistended bladder may function poorly. The catheter is left in place until the patient can void spontaneously. During this time, efforts are made to determine the cause of the retention. To test a patient's voiding, the catheter should be removed early in the day so voiding can be observed during that day. If the patient then voids normally, she should be followed over the ensuing few weeks to ensure that she is voiding completely. Women unable to void completely after an acute event should be taught clean ISC or their bladders should be drained with a urethral Foley catheter while an evaluation is conducted.

Women with mild voiding dysfunction may benefit from a variety of maneuvers aimed at augmenting their current voiding mechanism. Double voiding, Crede maneuver, Valsalva maneuver, and positional changes during voiding are techniques that may improve emptying.

Increasing patient awareness and control of the pelvic floor and urethral striated musculature with biofeedback may be helpful for patients with detrusor-sphincter dyssynergia or voiding dysfunction caused by inability to relax these muscles.

### Pharmacologic Management

Detrusor underactivity or areflexia is difficult to treat effectively. Pharmacologic therapy has produced mixed results. Cholinergic agents such as bethanechol chloride have been the backbone of treatment for more than 30 years. However, controlled studies have demonstrated that both subcutaneous and oral bethanechol have no effect on flow rate or residual volume. Similarly, oral bethanechol has no

beneficial effects in paralyzed patients with neuropathic bladders. Khanna (1979) suggested that poor therapeutic results with bethanechol chloride are caused by its nicotinic effects on urethral smooth muscle. Overall, there is no proven benefit to the use of bethanechol in patients with voiding dysfunction.

Alpha-adrenergic blockers such as phenoxybenzamine have been used to decrease urethral resistance. Khanna (1976) reported a significant improvement in 26 of 31 patients treated with both bethanechol and phenoxybenzamine. In contrast, Murray (1990) stated that women, unlike men, have no evidence of adrenergic innervation of the bladder neck, and that alpha-adrenergic blockers are of no help in clinical practice.

Prostaglandin $F_2$ ($PGF_2$) and prostaglandin $E_2$ ($PGE_2$) cause contraction of isolated strips of detrusor muscle in animals. The clinical effectiveness of $PGF_2$ and $PGE_2$ in humans is controversial. Bultitude et al. (1976) and Desmond et al. (1980) reported improved voiding in women with detrusor failure after a single intravesical instillation of $PGE_2$. Intravesical instillation of $PGF_2$ postoperatively also was shown to reduce urinary retention, urinary tract infection, and required hospital days with no side effects. In contrast, Andersson et al. (1978) were unable to show that $PGE_2$ had any beneficial effects in women with voiding disorders. Likewise, Delaere et al. (1981) could not demonstrate a significant benefit with use of either $PGE_2$ or $PGF_2$.

In postmenopausal women the urethra may become atrophic or stenotic because of inadequate levels of endogenous estrogens. Proof of intraurethral estrogen receptors and cytologic changes in urethral epithelium after estrogen therapy supports the use of estrogen for relief of urinary symptoms in postmenopausal women. A significant decrease in dysfunctional voiding symptoms was found by Hilton and Stanton (1983) using intravaginal estrogen cream and by Versi et al. (1990) with estradiol implants.

### Surgery

Cystoscopy and urethral dilation remain the primary surgical treatments for women with voiding dysfunction. Extreme dilation is not required and may cause urinary incontinence. Massey and Abrams (1988) showed that dilation to 36 French with estrogen replacement as needed resolved voiding dysfunction in 76% of women with intramural causes of dysfunction. In patients with neuropathic sphincter obstruction, Otis urethrotomy and sphincterotomy proved beneficial in less than 50% of patients treated with this modality. With the advent of clean ISC, there are few indications for more radical procedures because they may lead to incontinence.

### Catheterization

Clean ISC, introduced by Lapides et al. in 1972, has become the mainstay of treatment for patients with severe dysfunction. Patients are taught to catheterize themselves using a clean (not sterile) catheter. Sterile urine is maintained in 45% to 90% of patients using sterile technique and in 39% to 65% using a clean technique. Urinalysis and urine culture of 37 patients using ISC showed that 67% had more than 10 white blood cells per high-power field, 14% were sterile, 43% had nonsignificant growth, and 43% had significant bacterial growth. Suppressive antibiotics are not used, and infection is treated as it occurs. It is imperative that ISC be introduced to the patient in a positive and supportive manner; the benefits of avoiding surgery, the elimination of an external device, and preservation of renal function should be stressed. This technique is discussed in detail in Chapter 33.

Continuous suprapubic drainage can be established in patients for whom intermittent self-catheterization is impractical or impossible. A suprapubic catheter can be placed by the desired method and secured in place. The catheter tract epithelializes in 6 to 8 weeks, allowing for easy catheter replacement. The primary problems associated with long-term suprapubic drainage are infection, decreased bladder capacity over time, increased mucous production in response to the indwelling catheter, and calcification of the catheter. Acidifying the urine with oral vitamin C supplementation (3 g every 8 hours) or irrigating the bladder may be helpful.

A permanent transurethral catheter is the last resort in nonsurgical treatment because it carries the often inevitable risks of bladder and urethral irritation, bladder calculi formation, and urinary tract infection that can lead to fatal sepsis in debilitated patients.

## Voiding Dysfunction After Bladder Neck Surgery

Voiding dysfunction and urinary retention are often seen after antiincontinence operations; the estimated incidence ranges from 2.5% to 24% with different procedures. The cause of voiding difficulty after these operations is usually obstruction. Management is complicated by difficulty in establishing the diagnosis and determining the optimal treatment.

The presentation of patients with postoperative obstruction varies. Patients may complain of classic obstructive symptoms such as straining to void, hesitancy, incomplete emptying, or complete urinary retention. Patients also may complain of urinary frequency with small volumes, new-onset urge incontinence, or recurrent urinary tract infections. Patients with elevated postvoid residual urine volumes and total retention create a diagnostic dilemma because this may be the manifestation of a poorly contractile bladder or bladder neck obstruction. Likewise, patients with irritative symptoms may have other causes than obstruction.

Women with postoperative obstruction should be treated conservatively with ISC. Patients often are not satisfied with this outcome, however, and ISC may not provide sufficient relief for those with irritative symptoms. Nitti

and Raz (1994) evaluated 41 patients with postoperative obstruction and treated them with transvaginal urethrolysis and needle suspension. They were able to define three distinct patient groups: obstructed only, poorly contractile bladder, and obstructed and incontinent. They concluded that transvaginal urethrolysis with needle suspension was beneficial for the obstructed only and the obstructed/incontinent groups. Women with poorly contractile bladders may benefit from urethrolysis alone if they were voiding normally before the initial bladder neck surgery; however, they have a higher risk of continued self-catheterization after urethrolysis. The only variable that had any significant correlation with a successful surgical outcome was postvoid residual volumes, in that patients with high postvoid residual volumes had a decreased success rate after urethrolysis. Surgical outcome was independent of the presence or absence of a detrusor contraction during voiding, voiding pressure, flow rate, or time passed since bladder neck surgery. Therefore, Nitti and Raz (1994) questioned the value of urodynamic testing in the evaluation of patients presenting with urinary retention, although they did believe that urodynamic testing, cystoscopy, and radiographic studies may be beneficial in evaluating patients with irritative symptoms.

McGuire et al. (1989) evaluated the use of transvaginal urethrolysis after obstructive urethral suspension procedures in 13 women. They also commented on the difficulty in determining whether the primary problem was obstruction or a poorly contractile bladder. Transvaginal urethrolysis alone was done on obstructed-only patients and urethrolysis with a secondary procedure for stress incontinence was done in obstructed/incontinent patients, with good overall results.

Carr and Webster (1997) evaluated urethrolysis in 51 women with postoperative bladder neck obstruction. They noted a successful outcome in 86% of patients approached retropubically and 73% of patients approached vaginally. The most common symptoms in their patients were irritative, and only 12 patients were actually in retention. No preoperative urodynamic parameter, including postvoid residual volume, was helpful in predicting outcome. In view of their results, they recommend transvaginal urethrolysis or retropubic takedown in patients whose symptoms have a clear temporal relationship to previous cystourethropexy.

The technique of transvaginal urethrolysis involves placing a large Foley catheter with a 30-ml balloon in the bladder. A midline anterior vaginal wall incision is made at the level of the proximal urethra and bladder neck. Sharp dissection is used to separate vaginal epithelium from the underlying tissue. The dissection is extended laterally to the inferior ramus of the pubic bone. The urogenital diaphragm is then penetrated with the goal of creating some bladder neck mobility. This is subjectively guided by traction on the Foley balloon. We have not found it necessary to perform an antiincontinence operation in this setting.

If the desired approach to urethrolysis is via a retropubic approach, the retropubic space is entered in a conventional fashion. Again, with a large Foley catheter in the bladder, sharp dissection is performed along the back of the pubic bone to reach the periurethral area. Many times, this is best accomplished by making a high cystotomy and dissecting with a finger on the inside of the bladder wall. The dissection is then extended laterally with the goal of mobilizing the bladder neck and proximal urethra. Resuspension operations are used to correct anterior vaginal wall prolapse, or if the original suspension sutures were not placed in the appropriate periurethral area.

## CONCLUSION

Our understanding of voiding dysfunction and urinary retention in women is far from complete. A careful, thorough evaluation is essential, remembering that voiding dysfunction may be a harbinger of another disease process. Treatment depends on the cause of dysfunction. If voiding dysfunction is attributed to obstruction, relief of the obstruction or urethral dilation will improve symptoms. However, when voiding dysfunction or retention is secondary to an underactive or areflexic detrusor and treatment of the primary disease does not improve voiding function, then management usually consists of ISC. Clean intermittent self-catheterization should be considered for all women with chronic voiding dysfunction and retention.

## BIBLIOGRAPHY

Andersson KE, Hendriksson L, Ulmsten U: Effects of prostaglandin $E_2$ applied locally on intravesical and intra-urethral pressures in women, *Eur Urol* 4:366, 1978.

Austin P, Spyropoulos E, Lotenfoe R, et al: Urethral obstruction after anti-incontinence surgery in women: evaluation, methodology, and surgical results, *Urology* 47:890, 1996.

Barrett DM: The effect of oral bethanechol chloride on voiding in female patients with excessive residual urine: a randomized double-blind study, *J Urol* 126:640, 1981.

Bauer SB: Neurogenic dysfunction of the lower urinary tact in children. In Walsh PC, Retik AB, Vaughan ED, et al, eds: *Campbell's urology*, ed 7, Philadelphia, 1998, WB Saunders.

Bhatia NN, Bergman A: Urodynamic predictability of voiding following incontinence surgery, *Obstet Gynecol* 63:85, 1984.

Bultitude MI, Hills NH, Shuttleworth KE: Clinical and experimental studies on the action of prostaglandins and their synthesis inhibitors on detrusor muscle in vitro and in vivo, *Br J Urol* 48:631, 1976.

Carr LK, Webster GD: Voiding dysfunction following incontinence surgery: diagnosis and treatment with retropubic or vaginal urethrolysis, *J Urol* 157:821, 1997.

Cross CA, Cespedes RD, English SF, et al: Transvaginal urethrolysis for urethral obstruction after anti-incontinence surgery, *J Urol* 159: 1199, 1998.

Dean AM, Worth PHL: Female chronic urinary retention, *Br J Urol* 57:24, 1985.

Delaere KPJ, Thomas CMG, Moonen WA, et al: The value of intravesical prostaglandin $E_2$ and $F_2$ in women with abnormalities of bladder emptying, *Br J Urol* 53:306, 1981.

Desmond AD, Bultitude MI, Hills NH, et al: Clinical experience with intravesical prostaglandin $E_2$, *Br J Urol* 53:357, 1980.

Doran J, Roberts M: Acute urinary retention in the female, *Br J Urol* 47:793, 1976.

Greenstein A, Matzkin H, Kaver I, et al: Acute urinary retention in herpes genitalis infection, *Urology* 31:453, 1988.

Hemrika DJ, Schutte MF, Bleker OP: Elsberg syndrome: a neurologic basis for acute urinary retention in patients with genital herpes, *Obstet Gynecol* 68:37S, 1986.

Hilton P, Stanton SL: The use of intravaginal oestrogen cream in genuine stress incontinence, *Br J Obstet Gynaecol* 90:940, 1983.

Jaschevatzky OE, Anderman S, Shalit A, et al: Prostaglandin $F_2$ for prevention of urinary retention after vaginal hysterectomy, *Obstet Gynecol* 66:244, 1985.

Khan Z, Starer P, Yang EC, et al: Analysis of voiding disorders in patients with cerebrovascular accidents, *Urology* 25:265, 1990.

Khanna OP: Disorders of micturition: neuropharmacologic basis and results of drug therapy, *Urology* 8:316, 1976.

Khanna OP: Non-surgical therapeutic modalities. In Krane RJ, Siroky MB, eds: *Clinical neurourology,* Boston, 1979, Little, Brown.

Krane RJ, Siroky MB, eds: *Clinical neurourology,* ed 2, Boston, 1991, Little, Brown.

Lapides J, Diokno AC, Silber SJ, et al: Clean intermittent self-catheterization in the treatment of urinary tract disease, *J Urol* 107:458, 1972.

Lazzeri M, Beneforti P, Benajm G, et al: Vesical dysfunction in systemic sclerosis (scleroderma), *J Urol* 153:1184, 1995.

Massey JA, Abrams PH: Obstructed voiding in the female, *Br J Urol* 61:36, 1988.

McGuire EJ, Letson W, Wang S: Transvaginal urethrolysis after obstructive urethral suspension procedures, *J Urol* 142:1037, 1989.

Mundy AR: An anatomical explanation for bladder dysfunction following rectal and uterine surgery, *Br J Urol* 54:501, 1982.

Murray K: Medical and surgical management of female voiding difficulty. In Drife JO, Hilton P, Stanton SL, eds: *Micturition,* London, 1990, Springer-Verlag.

Nitti VW, Raz S: Obstruction following anti-incontinence procedures: diagnosis and treatment with transvaginal urethrolysis, *J Urol* 152:93, 1994.

Paviakis A, Wheeler JS, Krane RJ, et al: Functional voiding disorders in females, *Neurourol Urodyn* 5:145, 1986.

Philip NH, Thomas DG, Clarke SJ: Drug effects on the voiding cystometrogram: a comparison of oral bethanechol and carbachol, *Br J Urol* 52:484, 1980.

Preminger GM, Steinhardt JM, Fried FA, et al: Acute urinary retention in female patients: diagnosis and treatment, *J Urol* 130:112, 1982.

Resnick NM, Yalla SV: Detrusor hyperactivity with impaired contractile function, *JAMA* 257:3076, 1987.

Roberts M, Smith P: Non-malignant obstruction of the female urethra, *Br J Urol* 40:694, 1968.

Rudy DC, Woodside JR: Non-neurogenic neurogenic bladder: the relationship between intravesical pressure and the external sphincter electromyogram, *Neurourol Urodyn* 10:169, 1991.

Silva PD, Berberich W: Retroverted impacted gravid uterus with acute urinary retention: report of two cases and a review of the literature, *Obstet Gynecol* 69:121, 1986.

Smith PH, Turnbull MB, Currie DW, et al: The urological complications of Wertheim's hysterectomy, *Br J Urol* 41:685, 1969.

Stanton SL, Ozsoy C, Hilton P: Voiding difficulties in the female: prevalence, clinical and urodynamic review, *Obstet Gynecol* 61:144, 1983.

Tammela T, Kontturi M, Kaar K, et al: Intravesical prostaglandin $F_2$ for promoting bladder emptying after surgery for female stress incontinence, *Br J Urol* 60:43, 1987.

Tanagho EA, Miller ER: Initiation of voiding, *Br J Urol* 42:175, 1970.

Versi E, Cardozo L, Studd J: Long-term effects of estradiol implants on the female urinary tract during the climacteric, *Int Urogynecol J* 1:87, 1990.

Wein AJ: Neuromuscular dysfunction of the lower urinary tract and its treatment. In Walsh PC, Retik AB, Vaughan ED, et al, eds: *Campbell's urology,* ed 7, Philadelphia, 1998, WB Saunders.

Wein AJ, Barrett DM: *Voiding function and dysfunction,* Chicago, 1988, Year Book Medical Publishers.

Wein AJ, Mallory TR, Shoder F, et al: The effects of bethanechol chloride on urodynamic parameters in normal women and in women with significant residual urine volumes, *J Urol* 124:397, 1980.

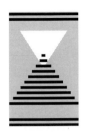

CHAPTER *27*

# *Lower Urinary Tract Infection*

Mickey M. Karram and Padma K. Mallipeddi

Urinary tract infections are a significant health care problem affecting an estimated 10% to 20% of women during their lifetimes and accounting for approximately 5.2 million office visits per year. Management of a single episode of cystitis costs an estimated $140 and the annual health care costs of urinary tract infections in women are estimated to exceed $1 billion.

In the past 30 years, there have been significant developments in our understanding of the pathogenesis and management of urinary tract infections. These include recognition that about one third of women with cystitis have bacterial counts lower than 100,000 colony-forming units (CFU) per milliliter of urine, realization that bacteria infecting the urinary tract usually come from fecal flora, documentation that most recurrent urinary tract infections are reinfections

caused by fecal bacteria and can be successfully managed by low-dose prophylaxis, introduction of newer antimicrobial therapy, and the understanding that certain women with cystitis-like symptoms have sterile urine and their conditions will ultimately be diagnosed as sensory urgency, urethral syndrome, or interstitial cystitis.

## EPIDEMIOLOGY

Urinary tract infections are more prevalent among women than among men (ratio of 20:1), probably secondary to an anatomically short urethra and its close proximity to the vagina and rectum. Approximately 5 million cases of cystitis occur annually in the United States, and over 100,000 patients are hospitalized every year for renal infection. At least 50% of women experience an episode of cystitis at some time during their lives and about 5% have frequent episodes.

The prevalence of urinary tract infections increases with age. At 1 year, 1% to 2% of female infants demonstrate bacteriuria. In this age group, there is a direct correlation between cystitis and upper urinary tract infection. As many as 50% of these patients demonstrate abnormalities on intravenous pyelograms, such as scarring, ipsilateral reflux, or some obstructive disease. After 1 year of age, the infection rate decreases to approximately 1% and remains low until puberty. Between ages 15 and 24, the prevalence of bacteriuria is about 2% to 3% and increases to about 15% at age 60, 20% after age 65, and 25% to 50% after age 80 (Fig. 27-1). Sexual activity and pregnancy are major factors in younger age groups, whereas pelvic relaxation, systemic illnesses, and hospitalization play major roles in older women. However, the prevalence of underlying urologic abnormalities decreases dramatically with age.

Approximately 2% of all patients admitted to a hospital acquire a urinary tract infection, which accounts for 500,000 nosocomial infections per year. One percent of all these infections become life-threatening. Instrumentation or catheterization of the urinary tract is a precipitating factor in at least 80% of these infections. Asymptomatic bacteriuria occurs in 2% to 8% of adult females, the likelihood of which increases with increasing age, diabetes mellitus, and a history of symptomatic urinary tract infection.

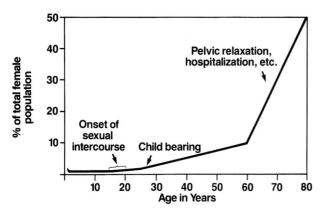

**Fig. 27-1** Prevalence of bacteriuria in females as a function of age.

From Karram MM: Lower urinary tract infection. In Ostergard DR, Bent AE, eds: *Urogynecology and urodynamics,* Baltimore, 1991, Williams & Wilkins.

## MICROBIOLOGY

Gram-negative bacilli of the family Enterobacteriaceae are responsible for 90% of urinary tract infections. *E. coli* is the single most important organism and accounts for 80% to 90% of uncomplicated infections. Others include *Klebsiella, Enterobacter, Serratia, Proteus, Pseudomonas, Providencia,* and *Morganella* species. *Pseudomonas aeruginosa* infection is almost always secondary to urinary tract instrumentation. *Staphylococcus saprophyticus* is the second most common cause of cystitis and causes 10% of infections in sexually active females. *Staphylococcus epidermidis* is a nosocomial pathogen identified in patients with indwelling catheters. *Staphylococcus aureus* is less commonly isolated and is often secondary to hematogenous renal infection. Other gram-positive organisms such as enterococci and *Streptococcus agalactiae* cause about 3% of episodes of cystitis. *Enterococcus fecalis* causes about 15% of nosocomial urinary infections, and *Streptococcus agalactiae* is more commonly the cause in patients with diabetes mellitus. Anaerobic bacteria, although abundant in fecal flora, rarely cause urinary tract infections. The oxygen tension in the urine probably prevents their growth and persistence in the urinary tract.

Candida albicans and other fungal organisms can cause lower urinary tract infections in patients with diabetes mellitus or indwelling urinary catheters. Immunocompromised patients and recipients of renal transplantation are vulnerable to candidal urinary tract infections. *Torulopsis glabrata* is second in frequency to *C. albicans.* Viruria has been documented with many viruses, but generally in association with viremia. Viral urinary tract infections occur as acute illnesses (acute hemorrhagic cystitis in children, polyoma virus infection after bone marrow transplant), during convalescence from viral infections (mumps, cytomegalovirus), and in asymptomatic patients (cytomegalovirus).

**Box 27-1**

### KNOWN RISK FACTORS FOR URINARY TRACT INFECTION

Advanced age
Inefficient bladder emptying
    Pelvic relaxation
        Large cystocele with high residuals
        Uterovaginal prolapse resulting in obstructive voiding
    Neurogenic bladder (i.e., diabetes mellitus, multiple sclerosis, spinal cord injury)
    Drugs with anticholinergic effects
Decreased functional ability
    Dementia
    Cardiovascular accidents
    Fecal incontinence
    Neurologic deficits
Nosocomial infections
    Indwelling catheters
    Hospitalized patients
Physiologic changes
    Decreased vaginal glycogen and increased vaginal pH in women
Sexual intercourse
    Diaphragm use

## PATHOGENESIS

Although the normal female urinary tract is remarkably resistant to infection, certain risk factors for developing urinary tract infections have been identified (Box 27-1). The majority of urinary tract infections are ascending infections wherein the fecal flora initially colonize the vaginal introitus, then the periurethral tissues, and eventually gain entry into the bladder (Fig. 27-2). The development of urinary tract infection requires the interaction of appropriate host susceptibility and pathogen virulence factors (Fig. 27-3).

### Host Factors

Several important host defense mechanisms are instrumental in the prevention of urinary tract infections. The normal acidic pH of the vaginal secretions in a premenopausal woman inhibits the growth of enterobacteria such as *E. coli* and promotes the growth of lactobacilli, diphtheroids, and other gram-positive bacteria, organisms that replicate poorly in urine. Normal periodic voiding with its dilutional effects and the high urea and organic acid concentrations of urine in a setting of a low pH serve as important bladder defense mechanisms. The glycosaminoglycans in the bladder lining and immunoglobulins in the urine are important factors that block bacterial adherence. The deficiency of glycosaminoglycans probably plays a role in recurrent urinary tract infections. In addition, the ascending loop of Henle secretes

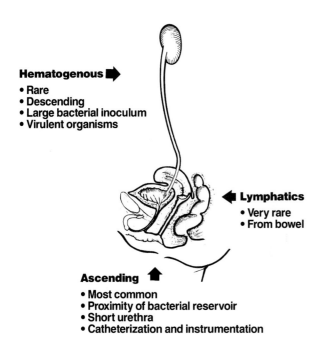

**Fig. 27-2** Pathways of bacterial entry into the urinary tract.

From Karram MM: Lower urinary tract infection. In Ostergard DR, Bent AE, eds: *Urogynecology and urodynamics,* Baltimore, 1991, Williams & Wilkins.

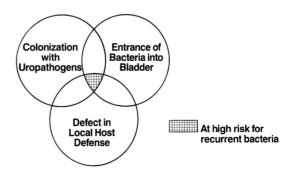

**Fig. 27-3** Factors determining host risk and susceptibility to bacterial cystitis in normal females with anatomically normal urinary tracts.

From Karram MM: Lower urinary tract infection. In Ostergard DR, Bent AE, eds: *Urogynecology and urodynamics,* Baltimore, 1991, Williams & Wilkins.

Tamm-Horsfall protein, a mannose-rich uromucoid that may inhibit bacterial adherence to epithelial cells and trap bacteria in the urine, thereby allowing them to be flushed from the urinary tract.

Studies have shown that women of blood groups B and AB, who are nonsecretors of blood-group substances, are at a greater risk for urinary tract infections, suggesting a possible genetic link. Similarly, a higher prevalence of HLA-A3 subtype was noted among women with recurrent urinary tract infections.

Factors such as sexual activity and diaphragm use are significantly associated with the development of lower urinary tract infections. The frequency and recency of sexual intercourse increase the risk of cystitis. This increase appears to occur through inoculation of periurethral bacteria into the bladder during intercourse. The increased risk associated with diaphragm use may be related to urethral obstruction caused by it as well as the propensity for vaginal colonization by coliforms.

## Bacterial Virulence Factors

The adherence of bacteria to mucosal cells appears to be a necessary step for colonization and pathogenicity. *E. coli,* the most common uropathogen, is the most extensively studied. Three different types of adhesins have been identified: type 1 pili (or fimbriae), P-fimbriae, and X-adhesins. Type 1 pili have a strong affinity for mannose-containing compounds, including Tamm-Horsfall protein, and facilitate attachment of *E. coli* to vaginal, periurethral, and bladder epithelial cells. P-fimbriae and the less well-studied X-adhesins are important in ascending infections of the kidney. P-fimbriae have a high affinity for P blood group antigens found on erythrocytes and uroepithelial cells. Type 1 pili and P-fimbriae are often possessed by the same bacterium and, after gaining entry to the kidney, the expression of Type 1 pili is turned to avoid phagocytosis.

Bacteria possess a variety of other virulence factors, of which multidrug resistance is most clinically significant. Uropathogens develop resistance primarily through the resistance transfer plasmid. Plasmid resistance has been found for beta-lactams, sulfonamides, aminoglycosides, and trimethoprim. So far, no plasmid-mediated resistance has been identified to fluoroquinolones, which makes these agents valuable in treating infections caused by multidrug-resistant bacteria. Other virulence factors include production of hemolysins and colicin V by some enterobacteria and urease by *Proteus* species.

## DEFINITIONS

When discussing urinary tract infections, an understanding of the generally accepted definitions is essential.

*Bacteriuria* implies the presence of bacteria in the urine. The term includes both renal and bladder bacteriuria. Symptomatic bacteriuria can have as few as 100 CFU/ml, whereas asymptomatic bacteriuria requires the growth of 100,000 CFU/ml.

*Urethritis* is inflammation of the urethra and requires an adjective for modification (e.g., nongonococcal, nonspecific). In women, symptoms of urethritis are indistinguishable from those of cystitis, and pure urethritis is exceedingly rare.

*Trigonitis* is inflammation or localized hyperemia of the trigone. Unfortunately, this term is often misused to describe the normal cobblestone or granular appearance of the trigone seen on cystoscopy. Embryologically, this represents squamous metaplasia because the trigone is a derivative of the müllerian system, unlike the rest of the bladder.

*Cystitis* indicates inflammation of the bladder and can be used as a histologic, cystoscopic, bacteriologic, or clinical term. Bacterial cystitis must be differentiated from nonbacterial cystitis (i.e., radiation or interstitial cystitis).

*Pyelonephritis* is a clinical term that refers to a syndrome of chills, fever, and flank pain accompanied by bacteriuria and pyuria.

*Uncomplicated* is a term used to describe an afebrile infection in a patient with a structurally and functionally normal urinary tract. The majority of episodes of isolated or recurrent cystitis in women are uncomplicated and can be eradicated easily by a short course of inexpensive antimicrobial therapy.

*Complicated infections* are those in patients with pyelonephritis or a urinary tract with structural or functional abnormality. These infections are often caused by bacteria that demonstrate multiple drug resistance.

*Chronic,* as it pertains to infection, is a poorly defined term that is best avoided.

*Prophylactic antimicrobial therapy* is the use of antimicrobial drugs for the prevention of reinfection of the urinary tract. It assumes that bacteria have been completely eliminated before the initiation of prophylaxis.

*Suppressive antimicrobial therapy* refers to suppression of an existing infection that the clinician is unable to eradicate. Suppression may result in abacteriuric urine or may reduce the bacterial load without achieving sterile urine.

*Reinfection* describes recurrent infection with different bacteria from outside the urinary tract. This is essentially a new event, with the urine showing no growth after the preceding infection. Reinfections are often caused by the same species, such as *E. coli,* that continue to colonize the vaginal introitus.

*Relapse* refers to consecutive urinary tract infections caused by the same bacterial strain from a focus within the urinary tract such as a stone. Unfortunately, some investigators use the term with a 2-week or shorter limitation between recurrences, implying that the kidney is the site of bacterial relapse when ascending reinfections from the urethra or vagina can also readily recur within 2 weeks.

*Persistence of bacteria* implies the continued presence of the same infecting microorganisms isolated at the start of treatment. This can be caused by several factors, including an underlying structural or functional abnormality, bacterial resistance, inadequate drug dosage, or poor patient compliance.

## CLINICAL PRESENTATION

The symptoms and signs of urinary tract infections in women are diverse. Lower urinary irritative symptoms associated with cystitis are dysuria, frequency, urgency, nocturia, and suprapubic discomfort. Occasionally, mild incontinence and hematuria may occur. Gross hematuria is rare. Systemic symptoms are usually absent. Upper urinary tract infections commonly present with fever, chills, malaise, and occasionally nausea and vomiting. Flank pain and costovertebral angle tenderness are usually present. The pain is colicky if acute pyelonephritis is complicated by a renal calculus or a sloughed renal papilla secondary to diabetic or analgesic nephropathy.

## DIAGNOSIS
### Urine Collection Methods

Considerable care should be taken when collecting urine from ambulatory patients. To minimize contamination, women should be instructed to spread the labia, wipe the periurethral area from front to back with clean, moistened gauze sponge, and collect a midstream urine sample holding labia apart. Certain patients with physical disability or obesity are unable to obtain a clean voided specimen. In such women, urethral catheterization or suprapubic aspiration of the bladder can be performed. However, urethral catheterization is not without risks. Catheter infection rates range from 1% in healthy young women to 20% in hospitalized patients.

### Urine Microscopy

Microscopic examination of urine adds valuable information to the diagnosis and evaluation of urinary tract disorders. A thorough microscopic examination of an uncentrifuged sample of urine can detect the presence of significant bacteria, leukocytes, and red blood cells. In a random urine sample, pyuria is defined as more than 10 white blood cells per milliliter of urine and is assessed using a hemocytometer. In a clinical setting with symptoms suggestive of urinary tract infection, pyuria and hematuria offer sufficient supportive evidence to warrant empiric antibiotic therapy. In the absence of pyuria, the diagnosis of urinary tract infection should be questioned. Some examples of abacterial or sterile pyuria are tuberculosis, renal calculi, glomerulonephritis, interstitial cystitis, and chlamydial urethritis.

Microscopic hematuria is found in 40% to 60% of cases of acute cystitis and is specific for cystitis in women with dysuria. Microscopic bacteriuria, using uncentrifuged Gram-stained urine, is found in over 90% of urinary tract infections with colony counts of 100,000 CFU/ml or more and is a highly specific finding. However, bacteria are not readily detectable in lower colony-count infections, such as 100 to 10,000 CFU/ml. Thus, microscopic hematuria and bacteriuria lack sensitivity but are highly specific for urinary tract infections.

### Rapid Diagnostic Tests

Rapid diagnostic tests are generally less accurate than urine microscopy but are convenient and cost-effective. The most common rapid detection test is the nitrite test, based on the bacterial conversion of nitrates to nitrite. Often integrated with it is the esterase test, which detects the presence of leukocyte esterase, suggesting pyuria. The sensitivity of these tests is 60% in bacterial counts greater than 100,000 CFU/ml and only 22% in infections with bacterial counts of 10,000 to 100,000 CFU/ml. The test is ideally performed on first morning voided specimens to minimize false negative results. False negative results can also occur in enterococcal infections and in the presence of certain dyes such as bilirubin, methylene blue, and phenazopyridine.

Other rapid detection methods include filtration stain tests that concentrate a specific quantity of urinary sediment on a filter of controlled pore size. This test is a good screening method because it offers a more reliable detection of smaller numbers of bacteria but has a lower specificity.

## Urine Culture

Once recommended universally, pretherapy cultures are no longer deemed necessary or cost-effective in uncomplicated cystitis. With the advent of single-dose and short-course antimicrobial therapies, treatment decisions are made and therapy is often completed before culture results are known. In patients with symptoms and signs suggestive of urinary tract infection in whom no complicating factors are present, a positive urine analysis or an office rapid diagnostic test is sufficient evidence to start antibiotic therapy. A urine culture should be obtained for patients in whom the diagnosis of cystitis is questionable or an upper-tract infection is suspected and for those in whom complicating factors are present. Urine culture can also be used to differentiate recurrent from persistent infection.

Traditionally, bacterial growth of more than 100,000 CFU/ml was considered a positive culture. However, the use of this value is limited by the fact that 20% to 40% of women with symptomatic urinary tract infections have lower colony counts and a single culture of 100,000 CFU/ml has a 20% chance of representing contamination. Stamm et al. (1982) proposed that the best diagnostic criterion for culture detection in young symptomatic women is 100 CFU/ml. The office methods currently available for urine culture are dipslides and direct surface plating on split-agar; the latter is more accurate. Clinicians using commercial laboratories for urine cultures should be aware that they often report only the predominant organism in mixed cultures, and some report any culture with bacterial counts lower than 100,000 CFU/ml as negative.

## Radiologic Studies

The overwhelming majority of patients with acute cystitis do not need a full urologic workup. The low yield (1% to 2%) of the intravenous pyelogram makes it an inefficient method of identifying underlying disease. However, radiologic studies can be useful in certain circumstances. These include poor response to appropriate antimicrobial therapy; evidence of bacterial persistence; infections caused by urea-splitting microbes (e.g., *Proteus*) and unusual organisms; history of calculi; potential ureteral obstruction; upper urinary tract symptoms or a history of previous nonpregnant

pyelonephritis; history of childhood urinary tract infections; and unexplained hematuria. When a suburethral diverticulum is suspected as the source of recurrent urinary tract infections, urethroscopy and a voiding cystourethrogram or double-balloon catheter study should be performed.

## Cystourethroscopy

Indications for cystourethroscopy in women with urinary tract infection are controversial. Fowler and Pulaski (1981) noted that the only abnormality that altered treatment was a urethral diverticulum, and it was found in 3 patients out of a total of 74 cystoscopies they performed in women with two or more previous infections. Thus, many of the abnormalities detected on cystoscopy have no impact on the management of urinary tract infection. However, cystoscopy is helpful in older patients with cystitis to eliminate the possibility of a bladder tumor. It is also indicated in women with gross hematuria and bacterial persistence.

## Urodynamic Studies

Urodynamic studies are useful in patients with abnormal voiding patterns that might be the cause of recurrent infections. They can also be diagnostic in women with the possibility of a neurogenic bladder (e.g., history of pelvic or spinal surgery).

## DIFFERENTIAL DIAGNOSIS

The symptoms of lower urinary tract infections can be mimicked by some genital conditions such as candidiasis, *Trichomonas* vaginitis, and other sexually transmitted diseases. Dysuria can be a presenting symptom in infections caused by chlamydia, gonococci, and herpes simplex virus. Frequency, urgency, and small voiding volumes are also common in sexually transmitted diseases. Pyuria occurs in patients with chlamydial urethritis. Hematuria is not a feature of vaginitis or sexually transmitted diseases, and its presence should strongly suggest a urinary tract infection. Postmenopausal atrophy caused by estrogen deficiency could lead to irritative bladder symptoms. The term *urethral syndrome* has been used to describe a condition in women who are not estrogen deficient and who complain of persistent lower urinary tract symptoms despite negative urine, vaginal, and urethral cultures. A suggested approach to the evaluation and treatment of women with dysuria is shown in Fig. 27-4.

## MANAGEMENT OF LOWER URINARY TRACT INFECTION

General measures such as rest and hydration should always be emphasized in women with urinary tract infection. Hydration dilutes urine and with frequent urination can lower bacterial counts. Acidification of urine is helpful only in recurrent infections and in patients taking methenamine compounds because the antibacterial activity of these

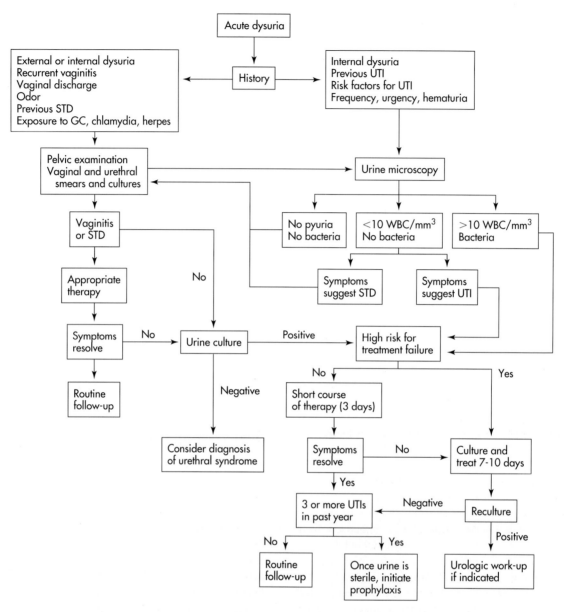

**Fig. 27-4**  Algorithm for diagnosis and management of acute dysuria in women.

agents is maximal at a pH of 5.5 or less. Urinary analgesics such as phenazopyridine hydrochloride (Pyridium) help relieve pain and burning on urination. When prescribed, they should be used for only 2 to 3 days along with a specific antibacterial agent.

General factors that influence the selection of antimicrobial agents for treatment of urinary tract infections include efficacy, cost of the agent, anticipated incidence and severity of adverse effects, and dosing interval. Ideally, the antimicrobial agent prescribed should have minimal or no effect on fecal flora so as to minimize the risk of emergence of more pathogenic or resistant strains. A drug can alter bacteria in the bowel either by passing unabsorbed through the gastrointestinal tract or by having a high serum level. It is also important that a drug maintain a low serum level and

not disrupt the flora in other parts of the body, such as the vagina. Drugs that cause yeast vaginitis add significantly to the patient morbidity and the overall cost of the treatment. In addition, vaginitis precipitated by the antibiotic could lead to a vaginitis-cystitis cycle that may be difficult to treat.

Trimethoprim with sulfamethoxazole (TMP-SMX, Cotrimoxazole, Bactrim, Septra) is one of the most effective agents available for oral administration. It has a broad range of activity against uropathogens and infrequent occurrence of bacterial resistance. However, the sulfamethoxazole component of TMP-SMX is a common cause of adverse drug reactions. Because the antibacterial efficacy of TMP-SMX in the urinary tract results primarily from the trimethoprim component, it is rational to use trimethoprim alone. Amoxicillin, once a popular antibiotic for cystitis, is

**Table 27-1**  Dosage and Toxicity of Antibiotics Commonly Used in the Treatment of Urinary Tract Infections

| Drug | Oral dose and frequency | Minor toxicity | Major toxicity |
|---|---|---|---|
| Trimethoprim-sulfamethoxazole | 1 tab BID | Allergic | Serious skin reactions, blood dyscrasia |
| Nitrofurantoin | 50-100 mg q 6-8 hr | GI upset | Peripheral neuropathy, pneumonitis |
| Ampicillin | 250-500 mg q 6 hr | Allergic, candidal overgrowth | Allergic reactions, pseudomembranous colitis |
| Tetracycline | 250-500 mg q 6 hr | GI upset, skin rash, candidal overgrowth | Hepatic dysfunction, nephrotoxicity |
| Cephalexin | 250-500 mg q 6 hr | Allergic | Hepatic dysfunction |
| Norfloxacin | 400 mg q 12 hr | Nausea, vomiting, diarrhea, abdominal pain, skin rash | Convulsions, psychoses, joint damage |
| Ciprofloxacin | 250 mg q 12 hr | Nausea, vomiting, diarrhea, abdominal pain, headache, skin rash | Arrhythmias, angina, convulsions, gastrointestinal bleeding, nephritis |

a poor choice as first line of treatment because of the widespread emergence of resistant *E. coli* and a high incidence of candidal vaginitis. Amoxicillin remains the drug of choice for treating *Enterococcus fecalis*. Nitrofurantoin is a valuable drug and has excellent activity against *E. coli*. It is completely absorbed in the upper gastrointestinal tract, has a 19-minute serum half life, and is metabolized in every tissue of the body, resulting in no significant changes in fecal or vaginal flora. For this reason, no increase in bacterial resistance to nitrofurantoin has occurred even after 30 years of use in the United States. Although nitrofurantoin continues to be prescribed in doses of 100 mg every 6 hours, it is equally efficacious at doses of 50 mg every 8 hours, with fewer side effects. Macrocrystalline formulations of nitrofurantoin (Macrodantin and Macrobid, Procter & Gamble, Cincinnati, OH) are available and are associated with fewer gastrointestinal side effects. Macrobid has a convenient twice-daily dosage.

Use of nalidixic acid and oxolinic acid has been largely superseded by the new fluoroquinolones such as norfloxacin, ciprofloxacin, ofloxacin, enoxacin, pefloxacin, fleroxacin, and lomefloxacin. These orally absorbed, broad-spectrum synthetic compounds are highly effective against a wide range of pathogens. However, these drugs are expensive and have no advantage over conventional agents such as nitrofurantoin or TMP-SMX in the management of uncomplicated infections. They should be reserved for use in patients with resistant infections or as an alternative to parenteral antibiotics in complicated infections. Cephalosporins such as cephalexin, cephradine, and cefaclor are useful in patients with renal insufficiency. Tables 27-1 and 27-2 list the dosages, toxicities, and spectra of antimicrobial activity for commonly prescribed antibiotics.

## First Infections or Infrequent Reinfections

Cystitis is a superficial infection of the bladder mucosa that rarely invades the lamina propria. Studies have shown that 30% of patients with simple cystitis can be cured by bladder irrigation with 10% neomycin solution. There is now considerable evidence that a single oral dose of an antibiotic is as effective as a conventional 7-day course therapy for the treatment of uncomplicated cystitis. Single-dose therapy is cost-effective, ensures compliance, has fewer adverse effects (rashes, gastrointestinal upset, vaginal candidiasis), and is less likely to cause bacterial resistance. Single-dose therapy should be considered for initial treatment of acute bacterial cystitis and asymptomatic bacteriuria and for girls with cystitis who are known to have radiologically normal urinary tracts. Use of single-dose treatment does not predispose to earlier, more severe, or more frequent recurrences.

The first drug to be evaluated in detail for single-dose therapy was amoxicillin (3 g orally). A single dose of trimethoprim (400 to 600 mg) or TMP-SMX (1.92 mg) was shown to be more effective than amoxicillin and equivalent to a 3- to 5-day course of either preparation. Some of the drugs recommended for single-dose treatment include trimethoprim 400 mg, TMP-SMX 1.92 mg, nitrofurantoin 200 mg, norfloxacin 800 mg, ciprofloxacin 500 mg, enoxacin 400 mg, pefloxacin 800 mg, and a novel compound fosfomycin trometamol 3 g. Single doses of tetracycline, doxycycline, pivmecillinam, sulfamethizole, and a range of cephalosporins have been shown to be efficacious but generally less so than trimethoprim or TMP-SMX. Amoxicillin and the cephalosporins are no longer recommended for single-dose regimens. Single-dose therapy is therefore the treatment of choice in community-acquired uncomplicated urinary tract infections. At present, there are no large randomized trials that evaluate single-dose therapy in hospitalized patients.

An alternative to single-dose therapy for women with bacterial cystitis is a 3-day course of treatment. The symptoms of dysuria and frequency in patients with cystitis typically last for 2 to 3 days. The 3-day treatment, unlike the single-dose therapy, obviates reassuring patients that they need no further therapy. Three-day therapy is probably

**Table 27-2**  Spectrum of Antimicrobial Activity Against Common Lower Urinary Tract Pathogens

| Organisms | TMP-SMX | Nitrofurantoin | Ampicillin | Tetracycline | Cephalexin | Carbenicillin | Gentamicin | Norfloxacin |
|---|---|---|---|---|---|---|---|---|
| *E. coli* | ++ | ++ | ++ | + | ++ | ++ | ++ | ++ |
| *Pseudomonas* | − | − | − | − | − | ++ | ++ | ++ |
| *Klebsiella* | ++ | ± | − | ± | ++ | − | ++ | ++ |
| *Proteus* | ++ | − | ++ | − | ++ | ++ | ++ | ++ |
| *Enterobacter* | ++ | − | − | − | − | ++ | ++ | ++ |
| *Enterococcus* | − | ± | ++ | ++ | ± | − | − | ++ |
| *Staphylococcus* | − | ± | ++ | + | ++ | ++ | + | ++ |
| *Serratia marcescens* | + | − | − | − | − | − | ++ | ++ |

*TMP-SMX,* Trimethoprim-sulfamethoxazole.
++ Excellent.
+ Good.
± Occasionally effective.
− Resistant.

more effective than single-dose treatment in patients with unrecognized complicating factors. Numerous studies have shown that there is no benefit in extending treatment beyond 3 days.

Posttherapy urine cultures are no longer recommended after completion of treatment, assuming the patient's symptoms resolve, because it is rare for a patient to become asymptomatic after therapy but continue to colonize bacteria in the urine. It has been estimated that the routine use of cultures to detect the infrequent cases of asymptomatic bacteriuria after therapy for simple cystitis can cost up to $2000 per case. Few of these cases, when left undetected, will result in pyelonephritis. Therefore, cultures can be safely omitted in first infections or infrequent recurrences if symptoms have resolved completely.

Posttherapy cultures should be obtained in all patients with persisting symptoms. Persistence of symptoms suggests that the initial diagnosis of cystitis was incorrect, the patient's infection was secondary to a resistant organism that was present at the onset of therapy or has developed during initial treatment, or the patient was not compliant in taking her medication. In cases of resistance, a 7- to 14-day course of an appropriate antibiotic should be prescribed. A prolonged course of antibiotic therapy should also be given to patients who are febrile, have structural or functional abnormalities of the urinary tract, remain bacteriuric on antimicrobial therapy, have systemic diseases such as diabetes mellitus, and have abnormal host defenses.

## Recurrent Infections

Twenty-five percent of women who develop urinary tract infections have almost three infections per year, and these women make up 50% of all women presenting with acute cystitis. Once the urine has been sterilized by appropriate antimicrobial therapy, the pattern of culture-documented recurrence is helpful in the subsequent treatment of these patients (Fig. 27-5). It can also be used to identify those who require further urologic evaluation and to plan specific, predictable, appropriate therapy. The most common type of

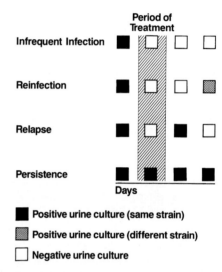

**Fig. 27-5**  Natural history of urinary tract infection.
From Karram MM: Lower urinary tract infection. In Ostergard DR, Bent AE, eds: *Urogynecology and urodynamics,* Baltimore, 1991, Williams & Wilkins.

recurrence is a reinfection by bacteria different from the initially infecting strain. Although the infections can be caused by the same species (*E. coli*), the organisms can usually be differentiated on the basis of colonial morphology and antimicrobial sensitivities. These infections are almost invariably caused by an ascending infection from the vaginal introital area. The same organism can also cause reinfection because the same strain can exist in the introital area for several months and cause multiple reinfections. Sexual intercourse and undiagnosed urinary tract abnormalities may also facilitate reinfection and must always be considered.

As previously mentioned, infection relapse is characterized by reappearance of the original infecting strain in the urine, usually but not necessarily within 2 weeks of finishing therapy. Relapsing infections can be caused by inadequately treated upper urinary tract infections or reinfection from the vaginal introital area. Relapsing infec-

**Box 27-2**

## CORRECTABLE URINARY TRACT ABNORMALITIES CAUSING PERSISTENT BACTERIURIA

Urethral diverticulum
Infected stone
Significant anterior vaginal wall relaxation
Papillary necrosis
Foreign body
Duplicated or ectopic ureter
Atrophic pyelonephritis (unilateral)
Medullary sponge kidney

**Table 27-3** Oral Antimicrobial Agents Useful for Prophylactic Prevention of Recurrent Urinary Tract Infections

| Agent | Dosage |
| --- | --- |
| Nitrofurantoin | 50 mg |
| Trimethoprim-sulfamethoxazole | 240 mg |
| Trimethoprim | 100 mg |
| Norfloxacin | 200 mg |

tion from an upper urinary tract source or an infected stone should be suspected if the same organism is repeatedly isolated 7 to 10 days after treatment with an antimicrobial agent to which the organism is sensitive. In patients in whom one cannot obtain sterile urine, these infections are called bacterial persistence (Box 27-2). Endoscopic and radiographic evaluations must be selectively performed in cases of relapse or persistence of infection.

Fecal flora is the ultimate source of the majority of recurrent urinary tract pathogens. Oral antimicrobial agents used to treat these patients should not alter rectal flora. Sulfonamides, penicillins, tetracyclines, and cephalosporins in full dosages can cause fecal flora to become rapidly resistant, not only to the original drug, but also to other antimicrobial agents by means of transfer of extrachromosomal plasmids. Quinolones and nitrofurantoin have minimal effects on fecal flora and cause very little resistance. The goal of management of reinfections is to achieve sterile urine; therefore, antimicrobial agents should be prescribed in dosages sufficient to exceed by a wide margin the minimum concentration required to inhibit growth. If the dosage is inadequate, resistant organisms can develop in up to 10% of patients.

Most patients with recurrent urinary tract infections can be treated successfully with continuous low-dose prophylaxis. This regimen is cost-effective and is recommended in women with frequent reinfections. Once the urine has been completely sterilized by a full-dose course of therapy, nightly prophylaxis can be initiated with one of many different drugs (Table 27-3). In general, the drugs should be taken before bedtime after emptying the bladder. In addition to the drugs listed in Table 27-3, satisfactory results have been obtained with methenamine hippurate 1 g and, in patients with renal insufficiency, cephalexin 125 mg. Trials have shown that medication on alternate nights or even 3 nights a week is just as effective. The treatment of atrophic vaginitis should be considered in postmenopausal women with recurrent cystitis. In a randomized,

double-blind, placebo-controlled trial of intravaginal estriol cream in 93 postmenopausal women, Raz and Stamm (1993) showed a significant reduction in the incidence of recurrent urinary tract infections. Using vaginal cultures, they demonstrated that estrogen promotes growth of lactobacillus species causing acidification of vaginal secretions, and decreases the rate of vaginal colonization with Enterobacteriaceae.

The majority of patients continue to maintain sterile urine while on prophylactic therapy, although breakthrough infections can occur occasionally and should be treated with full-dose antimicrobial therapy. We continue the prophylactic therapy for approximately 6 months and then follow the patient off therapy with frequent cultures. Approximately 30% of women are free of infection for at least the next 6 months. If reinfection occurs, it should be managed by reinstitution of nightly prophylaxis.

Self-start intermittent therapy is a useful adjunct in selected patients with frequent episodes of bacterial cystitis who are unwilling to take long-term, low-dose prophylaxis. With this form of treatment, the patient is given a dipslide and instructed to perform a urine culture when she has symptoms of a recurrent urinary tract infection. She then empirically begins a 3-day course of antimicrobial therapy. Norfloxacin, ciprofloxacin, nitrofurantoin, or TMP-SMX is usually effective for self-start intermittent therapy. Fluoroquinolones seem to be an ideal choice, with a broad spectrum of antimicrobial activity and low rate of spontaneous mutation to resistant organisms.

If the patient's symptoms do not respond to the initial antimicrobial drug, a repeat culture and sensitivity are performed, and therapy is adjusted accordingly. If the initial culture was negative, other causes of lower urinary tract symptoms must be pursued. This technique is particularly attractive for women with less frequent infections who are willing to play an active role in their diagnosis and management.

Finally, a small percentage of patients with recurrent urinary tract infections are at high risk for serious morbidity and renal scarring from bacteriuria because of pregnancy, diabetes mellitus, congenital abnormalities, or obstructive uropathy. The physician should identify such patients; prompt therapy, appropriate referral, and careful follow-up are essential.

## Asymptomatic Bacteriuria

Asymptomatic bacteriuria is defined as growth of more than 100,000 CFU/ml of a single bacterial species in two consecutive clean-catch urine specimens in the absence of clinical symptoms. Although 80% of patients with this condition can be cured by a 7-day course of antibiotic therapy, long-term eradication rates are no better than placebo therapy because of frequent reinfections and spontaneous remissions. Moreover, the treatment of asymptomatic bacteriuria often replaces *E. coli* that lack surface O antigens with *E. coli* with intact O antigens that could cause acute symptoms. The natural history of these infections is not completely known, but there seems to be no association with renal scarring, hypertension, or chronic renal disease. In general, treatment is not necessary. However, in certain situations (e.g., pregnant women, infections caused by *Proteus* species, and severe diabetes) antimicrobial therapy has proved beneficial. Treatment of asymptomatic bacteriuria in elderly women is controversial.

## SEXUAL INTERCOURSE AND DIAPHRAGM USE

Recurrent urinary tract infections are a particular problem in young, sexually active women. Many of these women are helped by simple measures such as completely emptying their bladders after intercourse and applying an antiseptic cream (e.g., cetrimide 0.5%) to the periurethral area before intercourse. Single-dose prophylaxis after intercourse is an effective way to prevent infections in women whose recurrences are related to sexual intercourse. Nitrofurantoin, TMP-SMX, nalidixic acid, and sulfonamides were all shown to be effective in preventing recurrent urinary tract infections in young, sexually active women. Compared with continuous low-dose prophylaxis, this approach may reduce medication costs and side effects and lessen the emergence of resistant bacterial strains.

Women with recurrent urinary tract infections using a diaphragm should consider another method of contraception. If such a change is not feasible, it should be determined whether symptoms of urinary obstruction occur with the diaphragm in place. Obstruction suggests that the diaphragm may be too large. Women in this category should be tried on a smaller diaphragm and be advised to void as soon as possible after intercourse.

## CATHETER-ASSOCIATED INFECTION

The urinary tract is the most common source of bacteremia and nosocomial infection in hospitalized patients. The most common predisposing factor for these infections is urethral instrumentation. Between 10% to 15% of hospitalized patients have indwelling catheters. The incidence of urinary tract infection in patients with indwelling catheters is directly related to the duration of catheterization. The

**Box 27-3**

## PREVENTION OF BLADDER INFECTION IN ELDERLY PATIENTS WITH LONG-TERM CATHETERIZATION

Monitor urine level in bag every 4 hours. Exchange catheter if cessation of flow for 4 hours.
Fluid intake of 1.5 L/day.
Avoid catheter manipulations.
Exchange catheter if infection is suspected.
Exchange catheter every 8 to 12 weeks.

incidence of bacteriuria is about 5% per day of catheterization, and the patient has only a 50% cumulative probability of remaining free of infection after 4 to 5 days of catheterization.

The pathogenesis of catheter-associated urinary infections has not been well studied, but points of bacterial entry have been identified. These include introduction of urethral bacteria into the bladder at the time of catheterization, subsequent entry of bacteria colonizing the urethral meatus along the mucus sheath external to the catheter, and ascent of bacteria along the catheter lumen itself. In 70% of women, the organisms causing catheter-related infections can be identified in the urethral and rectal flora 2 to 4 days before the onset of bacteriuria. Until more is known about the pathogenesis of nosocomial bacteriuria, the bulk of preventive efforts should continue to focus on the aseptic care of the catheter (Box 27-3). Use of local antiseptic ointments and antimicrobial irrigations has largely proved ineffective in reducing the prevalence of bacteriuria with catheterization. Although systemic antimicrobial agents reduce the occurrence of bacteriuria for the first few days of catheterization, their use is not widely recommended because of the attendant risk of development of resistant organisms.

Ten percent of elderly patients with indwelling catheters develop bacteremia and gram-negative septicemia, a serious disease with significant mortality. These patients require prompt hospitalization and vigorous antibiotic therapy. A traumatic event consisting of obstruction, manipulation, or removal of an inflated indwelling catheter often precedes the onset of urosepsis. In addition to antibiotic therapy, it is essential to establish free flow of urine in patients with acute urosepsis. The complications of septicemia, such as shock, disseminated intravascular coagulation, and adult respiratory distress syndrome, should be recognized and treated. Again, the most important preventive measure is complete asepsis in the insertion of the catheter and in the care of patients with chronic indwelling catheters.

## LOWER URINARY TRACT INSTRUMENTATION

Antibiotic prophylaxis against infective endocarditis should be given to all patients with prosthetic valves or valvular heart disease before genitourinary manipulation. However, the value of antimicrobial prophylaxis in patients who do not have cardiac valvular disorders is unclear. A prospective, double-blind, placebo-controlled study by Bhatia et al. (1992) noted that during cystoscopy, urodynamic evaluation or urethral dilation, patients receiving placebo had a significantly higher rate of infection than did those receiving one to three doses of antibiotic therapy. Cundiff et al. (1997) in a similar, more recent study, randomized 142 women to receive two doses of nitrofurantoin or two doses of a placebo following urodynamic and cystourethroscopic evaluation and found no significant difference in infection rates. We no longer administer prophylactic antibiotics routinely to patients after lower urinary tract instrumentation.

## PYELONEPHRITIS

A comprehensive discussion of pyelonephritis is beyond the scope of this chapter. It is sufficient to say that certain patients who appear to have typical symptoms of acute cystitis harbor upper urinary tract infection. These patients require aggressive therapy, usually a minimum of 10 days of antimicrobial treatment. As in cystitis, most cases of pyelonephritis are secondary to *E. coli* infection. Patients with acute pyelonephritis usually have high-titer bacteriuria; unless obstruction is present, microscopic examination of urine should demonstrate bacteria and leukocytes.

If the patient is compliant and if symptoms are mild, pyelonephritis can be managed on an outpatient basis with oral antimicrobial therapy. There is no evidence that parenteral therapy is more effective than oral therapy. TMP-SMX is an excellent drug for oral therapy in patients with pyelonephritis because of its broad antimicrobial spectrum and its ability to achieve high tissue concentrations. Other antibiotics that can be used orally include ciprofloxacin (500 mg every 12 hours) and norfloxacin (400 mg twice daily). Patients who exhibit toxicity, are unable to tolerate oral medications, have complicating factors, or are not entirely reliable should be hospitalized. They are treated initially with parenteral antibiotics and, when stable, switched to oral therapy to complete the 7- to 14-day course.

## BIBLIOGRAPHY
### Epidemiology

Cypress BK: Patients' reasons for visiting physicians: national ambulatory medical care survey, United States, 1977-78, *Vital and Health Statistics,* series 13, No. 56, 1981.

Mulholland SG: Controversies in management of urinary tract infection, *Urology* 27(suppl):3, 1986.

Rolleston GL, Shannon FT, Utley WLF: Relationship of infantile vesicoureteric reflux to renal damage, *BMJ* 1:460, 1970.

Winberg J, Anderson HJ, Bergstrom T, et al: Epidemiology of symptomatic urinary tract infection in childhood, *Acta Paediatr Scand* 252(suppl):3, 1974.

### Pathogenesis

Eden CS, Eriksson B, Hanson LA: Adhesions of *Escherichia coli* to human uroepithelial cells in vitro, *Infect Immun* 18:7657, 1977.

Fihn SD, Johnson L, Pinkstaff C, et al: Diaphragm use and urinary tract infection. Analysis of urodynamic and microbiologic factors, *J Urol* 136:853, 1986.

Fihn SD, Latham RH, Roberts P, et al: Association between diaphragm use and urinary tract infection, *JAMA* 253:240, 1985.

Foxman B, Frerichs RR: Epidemiology of urinary tract infection: I. Diaphragm use and sexual intercourse, *Am J Public Health* 75:1308, 1985.

Iwahi T, Abe Y, Nakao M, et al: Rule of type I fimbriae in the pathogenesis of ascending urinary tract infection induced by *Escherichia coli* in mice, *Infect Immun* 39:307, 1983.

Kinane DF, Blackwell CC, Brettle, et al: ABO blood group, secretor state and susceptibility to recurrent urinary tract infection in women, *BMJ* 285:7, 1982.

Nicolle LE, Harding GKM, Preiksaitis J, et al: The association of urinary tract infection with sexual intercourse, *J Infect Dis* 146:579, 1982.

Orskov I, Ferencz A, Orskov F: Tamm-Horsfall protein or uromucoid is the normal urinary slime that traps type I fimbriated *Escherichia coli.* Letter to the editor, *Lancet* 1:887, 1980.

Parsons CL: Prevention of urinary tract infection by the exogenous glycosaminoglycar sodium pertosan polysulfate, *J Urol* 127:167, 1982.

Parsons CL, Greenspan C, Moore SW, et al: Role of surface mucin in primary antibacterial defense of bladder, *Urology* 9:48, 1977.

Parsons DL, Schmidt JD: Control of recurrent lower urinary tract infections in postmenopausal women, *J Urol* 128:1224, 1982.

Reid G, Sobol JD: Bacterial adherence in the pathogenesis of urinary tract infection: a review, *Rev Infect Dis* 9:470, 1987.

Schaeffer AJ: Recurrent urinary tract infections in women: pathogenesis and management, *Postgrad Med* 81:51, 1987.

Schaeffer AJ, Amundsen SK, Schmidt LN: Adherence of *Escherichia coli* to human urinary tract epithelial cells, *Infect Immunol* 24:753, 1979.

Schaeffer AJ, Jones JM, Dunn JK: Association of in vitro *Escherichia coli* adherence to vaginal and buccal epithelial cells with susceptibility of women to recurrent urinary-tract infections, *N Engl J Med* 304:1062, 1981.

Schaeffer AJ, Radvany RM, Chmiel JS: Human leukocyte antigens in women with recurrent urinary tract infections, *J Infect Dis* 148:604, 1983.

Stamey TA, Sexton CC: The role of vaginal colonization with enterobacteriaceae in recurrent urinary infections, *J Urol* 113:214, 1975.

Stamey TA, Timothy MM: Studies of introital colonizations in women with recurrent urinary infections. I. The role of vaginal pH, *J Urol* 114:261, 1975.

Strom BL, Collins S, West SL, et al: Sexual activity, contraceptive use, and other risk factors for symptomatic and asymptomatic bacteriuria, *Ann Intern Med* 107:816, 1987.

Vaisanen V, Elo J, Tallgreen LG, et al: Mannose-resistant haemagglutination and P antigen recognition are characteristic of *Escherichia coli* causing primary pyelonephritis, *Lancet* 2:1366, 1981.

### Microbiology

Hoeprich PD, Jordan MC, Ronald AR, eds: *Infectious diseases: a treatise of infectious processes,* ed 5, Philadelphia, 1994, JB Lippincott.

Hovelius B: Urinary tract infections caused by *Staphylococcus saprophyticus* recurrences and complications, *J Urol* 122:645, 1979.

Lewis JF, Brake SR, Anderson DJ, et al: Urinary tract infection due to coagulase-negative staphylococcus, *Am J Clin Pathol* 77:736, 1982.

Marrie T, Kwan C, Noble M, et al: *Staphylococcus saprophyticus* as a cause of urinary tract infections, *J Clin Microbiol* 6:427, 1982.

Nicolle LE, Hoban SA, Harding GKM: Characterization of coagulase-negative staphylococci from urinary isolates, *J Clin Microbiol* 17:267, 1983.

Schaeffer AJ: Recurrent urinary tract infections in women. Pathogenesis and management, *Postgrad Med* 81:51, 1987.

Wallmark G, Arremark I, Telander B: *Staphylococcus saprophyticus:* a frequent cause of acute urinary tract infection among female outpatients, *J Infect Dis* 138:791, 1978.

### Diagnosis

Bixler-Forell E, Bertram MA, Bruckner DA: Clinical evaluation of three rapid methods for the detection of significant bacteriuria, *J Clin Microbiol* 22:62, 1985.

DeLange HE, Jones B: Unnecessary intravenous urography in young women with recurrent urinary tract infections, *Clin Radiol* 34:551, 1983.

Engel G, Schaeffer AJ, Grayhack JT, et al: The role of excretory urography and cystoscopy in the evaluation and management of women with recurrent urinary tract infection, *J Urol* 123:190, 1980.

Fair WR, McClennan BL, Jost RG: Are excretory urograms necessary in evaluating women with urinary tract infections? *J Urol* 121:313, 1979.

Fowler JE Jr, Pulaski T: Excretory urography, cystography, and cystoscopy in the evaluation of women with urinary tract infection, *N Engl J Med* 304:462, 1981.

Free AH, Free HM: Urinalysis: its proper role in the physician's office, *Clin Lab Med* 6:253, 1986.

Johnson JR, Stamm WE: Diagnosis and treatment of acute urinary tract infection, *Infect Dis Clin North Am* 1:773, 1987.

Johnson JR, Stamm WE: Urinary tract infection in women: diagnosis and treatment, *Ann Intern Med* 111:906, 1989.

Komaroff AL: Urinalysis and urine culture in women with dysuria, *Ann Intern Med* 104:212, 1986.

Kraft JK, Stamey TA: The natural history of symptomatic recurrent bacteriuria in women, *Medicine* 56:55, 1977.

Kunin CM: *Detection, prevention and management of urinary tract infection,* ed 4, Philadelphia, 1987, Lea & Febiger.

Mogensen P, Hansen LK: Do intravenous urography and cystoscopy provide important information in otherwise healthy women with recurrent urinary tract infection? *Br J Urol* 55:261, 1983.

Needham CA: Rapid detection methods in microbiology: are they right for your office? *Med Clin North Am* 71:591, 1987.

Newhouse JH, Rhea JT, Murphy RX, et al: Yield of screening urography in young women with urinary tract infection, *Urol Radiol* 4:187, 1982.

Pezzlo M: Detection of bacteriuria by automated methods, *Lab Med* 15:539, 1984.

Reid G: The office microbiology laboratory, *Urol Clin North Am* 13:569, 1986.

Schaeffer AJ: The office laboratory, *Urol Clin North Am* 7:29, 1980.

Stamm WE: Measurement of pyuria and its relation to bacteriuria, *Am J Med* 75:53, 1983.

Stamm WE: Quantitative urine cultures revisited (editorial), *Eur J Clin Microbiol* 3:279, 1984.

Stamm WE, Counts GW, Running KR, et al: Diagnosis of coliform infection in acutely dysuric women, *N Engl J Med* 307:463, 1982.

Wu TC, Williams EC, Koo SY, et al: Evaluation of three bacteriuria screening methods in a clinical research hospital, *J Clin Microbiol* 21:796, 1985.

### Management

Bailey RR: Management of lower urinary tract infections, *Drugs* 45(suppl 3):139, 1993.

Bailey RR, Abbott GD: Treatment of urinary tract infection with a single dose of amoxicillin, *Nephron* 18:316, 1977.

Bhatia NN, Karram MM, Bergman A, et al: Antibiotic prophylaxis following lower urinary tract instrumentation, *Urology* 39:583, 1992.

Buckwold FJ, Ludwid P, Godfrey KM, et al: Therapy for acute cystitis in adult women: randomized comparison of single-dose sulfasoxazole vs trimethoprim-sulfamethoxazol, *JAMA* 247:1839, 1982.

Burke JP, Garibaldi RA, Britt MR, et al: Prevention of catheter-associated urinary tract infections, *Am J Med* 70:655, 1981.

Burke JP, Jacobson JA, Garibaldi RA, et al: Evaluation of daily meatal care with poly-antibiotic ointment in prevention of urinary catheter-associated bacteriuria, *J Urol* 129:331, 1983.

Childs SJ, Goldstein EJ: Ciprofloxacin as treatment for genitourinary tract infection, *J Urol* 141:1, 1989.

Cundiff GW, McLennan MT, Bent AE: Double-blinded randomized evaluation of nitrofurantoin prophylaxis for combined urodynamics and cystourethroscopy, *Int Urogynecol J* 8:245, 1997.

Evans DA, Kass EH, Hennekens CH, et al: Bacteriuria and subsequent mortality in women, *Lancet* 1:156, 1982.

Fang LST, Tolkoff-Rubin NE, Rubin RH: Efficacy of single-dose and conventional amoxicillin therapy in urinary tract infection localized by the antibody-coated bacteria technic, *N Engl J Med* 298:413, 1978.

Fihn SD: Single-dose antimicrobial therapy for urinary tract infections: "less is more"? or "reductio ad absurdum"? *J Gen Intern Med* 1:62, 1986.

Fihn SD, Johnson C, Roberts PL, et al: Trimethoprim sulfamethoxazole for acute dysuria in women: a double-blind, randomized trial of single-dose versus 10-day treatment, *Ann Intern Med* 108:350, 1988.

Garibaldi RA, Burke JP, Dickman ML, et al: Factors predisposing to bacteriuria during indwelling urethral catheterization, *N Engl J Med* 291:215, 1974.

Goldstein EJ, Alpert ML, Najem A: Norfloxacin in the treatment of complicated and uncomplicated urinary tract infections: a comparative multicenter trial, *Am J Med* 82:65, 1987.

Greenberg, RN, Sanders CV, Lewis AC, et al: Single-dose cefaclor therapy of urinary tract infection: evaluation of antibody-coated bacteria test and C-reactive protein assay as predictors of cure, *Am J Med* 71:841, 1981.

Harding GK, Buckwold FJ, Marrie TJ, et al: Prophylaxis of recurrent urinary tract infection in female patients: efficacy of low-dose, thrice weekly therapy with trimethoprim-sulfamethoxazole, *JAMA* 242:1975, 1979.

Hoener B, Patterson SE: Nitrofurantoin disposition, *Clin Paramcol Ther* 29:808, 1981.

Hooper DC, Wolfson JS: The fluroquinolones: pharmacology, clinical uses and toxicities in humans, *Antimicrob Agents Chemother* 28:716, 1985.

Kalowski S, Rudford N, Kincaid-Smith P: Crystalline and macrocrystalline nitrofurantoin in the treatment of urinary tract infection, *N Engl J Med* 290:385, 1974.

Kraft JK, Stamey TA: The natural history of symptomatic recurrent bacteriuria in women, *Medicine* 56:55, 1977.

Lee C, Ronald AN: Norfloxacin: its potential in clinical practice, *Am J Med* 82:27, 1987.

Martinez FC, Kindrachuk RW, Thomas E, et al: Effect of prophylactic low dose cephalexin on fecal and vaginal bacteria, *J Urol* 133:994, 1985.

Mayer TR: UTI in the elderly: how to select treatment, *Geriatrics* 35:67, 1980.

Mayrer AR, Andriole VT: Urinary tract antiseptics, *Med Clin North Am* 66:199, 1982.

Neu HC: Quinolones: a new class of antimicrobial agents with wide potential uses, *Med Clin North Am* 72:623, 1988.

Parsons CL: Urinary tract infections in the female patient, *Urol Clin North Am* 12:355, 1985.

Pfau A, Sacks T, Englestein D: Recurrent urinary tract infections in premenopausal women. Prophylaxis based on an understanding of the pathogenesis, *J Urol* 129:1152, 1983.

Platt R: Adverse consequences of acute urinary tract infections in adults, *Am J Med* 82(suppl 6B):47, 1987.

Platt R, Polk BF, Murdock B, et al: Mortality associated with nosocomial urinary tract infection, *N Engl J Med* 307:736, 1982.

Raz R, Stamm WE: A controlled trial of intravaginal estriol in postmenopausal women with recurrent urinary tract infections, *N Engl J Med* 329:753, 1993.

Reed MD, Blumer JL: Urologic pharmacology in the office setting, *Urol Clin North Am* 15:737, 1988.

Rubin RH, Fang LST, Jones SR, et al: Single-dose amoxicillin therapy for urinary tract infection, *JAMA* 244:561, 1980.

Sabbaj J, Hoagland VL, Shih WJ: Multiclinic comparative study of norfloxacin and trimethoprim-sulfamethoxazole for treatmet of urinary tract infections, *Antimicrob Agents Chemother* 27:297, 1985.

Schaeffer AJ: Recurrent urinary tract infections in women. Pathogenesis and management, *Posgrad Med* 81:51, 1987.

Schultz HJ, McCaffrey LA, Keys TF, et al: Acute cystitis: a prospective study of laboratory tests and duration of therapy, *Mayo Clin Proc* 59:391, 1984.

Stamey TA, Condy M, Mihara G: Prophylactic efficacy of nitrofurantoin macrocrystals and trimethoprim-sulfamethoxazole in urinary infections: biologic effects on the vaginal and rectal flora, *N Engl J Med* 296:780, 1977.

Stamm WE, Counts GW, McKevitt M, et al: Urinary prophylaxis with trimethoprim and trimethoprim-sulfamethoxazole: efficacy, influence on the natural history of recurrent bacteriuria, and cost control, *Rev Infect Dis* 4:450, 1982.

Stamm WE, McKevitt, Counts GW, et al: Is antimicrobial prophylaxis of urinary tract infections cost effective? *Ann Intern Med* 94:251, 1981.

Tolkoff-Rubin NE, Weber D, Fang LST, et al: Single dose therapy with trimethoprim-sulfamethoxazole for urinary tract infection in women, *Rev Infect Dis* 4:443, 1982.

Vosti KL: Recurrent urinary tract infections: prevention by prophylactic antibiotics after sexual intercourse, *JAMA* 231:934, 1975.

Wise R, Griggs D, Andrews JM: Pharmacokinetics of the quinolones in volunteers: a proposed dosing schedule, *Rev Infect Dis* 10(suppl 1):S83, 1998.

Wolfson JS, Hooper DC: The fluoroquinolones: structures, mechanisms of action and resistance, and spectra of activity in vitro, *Antimicrob Agents Chemother* 28:581, 1985.

Wong ES, Hooton TM: Guidelines to prevention of catheter-associated urinary tract infection, *Infect Control* 2:125, 1980.

Wong ES, McKevitt M, Running K, et al: Management of recurrent urinary tract infections with patient-administered single-dose therapy, *Ann Intern Med* 102:302, 1985.

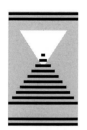

CHAPTER **28**

# Lower Urinary Tract Fistulas

Thomas E. Elkins† and Jason R. Thompson

## HISTORICAL PERSPECTIVES

The earliest evidence of a vesicovaginal fistula was reported by Derry (1935) in the mummified remains of Queen Henhenit, one of the wives of King Mentuhotep II of Egypt (11th Dynasty, circa 2050 BC). In his dissection of the mummy at the Cairo School of Medicine in 1923, Derry noted a large vesicovaginal fistula in the presence of a severely contracted pelvis; he concluded that the fistula was a consequence of obstructed labor. Hippocrates (460-377 BC) recognized the problem of urinary incontinence after confinement but offered no clue as to its cause. In his textbook, *Al Kanoun,* celebrated Persian physician Avicenna (980-1037) was the first to recognize that urinary incontinence after difficult labor was caused by communication between the bladder and vagina.

No further reference to vesicovaginal fistula appeared until 1597, when both Felix Platter of Basle and Luiz de Mercado of Valladolid separately reviewed the problem but offered no constructive therapeutic advice. Zacharin (1988) states that the term *fistula* was first used by de Mercado instead of the usual term *ruptura.*

In 1663, Hendrik Von Roonhuyse of Amsterdam published *Medico-Chirurgical Observations About the Infirmities of Women.* Commonly thought of as the first textbook on operative gynecology, this text was translated into English in 1676. The fourth chapter is titled "Rupture of the Bladder: The Signs, Causes, Prognostics and Cure Thereof." Von Roonhuyse proposed a revolutionary surgical technique for the closure of vesicovaginal fistulas based on the following principles: lithotomy position, good exposure of the fistula with a vaginal speculum, marginal denudation of the fistula edge using a fine scissors or knife, and approximation of the denuded edges with "stitching needles of stiff swans' quills." There is no record that Von Roonhuyse operated on patients using this technique. In 1752, a medical text by Swiss physician Johann Fatio was posthumously published. In it were recorded two successful fistula repairs performed by Fatio in 1675 and 1684 using Von Roonhuyse's technique.

Volter in 1687 suggested that sutures should be interrupted, and he introduced the use of a retention urinary catheter. During this same period Pietro DiMarchettis claimed complete cures using cautery. In later years Monteggia, Dupuytren, and others also recommended cautery.

The nineteenth century was the dawn of a new era in the surgical treatment of vesicovaginal fistula. In 1834, Jobert de Lamballe successfully repaired a small number of fistulas using pedicled skin flaps *(autoplastie vaginale par la methode indienne).* A second technique *(autoplastie par glissment ou par locomotion)* later enabled him to close a greater number of fistulas. This technique involved dissecting the bladder from the cervix and vagina with the additional use of curved releasing incisions in the vagina to facilitate mobilization and closure without tension.

In a letter to the *Boston Medical and Surgical Journal* in August 1838, John Peter Mettauer of Virginia stated that he had repaired a vesicovaginal fistula about the size of a half dollar piece using lead wire, with good results. This was the first successful repair in the United States.

†Deceased

On June 21, 1849, in an eight-bed infirmary on Perry Street in Montgomery, Alabama, James Marion Sims operated on a young slave woman named Anarcha for the thirtieth time. Using the genupectoral position, a bent pewter spoon as a vaginal speculum, and reflected light from a mirror, Sims denuded the fistula edge, closing the defect in one layer with fine silver wire applied with leaden bars and perforated shot. On the eighth day, Sims reexamined the patient and noted that the wound was well healed. In 1852, he published his classic paper "On the treatment of vesicovaginal fistula" in the *American Journal of Medical Sciences*. He deprecated both cautery as advocated by Dupuytren for small fistulae and obturation of the vulva as practiced by Vidal De Cassis (whereby the bladder and vagina are converted into a common reservoir for urinary and menstrual discharge). Sims insisted on liberal use of opium for perioperative analgesia and stressed the importance of postoperative bladder drainage with a urethral catheter. He later designed a silver sigmoid-shaped, self-retaining catheter for this purpose. In 1853 Sims moved to New York and in 1855 he became chief surgeon in the newly built Woman's Hospital, where he was later joined by a brilliant young assistant, Thomas Addis Emmet. Sims and Emmet worked closely together, Emmet perfecting many of his mentor's techniques.

In his text *Vesico-Vaginal Fistula from Parturition and Other Causes with Cases of Recto-Vaginal Fistula* (1868), dedicated to Sims, Emmet reported on 270 consecutive patients treated in the Woman's Hospital: 200 were cured, 65 were improved, and 5 were considered incurable. Emmet eventually succeeded Sims at the Woman's Hospital. Probably his greatest contribution to obstetric care was his insistence that frequent catheterization of the bladder in labor, together with the judicious use of forceps for second-stage delay, would prevent the majority of labor-related vesicovaginal fistulas.

In 1861, Maurice Collis of Dublin advocated the flap-splitting technique, whereby the anterior vaginal wall is widely dissected from the bladder with separate closure of the two defects. This method was later popularized by Mackenrodt (1894) in Berlin.

In the 1880s and 1890s, Trendelenburg and Von Dittel reported failed attempts at fistula repair using extraperitoneal and suprapubic approaches, respectively. Schuchardt (1893) also devised a parasacral incision, which permitted better access to high fistulas, particularly when associated with vaginal stenosis.

The discovery of antibiotics and the development of general and regional anesthesia contributed significantly to the surgical treatment of vesicovaginal fistulas in the twentieth century. Other notable milestones included urethral reconstruction using lateral vaginal flaps and labium minus grafts (Noble, 1901), suprapubic intraperitoneal repair of posthysterectomy, high vesicovaginal and rectovaginal fistulas (Kelly, 1902), partial colpocleisis for posthysterectomy vesicovaginal fistulas (Latzko, 1914, 1942), urethral reinforcement using pelvic floor muscles (Martius, 1928), pedicled gracilis muscle flap (Garlock, 1928), bulbocavernosus flaps (Martius, 1942), pubococcygeus, bulbocavernosus, rectus abdominis, and gracilis flaps (Ingleman-Sundberg, 1960), the use of pedicled omental flaps in the repair of extensive vesicovaginal fistulas (Kiricuta and Goldstein, 1972), and urethral reconstruction (Symmonds and Hill, 1978; Tanagho and Smith, 1972). Knowledge of effective repair of genitourinary fistulas became more widely disseminated with publication of *The Vesico-Vaginal Fistula* (Moir, 1961). Greater international attention was brought to the immense problem of genitourinary fistulas in developing countries with the foundation of the Second Fistula Hospital in Addis Ababa, Ethiopia, in 1975, and the report of 1789 fistulas repaired over an 11-year period from Nigeria (Ward, 1980).

## EPIDEMIOLOGY AND ETIOLOGY

To understand the cause of fistulas one must understand wound healing because it is a defect or vulnerability in this process that results in fistula development. Wounded tissue undergoes four phases of healing: coagulation, inflammation, fibroplasia, and remodeling. These phases do not occur independently but overlap each other like runners in a baton relay. During the fibroplastic phase collagen is laid down, reaching its peak on the seventh day after injury and continuing for 3 weeks. Between the first and third weeks healing is most vulnerable to hypoxia, ischemia, malnutrition, radiation, and chemotherapy, so this is the time when most fistulas present. Conditions known to interfere with wound healing are associated with increased risk of fistula formation, including diabetes mellitus, smoking, infection, peripheral vascular disease, chronic steroid use, malignancy, or previous tissue injury.

### Obstetric Fistulas

The vast majority of vesicovaginal fistulas that occur in developing countries are caused by obstetric trauma. Of 377 cases reported by Lawson (1989) from Ibadan, Nigeria, 369 (97.9%) were obstetric and 343 were a consequence of obstructed labor. Demographic characteristics of women affected by vesicovaginal fistulas speak to the sociocultural climate in which they occur and to the terrible consequences. Childbearing at a young age may occur before full growth and development of the pelvis; in a 1989 report from Nigeria, 41% of patients with vesicovaginal fistulas were under 15 year of age. All were primiparas whose labors had resulted in stillborn infants. All had been ostracized by their husbands, families, and communities. Many had waited 5 years or more for primary surgical repair.

Because knowledge of vesicovaginal fistulas in the developing world is based on women treated in hospitals, the prevalence is probably underestimated considerably.

Many women are unaware that the condition is treatable, and are prevented from learning about appropriate care by severe social isolation as a result of their incontinence. Few area hospitals have the staff, equipment, or expertise to manage the overwhelming problem. Poverty, long distances, and long waiting lists deter women from traveling to major centers.

Obstructed labor remains the most important cause of vesicovaginal fistulas in developing countries. Absent or untrained birth attendants, reduced pelvic dimensions (caused by early childbearing, chronic disease, malnutrition, and rickets), uncorrected inefficient uterine action, malpresentations, hydrocephalus, and introital stenosis secondary to tribal circumcision all contribute to obstructed labor. Prolonged impaction of the presenting fetal part against a distended edematous bladder eventually leads to pressure necrosis and fistula formation. Fistulas may be caused by trauma from forceps, instruments used to dismember and deliver stillborn infants, and surgical abortion. They are also associated with symphysiotomy, the practice of Gishiri cuts (i.e., an incision in the anterior vaginal wall, made for a variety of obstetric and gynecologic disorders), and the use of traditional postpartum vaginal caustics.

Obstetric fistulas are characterized by considerable necrosis, sloughing, tissue loss, and cicatrization. Vesicovaginal fistulas commonly occur in the setting of a wide range of other immediate problems, such as stillbirth, ruptured uterus, third- and fourth-degree perineal lacerations with resultant rectovaginal fistulas and anal incontinence, and pelvic infection. Longer-term conditions contribute to ongoing morbidity from vaginal stenosis, bladder calculi, symphyseal chondritis and osteitis, and foot-drop caused by nerve injury. The social consequences of ostracism take an enormous toll on affected women; divorce is common, and depression and suicide may follow.

In modern obstetrics, most of these conditions do not exist; however, genitourinary fistulas still occur. Vesicovaginal fistulas can follow cesarean delivery or peripartum hysterectomy, particularly in the presence of distorted anatomy (e.g., massive fibroids) and surgical inexperience. Unusual cases have been reported of a ureterouterine fistula after cesarean delivery and a vesicouterine fistula following vaginal birth after previous cesarean.

## Gynecologic Fistulas

In developed countries, abdominal surgery, particularly total abdominal hysterectomy, is the major cause of genitourinary fistulas. Of 166 cases from the United Kingdom, 116 (69.9%) were related to surgery and only 21 (12.6%) to obstetrics. Fistulas related to surgery performed by obstetrician-gynecologists account for approximately 80% of all urogenital fistulas. The remaining 20% is divided among urologists and colorectal, vascular, and general surgeons. Because gynecologic surgery is the cause of the

majority of urogenital fistulas, gynecologic surgeons should be skilled in their identification and management. Most genitourinary fistulas resulting from gynecologic surgery occur secondary to urinary tract injuries. These injuries can occur with pelvic surgery performed by even the most experienced surgeons. Although some series have documented ureteral injury in 0.5% to 2.5% of patients undergoing hysterectomy, others have reported a much lower rate of injury to either the bladder or ureter in 0.05% of 35,000 pelvic operations.

In the United States, vesicovaginal fistulas are caused by benign gynecologic surgery (80%), obstetric events (10%), surgery for malignancies of the cervix, uterus, or ovary (5%), and pelvic radiotherapy (5%). Uncommon causes of vesicovaginal fistulas include lymphogranuloma venereum, tuberculosis, syphilis, bladder calculus, retained vaginal foreign body, and trauma. Although schistosomiasis rarely causes fistula formation, this infection may make fistula closure more difficult and healing less certain.

Lee et al. (1988) reviewed 303 women with genitourinary fistulas treated at the Mayo Clinic. Gynecologic surgery was responsible for 82%, obstetric events 8%, radiation therapy 6%, and trauma or fulguration 4%. Seventy-four percent of fistulas resulted from gynecologic surgery for benign conditions, most commonly fibroids, dysfunctional uterine bleeding, prolapse, incontinence, carcinoma in situ, and endometriosis. Fistulas occurred after surgery for malignancy in 42 patients (14%). This review included 53 patients with urethrovaginal fistulas, 10 of whom also had vesicovaginal fistula. Antecedent events included vaginal surgery for incontinence or cystocele, urethral diverticulum repair, treatments for gynecologic cancer, and the use of forceps.

Vesicovaginal fistulas as a consequence of simple hysterectomy are most often caused by faulty dissection of the bladder from the uterus and cervix, resulting in an unrecognized laceration. Necrosis from crush injury by clamping or suture may also be responsible. Although suture ligation causing necrosis may lead to a fistula, the mere presence of suture probably does not. Using a rabbit model, Meeks et al. (1997) demonstrated that suture placed through the vaginal cuff and bladder was not associated with the development of vesicovaginal fistula. Posthysterectomy fistulas are usually located above the interureteric ridge, medial to both ureteral orifices. Unlike obstetric fistulas, massive tissue loss is uncommon.

Fistulas caused by radiotherapy are secondary to slowly progressive endarteritis, which ultimately leads to tissue necrosis, and may be further complicated by urethral dysfunction, detrusor muscle fibrosis, vesicoureteral reflux, and renal deterioration. Patients may present with urinary symptoms several years after treatment. It is essential to rule out recurrent cancer with appropriate biopsies and histologic study. Surgical management is fraught with difficulty because of marked tissue fibrosis, contracture, fixity, and

**Box 28-1**

## FUNCTIONAL CLASSIFICATION OF DIFFICULT OR HIGH-RISK OBSTETRIC FISTULAS

More than 4-5 cm in diameter
Involvement of:
    Urethra
    Ureter(s)
    Rectum
Juxtacervical fistulas with incomplete visualization of the
    superior edge
Previous failed repairs

**Box 28-2**

## SUGGESTED CLASSIFICATION OF GYNECOLOGIC VESICOVAGINAL AND URETHROVAGINAL FISTULAS

**Vesicovaginal**

*Simple*
Less than 2-3 cm in size and near the cuff (supratrigonal)
No history of radiation or malignancy
Normal vaginal length
*Complicated*
Previous radiation therapy
Pelvic malignancy
Compromised vaginal depth
More than 3 cm in size
Away from the cuff or involving the trigone

**Urethrovaginal**

*Simple*
Involves distal third of urethra
*Complicated*
Involves proximal two thirds of urethra
Previous radiation
Circumferential fistula
Involves continence mechanism

devascularization that may interfere with initial and subsequent repair attempts.

Ureterovaginal fistulas are preceded by benign gynecologic surgery in 90% of cases. The remaining 10% are divided between surgery for malignant disease, pelvic radiotherapy, and obstetrics.

Most patients with urethrovaginal fistulas fall into one of three groups based on history: postpartum, especially after operative vaginal delivery; surgical repair for urethral diverticulum, cystocele, or urinary incontinence; and radiation therapy.

## CLASSIFICATION
### Obstetric Fistulas

Obstetric vesicovaginal fistulas may be classified in a number of ways, depending on their location, cause, or complexity. One anatomic classification is as follows:

*Juxtaurethral:* involving the bladder neck and proximal urethra, with damage to the sphincteric mechanism, occasionally with total urethral loss and fixity to bone

*Mid-vaginal:* without involvement of the bladder neck or trigone

*Juxtacervical:* opening into the anterior vaginal fornix or cervical canal, with possible distal ureteral involvement

*Massive:* a combination of the first three fistulas, with dense scarring and fixity to bone and often with ureteral involvement at the fistula margins and bladder prolapse through the large defect

*Compound:* involving rectovaginal or ureterovaginal as well as vesicovaginal fistulas

*Vesicocervical or vesicouterine:* tracts between bladder and uterus or cervix, usually following cesarean delivery

Another classification of obstetric fistulas, proposed by Mahfouz (1938), considers the site of obstruction during labor. Juxtacervical fistulas result from obstruction at the pelvic inlet, mid-vaginal fistulas at the level of the ischial spines, and suburethral or urethral fistulas from pelvic outlet obstruction.

A newer classification for obstetric fistulas allows triage of fistulas based on the anticipated complexity of repair (Box 28-1). This classification identifies characteristics of difficult repairs more likely to have significant complications. This approach targets cases for appropriate referrals to specialty centers and encourages general repair efforts of simple fistulas to expand among nonspecialists.

### Gynecologic Fistulas

Gynecologic urethrovaginal and vesicovaginal fistulas are separated into those resulting from radiation therapy and those that are postsurgical and described by their anatomic location. A useful classification to remember is based on location as well as associated risk factors (Box 28-2).

## PRESENTATION AND INVESTIGATION

Patients present with genitourinary fistulas in many ways. Gross hematuria or abnormal intraperitoneal fluid accumulation (urinoma) noted during or after surgery should raise suspicion of an unrecognized urinary tract injury and dictates immediate investigation. In the postoperative period, symptoms may develop after an interval of days, weeks (surgical and obstetric fistulas), months, or even years (radiotherapy-related fistulas). Postsurgical fistulas usually present 7 to 21 days after surgery. Most patients have urinary incontinence or persistent vaginal discharge. If the fistula is very small, leakage may be intermittent, occurring only at maximal bladder capacity or with particular body positions. Other signs and symptoms include unexplained fever; hematuria; recurrent cystitis or pyelonephritis; vaginal, suprapubic, or flank pain; and abnormal urinary stream.

The initial evaluation of all patients with symptoms of genitourinary fistulas starts with a complete physical examination. A thorough speculum examination of the vagina may reveal the source of fluid, which can then be collected; measurement of its urea concentration may identify it as urine. Urine should be examined microscopically and cultured, and appropriate treatment instituted for infection. Urethrovaginal fistulas are usually easily diagnosed on physical examination. Further office evaluation, cystourethroscopy, and intravenous urogram permit the physician to localize the fistula, determine adequacy of renal function, and exclude or identify other types of urinary tract injury.

Office testing is often able to distinguish between fistulas involving the bladder or ureters. Instillation of methylene blue or sterile milk into the bladder stains vaginal swabs or tampons in the presence of a vesicovaginal fistula. If this test is not diagnostic, a transurethral Foley catheter should be placed to prevent any staining of the distal tampon from the urethral meatus. Unstained but wet swabs may indicate a ureterovaginal fistula. Intravenous indigo carmine can be given and the tampon observed for blue staining. Use of methylene blue intravenously must be chosen with caution because of the risk of methemoglobinemia, a rare but serious complication. If leakage is not demonstrated, the bladder is filled to maximum capacity and provocative maneuvers such as Valsalva or manual pressure over the bladder used to reproduce and confirm the patient's symptoms.

Radiologic imaging is recommended in most cases, either intravenous urography or cystoscopic retrograde urography. Renal ultrasound may miss up to 20% of ureteral injuries. A Tratner catheter may be useful in cases of suspected urethrovaginal fistula.

Cystourethroscopy is also indicated in most cases. The size, site, and number of fistulas and condition of local tissues are carefully noted. Key observations include the fistula's proximity to the bladder neck, urethral sphincter, and ureteral orifices as well as the presence of tissue edema, slough, infection, induration, scarring, and fixity to bone. Water cystoscopy may be impossible with large fistulas. Placing the patient in the genupectoral position allows the bladder to fill with air, thus permitting dry cystoscopy. Bladder calculi and nonabsorbable sutures should be removed. In areas of endemic schistosomiasis, cystoscopic biopsies may be needed to confirm the diagnosis. Associated problems such as rectovaginal fistulas, anal sphincter disruption, and vaginal stenosis must be identified and plans made for appropriate treatment.

# PRESURGICAL MANAGEMENT

Patients awaiting surgical repair need considerable psychologic support. Leakage from small fistulas may be controlled by frequent voiding and the use of tampons, perineal pads, or silica-impregnated incontinence pants. A vaginal diaphragm with a watertight attachment to a urinary catheter can collect urine from larger fistulas into a leg bag. Long-term indwelling catheters should be avoided.

Ammoniacal dermatitis is treated with sitz baths and zinc oxide barrier ointment. Before surgical repair, oral or vaginal estrogen should be given to women who are surgically or naturally postmenopausal to improve urogenital tissue integrity. In malnourished patients, a high-protein diet, vitamin and trace element supplements, and correction of anemia are essential before surgical repair. Surgery should not be performed during menstruation because of the increased tissue vascularity at that time.

## Vesicovaginal Fistulas

If a vesicovaginal fistula is diagnosed within 7 days of occurrence, is less than 1 cm in diameter, and is unrelated to malignancy or radiation, bladder drainage alone for up to 4 weeks allows spontaneous healing in 12% to 80% of cases, but the outcome is unpredictable. Cystoscopic cauterization of small lesions may also be successful. Standard management of vesicovaginal fistula dictates an interval from injury to repair of 3 to 6 months in surgical and obstetric fistulas and up to 1 year in radiation-induced fistulas to allow for resolution of necrosis and inflammation. If there is an associated rectovaginal fistula, a transverse colostomy performed 2 to 3 months before fistula repair may be helpful.

Some pelvic surgeons have championed the early closure of small fistulas as soon as they are identified postoperatively. Fearl and Keizur (1969) used serial cystoscopy in 20 patients to determine suitability for fistula repair; surgery was performed an average of 2 to 4 months earlier than if they had used empiric intervals, with no decrease in success rates. Herbert and Vaughn (1985) recommended that the time for repair should be individualized based on endoscopic evidence of healing. When the fistula site and adjacent tissues are pliable, noninflamed, epithelialized, and free of granulation tissue and necrosis, little is gained by waiting longer. Corticosteroids and nonsteroidal antiinflammatory drugs have been used by some to facilitate early surgery but their efficacy has not been proven.

## Ureterovaginal Fistulas

Once the diagnosis of ureterovaginal fistula is confirmed, recommended initial management is ureteral stenting (deBaere et al., 1995; Selzman et al., 1995). Stenting is more successful when performed sooner rather than later; in one study, 82% of attempts in patients whose fistulas were less than 1 month old were successful, compared to 33% with older fistulas. High success rates of stenting and complete resolution of fistulas have been reported when both ante-grade and retrograde techniques were used together.

Stents are usually made of silastic, with length measured in centimeters and diameter in French units, with single-J or double-J ends. Double-J stents are preferred because there is less risk of migration out of the renal pelvis and the distal J tip in the bladder is atraumatic. Ureteral stenting is best accomplished in a suite that can accommodate anesthesia, fluoroscopy, and cystoscopy. Epidural anesthesia is ideal. The first step is placement of a guidewire from the kidney to the bladder (antegrade), then antegrade stent placement is attempted. If this fails, retrograde guidewire and stenting may be attempted. Occasionally a guidewire can be passed but a stent cannot. This may be caused by a stricture, which can be dilated using angioplasty. Another technique that may aid in stent placement is ureteroscopy.

If a stent is placed successfully, it should be left in for 6 to 8 weeks. The risk of infection, stone formation, and ureteral occlusion increases with time. After 4 to 6 weeks, intravenous or retrograde pyelogram should be performed to evaluate for persistence of the fistula. If the fistula has healed, the stent may be removed via cystoscopy and intravenous pyelograms should be performed at 3, 6, 12, and 24 months to rule out subsequent stricture formation. If the fistula has not healed at 6 weeks, a repeat examination may be performed at 8 weeks, with preparation to proceed with surgical repair if the fistula still has not healed.

If stenting is not possible, then it is helpful to subdivide the patient population for subsequent treatment. Surgical management of ureteroneocystostomy should be reserved for those whose fistulas have been diagnosed within the first 2 or after 12 postoperative weeks. Interval management with percutaneous nephrostomy should be used when fistulas are diagnosed between 2 and 12 weeks postoperatively and also in patients who are poor surgical candidates or in the presence of previous radiation therapy, radical pelvic surgery, or pelvic malignancy. If the fistula has failed to heal after 12 weeks of percutaneous nephrostomy drainage, then surgery should be considered.

## SURGICAL REPAIR
### Anesthesia and Patient Positioning

Suitable methods of anesthesia include epidural, low spinal, and general. Small fistulas may be repaired under local anesthesia with or without sedation. For proximal urethral or bladder neck fistulas, Lawson's position may be used. The patient is placed prone on the operating table with her knees apart and her ankles raised and supported in stirrups, with the table in reversed Trendelenburg position. Alternatively, a jackknife position may be used in which the patient is placed prone with the hips abducted and well flexed, the table being "jackknifed" at this point. For higher fistulas, an exaggerated lithotomy position with standard Trendelenburg

provides optimal access; we prefer this position for all vaginal approaches. Labial retraction sutures and, if necessary, an episiotomy or Schuchardt incision may improve exposure. For abdominal repairs, steep Trendelenburg position may be helpful.

## Instruments and Materials

Adequate light and appropriate instruments and materials are mandatory. Instruments most useful include Chassar Moir, Church, Kelly fistula scissors, fine Allis forceps, Sims skin hooks, Sims or Breisky retractors, fine-tipped suction tips, and long-handled scalpels with No. 11 and No. 15 blades. Although no single suture material has proven superiority, the use of No. 2-0 and 3-0 polyglycolic acid on CT-2 needles is favored by many for closure of all layers. The use of fine monofilament nylon for vaginal closure (with delayed removal at 3 to 4 weeks) also remains popular. In developing countries the choice of instruments and materials in many centers is strongly influenced by local supplies and financial constraints.

## Vaginal Repair of Vesicovaginal and Urethrovaginal Fistulas

Examination under anesthesia may be necessary to identify tissue edges and plan surgical approaches in the case of large or obscure vesicovaginal fistulas. The majority of vesicovaginal fistulas can be closed transvaginally. Simple vesicovaginal fistulas are usually repaired with the Latzko technique; more complex fistulas should undergo individualized repairs. In the series of 303 cases reported by Lee et al. (1988), 80% were repaired transvaginally irrespective of fistula size, number, or history of previous repairs.

The use of stay sutures close to the fistula margin or the insertion and inflation of a pediatric-sized Foley catheter through the fistula tract into the bladder helps to evert the fistula edges and improves descent and stability for dissection. Very small fistulas may require gentle dilation using lacrimal duct probes and small dilators to allow insertion of the catheter through the fistula tract (Fig. 28-1). Infiltration of tissues with normal saline or dilute solution of epinephrine (1:200,000) may aid dissection and reduce oozing. There is some concern about increased infection rates after epinephrine use in vaginal surgery, so many surgeons use only saline.

If the fistula encroaches on one or both ureteral orifices, the ureters should be catheterized at the outset of surgery. If identification proves difficult, intravenous indigo carmine with or without furosemide may be helpful.

The classic method of fistula repair involves split-flap dissection, mobilization of tissue planes, absolute hemostasis, and closure without tension (Fig. 28-2). A circumscribing vaginal (usually vertical) incision is made along the long axis of the fistula. The subvaginal plane is dissected in all directions, taking care to avoid excessive

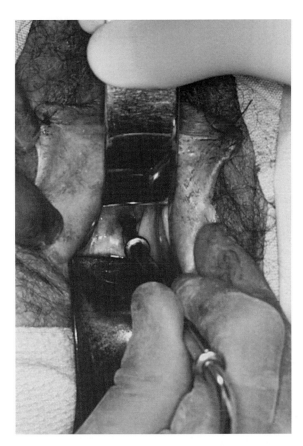

**Fig. 28-1** The vesicovaginal fistula is dilated to allow insertion of a pediatric Foley catheter through the fistula and into the bladder. Use of a catheter helps to evert the fistula edge, thus improving descent and stability for dissection.

dissection, which may result in avascular necrosis. If the fistula tract is small, it can be excised; if large and fibrotic, the edges can be freshened. Overexcision of fistula edges may enlarge the defect excessively and increase the risk of intracystic hemorrhage from bladder edges postoperatively. This can cause catheter blockage, bladder distention, and failure of the repair. If mobilization proves difficult, radial or circumferential vaginal incisions, made at a distance from the fistula, may facilitate mobilization and low-tension closure. Once hemostasis is achieved, these incisions are left open to heal.

Bladder closure in the trigonal area should be in a transverse direction; vertical closure may draw the ureteral orifices toward the midline and cause obstruction. Before closure of large defects, Zacharin (1988) recommends bilateral attachment of healthy bladder wall to the ischiopubic periosteum to stabilize the bladder and thereby protect the repair postoperatively. The bladder is closed using submucosal interrupted Lembert sutures, placed 3 mm apart and at a similar distance from fistula edge. Sutures should be tied gently to approximate the tissue edges without strangulation. Pursestring closure may compromise blood supply

at tissue edges and is not recommended. A second layer of interrupted sutures closes the bladder muscularis and reduces tension on the first layer. The vagina may be closed in one or two layers using interrupted sutures, the outside layer being mattressed.

If the fistula is recurrent or large, resulted from radiotherapy, or involves the bladder neck and urethra, a flap of rectus or gracilis muscle or an omental J-flap may be tunneled subcutaneously and anchored between the bladder and vaginal walls. Alternatively, a graft using the Martius technique can be used. The function of these grafts is to introduce a new blood supply, separate the bladder and vaginal suture lines, provide support, and obliterate dead space. A modified Martius graft technique is shown in Fig. 28-3.

The integrity of the repair may be tested by the instillation of methylene blue or indigo carmine into the bladder, but care must be taken to avoid overdistention. A vaginal pack may be inserted for 24 hours postoperatively, particularly if vaginal relaxing incisions are used. The bladder is drained for 10 to 14 days, depending on the fistula size. If some leakage persists at 14 days, further drainage for 7 more days may occasionally result in fistula closure. Placing the patient in the prone position for 24 to 48 hours after surgery may prevent pressure from the catheter on the suture line before bladder mucosal integrity is restored. Fixation of the transurethral catheter externally is important, especially in suburethral fistulas, to avoid undue tension from the Foley balloon against the bladder neck. Extreme efforts to hydrate the patient are important postoperatively to autoirrigate the bladder, which avoids clot formation, catheter obstruction, bladder distention, and repair disruption. While catheterized, the patient is maintained on prophylactic antibiotics.

The Latzko technique of partial colpocleisis may be used for repair of posthysterectomy vesicovaginal fistulas, with reported cure rates between 93% and 100% for the first attempt (Fig. 28-4). A simple procedure, it has the advantage of short operating time, minimal blood loss, and low postoperative morbidity. Inadequate vaginal length is not a problem unless the vagina is already shortened. The technique is significantly different from the classic method of fistula repair described earlier. In the Latzko operation, the vaginal mucosa is mobilized around the fistula margin in the shape of an ellipse, at least 2.5 cm in all directions, with closure of the subvaginal tissue and vaginal mucosa in layers using No. 2-0 or 3-0 interrupted sutures. The vaginal wall in contact with the bladder reepithelializes with transitional epithelium.

Juxtacervical fistulas may be repaired vaginally if the cervix can be drawn down to provide access; if not, an abdominal approach is warranted. Although rarely necessary, repair may be facilitated by concomitant hysterectomy.

Simple urethrovaginal fistulas may be repaired by a double-breasted closure technique or excision of mucosa,

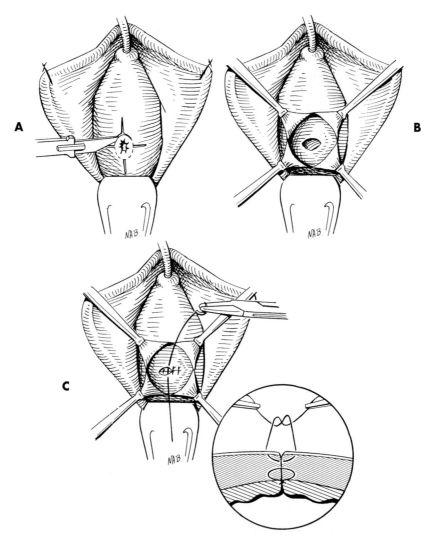

**Fig. 28-2**   Vaginal approach to vesicovaginal fistula repair. **A,** The vaginal epithelium around the fistula is sharply excised. **B,** The vaginal wall is mobilized off the bladder in preparation for layered closure. **C,** The bladder wall is closed transversely in two layers, using interrupted sutures.

with closure of the fistula using No. 3-0 running absorbable suture followed by a Lembert row of sutures. When urethrovaginal fistulas are accompanied by sphincter destruction, achieving postoperative continence remains a considerable challenge. Noble (1901) originally described urethral reconstruction using bilateral vaginal flaps tubularized around a catheter, with labial skin grafts to cover the resultant defects. Moir (1961) used suburethral buttress sutures to improve continence. Symmonds and Hill (1978) achieved continence in 37 of 50 patients with significant urethral destruction by constructing a urethra using contractile tissues that had retracted into the urethral roof and using Martius grafting and retropubic suspension at a later date if necessary. Morgan et al. (1978) reported success in 8 of 9 patients using a combined abdominovaginal approach with urethral reconstruction from residual urethral tissue, Martius

grafting, Marlex suburethral sling, and labial skin flaps. Tubularized anterior bladder flaps also have been used with some success to achieve continence. Tanagho and Smith (1972) have convincingly shown that the concentrically arranged muscle fibers in the bladder directly adjacent to the internal urethral meatus can be used to create a neosphincter. Our choice of repair is wide mobilization of the fistula tract, as in a split-flap technique. The urethra and bladder neck are closed in two or three layers. A Martius graft is brought over the fistula repair, a fascial sling is placed, and the vaginal flaps are then closed.

Use of transurethral versus suprapubic drainage after surgery is controversial, with neither method having proven superiority. We usually place a transurethral Silastic Foley catheter for 14 days. Postoperatively, patients should have strict pelvic rest for 3 months.

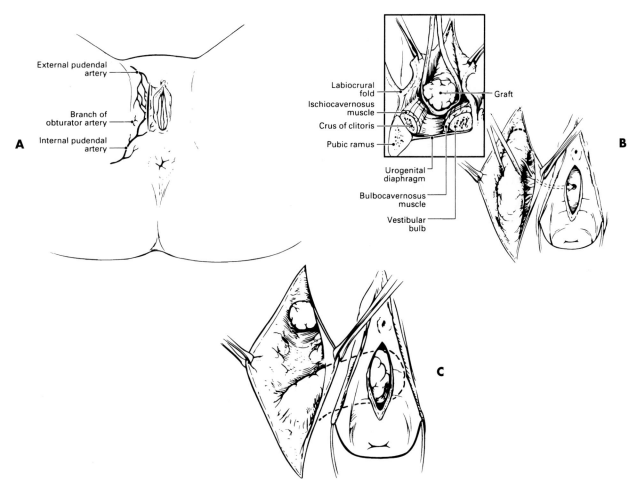

**Fig. 28-3** Technique of modified Martius graft for vesicovaginal fistula repair. **A,** Blood supply of the Martius graft region. **B,** Anatomic structures adjacent to the Martius graft. **C,** Tunneling of the Martius graft into position over the closed fistula.

From Elkins TE, DeLancey JOL, McGuire EJ: *Obstet Gynecol* 75:727, 1990.

## Abdominal Repair of Vesicovaginal Fistulas

The indications for abdominal repair of vesicovaginal fistulas include high inaccessible fistulas, multiple fistulas, involvement of the uterus or bowel, and the need for ureteral reimplantation. A midline abdominal incision facilitates omental grafting when needed. The peritoneal cavity should be opened, both to exclude adherent bowel and omentum and to allow omental grafting. O'Conor (1980) recommends bivalving the bladder. The ureteral orifices and fistula are identified; the fistula is mobilized and closed using peritoneal or preferably omental grafts interposed between the bladder and vaginal suture lines. The omental graft can be mobilized and lengthened by division and ligation of the omental attachments to the hepatic flexure and right half of the transverse colon, preserving enough branches of the gastroepiploic vessels to provide adequate blood supply.

Rarely, a combined abdominovaginal repair is necessary. The procedure is most commonly necessary with high juxtacervical fistulas, in which the distal edge cannot be visualized by the vaginal approach. The omentum can be sufficiently mobilized to allow paraurethral grafting into the vaginal operative field.

## URINARY DIVERSION

Most patients requiring urinary diversion because of genitourinary fistulas have had previous radiation therapy. Bladder capacity is usually severely compromised from fibrosis. Urinary conduits can be constructed from small or large bowel; they may be continent or incontinent. The major continent conduits are the Kock pouch and the Miami pouch. The Kock pouch uses ileum with intussusception techniques, and the Miami pouch uses right hemicolon and a tapered terminal ileum. Both continent conduits have similar continence rates of 93% to 94%. Patients must be able and motivated to catheterize the stoma every 4 to 8

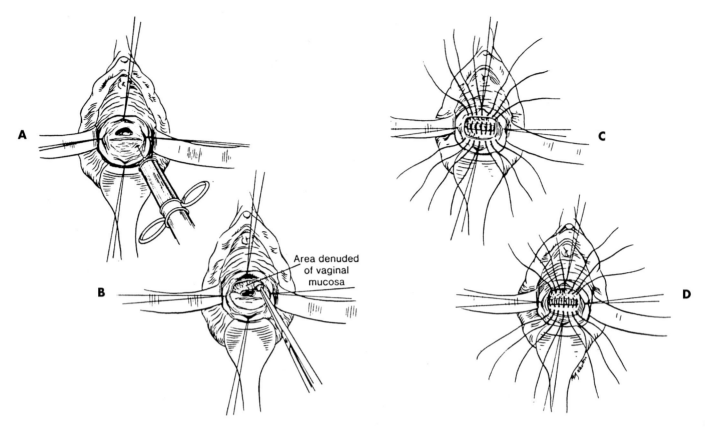

**Fig. 28-4** The Latzko procedure and closure. **A,** The fistulous site after application of four traction sutures, showing typical location of the fistula and injection of a hemostatic solution. **B,** The vaginal mucosa around the fistula is removed. **C,** The submucosa is closed in layers with interrupted sutures. **D,** The vaginal wall is similarly closed.

From Robertson JR: Vesicovaginal fistula: vaginal repair. In Ostergard DR, Bent AE, eds: *Urogynecology and urodynamics,* ed 4, Baltimore, 1996, Williams & Wilkins.

hours. Complications include stone formation, conduit leak and reflux, and metabolic disturbances. Early and late complications in continent diversions occur in 13% to 15%; reoperation is necessary in 1% to 4%.

## COMPLICATIONS

The surgical repair of genitourinary fistulas may be complicated by risks common to all surgeries, such as hemorrhage, infection, and thromboembolism. If tissue breakdown occurs at the vaginal or bladder suture lines, the fistula may persist or recur. Other delayed surgical complications include vaginal stenosis and small-bladder syndrome, osteitis pubis, and urinary incontinence (stress and urge). Dyspareunia caused by tenderness over the site of Martius grafts has been reported. Metabolic disturbances and recurrent pyelonephritis may develop after ureterosigmoidostomy. After successful fistula repair, elective cesarean delivery is strongly recommended for all subsequent births.

## PREVENTION

Every year 500,000 women die in developing countries from complications of pregnancy. For every mother who dies, 10 to 15 are permanently injured, many as a result of vesicovaginal fistula (World Health Organization, 1987). Epidemiologic research is urgently needed to identify communities with a high prevalence of fistulas and to determine the characteristics of women at high risk for bladder or urethral injury during childbirth. Preventive strategies must be directed at several levels to achieve meaningful reduction in the occurrence of genitourinary fistulas caused by neglected obstructed labor. Economic gains will lead to improved nutritional status and decreased prevalence of pelvic contracture. Sociocultural changes are necessary to delay childbearing until pelvic maturity. Increased availability of prenatal care and establishment of maternity waiting homes would improve care during pregnancy and identify conditions such as abnormal fetal presentation before labor. Trained birth attendants could perform bladder drainage in labor and identify abnormal labor patterns using partographs. Emergency transport for women in prolonged labor to centers staffed by skilled personnel could enable abdominal delivery when vaginal delivery is impossible. Until all these goals and more can be realized, genitourinary fistulas will continue to occur and women will need advanced care for surgical management. Generalists should be trained to repair simple fistulas, with referral of complex cases to specialized fistula hospitals.

In developed countries, the majority of vesicovaginal fistulas could be prevented by careful dissection of the bladder from the uterus and cervix at the time of hysterectomy, careful placement of sutures and clamps during vaginal cuff closure, and the intraoperative recognition and repair of bladder trauma. Studies by Pettit and Petrou (1994) and Wiskind and Thompson (1995) have shown a significant prevalence of unsuspected ureteral injuries (0.1% to 2%) and advocate routine cystoscopy at all pelvic operations. This would allow immediate diagnosis and appropriate management of bladder and ureteral injury, thus preventing sequelae such as fistula formation.

Careful dosage calculation, administration, source insertion, and shielding, together with appropriate bladder drainage, can reduce the risk of radiation-induced lower urinary tract fistulas. This complication may nonetheless arise many years after a symptom-free interval and may not be completely preventable.

## BIBLIOGRAPHY
### Historical Perspectives

Collis MH: Further remarks upon a new and successful mode of treatment for vesicovaginal fistula, *Dublin Q J Med Sci* 31:302, 1861.

Derry DE: Note on five pelves of women in the eleventh dynasty in Egypt, *J Obstet Gynaecol Br Emp* 42:490, 1935.

DiMarchettis P: *Observationum medico-chirurgacarum rariorum sylloge,* Patave, 1675.

Emmet TA: *Vesico-vaginal fistula from parturition and other causes with cases of recto-vaginal fistula,* New York, 1868, William Wood.

Falk HC: *Urological injuries in gynecology,* ed 2, Philadelphia, 1964, FA Davis.

Fatio J: *Helvetisch-vernunstige Wehemutter,* Basel, 1752.

Garlock JH: The cure of an intractable vesicovaginal fistula by the use of pedicled muscle graft, *Surg Gynecol Obstet* 47:255, 1928.

Ingelman-Sundberg A: Pathogenesis and operative treatment of urinary fistula in irradiated tissue. In Youssef AF, ed: *Gynecological urology,* Springfield, 1960, Charles C Thomas.

Jobert de Lamballe A-J: *Traite des fistules vesico-uterines,* Paris, 1852, Balliere et Fils.

Kelly HA: The treatment of vesico-vaginal and recto-vaginal fistulae high up in the vagina, *Johns Hopkins Hosp Bull* 13:73, 1902.

Kiricuta I, Goldstein AM: The repair of extensive vesicovaginal fistulas with pedicled omentum: a review of 27 cases, *J Urol* 108:724, 1972.

Latzko W: Postoperative vesicovaginal fistulae: genesis and theory, *Am J Surg* 58:211, 1942.

Mackenrodt A: Die operative Heilung grosser Blasenscheidenfisteln, *Zentralbl Gynakol* 8:180, 1894.

Martius H: Die operative Wiederher-stellung der Volkommen fehlenden Harnrohre und des Schliessmuskels derselben, *Zentralbl Gynakol* 8:480, 1928.

Martius H: Zur Auswahl der harnfistel-und inkontinenz Operation, *Zentralbl Gynakol* 32:1250, 1942.

Mettauer JP: Vesico-vaginal fistula, *Boston Med Surg J* 22:154, 1840.

Moir JC: *The vesico-vaginal fistula,* London, 1961, Balliere Tindall.

Noble CP: The new formation of the female urethra with report of a case, *Am J Obstet Gynecol* 43:170, 1901.

Schuchardt K: Eine neue Methode der Gebarmutterexstirpation, *Zentralbl Chir* 20:1121, 1893.

Sims JM: On the treatment of vesico-vaginal fistula, *Am J Med Sci* 23:59, 1852.

Ward A: *Vesicovaginal fistulas: a report of 1789 cases.* Paper presented to the meeting of the Federation of International Gynaecology and Obstetrics World Congress, San Francisco, 1980.

### Epidemiology and Etiology

Cohen IK, Diegelmann R, Couss M: Wound care and wound healing. In Schwartz S, Shiver GT, Spencer F, eds: *Principles of surgery,* New York, 1994, McGraw-Hill.

Freda VC, Tacchi D: Ureteral injury discovered after pelvic surgery, *Am J Obstet Gynecol* 83:406, 1962.

Gerber GS, Schoenberg HW: Female urinary tract fistulas, *J Urol* 149:229, 1993.

Lawson J: Tropical obstetrics and gynaecology III. Vesico-vaginal fistula: a tropical disease, *Trans R Soc Trop Med Hyg* 83:454, 1989.

Lee RA, Symmonds RE, Williams TJ: Current status of genitourinary fistula, *Obstet Gynecol* 72:313, 1988.

Meeks GR, Sams JO, Field KW, et al: Formation of vesicovaginal fistula: the role of suture placement into the bladder during closure of the vaginal cuff after transabdominal hysterectomy, *Am J Obstet Gynecol* 177:1298, 1997.

Miklos JR, Sze E, Parobeck D, et al: Vesicouterine fistula: a rare complication of vaginal birth after cesarean, *Obstet Gynecol* 86:638, 1995.

Nnabugwu-Otensanya BE: *Social consequences of vesico-vaginal fistulae: Zaria experiences,* Society of Obstetrics and Gynecology of Nigeria Conference, Calabar, September 5-8, 1989.

Saltutti C, Di Cello V, Costanzi A, et al: Ureterouterine fistula as a complication of Cesarean section, *J Urol* 152:1199, 1994.

Solomons E, Levin EJ, Bauman JS, et al: A pyelographic study of ureteric injuries sustained during hysterectomy for benign conditions, *Surg Gynecol Obstet* 111:41, 1960.

Symmonds RE: Incontinence: vesical and urethral fistulas, *Clin Obstet Gynecol* 27:499, 1984.

### Classification

Elkins TE, Mahama E, O'Donnell P, et al: Recognition and management of patients with high-risk vesicovaginal fistulas: implications for teaching and research, *Int J Urogynecol* 5:183, 1994.

Hamlin RH, Nicholson EC: Reconstruction of urethra totally destroyed in labour, *BMJ* 1:147, 1969.

Lawson JB: Tropical gynaecology. Birth-canal injuries, *Proc R Soc Med* 61:368, 1968.

Mahfouz NB: Urinary and faecal fistulae, *J Obstet Gynaecol Br Emp* 45:405, 1938.

### Presentation, Investigation, and Preoperative Preparation

Collins CG, Pent D, Jones FB: Results of early repair of vesicovaginal fistula with preliminary cortisone treatment, *Am J Obstet Gynecol* 80:1005, 1960.

deBaere T, Roche A, Lagrange C: Combined percutaneous antegrade and cystoscopic retrograde approach in the treatment of distal ureteral fistulae, *Cardiovasc Intervent Radiol* 18:349, 1995.

Falk HC: *Urological injuries in gynecology,* Philadelphia, 1984, FA Davis.

Falk HC, Orkin LA: Nonsurgical closure of vesicovaginal fistulas, *Obstet Gynecol* 9:538, 1957.

Fearl CL, Keizur LW: Optimum time interval from occurrence to repair of vesicovaginal fistula, *Am J Obstet Gynecol* 104:205, 1969.

Herbert DB, Vaughn ED: Vesicovaginal fistula: a therapeutic challenge, *Infect Surg* February:130, 1985.

O'Conor VJ: Review of experience with vesico-vaginal fistula repair, *J Urol* 123:367, 1980.

Persky L, Herman G, Guerrier K: Nondelay in vesicovaginal fistula repair, *Urology* 13:273, 1979.

Selzman AA, Spirnak JP, Kursh ED: The changing management of ureterovaginal fistulas, *J Urol* 153:626, 1995.

Taylor JS, Hewson AD, Rachow P, et al: Synchronous combined transvaginal-transvesical repair of vesicovaginal fistulas, *Aust NZ J Surg* 50:23, 1980.

Thompson JD: Operative injuries to the ureter: prevention, recognition and management. In Rock JA, Thompson JD, eds: *TeLinde's operative gynecology,* Philadelphia, 1997, JB Lippincott.

## Surgical Repair

Bissada NK, McDonald D: Management of giant vesicovaginal and vesicourethrovaginal fistulas, *J Urol* 130:1073, 1983.

Elkins TE: Surgery for the obstetric vesicovaginal fistula: a review of 100 operations in 82 patients, *Am J Obstet Gynecol* 170:1108, 1994.

Elkins TE, DeLancey JOL, McGuire EJ: The use of modified Martius graft as an adjunctive technique in vesicovaginal and rectovaginal fistula repair, *Obstet Gynecol* 75:727, 1990.

Elkins TE, Drescher C, Martey JO, et al: Vesicovaginal fistula revisited, *Obstet Gynecol* 72:307, 1988.

Elkins TE, Ghosh TS, Tagoe GA, et al: Transvaginal mobilization and utilization of the anterior bladder wall to repair vesicovaginal fistulas involving the urethra, *Obstet Gynecol* 79:455, 1992.

Falk HC, Bunkin IA: The management of vesico-vaginal fistula following abdominal total hysterectomy, *Surg Gynecol Obstet* 93:404, 1951.

Hanash KA, Sieck U: Successful repair of a large vesicovaginal fistula with associated urethral loss using the anterior bladder flap technique, *J Urol* 130:775, 1983.

Lawson JB: Vesical fistulae into the vaginal vault, *Br J Urol* 44:623, 1972.

Margolis T, Elkins TE, Seffah J, et al: Full-thickness Martius grafts to preserve vaginal depth as an adjunct in the repair of large obstetric fistulas, *Obstet Gynecol* 84:148, 1994.

Miller NF: The surgical treatment and postoperative care of vesicovaginal fistula, *Am J Obstet Gynecol* 44:873, 1942.

Morgan JE, Farrow GA, Sims RH: The sloughed urethra syndrome, *Am J Obstet Gynecol* 130:521, 1978.

Nichols DH, Randall CL: *Vaginal surgery,* ed 3, Baltimore, 1989, Williams & Wilkins.

O'Conor VJ: Repair of vesicovaginal fistula with associated urethral loss, *Surg Gynecol Obstet* 146:251, 1978.

Robertson JR: Vesicovaginal fistulas. In Slate WG, ed: *Disorders of the female urethra and urinary incontinence,* Baltimore, 1982, Williams & Wilkins.

Robertson JR: Vesicovaginal fistula: vaginal repair. In Ostergard DR, Bent AE, eds: *Urogynecology and urodynamics,* ed 4, Baltimore, 1996, Williams & Wilkins.

Symmonds RE, Hill LM: Loss of the urethra: a report on 50 patients, *Am J Obstet Gynecol* 130:130, 1978.

Tanagho EA, Smith DR: Clinical evaluation of a surgical technique for the correction of complete urinary incontinence, *J Urol* 107:402, 1972.

Zacharin RF: *Obstetric fistula,* New York, 1988, Springer Verlag Wien.

Zoubek J, McGuire EJ, Noll F, et al: The late occurrence of urinary tract damage in patients successfully treated by radiotherapy for cervical carcinoma, *J Urol* 141:1347, 1989.

## Prevention

American College of Obstetricians and Gynecologists: *Genitourinary fistulas,* ACOG Technical Bulletin No. 53, Jan 1985.

Pettit PD, Petrou SP: The value of cystoscopy in major vaginal surgery, *Obstet Gynecol* 84:318, 1994.

Thornton JG: Should vesicovaginal fistula be treated only by specialists? *Trop Doct* 16:78, 1986.

Wiskind AK, Thompson JD: Should cystoscopy be performed at every gynecologic operation to diagnose unsuspected ureteral injury? *J Pelvic Surg* 1:134, 1995.

World Health Organization: *Call to Action: Safe Motherhood Conference,* Nairobi, Feb 10-13, 1987.

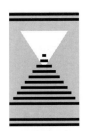

CHAPTER **29**

# *Suburethral Diverticula*

Laszlo Sogor

The female urethra is a 4-cm-long, narrow, membranous canal that extends from the bladder to the external orifice on the vulvar vestibule. Dysfunction of this tube leads to major disability, as has been recognized since ancient times. Obstruction of the urethra is life-threatening. Incontinence produces psychologic, emotional, and social consequences.

This chapter describes diseases of the urethra. It traces the history from antiquity to the present and offers insight into etiology. After the classic diagnostic methods are reviewed, newer diagnostic modalities are presented. Three effective methods of surgical repair are described.

## HISTORICAL PERSPECTIVES ON DISEASES OF THE URETHRA

The first recorded evidence of interest in and treatment of the urethra is in the *Ayuveda of Sucrutu,* a Hindu treatise written around 500 BC. The Hindus at this time were treating strictures of the urethra by graduated dilators made of wood or metal, as well as treating other diseases of the urethra by injections. Hippocrates, in 400 BC, was the first to write about urethral abscesses. Cornelius Celcus at the beginning of the first century was the next to write definitively of urethral conditions.

Aside from the mention of urethral strictures and abscesses in the ancient literature, the first specific mention of urethral pathology in Western literature occurred in Ambrose Pare's collected works (1575), wherein he wrote about the "skinny caruncles of women's privies." This condition also was observed by Morgagni during postmortem examination in a young girl. He described "from the orifice of the urethra a small reddish body was vominant and this one cut into longitudinally I perceived to be nothing else, but the internal code at that meatus." In 1750, Samuel Sharp noted "the excruciating torment and violent disorders caused by caruncles and I excised one with complete relief of symptoms."

The first description of an operation to treat diverticula in the English literature was published in 1786 (Hey, 1805). In this report, a vaginal incision was made into the diverticulum cavity. The cavity was packed with lint, resulting in a cure. A century later, Cullen (1894) reviewed the literature of the time and presented his first case (from Prof. H. Kelly's service at Johns Hopkins Hospital). Thirty-eight cases were summarized and possible causes of the various types of suburethral sacs were discussed. During the intervening years, many different terms were used to describe what we now consider suburethral diverticulum. These included urethrocele, urethral diverticulum, suburethral abscess, suburethral diverticulum, and urethrovaginal urinary pocket.

## PERTINENT ANATOMY

The urethra is dorsal to the symphysis pubis and is embedded in the anterior wall of the vagina. The diameter, when undilated, averages 6 mm. It perforates through the perineal membrane, with its external orifice directly above the vaginal opening. The lining membrane has longitudinal folds and many small urethral glands that open into the urethra throughout its entire length. The largest of these are the periurethral glands of Skene. Skene's ducts open just within the urethral orifice, although the exact anatomic location varies. The mucous coat is continuous externally with that of the vulva and internally with that of the bladder. It is primarily a stratified squamous epithelium, which becomes transitional near the bladder.

# PATHOPHYSIOLOGIC CONSIDERATIONS
## Definition

For practical considerations, a suburethral diverticulum is any fluid-filled mass along the anterolateral portions of the vagina that can be shown to have direct communication with the urethra.

## Etiology
### Congenital Causes

Suburethral diverticula have been diagnosed in female patients from age 5 through menopause. This fact, and case descriptions of male newborns with diverticula, makes a compelling case for congenital origin. Further support stems from histologic studies of dissected diverticular walls wherein mucosa, submucosa, and a muscular coat can be found.

The specific congenital origin cannot be ascertained; however, several known structures may be involved, including remnants of Gartner's or wolffian duct cysts that rupture into the urethra. In addition, a faulty union of the longitudinal folds of the urethra may lead to suburethral diverticular cysts. Other theories have implicated cell rests that become cystic and ultimately perforate into the urethra.

Despite these theories, one must be careful in assigning congenital cause based simply on histology because a suburethral abscess that becomes sterile can become entirely reepithelialized from the urethra. If the patient is evaluated late in the course of events, a congenital cause might be assigned although the condition was acquired.

### Acquired Causes

In this category, birth trauma, infection, instrumentation, and urethral stones are of primary consideration. Many patients with diverticula give a history of prolonged, difficult labor. The presumption is that the inferior wall of the urethra is damaged by the descending fetal head. The mechanism of damage may be related to necrosis and obstruction of Skene's duct. Some authors of older gynecologic texts, including TeLinde (1953), mention infection as the primary cause of suburethral diverticula. The most notable organism mentioned is gonococcus. The mechanism is identical to that seen with Bartholin's abscess (i.e., infection with subsequent suppuration of the periurethral and paraurethral glands). Because of the delicate nature of the urethral folds, any instrumentation can tear through the epithelium and create false channels and pockets, which, over time, may become reepithelialized and filled with fluid, thus meeting criteria for suburethral diverticulum. Numerous reports in the literature note the presence of stones in suburethral diverticula. One thought is that the passage of stones through the urethra can lead to an erosion through the mucosal wall, with incomplete reepithelialization of the erosion. A suburethral diverticulum with a stone could form. Alternatively, the presence of a stone in a diverticulum may simply be a precipitate that forms after the diverticulum has formed from other causes.

## Summary

Skene (1880) described two large ducts lying on each side of the urethra and related them to clinical problems. Although these structures were described as early as 1672 by deGraaf, our anatomic understanding of them and their potential role in diseases of the urethra became evident only after Huffman (1943) performed detailed studies of the development of periurethral glands in the human female. In his initial studies, Huffman (1943, 1948) performed wax model reconstructions of portions of the urethra and the uterovaginal anlage in fetuses from 50 to 224 mm and in six women. From these studies, the anlagen of periurethral glands were observed for the first time in a 50-mm fetus. These small buds arise from the ventral and lateral surfaces of the urethra above the müllerian tubercle. In adult urethras, the orifices of all paraurethral and periurethral glands arise from the urethral mucosa itself. No glandular structures were observed arising from the urogenital sinus in the vaginal epithelium or the vestibule. From the histologic appearance of these glands, one can conclude that they are homologues to the portion of the male prostate that develops cranial to the mesonephric duct/urogenital sinus union.

Huffman (1951) continued his work using wax models of the duct systems surrounding the urethra (Fig. 29-1). From this work we conclude that the distinction between paraurethral and periurethral glands is meaningless.

Everett (1944) pointed out the importance of gonococci in infections of the periurethral ducts and glands. Periurethral ducts and glands may play an important role in many cases of urethritis by acting as a nidus for chronic infections of the female urethra and vagina. Organisms involved include gonococci, *Chlamydia trachomatis,* and *Trichomonas vaginalis.* The latter organism can use the urethral glands as a source for recurrent vaginal infections. Other opportunistic organisms can also be involved. Whenever these glands become obstructed, small abscesses can form from which putrid material can be expressed through the urethra. These abscesses then point into the urethra and rupture into it, thereby forming a suburethral diverticulum. Therefore, the majority of cases of suburethral diverticula probably arise from infections.

Primary cysts of the periurethral duct system do occur. They are seen in histologic preparations but usually are microscopic. If these cysts do enlarge, they generally produce small, fluctuant tumors of the anterior vaginal wall, generally no larger than 2 or 3 cm. They usually are asymptomatic and not appreciated on physical examination. Rarely, they may cause dyspareunia. Anterior and anterolateral wall cysts must be differentiated from cysts of mesonephric or paramesonephric origin.

Netter (1974), presumably using the work of Huffman (1948) and Krantz (1951), made color drawings of his conceptualization of periurethral and paraurethral gland structures. He noted that the majority of the glands tend to form an interdependent conducting system terminating in the large Skene's duct, which opens on either side of the

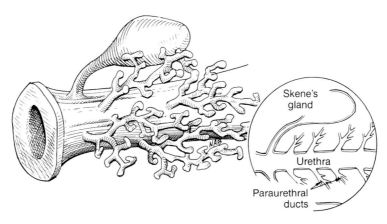

**Fig. 29-1**  Schematic diagram of the paraurethral glands and Skene's gland (after Huffman, 1951).

midline just dorsal to the urethral meatus. He believed that these are remnant structures that serve no specific purpose. Netter also pointed out that their position predisposes them to infection, especially by gonococci. Their poor drainage fosters the tendency of such infections to become chronic.

Our model for cyst or abscess formation is shown in Fig. 29-2.

## INCIDENCE

Wharton and Kearns (1950) discussed 30 cases of urethral diverticula in women at the Johns Hopkins Hospital between 1890 and 1949. The incidence of this condition was 1 in 2300 gynecologic admissions. The majority of these diverticula were reported between 1939 and 1949. Johnson (1938) reported no observations of a suburethral diverticulum in 140,000 admissions over a period of 10 years. After the lesion was called to the attention of the staff, nine proven cases were found in the following year. MacKinnon et al. (1959) reported 204 cases of suburethral diverticula between 1935 and 1955. Interestingly, they lamented that the standard urologic text failed to list suburethral diverticulum as a condition found in female patients. Furthermore, they noted that many teaching programs in urology and gynecology overlooked this subject. No incidence figures were given in this publication. Davis and TeLinde (1958) reported an 8% rate. Bruning (1959) found 3 diverticula in 500 autopsy specimens (0.6% incidence). In response to this study, Anderson (1967) evaluated patients in Aarhus, Denmark, using injection urethrography. He reported a 3% incidence of suburethral diverticula. Despite the approximate incidence of at least 3%, several modern gynecologic textbooks do not mention this entity.

A recent study from the University of Copenhagen (Jensen et al., 1996) reports only 15 women referred during a 9-year period. In our practice we also have seen a progressive decline in the prevalence of this condition. This may be related to earlier diagnosis and treatment of sexually transmitted diseases.

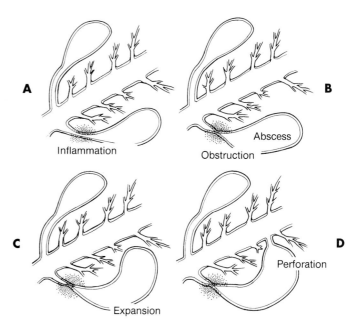

**Fig. 29-2**  Hypothetical mechanism of acquired suburethral diverticulum. **A,** An initial inflammatory response occurs in Skene's duct or one of the paraurethral ducts. **B,** An abscess forms within the gland or duct, leading to obstruction of the gland neck. **C,** Expansion of the abscess. **D,** Perforation of the abscess into the urethra, leading to diverticulum formation.

## CLINICAL DIAGNOSIS

Patients with suburethral diverticula can be asymptomatic or can have symptoms of chronic recurring cystitis with pain, burning, frequency, and dyspareunia. The main feature of these episodes is refractoriness to medical treatment. In addition, a significant percentage of patients complain of difficulty voiding, postvoid dribbling, urinary incontinence, or gross hematuria. Some patients notice a protruding tender vaginal mass. Rarely, obstruction of the urethra can ensue. Interestingly, the duration of symptoms is often quite long. Table 29-1 summarizes the clinical manifestations in several of the larger published series.

**Table 29-1** Frequency of Symptoms in Women With Urethral Diverticula

| Symptom | Wharton and Kearns (1950) | MacKinnon et al. (1959) | Hoffman and Adams (1965) | Davis and Robinson (1970) |
| --- | --- | --- | --- | --- |
| Frequency | 63% | 66% | — | 70% |
| Burning | 63% | 79% | 35% | 35% |
| Pain | 40% | 29% | 30% | 36% |
| Incontinence | 30% | 25% | 42% | 49% |
| Dyspareunia | 13% | 14% | 12% | 14% |
| Retention | 6% | — | — | 3% |
| Difficulty voiding | 20% | 32% | — | — |
| Hematuria | — | 17% | 11% | 20% |
| Vaginal mass | — | 12% | 27% | — |

The most commonly described signs of suburethral diverticula are the presence of an anterior vaginal mass and the ability to express pus or urine from the mass via the urethral orifice. Using these signs, Davis and TeLinde (1958) diagnosed diverticula correctly in 63% of their cases. Ancillary techniques were required for diagnosis because of failure to express fluid in the remainder of cases with an anterior vaginal mass.

## DIAGNOSTIC TECHNIQUES
### Radiography

The objective of all diagnostic methods is to demonstrate a urethral communication to a diverticular sac. Thomas (1930) described a technique for female urethrography using retrograde injection of iodized oil into the urethra. He used a simple syringe inserted into the urethral meatus. A variation on this technique was discussed by Taylor (1950), who used a Foley catheter with a distal silk ligature to tamponade the vesicourethral sphincter and prevent reflux. Other authors catheterized the diverticular orifice with ureteral catheters during urethroscopy and installed radiopaque media. This procedure was difficult and often unsuccessful and led to failure of diagnosis in up to one third of the cases.

Davis and Cian (1956) reported a new technique—positive-pressure urethrography—for the diagnosis of urethral diverticula, for which they constructed a special catheter. This system is similar to the one devised by Taylor (1950) to prevent bladder reflux; however, a sliding balloon was added to maintain the catheter in position and to tamponade the external meatus. In this fashion, the urethra became a closed tube, which could be injected with contrast medium under moderate pressure, permitting visualization of diverticula even with minute sinus tracks (Fig. 29-3). They reported four cases using this system and recommended that a urethrogram be obtained in any case of chronic urinary tract infection or suspected diverticulum. They noted that several diverticula may be present concurrently, and that some diverticula may have more than one urethral orifice.

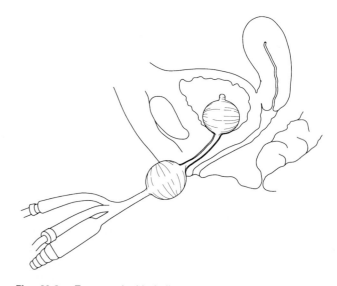

**Fig. 29-3** Trattner double-balloon catheter. Proximal balloon inflates within bladder neck, anchoring catheter, and distal balloon occludes external meatus. Contrast fills urethra through slit between balloons.

From Greenberg M, Stone D, Cochran ST, et al: *AJR* 136:259, 1981.

Voiding cystourethrograms done under cinefluoroscopy have improved the diagnostic yield by 40%. No comparative studies between cinefluoroscopy and positive-pressure urethrography are available.

### Endoscopy

Cystourethroscopy is the time-honored method of diagnosis for suburethral diverticula. Most urogynecologic articles recommend this diagnostic modality. However, Hoffman and Adams (1965) specifically note that endoscopic diagnosis has not been a routine part of their evaluation because many times the diverticular opening into the urethra is too small to be seen endoscopically. Cystourethroscopy alone is inadequate to establish the diagnosis because of the 30% to 40% false negative rate.

Recently we have used indigo carmine dye injection to increase the diagnostic accuracy of endoscopy. In this technique, a 25- to 27-gauge needle is used to inject the suspected suburethral diverticulum transvaginally with indigo carmine dye while observing the urethra endoscopically. Although this may improve diagnosis, a radiographic procedure is still recommended in all suspected cases.

## Sonography

With the advent of vaginal probe sonography, the evaluation of vaginal masses has become feasible. We have used vaginal ultrasound to evaluate cases of proven suburethral diverticula. Although ultrasound evaluates these cystic lesions satisfactorily, especially when they are distended, it cannot prove that they are true suburethral diverticula because of inadequate visualization of the connection into the urethra.

Martensson and Ducheck (1994) reported on the use of translabial sonography as an improved diagnostic modality. With this technique they were able to visualize the entire urethra and diverticula satisfactorily in five patients. In addition, the use of color doppler enabled the evaluation of blood vessels within the diverticulum, which might improve the diagnosis of associated malignant tumors. Chancellor et al. (1995) described an intraoperative endoluminal ultrasound to aid the surgeon during diverticulectomy and described the use of this technique in seven women. Comparison of this newer technique to traditional techniques indicated two false negative and one false positive voiding cystourethrograms, one false negative transvaginal ultrasound, and one false negative double-balloon urethrogram. The endoluminal ultrasound was felt to provide excellent visualization of all the diverticula. This could enhance the accuracy of surgical repair and help to prevent inadvertent urethral and bladder neck injuries.

## Magnetic Resonance Imaging

Kim et al. (1993) reported the utility of magnetic resonance technology in 20 women undergoing surgery for suburethral diverticula. Magnetic resonance imaging depicted 14 of the 20 cases of diverticula, although the ostia of the diverticula could not be identified in any of the images. Concomitant urethrography and urethroscopy depicted only 11 of the 20 cases.

## Urethral Pressure Profilometry

Suburethral diverticula can sometimes show a dip in urethral pressure on urethral pressure profile. This finding can be used to localize suburethral diverticular openings in relation to the area of maximal urethral closure pressure (MUCP). If the openings are distal to the MUCP, then diverticulectomy or marsupialization can be used for treatment with little risk of damage to the continence mechanism. If the openings are proximal to or at the MUCP, then diverticulectomy or partial ablation should be used, with the attendant risk of urinary incontinence in cases complicated by noncure or fistula formation. Unfortunately,

the biphasic pattern often is not observed in patients with proven diverticula.

## Summary

We perform positive-pressure urethrography or voiding cystourethrography after physical examination raises suspicion for suburethral diverticulum. In this manner, adequate evaluation of the size and complexity of the diverticular sacs and the location of all orifices can be gleaned. We do not believe that cystourethroscopy offers additional benefits before surgical resection. It is important to recognize that all modalities have both false positive and false negative rates. Clearly, any symptomatic suburethral mass should be explored surgically. Endoluminal sonography may be of value intraoperatively in complex cases. The clinician should be aware that both historical and recent accounts indicate that carcinoma can arise in Skene's gland and be mistaken for simple diverticula.

## SURGICAL TREATMENT
### Historical Review

We do not know how the barbers of Europe approached acute suburethral diverticulum, but we suspect that they practiced simple incision and drainage. As discussed previously, Hey (1805) opened the sac per vaginum and then packed the diverticulum. It is fascinating that two papers in *Urologic and Cutaneous Reviews* in 1937 and 1938 came to opposite conclusions about the preferred method of surgical treatment. Young and McCrea (1937) concluded that simple vaginal incision of the pouch usually results in complete recovery in 2 to 4 weeks. Hunner (1938) recommended a diverticulectomy. He initiated the procedure by removing an oval piece of redundant vaginal mucosa overlying the diverticulum, followed by resection of the diverticulum.

Hunner later modified his operation to involve a simple midline incision with subsequent resection of the right vaginal margin. A de facto vaginal flap then was created from the left to the right to prevent the final row of sutures from overlapping the first two lines of closure. A pursestring suture was used to close the fistulous opening in the urethral mucosa. Interrupted sutures brought the paraurethral fascial tissue together. The vagina was closed with silver wire. The bladder was catheterized and the vagina was packed with gauze.

Hoffman and Adams (1965) identified several important principles for successful suburethral diverticular repair. These included complete removal of the sac and identification and closure of all openings into the urethra. They made a longitudinal incision over the diverticulum with dissection of the sac, subsequent entry into the sac, excision, and layer closure. In their series of 60 patients, 55 achieved excellent results. Stress incontinence developed in three patients because the diverticula were located close to the bladder neck. Anterior colporrhaphy cured two of these patients.

O'Connor (1969) stressed several factors in repair of the diverticulum. Most notable was that the urethra is not readily separable from the anterior vaginal wall, so there is no anatomic plane of cleavage.

Davis and Robinson (1970) reported on 120 cases of urethral diverticulum. The majority (98) were treated by transvaginal diverticulectomy encompassing removal of the sacs with layer closure of the urethra and vagina. They reported no cases of vesicovaginal fistula, one recurrent diverticulum, and four patients with urethrovaginal fistula. Urethral strictures were not classified as a complication of the procedure because many of their patients had preoperative strictures related to the diverticulum or repair.

Spence and Duckett (1970) presented their observations on suburethral diverticula, initially stressing complete excision of the diverticulum. They pointed out the importance of the division of the communication between the diverticulum and the urethra and the reconstruction of the urethra in layers overlying a urethral catheter. They also emphasized the value of using methylene blue dye to distend the diverticular cavity before the surgical procedure.

Spence and Duckett (1970) described an alternative surgical procedure that became known as the Spence procedure. Basically, this procedure is a marsupialization procedure applicable only to distal diverticula. These authors reported resolution of the diverticula in all patients and no postoperative incontinence in seven of their nine patients. This procedure is one of the most common repair operations for distal diverticula because of its ease and success.

An interesting approach was presented by Sholem et al. (1974), who made a semilunar incision beneath the urethral orifice, dissected underneath the vaginal mucosa to the diverticulum, and excised it. This technique avoids an extensive vaginal incision and its attendant difficulties. The vaginal epithelium remains intact over the area of excision. These authors reported successful use of the method in 17 patients. They noted no difficulty in establishing an appropriate plane between the vagina and diverticulum. Although this procedure is an interesting variation on excision of the sac, it is difficult in practice, especially for proximal diverticula.

Proximal diverticula have a higher risk of bladder entry and its attendant propensity for vesicovaginal fistula formation and bladder neck damage, potentially resulting in stress incontinence. Because of these difficulties, Tancer et al. (1983) reported a partial ablation technique for these difficult diverticula. In this procedure, the diverticular sac is dissected out vaginally, incised longitudinally, and entered. The main body of the diverticulum is excised, but no effort is made to enucleate the sac at its neck. The opening is closed side to side using No. 3-0 suture. A second layer of sutures is placed, which imbricates the urethral incision. The periurethral fascia is then closed in a double-breasted fashion to bolster the previous closure and to obliterate the original cavity. Tancer et al. performed this operation on 34 women over a 10-year period and reported no cases of urinary incontinence or fistula formation. This procedure has become popular for proximal diverticula because of its high success rate and low frequency of urinary incontinence.

## Surgical Techniques

Because multiple operations are available to correct suburethral diverticula, the operation must be adjusted for the patient. Our primary operation is a diverticulectomy (Fig. 29-4). We use an inverted U-flap for the vaginal epithelium and a "vest-over-pants" closure of the periurethral fascia to avoid overlapping sutures and thereby reduce the incidence of urethrovaginal fistulas.

If the diverticulum is located in the proximal urethra near the bladder neck, we prefer to perform a partial ablation technique, as described by Tancer et al. (1983), to lower the risk of damage to the bladder neck and urethral sphincteric continence mechanism.

The Spence operation is indicated for diverticula in the distal urethra, distal to the area of maximal urethral closure pressure. This operation is very straightforward, but patients should be selected carefully to avoid the risk of postoperative incontinence.

The following are step-by-step descriptions of the three main operations for suburethral diverticula.

### Diverticulectomy

1. After regional or general anesthesia, the patient is placed in lithotomy position. One to three doses of prophylactic antibiotics generally are used. Urethroscopy is performed before the surgery to localize the diverticular opening(s) into the urethra and ensure that there are no other unsuspected findings.
2. A double-balloon catheter is placed into the urethra; the balloons are set at the proximal and distal urethra and inflated. Sterile milk or methylene blue dye is injected into the catheter to inflate the urethra and diverticulum. This catheter is kept in place until the sac is entered so that it can be inflated periodically during dissection. It is also necessary to ensure that the urethra and diverticular sac have not been entered inadvertently.
3. Hemostatic solution can be injected submucosally. An inverted U-shaped incision is made over the diverticulum through the vaginal epithelium, which is then dissected off the urethra and periurethral tissue (Fig. 29-4, A).
4. A longitudinal incision is made carefully over the diverticular sac. The fascial tissue overlying and surrounding the diverticulum is completely dissected and mobilized (Fig. 29-4, B and C).
5. Dissection is continued around the sac until the neck is visualized. If the entire neck of the diverticulum is isolated, the diverticulum is excised from the urethra (Fig. 29-4, D). If the entire sac cannot be mobilized, then the sac should be opened longitudinally and the inside of

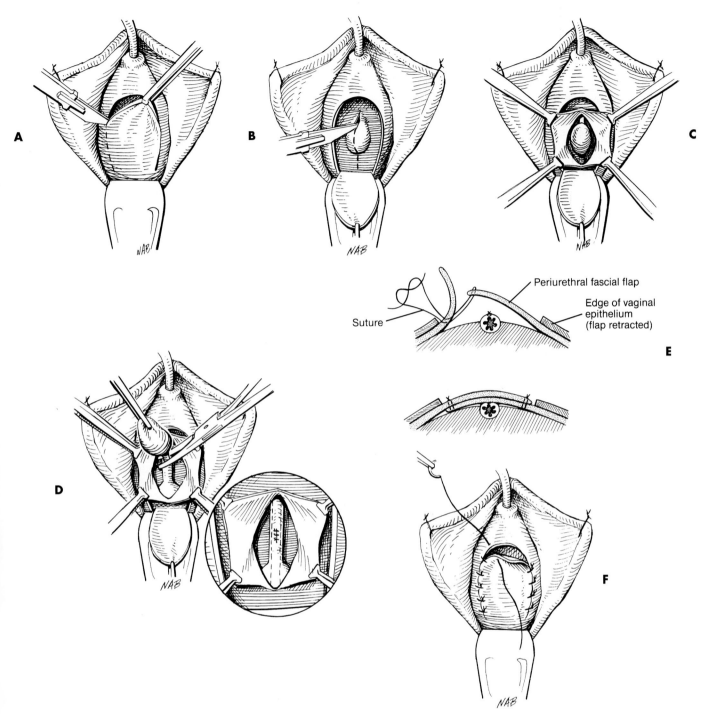

**Fig. 29-4** Suburethral diverticulectomy. **A,** Incision of the vaginal epithelium overlying the suburethral diverticulum, creating a U-shaped flap. **B,** Incision of the periurethral fascial tissue over the diverticular sac. **C,** Complete dissection and mobilization of the fascial tissue surrounding the suburethral diverticulum. **D,** Complete dissection of the suburethral diverticulum, with its attendant neck. The sac is excised at its neck. *Inset,* Defect in the urethra after closure with fine, absorbable interrupted sutures. **E,** The ''vest-over-pants'' technique of closure of periurethral fascial tissue. **F,** Closure of the vaginal flap with interrupted No. 2-0, absorbable suture. We prefer to use interrupted suturing techniques to avoid tissue shortening.

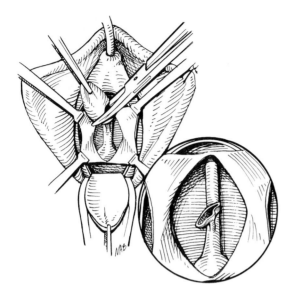

**Fig. 29-5** Demonstration of the partial ablation technique for proximal diverticulum (as described by Tancer et al., 1983). In this technique, the diverticulum is excised, and a portion of the base of the diverticulum and its neck are left intact and closed in an imbricating fashion with interrupted, fine absorbable suture.

the diverticulum explored to note the condition of the tissue and the presence of other diverticular openings or sacculations. The sac then is excised at its neck. The urethral opening is closed longitudinally over a Foley catheter with interrupted, fine, delayed-absorbable suture (Fig. 29-4, *D,* and *inset*).

6. The periurethral fascia, which previously was developed into flaps bilaterally, is closed in a "vest-over-pants" fashion over the urethra (Fig. 29-4, *E*). This maneuver avoids suture lines that overlap the urethral repair.

7. The flap of vaginal epithelium is repositioned and the incision is closed with No. 2-0, absorbable, interrupted sutures (Fig. 29-4, *F*).

8. The vagina is generally packed for 1 day. Continuous urinary drainage may be carried out with a transurethral silastic Foley catheter or suprapubic catheter for 5 to 7 days.

### *Partial Ablation Technique*

1. The surgical steps for the partial ablation technique are the same as for diverticulectomy up to the point of identification and dissection of the intact diverticular sac.

2. The diverticulum is incised longitudinally; the sac is entered and explored. The opening into the urethra is identified.

3. The easily excisable portion of the sac, not including the neck of the diverticulum, is excised (Fig. 29-5). No effort is made to enucleate the sac at its neck or at the juncture with the urethra. The base and neck of the diverticulum are then closed side to side, using fine, interrupted, absorbable suture. A second layer of similar sutures is

**Table 29-2** Complications Associated With Repair of Suburethral Diverticula

| Complication | Frequency of occurrence (%) |
|---|---|
| Recurrent urinary tract infection | 5 |
| Fistula | 4 |
| Recurrence | 4 |
| Stress incontinence | 2 |
| Stricture formation | 1 |

Modified from Ginsburg DS, Genadry R: *Obstet Gynecol Surv* 39:1, 1984.

placed, which further imbricates the previous urethral defect.

4. The "vest-over-pants" periurethral fascial closure and closure of the vaginal epithelium are completed as for a diverticulectomy.

5. A bulbocavernosus muscle transplant, as described in Chapter 28, is optional for diverticulectomy or partial ablation.

### *Spence Procedure*

1. The patient is positioned as for a diverticulectomy. A urethroscopy is performed to locate the diverticulum and its opening.

2. An Allis clamp is placed on the anterior vaginal wall opposite the diverticular orifice. One blade of the scissor is placed in the urethra and the other in the vagina. The scissor divides the floor of the diverticulum and the overlying vaginal epithelium, including the posterior urethra distal to the diverticulum.

3. Redundant flaps of diverticular sac and vaginal epithelium are trimmed.

4. A running, locking, delayed absorbable suture coapts the margins of the remaining lining of sac and adjacent vaginal epithelium. The bladder neck and the urethra proximal to the diverticular orifice are left untouched.

5. A vaginal pack and urethral catheter were used for 48 hours in the original article by Spence and Duckett (1970); however, they are probably not necessary. This procedure usually can be performed on an outpatient basis.

Certainly, no surgical procedure is without difficulties and complications, and excision of suburethral diverticula by any method falls within this general dictum. Ginsburg and Genadry (1984) reviewed the literature to 1984. Their complication and recurrence rates are summarized in Table 29-2.

## SUMMARY

The suburethral diverticulum has a long history as a clinical problem for women. Diagnosis clearly depends on a heightened index of suspicion because many of the symptoms can be attributed to other urogynecologic conditions. It is unfortunate that to some extent our instruments inhibit the diagnosis itself. For example, the anterior blade of a bivalve speculum may hide a suburethral diverticulum. Generally, careful palpation of the urethra and anterior vaginal wall is not included in the instruction of bimanual examination. Palpation should be performed because the incidence of diverticula can be up to 3% in the general female population and can be readily diagnosed by a careful physical examination in up to two thirds of patients. Radiologic, endoscopic, and urodynamic techniques also are used to diagnose and localize suburethral diverticula.

Variations on surgical procedures for this condition have been summarized. The major feature of the surgical procedures is careful dissection and excision of the sac with closure of the urethra and intervening spaces. With meticulous dissection and careful closure, success rates higher than 95% can be achieved with few complications.

## BIBLIOGRAPHY

Anderson MJF: The incidence of diverticula in the female urethra, *J Urol* 98:96, 1967.

Asmussen M, Miller A: *Clinical gynecologic urology,* Boston, 1983, Blackwell Scientific.

Benjamin J, Elliott L, Cooper JF, et al: Urethral diverticulum in adult female: clinical aspects, operative procedure and pathology, *Urology* 3:1, 1974.

Bruning EJ: *Die Pathologie der Weiblichen Urethra und des Paraurethreium,* Berlin, 1959, Stuttgart.

Butler WJ: The diagnosis of urethra diverticula in women, *J Urol* 95:63, 1966.

Chancellor MD, Liu JB, Rivas DA, et al: Intraoperative endo-luminal ultrasound evaluation of urethral diverticula, *J Urol* 153:72, 1995.

Cullen TS: Abscess in the urethro-vaginal septum, *Bull Johns Hopkins Hosp* 5:45, 1894.

Davis BC, Robinson DG: Diverticula of the female urethra: assay of 120 cases, *J Urol* 204:850, 1970.

Davis HJ, Cian LG: Positive pressure urethrography: a new diagnostic method, *J Urol* 75:753, 1956.

Davis HJ, TeLinde RW: Urethral diverticula: an assay of 121 cases, *J Urol* 80:34, 1958.

Edwards EA, Beebe RA: Diverticula of the female urethra, *Obstet Gynecol* 5:729, 1955.

Evans KJ, McCarthy MP, Sands JP: Adenocarcinoma of a female urethral diverticulum: a case report and review of the literature, *J Urol* 126:124, 1981.

Everett HS: *Gynecologic and obstetrical urology,* Baltimore, 1944, Williams & Wilkins.

Folsom AI: Diseases of the urethra and penis. In Bransford L, ed: *History of urology,* Baltimore, 1933, Williams & Wilkins.

Ginsburg DS, Genadry R: Suburethral diverticulum in the female, *Obstet Gynecol Surv* 39:1, 1984.

Greenberg M, Stone D, Cochran ST, et al: Female urethral diverticula: double-balloon catheter study, *AJR* 136:259, 1981.

Hey, W: *Practical observations in surgery,* Philadelphia, 1805, Humphreys.

Hoffman MJ, Adams WE: Recognition and repair of urethral diverticula, *Am J Obstet Gynecol* 92:106, 1965.

Huffman JW: The development of the periurethral glands in the human female, *Am J Obstet Gynecol* 46:773, 1943.

Huffman JW: The detailed anatomy of the paraurethral ducts in the adult human female, *Am J Obstet Gynecol* 55:86, 1948.

Huffman JW: Clinical significance of the paraurethral ducts and glands, *Arch Surg* 62:615, 1951.

Hunner GL: Calculus formation in a urethral diverticulum in women. Report of three cases, *Urol Cutan Rev* 42:336, 1938.

Jensen L, Aabech J, Lundval F, et al: Female urethral diverticulum. Clinical aspects and presentation of 15 cases, *Acta Obstet Gynecol Scand* 75:748, 1996.

Johnson CM: Diverticula and cysts of female urethra, *J Urol* 39:506, 1938.

Kim B, Hricak H, Tanagho EA: Diagnosis of urethral diverticulum in women: value of MR imaging, *AJR* 161:809, 1993.

Kistner RW: *Gynecology: principles and practice,* Chicago, 1983, Year Book Medical Publishers.

Krantz K: Anatomy of urethra and anterior vaginal wall, *Am J Obstet Gynecol* 62:374, 1951.

Kretschmer HL: Diverticula in the anterior urethra in male children, *Surg Gynecol Obstet* 62:634, 1936.

MacKinnon N, Pratt JH, Pool TL: Diverticulum of the female urethra, *Surg Clin North Am* 39:953, 1959.

Martensson O, Ducheck M: Translabial ultrasonography with pulsed color doppler in the diagnosis of female urethral diverticula, *Scand J Urol Nephrol* 28:101, 1994.

Moore TD: Diverticula of the female urethra with a new approach at surgical excision, *J Urol* 68:611, 1953.

Murphy LJT: *History of urology,* Springfield, Ill, 1972, Charles C Thomas.

Netter FH: *The CIBA collection of medical illustrations, vol 2, The reproductive system,* Summit, NJ, 1974, CIBA-GEIGY Corp.

O'Connor VJ: Surgery in the female urethra. In Glen JF, Boyce WH, eds: *Urologic surgery,* New York, 1969, Harper Norwell.

Pare A: *The works of that Famous Chirurgion, Ambrose Pare. Translated out of Latin and compared with the French. By Thomas Johnson; Whereunto are added three tractates out of Adrianus Spigelius of the veines, arteries, & nerves, with large figures,* London, 1649, Richard Cotes.

Pete LG, Ames BL: The female urethra. In Sciara JJ, ed: *Gynecology and obstetrics,* New York, 1987, Harper & Row.

Reid DE, Ryan KG, Benirschke K: *Principles and management of human reproduction,* Philadelphia, 1972, WB Saunders.

Sholem SL, Wechsler M, Roberts M: Management of the urethral diverticulum in women: a modified operative technique, *J Urol* 112:485, 1974.

Skene AJ: The anatomy and pathology of two important glands of the female urethra, *Am J Obstet Gynecol* 13:265, 1880.

Slate WG: Lesions of the female urethra. In Pratt JH, Malek RS, eds: *Disorders of the female urethra and urinary incontinence,* Baltimore, 1978, Williams & Wilkins.

Spence HM, Duckett JW: Diverticulum of the female urethra: clinical aspects and presentation of a simple operative technique for cure, *J Urol* 104:432, 1970.

Tancer ML, Mooppan MU, Pierre-Louis C, et al: Suburethral diverticulum treatment by partial ablation, *Obstet Gynecol* 62:511, 1983.

Taylor WN: *Urologists Correspondence Club Letters* 16:37, 1950.

TeLinde RW: Surgical conditions of the vulva and the vagina, In Mattingley RE, ed: *Operative gynecology,* ed 2, Philadelphia, 1953, JB Lippincott.

Thomas R: Examination of the female urethra, *Acta Radiol* 11:527, 1930.

Torres SA, Quattlebaum RB: Carcinoma in a urethral diverticulum, *South Med J* 65:1374, 1972.

Wershub LP, Green WH: *Urology: from antiquity to the 20th century,* St Louis, 1970, Green.

Wharton LR, Kearns W: Diverticula of the female urethra, *J Urol* 63:1063, 1950.

Young BR, McCrea LE: Urethrocele; urethral diverticulum; suburethral abscess in the female: roentgen appearance; treatment; review of the literature, report of a case, *Urol Cutan Rev* 41:91, 1937.

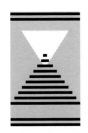

# CHAPTER 30

# Gynecologic Injury to the Ureters, Bladder, and Urethra
## Prevention, Recognition, and Management

W. Glenn Hurt

In the female body, the intimate anatomic relationship between the reproductive and lower urinary tracts predisposes the lower urinary tract to involvement by gynecologic disorders and places it at risk for injury during gynecologic surgery. Between 50% and 90% of all lower urinary tract injuries occur during gynecologic surgery. Some of these injuries cannot be avoided, but the majority are avoidable.

Reviews of the surgical literature reveal two disturbing facts: most lower urinary tract injuries occur during gynecologic surgery performed for benign and otherwise uncomplicated conditions and most lower urinary tract injuries are not recognized during the operative procedure in which they occur. For this reason, the emphasis in this chapter is on the prevention and recognition of lower urinary tract injuries.

## INCIDENCE

Injuries to the bladder or ureter occur in approximately 1% to 2% of all major gynecologic procedures. The true incidence is probably somewhat higher when one considers the number of unreported cases, the spontaneous resolution of partial ureteral obstructions, and the loss of some renal systems. Seventy-five percent of these injuries occur during a hysterectomy. Because about 500,000 hysterectomies are performed in the United States annually, it is estimated that 5000 women will experience a bladder or ureter injury each year as a result of this procedure.

Studies of genitourinary fistulas reveal that the ratio of bladder injury to ureteral injury is approximately 5:1. It is also apparent that most injuries that result in the formation of genitourinary fistulas are not recognized during surgery.

## PREVENTION OF INJURIES
### Preoperative Assessment

The patient's history, physical examination, and preoperative laboratory evaluation may suggest abnormal function of the urinary tract. The elective nature of most gynecologic surgery allows time for an evaluation that may include imaging, endoscopy, and consultation. When emergency surgery is performed on women with undiagnosed and untreated urinary tract abnormalities, it is accompanied by an increased incidence of perioperative and postoperative complications.

Because many gynecologic conditions are associated with an increased frequency of lower urinary tract infections, the urine should be tested for infection before surgery. If there is evidence of urinary tract infection, either asymptomatic or symptomatic, it should be treated until the urine is sterile. Most gynecologic procedures require catheterization of the bladder and many affect bladder function. Because bladder catheterization and gynecologic surgery may initiate or aggravate a urinary tract infection, the patient should go to the operating room with sterile urine.

Sonographic imaging of the urinary tract is useful in determining kidney size and detecting ureteral obstruction. Sonography also can be used to image the bladder and estimate urinary residual volumes. Intravenous urography documents anatomic abnormalities, further defines renal function, and localizes ureteric obstruction; it is important in the evaluation of genitourinary fistulas. Routine preoperative imaging studies have not been shown to reduce the incidence of operative injuries to the lower urinary tract.

Cystourethroscopy is indicated in the preoperative evaluation of hematuria, abnormal urine cytology, persistent or recurrent urinary tract infections, lower urinary tract fistulas, urethral or bladder diverticula, bladder and urethral pain, selected cases of urinary incontinence, and staging of gynecologic malignancies. Retrograde pyelograms are helpful in locating ureteral obstructions and fistulas.

Preoperative retrograde ureteral stent or catheter placement has not been shown to reduce the incidence of surgical injury to the ureter. The procedure itself may cause bleeding, edema, and perforation of the ureter. The stent is often difficult to feel within an area of fibrosis, and it may predispose the ureter to damage as a result of the immobility it imparts to the ureter. During surgery, when it is difficult to determine the course of the ureter or the integrity of its wall, placement of a ureteral catheter may be indicated. This may be done via cystoscopy or cystotomy. Ureteral catheter insertions also can be helpful during endoscopic surgery. If the endoscopic surgeon observes the ureter during the insertion of a catheter, the movement of the ureter will help define its retroperitoneal course.

## Intraoperative Care

In the operating room there is no substitute for good lighting, proper patient preparation and positioning, adequate exposure, and strict adherence to sterile techniques. Lighting can be improved by the use of headlamps, light-containing suction irrigators, or fiberoptic lighted retractors. During complicated cases, abdominal-perineal-vaginal preparation, drapes that permit access to the abdominal and vaginal areas, positioning of the patient in universal stirrups, and a transurethral three-way continuous irrigation balloon catheter (16 or 18 French) for emptying and filling the bladder are recommended. These measures give the surgeon the flexibility to operate abdominally or vaginally, to perform endoscopy, and to detect and repair lower urinary tract injuries.

During all surgical procedures, sharp dissection is preferable to blunt dissection, and taking small pedicles is preferred to taking large pedicles. When hemostasis is a problem, pressure should be applied until the bleeding vessel can be identified and selectively clamped. Many ureters are damaged by the application of clamps in a frantic effort to control pelvic hemorrhage.

## Abdominal Approach

Abdominal incisions should allow adequate exposure of the entire pelvis. Entry into the peritoneal cavity should be as high as possible to avoid direct cystotomy. The surgeon should be aware that the bladder may be pulled up beneath the anterior abdominal wall by its peritoneal reflection as a result of incomplete emptying, tumor, or previous surgery, especially cesarean section.

Entry into the peritoneal cavity should be followed by exploration of its contents, restoration of normal anatomic relationships, and exposure of the operative site. Attention should be given to the location and size of each kidney. With the patient in the Trendelenburg position, the bowel may be packed into the upper abdomen and retained by a retractor.

At this point, an effort should be made to identify both ureters and trace their pelvic courses. The ureters are most easily identified as they descend into the pelvis over the bifurcation of the common iliac arteries. They then follow the posterior boundaries of the ovarian fossae to pass beneath the uterine arteries and to course anteriorly and laterally about the cervix and upper vagina. Each ureter enters a separate tunnel within the base of the bladder. An alternative approach to the ureter is through an incision of the lateral broad ligament. Dissection of the pararectal space reveals the ureter on its medial margin as it approaches the uterine artery. Although palpation of the ureter between the forefinger and thumb imparts a "clicking" sensation and sound, these characteristics can also be obtained by palpating other retroperitoneal structures. To positively identify the ureter, it is best to observe its distinctive periodic peristalsis.

The ureter usually can be dissected away from or out of a gynecologic disease process. The aim is to do so with the least possible ureteral trauma. It is helpful to place the tips of a right-angle or Adson tonsil forceps between the adventitial sheath of the ureter and the adjacent tissue to guide the dissection. If at all possible, the ureter should not be separated from its overlying peritoneum. This attachment protects the ureter's blood supply, elevates it out of the depths of the pelvis (where it might be surrounded by blood and serum), and assists its peristalsis. If a portion of the ureter is invaded by endometriosis or cancer, it may have to be resected and a ureteroneocystostomy or ureteroureterostomy performed.

Likewise, it is important to determine the location and extent of the outer wall of the bladder. It is usually possible to dissect the bladder from adjacent pathologic conditions. Rarely, in some cases of endometriosis or cancer it is necessary to resect a portion of the bladder wall.

Increasingly, urogynecologists and reconstructive pelvic surgeons are encountering dense adherence of the bladder to the posterior symphysis when performing repeat retropubic procedures. Under these circumstances, it is best to perform an extraperitoneal cystotomy in the dome of the bladder and then to dissect the bladder and upper urethra from the posterior symphysis under direct vision. Experience has shown that this procedure reduces the extent of damage to both organs.

The pelvic surgeon should always be ureter-conscious. Throughout an abdominal procedure, it is important to know where the ureters are and to keep them out of harm's way. Care should be taken not to kink the ureters during obliteration of the cul-de-sac, plication of the uterosacral ligaments, or suspension of the vaginal apex.

## Vaginal Approach

In preparing the patient for vaginal surgery, we drain the bladder with a transurethral catheter, and then we often instill undiluted indigo carmine (5 ml) into the bladder. After this is done, the catheter is clamped or removed to keep the dye within the bladder. During surgery, if the bladder is partially or completely incised, the blue color of the indigo carmine is recognized, alerting the surgeon to the bladder injury.

During vaginal operations, the surgeon should avoid a cystotomy by identifying the trigone and base of the bladder. Their location may be determined by palpating the balloon of a transurethral catheter, inserting a probe or Kelly clamp and palpating its tip, or reaching through a posterior colpotomy incision around and in front of the lower uterine segment with a finger and seeing the tip of the finger between the bladder and the lower uterine segment. Once the base of the bladder has been dissected free of the lower uterine segment and the vesicoperitoneal fold has been incised, a vaginal retractor should be placed between the bladder and the uterus. This retractor is protective in that it elevates the bladder and lateralizes the ureters. However, care should be taken not to perforate the bladder with the tip of the retractor.

During vaginal surgery, visualization of the ureter is difficult and somewhat hazardous. When the pelvic cavity has been opened, it is possible, with experience, to palpate the ureters against an appropriately placed vaginal sidewall retractor. This is a very important maneuver when operating on patients with prolapse and when performing extensive culdeplasties. If there is any question about the integrity of the ureters or bladder, cystoscopy should be performed.

Dissection of the anterior vaginal wall exposes the urethra and the bladder trigone to injury. Most urethral injuries result from diverticulum repair, anterior colporrhaphy, or instrumentation of the urethra. Some urethral injuries are caused by urethropexies and sling procedures. Urethral injuries, both direct and indirect, may damage the organ's sphincter mechanism and cause stress urinary incontinence.

## Laparoscopic Approach

Urinary tract injuries occur in 1% to 2% of patients undergoing major laparoscopic surgery. The incidence of urinary tract complications appears to increase with the complexity of the procedure.

Endoscopic adnexectomy poses a higher risk of ureteral injury than does hysterectomy. This may be because of adhesions caused by endometriosis, pelvic inflammatory disease, or previous surgery. It may also result from the instrumentation involved.

Most bladder injuries result from sharp dissection, with or without cautery, during laparoscopically assisted vaginal hysterectomy. It is believed that the incidence of bladder injuries associated with laparoscopically assisted vaginal

hysterectomy can be reduced if the bladder dissection is done vaginally instead of laparoscopically. Most series of laparoscopic urinary continence and pelvic support procedures report some bladder and urethral injuries. The incidence of these injuries appears to be related directly to the surgeon's experience with these procedures.

During laparoscopy, urinary tract injury may be revealed by direct observation, injection of dye solution, presence of gas in the catheter bag, and detection of bubbles during cystoscopy. If urinary tract injury is suspected, cystoscopy should be performed and sometimes repeated. If ureteral injury is suspected, a ureteral catheter should be inserted. Other diagnostic tests might be required for the diagnosis of postoperative lower urinary tract injuries.

## RECOGNITION AND MANAGEMENT OF INJURIES

Several general principles apply to the management and repair of all lower urinary tract injuries. The administration of prophylactic antibiotics should be considered. The extent of the damage to the urinary tract must be explored. Devitalized tissues must be excised. Urinary tract repairs should be performed with small-caliber delayed absorbable (polyglactin or polyglycolic acid) or absorbable (chromic) suture. There must be absolutely no tension on the repair site. Extraperitoneal suction drainage should be placed adjacent to, but not in contact with, all retroperitoneal repairs. Bladder drainage is important to reduce tension within the wall of the bladder during the healing phase.

### Recognition of Ureteral Injury
#### Ureteral Dye Injection

The integrity of a single ureter can be demonstrated by injecting indigo carmine dye into the lumen of the ureter above the surgical site. This may be done using a 22-gauge needle and directing its tip in the direction of the bladder. Resistance to dye injection suggests ureteral obstruction; extravasation of dye suggests damage to the ureter wall. The passage of blue urine without resistance to the injection or the extravasation of urine is reassuring.

#### Intravenous Dye Injection

Intravenous injection of indigo carmine (slow infusion of 5 ml) normally results in the excretion of blue urine within 5 to 10 minutes. If the dye injection is accompanied by an increase in intravenous fluids or mannitol or the administration of a diuretic, dye excretion may be enhanced. In some women the excretion of dye is delayed. A second dose of indigo carmine (5 ml) may be administered; however, indigo carmine can be vasoactive and a third dose is not recommended.

When an intravenous dye such as indigo carmine is administered, the passage of blue urine means that at least one renal unit is functioning. To determine which renal unit is functioning, the surgeon must perform either cystoscopy (suprapubic or transurethral) or cystotomy. Leakage of blue urine into the operative field is evidence of lower urinary tract injury. This requires further investigation.

### Cystoscopy

Cystoscopy may be performed transurethrally or suprapubically. Transurethral cystoscopy is facilitated by the routine use of universal stirrups. Suprapubic cystoscopy is called teloscopy. When teloscopy is completed, the cystotomy site may be used for subsequent suprapubic bladder catheter drainage.

The intravenous injection of indigo carmine (5 ml) just before cystoscopy enables the examiner to determine ureteric function, as evidenced by the excretion of blue urine. When either ureter fails to excrete blue urine, the reason must be determined.

### Cystotomy

A cystotomy is another method of observing the inside of the bladder. Ideally, the cystotomy should be placed in the extraperitoneal portion of the dome of the bladder. If intravenous indigo carmine is administered, the excretion of blue urine helps determine the integrity of each renal unit.

### Ureteral Catheterization

Intraoperative ureteral catheterization is usually performed by cystoscopy or cystotomy. It also may be performed by ureterotomy. When cystoscopy or cystotomy is performed, the ureters may be catheterized using a small pediatric feeding tube, ureteral catheter, or ureteral stent (Fig. 30-1). The pediatric feeding tube is more easily passed through the ureteric tunnels. It is usually used intraoperatively to demonstrate ureteral patency, but it can be used for short-term postoperative ureteral drainage. Ureteral catheters and stents are somewhat more difficult to pass through the ureteric tunnels because of their stiffness. Ureteral catheters may be brought out of the urethra or through the dome of the bladder and abdominal wall for long-term drainage. Ureteral double-J stents are ideal for ureteral drainage because the upper J maintains the catheter within the renal pelvis and the lower J maintains the catheter within the bladder. These catheters are not exposed to the external environment.

Resistance to the passage of a ureteral catheter suggests kinking or obstruction of the ureter. The drainage of urine through the catheter documents renal function. Catheters and stents may be left in place when there are obstructions, crush injuries, or ureteric repairs in order to drain urine from the kidneys, help prevent stenosis of the ureter, and facilitate healing.

### Intravenous Urography

Intravenous urography may be performed intraoperatively to determine renal function and document the integrity of the lower urinary tracts. Radiologic imaging provides films

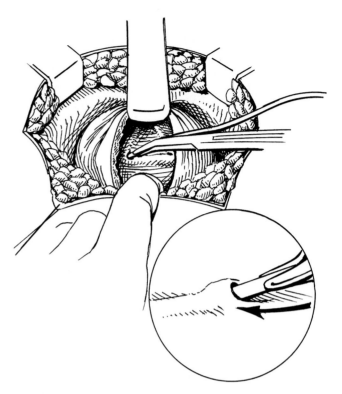

**Fig. 30-1**   Technique of ureteral catheter passage after cystotomy has been performed.

for documentation of findings. This method of testing is somewhat cumbersome intraoperatively, and it should be done in a manner that minimizes radiation exposure.

## Management of Ureteral Injury

Ureteral angulations and kinks should be released if they cause significant obstruction. A ligated ureter should have the ligating suture removed. Minor ureteral crush injuries may be managed with stenting; significant crush injuries require resection of the damaged segment and ureteroneocystostomy or ureteroureterostomy. On occasion, partial lacerations of a ureter can be repaired by appropriate placement of several absorbable or delayed absorbable sutures. Complete lacerations of the ureter and loss of a segment of ureter require definitive surgical repair.

The surgical procedures recommended for ureteral repair vary according to the ureteral segment that is involved (Fig. 30-2). Because most gynecologic injuries to the ureter involve its distal 4 to 5 cm, most can be repaired by ureteroneocystostomy. Injuries just below the pelvic brim may be repaired by ureteroureterostomy or ureteroneocystostomy. Ureteroneocystostomy is not recommended for injuries above the pelvic brim.

### Ureteroneocystostomy

Ureteroneocystostomy is the procedure of choice for injuries involving the terminal 4 to 5 cm of either ureter (Fig. 30-3). The distal ureteral segment is ligated with permanent suture at its entry into the bladder. If the proximal

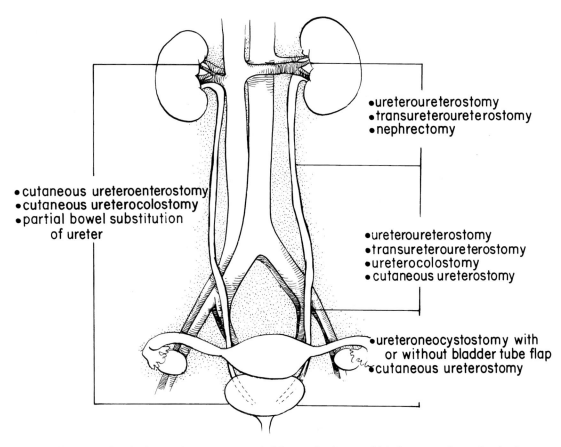

**Fig. 30-2** Surgical procedures recommended for repair of ureteral injuries, according to involved ureteral segment.

From Hurt WG, Dunn LJ: Complications of gynecologic surgery and trauma. In Greenfield LJ, ed: *Complications in surgery and trauma,* ed 2, Philadelphia, 1990, JB Lippincott.

ureter has a nonviable segment, this is excised. The end of the ureter is then tagged with a long through-and-through suture. The bladder may be mobilized by the release of its attachments to the posterior surface of the pubis. An extraperitoneal cystotomy is performed in the dome of the bladder, and the base of the bladder is displaced toward the end of the injured ureter. A Kelly clamp is used to make a direct puncture through the full thickness of the base of the bladder at an appropriate location to allow the tagged distal end of the ureter to be brought into the bladder. When this is accomplished and there is at least 1 cm of ureter inside of the bladder, the end of the ureter is spatulated bilaterally and its distal flaps are secured to the inside of the bladder with No. 3-0 chromic sutures. The adventitia of the ureter is anchored to the outside of the bladder with several No. 3-0 delayed absorbable sutures. It is most important that there be no tension on the ureter or the bladder at the site of ureteroneocystostomy. If there is tension on the anastomosis, it should be relieved by a vesicopsoas hitch procedure (Fig. 30-4). If a vesicopsoas hitch is needed, it is best to perform it before reimplantation or reanastomosis of the ureter. Surgeons differ on the need for ureteral stenting following ureteroneocystostomy. If there is any question about the use

of a stent, one should be used. The site of the anastomosis should be drained by an extraperitoneal suction drain. The cystotomy should be closed and the bladder should be drained continuously for at least 7 days.

### *Ureteroureterostomy*

The simplest ureteroureterostomy involves the tension-free reanastomosis of two cut ends of a ureter. When there is loss of a ureteral segment, there may be a need for bladder or kidney mobilization, a bladder extension procedure, transureteroureterostomy, or the interposition of an intestinal segment.

In performing a ureteroureterostomy, the viable cut ends of each ureteral segment are spatulated for a distance of about 0.5 cm to help prevent stenosis of the anastomosis. A ureteral catheter is inserted into the ureter to bridge the anastomotic site. Four to six interrupted full-thickness No. 4-0 chromic sutures are used to perform the anastomosis. The anastomotic site should be drained by an extraperitoneal suction drain to prevent the accumulation of blood, serum, or urine. This drain should remain in place until the ureteral catheter has been removed. The ureteral catheter should be left in place for at least 7 days. Postoperative bladder drainage is usually recommended.

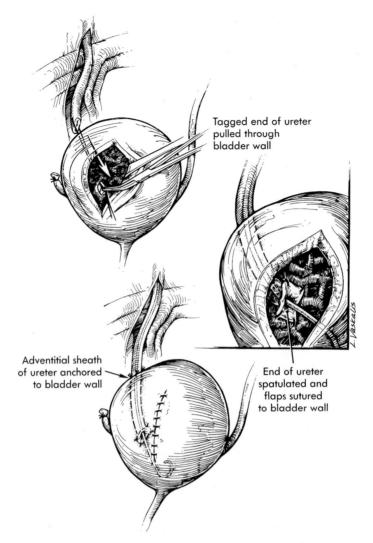

Tagged end of ureter
pulled through
bladder wall

Adventitial sheath
of ureter anchored
to bladder wall

End of ureter
spatulated and
flaps sutured
to bladder wall

**Fig. 30-3**  Ureteroneocystostomy. After ureter is divided and the distal segment ligated, an incision is made in the bladder wall near the old ureteral orifice, and the tagged end of the ureter is pulled through the bladder wall. The end of the ureter is spatulated, and the flaps are sutured to the bladder mucosa. The adventitial sheath of the ureter is anchored to the bladder wall.

From Hurt WG, Segreti EM: Intraoperative ureteral injuries and urinary diversion. In Nichols DH, Clarke-Pearson D, eds: *Gynecologic and obstetric surgery*, ed 2, St Louis, 1999, Mosby.

## Bladder Mobilization and Extension

When performing a ureteroneocystostomy or ureteroureterostomy, there must be no tension on the site of the anastomosis. Dissection of the retropubic space (of Retzius) frees the bladder from its attachments to the posterior symphysis and allows it to be mobilized toward the site of the repair. If this is done and there is still some tension on the anastomosis, the surgeon should consider performing a psoas hitch or bladder extension procedure.

The vesicopsoas hitch is performed by placing one or two fingers through an extraperitoneal cystotomy and pushing the bladder toward the psoas muscle on the side of the anticipated ureteral repair (see Fig. 30-4). When it is determined that the displacement of the bladder will allow a

tension-free repair, the outer muscular wall of the bladder is sutured to the psoas muscle with several interrupted No. 2-0 or 1-0 delayed-absorbable sutures. The attachment of the bladder to the psoas muscle must also be tension-free to prevent pressure necrosis around the sutures and premature detachment of the bladder.

If dissection of the retropubic space and a psoas hitch do not give enough mobility to the bladder to allow a satisfactory ureteral implantation or reanastomosis, the creation of a bladder flap made into a tubular structure and ureteral implantation should be considered. The Boari-Ockerblad bladder flap (Fig. 30-5) and the Demel bladder flap differ primarily in the direction of excision of the full-thickness bladder flap. In either case, the flap must

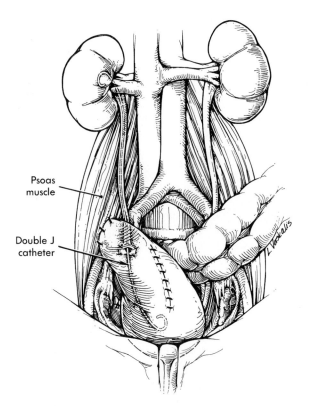

**Psoas muscle**

**Double J catheter**

**Fig. 30-4** Vesicopsoas hitch, used for distal ureteral injuries in which there is tension on a ureteroneocystostomy or uretero-ureterostomy. This technique brings the bladder cephalad to relieve tension on the suture site.

From Hurt WG, Segreti EM: Intraoperative ureteral injuries and urinary diversion. In Nichols DH, Clarke-Pearson D, eds: *Gynecologic and obstetric surgery*, ed 2, St Louis, 1999, Mosby.

have a wide base to ensure an adequate blood supply. The flap is made tubular by suturing together its lateral margins, and the cut end of the ureter is brought into the end of the flap in much the same way as one would perform a ureteroneocystostomy.

It is possible to bridge the gap between the cut end of a ureter and the bladder by performing an ileoureteroneocystostomy. A segment of ileum of sufficient length and with adequate blood supply is isolated from the bowel. Its distal end is sutured to a cystotomy site in the dome of the bladder and the cut end of the ureter is implanted into its proximal end. The continuity of the ileum is then reestablished.

### Transureteroureterostomy

When so much of the ureter has been lost that it is impossible to perform a ureteroneocystostomy or uretero-ureterostomy, a transureteroureterostomy should be considered. In performing a transureteroureterostomy, the proximal ureter is mobilized and passed retroperitoneally below the inferior mesenteric artery and in front of the great vessels to meet the opposite ureter. The recipient ureter is longitudinally incised and an end-to-side anastomosis is performed using full-thickness No. 4-0 absorbable sutures.

The anastomosis should be watertight but not ischemic. The anastomotic site should be drained by an extraperitoneal suction drain. Ureteral catheters usually are not necessary.

### Cutaneous Ureterostomy

A cutaneous ureterostomy should not be considered a permanent method of urinary diversion. It may be done when the patient's chances of survival are limited or in cases in which the surgeon is not prepared to perform a more definitive repair. It is performed by bringing the cut end of the ureter out retroperitoneally though the skin and performing a ureteral-skin anastomosis. Ureteral catheters usually are not necessary.

### Follow-Up of Ureteral Repairs

Extraperitoneal suction drains should be placed to the site of, but not in contact with, all internal ureteral anastomoses. These drains should remove all blood, serum, lymph, and urine that collects near the anastomosis. They usually are not removed until all ureteral catheters and stents have been removed.

Continuous bladder catheter drainage, either transurethrally or suprapubically, should be initiated whenever there is a cystotomy, ureteroneocystostomy, or ureteroureterostomy. In the latter case, when there is no cystotomy, the bladder catheter may be removed before the ureteral catheter or stent is removed.

All ureteric injuries should be followed by an intravenous urogram to determine the integrity of the repair and the presence or absence of a stenosis. This is done to detect fistulas or conditions that might cause kidney damage.

## Recognition of Bladder Injury
### Bladder Dye Instillations

If surgery is performed with an indigo carmine solution inside the bladder, partial lacerations of the bladder wall reveal the underlying blue mucosa. Penetrations and lacerations of the bladder are indicated by blue dye leaking onto the surgical field.

The integrity of the bladder wall cannot be tested thoroughly until the bladder is filled with 300 to 400 ml of an appropriate liquid distending medium (sterile water or normal saline containing indigo carmine dye or sterile milk or infant's formula). The bladder can be filled using a single-channel or double-channel transurethral catheter. In difficult cases, repetitive emptying and filling of the bladder is facilitated by the placement of an indwelling three-channel transurethral balloon catheter.

### Cystoscopy

Cystoscopy may be performed transurethrally or suprapubically as described under the section on the detection of ureteral injuries. A thorough examination of the bladder requires the use of different telescopic lenses. It is important to detect and remove any suture material and other foreign

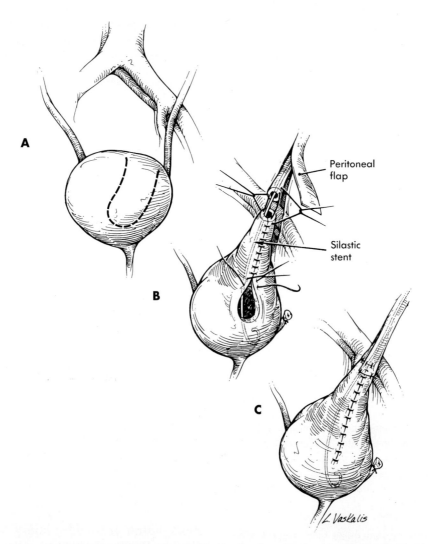

**Fig. 30-5** Boari-Ockerblad bladder flap. **A,** Bladder flap is outlined on the bladder. **B,** Bladder flap is created and ureter is sewn into its end. **C,** Bladder flap and ureteral anastomosis are completed.

From Hurt WG, Segreti EM: Intraoperative ureteral injuries and urinary diversion. In Nichols DH, Clarke-Pearson D, eds: *Gynecologic and obstetric surgery,* ed 2, St Louis, 1999, Mosby.

matter. It is also important to determine the location and extent of all bladder injuries and their relationship to each ureter and the urethra. The bladder must be distended to perform an adequate cystoscopic examination. This in itself may help identify lacerations of the bladder wall.

### Cystotomy

A cystotomy may be performed in the extraperitoneal portion of the dome of the bladder and the inside of the bladder may be examined thoroughly for injuries.

### Management of Bladder Injury

Intraoperative repair of bladder injuries varies slightly according to the location of the injury. Extraperitoneal lacerations in the dome of the bladder may be closed with one or two layers of No. 3-0 absorbable or delayed

absorbable suture. The suture may be placed in an interrupted or running fashion depending on the type and extent of the injury. Some extraperitoneal cystotomies in the dome of the bladder may be used for the insertion of a bladder catheter for postoperative suprapubic bladder drainage.

Transperitoneal lacerations of the bladder and lacerations of the base of the bladder should be repaired in two layers using No. 3-0 absorbable or delayed absorbable interrupted or running suture. These lacerations also should be covered by a layer of peritoneum or an omental flap. This procedure separates the injury from adjacent structures and cushions the repair by adding bulk. An omental flap brings in new tissue with its own separate blood supply.

Significant bladder repairs should have continuous bladder drainage for at least 7 days to facilitate healing.

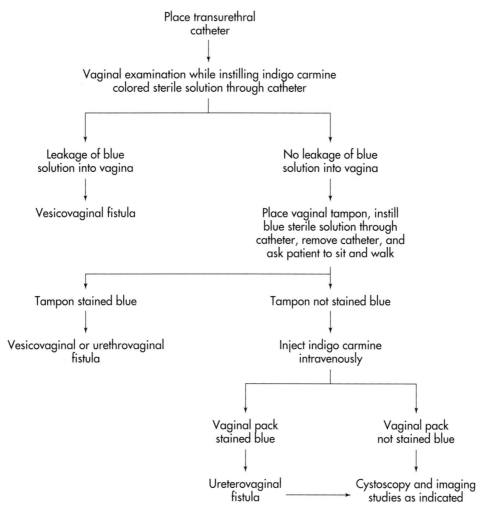

**Fig. 30-6**   Algorithm for the bedside or office evaluation of suspected vesicovaginal or ureterovaginal fistulas.

## Recognition of Urethral Injury
### Catheter Insertion

Intraoperatively, urethral injuries are most often diagnosed by the surgeon seeing the catheter through an incision in the wall of the urethra. Small clamps or probes may be used to confirm the injury.

### Urethroscopy

Urethroscopy is best performed with a special female urethroscope sheath and a 0-degree telescope lens. It can be used to detect suture material, foreign matter, and lacerations of the urethra.

## Management of Urethral Injury

Lacerations of the urethra should be repaired over a transurethral catheter in layers using No. 4-0 or 3-0 absorbable or delayed absorbable sutures. If the proximal urethra is involved, it is important to buttress the ure-

throvesical junction in an attempt to prevent the development of postoperative stress urinary incontinence. The use of a bulbocavernosus fat pad transplant should be considered if there is a need for additional tissue depth.

## POSTOPERATIVE EVALUATION OF SUSPECTED GENITOURINARY FISTULAS

Postoperative genitourinary fistulas may leak urine immediately or after several weeks. Any loss of urine from the vagina should be evaluated promptly. An algorithm for bedside or office evaluation of urine leakage from the vagina is shown in Fig. 30-6. If this examination suggests that the leakage is caused by a urethrovaginal, vesicovaginal, or ureterovaginal fistula, it is important to perform endoscopy. In women with vesicovaginal or ureterovaginal fistulas, an intravenous urogram must be done to document the function of both renal units and to determine whether the fistula involves more than one organ. Posthysterectomy vesico-vaginal fistulas are usually located just anterior to the vaginal cuff. On cystoscopy, they are usually located just above the interureteric ridge. Simple vesicovaginal fistulas that occur in the vaginal apex following an otherwise uncomplicated total hysterectomy are best treated by a partial apical colpocleisis (Latzko procedure).

## BIBLIOGRAPHY

American College of Obstetricians and Gynecologists: *Lower urinary tract operative injuries,* ACOG Technical Bulletin 238. Washington, DC: ACOG, 1997.

Boari A: Contributo sperimentale alla plastica dell' uretere, *Atti Acad Sci Med Nat Ferrara* 68:149, 1894.

Brubaker LT, Wilbanks GD: Urinary tract injuries in pelvic surgery, *Surg Clin North Am* 71:968, 1991.

Cruikshank SH: Surgical method of identifying the ureter during total vaginal hysterectomy, *Obstet Gynecol* 67:277, 1986.

Demel R: Ersatz des Ureters durch eine Plastik aus der Harnblase (Vorlaufige Mitteilung), *Zentralbl Chir* 51:2008, 1924.

Giberti C, Germinale F, Lillo M, et al: Obstetric and gynaecological ureteric injuries: treatment and results, *Br J Urol* 77:21, 1996.

Goodno JA Jr, Powers TW, Harris VD: Ureteral injury in gynecologic surgery: a 10-year review in a community hospital, *Am J Obstet Gynecol* 172:1817, 1995.

Hurt WG, Segreti EM: Intraoperative ureteral injuries and urinary diversion. In Nichols DH, Clarke-Pearson D, eds: *Gynecologic and obstetric surgery,* ed 2, St Louis, 1999, Mosby.

Lee RA, Symmonds RE, Williams TJ: Current status of genitourinary fistulas, *Obstet Gynecol* 71:313, 1988.

Mann WJ, Arato M, Pasatner B, et al: Ureteral injuries in an obstetric and gynecology training program: etiology and management, *Obstet Gynecol* 72:82, 1988.

Piscitelli JT, Simel DL, Addison WA: Who should have intravenous pyelograms before hysterectomy for benign disease? *Obstet Gynecol* 698:541, 1987.

Saidi MH, Sadler RK, Vancaillie TG, et al: Diagnosis and management of serious urinary complications after major operative laparoscopy, *Obstet Gynecol* 87:272, 1996.

Timmons MC, Addison WA: Suprapubic teloscopy: extraperitoneal intra-operative technique to demonstrate ureteral patency, *Obstet Gynecol* 75:137, 1990.

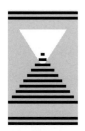

CHAPTER **31**

# The Effects of Gynecologic Cancer and Its Treatment on the Lower Urinary Tract

Paul P. Koonings

Cancer strikes approximately one third of Americans during their lifetimes. The American Cancer Society predicts close to 600,000 new cases of invasive cancer in women during 1997; genital cancers will account for 10% of this total. Furthermore, it has been predicted that 1 in 10 female deaths will occur secondary to a gynecologic malignancy. As the population continues to age, the gynecologist will see an increasing frequency of genital cancer. Hence, the gynecologist must have a working knowledge of the evaluation and treatment of female cancer and its urologic side effects.

The integral apposition of the urinary and genital tracts places the former at risk for dysfunction when genital malignancy develops, especially lower genital cancer. Urogenital dysfunction can result from the malignancy itself or from its treatment. The three major cornerstones of cancer therapy—chemotherapy, irradiation, and surgery—all have been implicated with both temporary and permanent urologic complications.

This chapter provides an overview of the effects of gynecologic cancer and its treatment on the urinary tract. The effects of genital cancer on the ureter, bladder, and urethra are discussed. Urogenital effects secondary to surgery, irradiation, chemotherapeutic agents, and hemorrhagic cystitis from a gynecologic cancer perspective are also described.

## UROLOGIC COMPLICATIONS OF GENITAL CANCER
### General Effects

The unique intimacy of the urinary and genital tracts accounts for the majority of urinary tract symptoms experienced when genital cancer occurs. Symptoms usually arise from one of two mechanisms: direct invasion or compression. Rarely do paraneoplastic syndromes cause urinary dysfunction. Usually, the primary site of disease is responsible for the effects demonstrated by the urinary system, although metastatic disease may be responsible in some circumstances.

In general, involvement of the urinary system secondary to genital cancer portends a poorer prognosis, which is reflected in the majority of staging schemes used for genital cancer. Pathologic confirmation documenting mucosal invasion must be demonstrated for the large number of staging systems.

It is beyond the scope of this chapter to completely discuss the risk factors and histologic types involved with genital cancer. The reader is directed to a textbook on gynecologic cancer. Generally 90% of the lower genital cancers are squamous in nature, with smoking and human papilloma virus representing the major risk factors.

### Cervical Cancer
#### Background and Staging

With the advent of the Papanicolaou smear, it was once hoped that routine screening would eliminate cervical cancer. Unfortunately, this scenario has not materialized, although routine cervical cancer screening apparently has decreased the incidence of this disease. Nevertheless, it is important to realize that in 1997 the American Cancer Society predicted close to 15,000 new cases of invasive cervical cancer.

**Box 31-1**

### DIAGNOSTIC TESTS ALLOWED BY FIGO FOR CERVICAL CANCER STAGING

Physical examination
Chest radiograph
Skeletal radiograph
Intravenous pyelogram
Barium enema
Biopsy
Cystoscopy
Proctoscopy

**Box 31-2**

### FIGO STAGING FOR CARCINOMA OF THE CERVIX UTERI

| | |
|---|---|
| Stage 0 | Carcinoma in situ; intraepithelial carcinoma. |
| Stage I | The carcinoma is strictly confined to the cervix (extension to the corpus should be disregarded). |
| Stage II | The carcinoma extends beyond the cervix but has not extended to the pelvic wall. The carcinoma involves the vagina, but not as far as the lower third. |
| Stage III | The carcinoma has extended to the pelvic wall. On rectal examination, there is no cancer-free space between the tumor and the pelvic wall. The tumor involves the lower third of the vagina. All cases with a hydronephrosis or nonfunctioning kidney are included unless known to result from other causes. |
| Stage IV | The carcinoma has extended beyond the true pelvis or has clinically involved the mucosa of the bladder or rectum. Bullous edema itself does not permit a case to be classified as stage IV. |

Evaluation of the urinary tract is necessary for cervical cancer staging. Today, cervical cancer staging is obtained from clinical evaluation alone. Under the auspices of the International Federation of Gynecology and Obstetrics (FIGO), the diagnostic tests listed in Box 31-1 are permitted for staging. These tests take into account the usual routes by which cervical cancer spreads, including local invasion into the vagina, parametrium, bladder, rectum, and lymphatic spread, both local and distant. Cystoscopy and proctoscopy are nonproductive in early stage disease.

Computed tomography (CT), ultrasound (US), and laparoscopy may not be used for FIGO staging. These tests should be used when clinically indicated to individualize therapy for each patient.

The current FIGO staging system is shown in Box 31-2. Involvement of the urinary tract usually allows for a step up in stage, with a resultant decrease in 5-year survival, as demonstrated in the 1988 FIGO report (Table 31-1).

### Effects on the Urinary Tract

The central location of the cervix places the ureter, bladder, and urethra at risk of involvement when cervical cancer develops. Urinary dysfunction develops insidiously from either the primary disease or its lymphatic metastasis. The ureters are particularly vulnerable to obstruction because their course through the pelvis brings them within millimeters of the cervix as they traverse the parametria, a favored path of cervical cancer extension.

Obstruction is caused by the mechanical effect of the adjacent tumor collapsing the tunnel. Direct ureteral invasion, as noted by van Nagell et al. (1982), is exceptional. Alternatively, ureteral obstruction occurs as the ureter enters the pelvis. Metastatic disease causes enlargement of lymph nodes, resulting in ureteral impingement. Henriksen (1949) reported on 356 necropsies secondary to both treated and untreated cases of cervical cancer. Ureteral obstruction with resulting uremia was responsible for at least 50% of the untreated cervical cancer deaths. Both mechanisms of ureteral obstruction were described.

Ureteral obstruction may be unilateral or bilateral. Unilateral obstruction may be completely asymptomatic. Other

**Table 31-1** FIGO Staging of Cervical Cancer

| Stage | N | 5-year survival (%) |
|---|---|---|
| I | 10,912 | 76 |
| II | 10,765 | 55 |
| III | 8,255 | 31 |
| IV | 1,386 | 7 |

patients may present with flank pain, fever, and uremia secondary to urinary infection. Unless the condition resolves, rapid deterioration of the affected kidney will occur.

Unrecognized ureteral obstruction results in destruction of the involved kidney. Urine continues to be formed, causing increased intraluminal pressure that damages the renal pelvis. Bricker (1980) and Crowley et al. (1990) demonstrated that the rapidity and extent of kidney damage result from several factors, such as the duration, level, and degree of obstruction; associated infection; and previous state of renal function. Therefore, once cervical cancer is suspected, ureteral involvement needs to be ruled out, especially with a bulky lesion (4 cm). Physical examination should include costovertebral palpation to detect renal tenderness or enlargement. Renal function tests should be obtained to rule out uremia. Electrolytes and an electrocardiogram will determine whether hyperkalemia and cardiac dysfunction are present. Previously, the intravenous pyelogram (IVP) was the method of choice for diagnosis of ureteral obstruction. Webb et al. (1984) showed that US is as sensitive in detecting ureteral obstruction as IVP. Because US is a less invasive diagnostic procedure not requiring dye administration, it should be the method of choice to diagnose ureteral obstruction. Furthermore, as Frolich et al. (1990) pointed out in a study of 210 new cases of cervical cancer, US examination of the kidneys and ureters requires no patient preparation. IVP dye administration in patients with compromised kidney function can precipitate renal failure. Thus, before any IVP dye administration, baseline renal function should be obtained.

Once diagnosed, ureteral obstruction demands prudent and timely intervention. Each case should be managed individually, especially those with prior pelvic irradiation. Optimally, patients should achieve relief of ureteral obstruction via the retrograde passage of double-J stents using cystoscopy. Once they are placed, their proper location should be confirmed with US or fluoroscopy. The urine should be evaluated at regular intervals for bacteriologic infection, which should be treated appropriately. Ureteral stents should be replaced according to the manufacturer's guidelines. Recommendations range from 3 to 12 months depending on stent composition.

Often, retrograde placement of ureteral stents is impossible. In these circumstances, percutaneous nephrostomy tubes are placed. US is the method of choice to assist placement. As Dudly et al. (1986) reported, nephrostomy tubes are not a panacea and can be associated with serious complications. Placement has been associated with pneumothorax, severe hemorrhage, and even death. Long-term nephrostomy use is complicated by infection, blockage, and accidental dislodgment. Fortunately, resolution of perinephric edema after nephrostomy tube use allows for placement of antegrade ureteral stents in a large number of cases. This approach is attempted 5 to 7 days after nephrostomy tube placement. Once performed, the percutaneous nephrostomy tubes are discontinued. The absence of a vesicovaginal fistula should be confirmed before ureteral stent placement. Otherwise, urinary incontinence will result.

Electrolyte abnormalities secondary to ureteral obstruction present a more difficult challenge. Hyperkalemia should be corrected by the judicious use of insulin, dextrose, and sodium bicarbonate to lower potassium levels, as well as the occasional use of calcium chloride to protect the heart from dysrhythmias. After these electrolyte imbalances have been recognized and treated appropriately, steps should be taken to alleviate ureteral obstruction as previously discussed.

Most patients with cervical cancer do not complain of bladder symptoms. However, when these symptoms are present, they can arise from either mass effect or direct invasion of the bladder. Mass effect causes compression of the bladder, resulting in nocturia, urge, and frequency. Direct invasion occasionally produces vesicovaginal fistulas associated with hematuria. Documented mucosal involvement is mandatory for FIGO upstaging. During cystoscopy, bladder washings should be obtained for cytologic evaluation. Punch biopsies of suspicious areas should be obtained. The number and location of the ureteral orifices should be noted and ureteral stents passed when appropriate. As

**Box 31-3**

**FIGO STAGING FOR CARCINOMA OF THE VULVA**

Stage 0 — Carcinoma in situ; intraepithelial carcinoma.

Stage I — Tumor confined to the vulva or perineum; 2 cm or less in greatest dimension; no nodal metastasis.

Stage II — Tumor confined to the vulva or perineum; more than 2 cm in greatest dimension; no nodal metastasis.

Stage III — Tumor of any size with adjacent spread to the lower urethra, vagina, or anus, or unilateral regional lymph node metastasis.

Stage IVA — Tumor invades any of the following: upper urethra, bladder mucosa, rectal mucosa, pelvic bone, or bilateral regional node metastasis.

Stage IVB — Any distant metastasis including pelvic lymph nodes.

previously mentioned, the presence of any fistulas must be addressed.

Rarely, subvaginal extension of cervical cancer may involve the urethra. Obstruction, fistula formation, and hematuria can result. Urethroscopy with appropriate biopsies is required. Urethral obstruction can be resolved with either suprapubic drainage or intermittent catheterization.

## Vulvar Cancer
### Background and Staging

Vulvar cancer represents approximately 5% of female genital cancers, although this proportion rises with age. The peak age is 70 years; only 15% of vulvar cancer patients are premenopausal, although this percentage appears to be rising.

Unlike cervical cancer staging, vulvar cancer staging is surgical. Previously, vulvar cancer staging was based on clinical examination alone. The body of evidence confirmed that clinical examination, compared to surgicopathologic staging, is notoriously inaccurate.

Involvement of the urinary tract is an integral component of the vulvar staging system (Box 31-3). Once again, invasion of the urinary tract usually allows for an upstage. Mucosal involvement should be confirmed in these situations.

### Effects on the Urinary Tract

Urinary symptoms rarely arise from vulvar cancer. Less than 10% of patients complain of dysuria. Urethral obstruction secondary to cancer is exceptional. Bladder invasion is usually caused by greatly advanced disease, which may result in incontinence and hematuria. However, other symptoms of vulvar cancer, including pain, discharge, and a mass, usually bring the patient to the attention of a physician.

**Box 31-4**

**FIGO STAGING FOR CARCINOMA OF THE VAGINA**

Stage 0     Carcinoma in situ; intraepithelial carcinoma.
Stage I     Carcinoma is limited to the vaginal wall.
Stage II     Carcinoma has involved the subvaginal tissue but has not extended to the pelvic wall.
Stage III     Carcinoma has extended to the pelvic wall.
Stage IV     Carcinoma has extended beyond the true pelvis or has clinically involved the mucosa of the bladder or rectum; bullous edema itself does not permit a case to be classified as stage IV.
Stage IVA     Spread to adjacent organs or direct extension beyond the true pelvis.
Stage IVB     Spread to distant organs.

**Box 31-5**

**FIGO STAGING FOR CARCINOMA OF THE CORPUS UTERI**

Stage IA     Tumor limited to endometrium.
Stage IB     Invasion to less than one half the myometrium.
Stage IC     Invasion to more than one half the myometrium.
Stage IIA     Endocervial glandular involvement only.
Stage IIB     Cervical stromal invasion.
Stage IIIA     Tumor invades serosa or adnexa, or positive peritoneal cytology.
Stage IIIB     Vaginal metastases.
Stage IIIC     Metastases to pelvic or paraaortic lymph nodes.
Stage IVA     Tumor invasion of bladder or bowel mucosa.
Stage IVB     Distant metastases including intraabdominal or inguinal lymph nodes.

## Vaginal Cancer
### Background and Staging

Vaginal cancer is the rarest female genital cancer. Malignancies that involve the cervix or vulva along with the vagina are not considered vaginal cancer by definition. Because vaginal cancer usually presents in the proximal and distal third of the vagina, it usually involves these structures.

Diethylstilbestrol (DES) exposure has been associated with vaginal adenocarcinoma. Since the discontinuation of DES use, the DES registry has recorded approximately 500 putative cases. Most patients with intrauterine DES exposure do not develop vaginal cancers.

Vaginal cancer staging is clinical, as shown in Box 31-4. Anterior lesions should be a signal to perform cystourethroscopy, including cytologic washings and biopsy of any suspicious lesions. As in the cervical and vulvar staging, involvement of the urinary tract allows upstaging.

### Effects on the Urinary Tract

The central position of the vagina between the vulva and cervix allows for varied presentations when malignancy develops. Upper vault involvement may mimic cervical cancer-related urogenital problems (e.g., ureteral and bladder dysfunction). Evaluation of these problems has been discussed previously. Similarly, lower vaginal malignancy may duplicate the symptoms associated with vulvar cancer. Malignancy involving the midportion of the vagina may simulate either proximal or distal vaginal cancer, depending on spread.

## Ovarian, Fallopian Tube, and Endometrial Cancer

The ovary is one of the five leading cancer sites causing mortality in women. Despite the pelvic location and propensity for intraabdominal spread of ovarian cancer, dysfunction of the urinary tract is uncommon. Occasionally, mass effect of the tumor may compromise bladder capacity and cause ureteral dilation; however, bladder or ureteral mucosal invasion is uncommon. Rarely, ovarian cancer compromises the ureters to the point of renal failure. Unlike in the majority of genital cancer staging systems, urinary tract involvement is not a consideration for staging. Fallopian tube cancer affects the urinary tract in a similar fashion.

Endometrial cancer is the most common female genital cancer in the United States. Early detection with a high index of suspicion has led to a decline in the cancer death rate. Involvement of the bladder mucosa allows for upstaging, as shown in Box 31-5. Symptomatic complaints arising from the urinary tract secondary to the malignancy are unusual unless a large mass is present or there is bladder invasion. If invasion is suspected, evaluation of the urinary tract with cystoscopy and US may be indicated to rule out an obstructive problem.

## UROLOGIC COMPLICATIONS OF SURGICAL THERAPY
### Radical Hysterectomy

Since Professor Wertheim (1912) published his monograph "The Extended Abdominal Operation for Carcinoma Uteri," radical hysterectomy has emerged as the premier technique for treating early stage cervical cancer. With early stage disease, cure rates are excellent: well over 85% 5-year cure rates in selected populations. The procedure is fraught with hazards and pitfalls that may lead to morbidity. Thus, before selecting this option, the surgeon should be experienced with this technically demanding operation.

The incidence of urogenital fistulas, both ureterovaginal and vesicovaginal, after radical hysterectomy had decreased dramatically over the last century. In Wertheim's (1912) series of 500 patients, 32 (6.4%) developed ureterovaginal fistulas and 34 (6.8%) developed postoperative vesicovaginal fistulas. Infection leading to necrosis was believed to be responsible for these complications.

In 1951, Meigs described 280 cases of radical hysterectomy. He reported a rate of ureterovaginal fistulas similar to Wertheim's. The ureterovaginal fistulas were attributed to compromised ureteral blood supply. Noteworthy is the low vesicovaginal fistula rate—only 2 instances in over 280 cases—a tremendous improvement over Wertheim's experience. No explanation was given for these disparate experiences.

Contemporary studies place the vesicovaginal and ureterovaginal fistula rates at approximately 1%. Larson et al. (1987) described 223 patients who underwent radical hysterectomy with pelvic lymphadenectomy. Two patients (0.8%) developed a ureteral fistula, and one developed a ureteral stricture. Other recent studies have documented similar experiences.

Intraoperative recognition and respect for the ureter and bladder are paramount in avoiding a urogenital fistula. The course of the ureter should be visualized directly from its entrance into the pelvis to its termination at the bladder. Therefore, complete familiarity with pelvic anatomy and exposure of the retroperitoneal spaces is mandatory. Injury via avulsion, transection, ligation, crushing, and fulguration must be avoided. The ureter should not be handled directly. Resultant damage to the blood supply may account for subsequent fistula formation. Indirect ("no-touch") handling is attempted in all instances.

A variety of approaches have been used in an effort to avoid fistula formation. Green et al. (1962) attached the ureter to the superior vesical artery. They believed that the artery would act as a stent for the ureter. Avoidance of hypogastric artery ligation has also been proposed as a method of decreasing fistula formation, although confirmatory data concerning efficacy are lacking. A comparison between these two techniques awaits study.

Immediate identification and treatment of intraoperative ureteral injuries yield excellent results. It is easier to correct the damage immediately than postoperatively. Classic teaching divides ureteral repairs into those above and those below the pelvic brim. If a suprapelvic repair is required, direct ureteral anastomosis is attempted, which is facilitated by placement of a ureteral stent. Moreover, a closed suction drain in the abdominal area is recommended. Examples are ureteroureterostomy and transureteroureterostomy.

Ureteroneocystostomy is the usual ureteral repair performed in the pelvis. A nonrefluxing type of anastomosis is recommended. Once again, use of a ureteral splint and closed suction drain for approximately 1 week is indicated. Longer drainage is recommended if the area has undergone irradiation.

If the bladder lumen is violated during surgery, early recognition with adequate repair usually results in an intact bladder. A two-layer closure using fine absorbable suture is indicated in most cases. If the laceration is near a ureteral orifice, cystoscopic evaluation for ureteral patency needs to be confirmed via direct visualization. Judicious passage of ureteral stents should be considered to ensure patency in select cases. Bladder drainage is facilitated with a transurethral or suprapubic catheter for approximately 1 week. A retroperitoneal drain usually is not needed.

The majority of unrecognized ureterovaginal and vesicovaginal fistulas present 1 to 2 weeks postoperatively. Location and identification of the fistulas are essential in subsequent management. Methylene blue, indigo carmine, or preferably sterile milk is instilled into the bladder to determine whether there is a vesicovaginal fistula. If no leak is identified, indigo carmine is given intravenously to determine whether a ureteral-vaginal fistula is present. IVP and cystoscopy also are used to locate the fistula.

Although the patient will want immediate correction, most authorities recommend waiting 3 to 6 months before attempting a repair to allow resolution of any inflammation and infection. An attempt at repair before inflammation resolves is a formula for surgical failure; subsequent repair will prove more difficult.

Several nonsurgical measures may be attempted during this waiting period. Occasionally, these measures alone result in permanent resolution of the problem. The use of bladder drainage may keep dry a patient with a vesicovaginal fistula. A trial of suprapubic or Foley catheter occasionally produces permanent continence because smaller fistulas occasionally heal with simple urinary diversion. The use of prophylactic antibiotics during bladder drainage is controversial because resistant organisms emerge. Treatment of a specific bladder infection is recommended in most cases; however, no study has compared these two approaches in depth.

Retrograde placement of ureteral stents should be attempted in the presence of ureterovaginal fistulas. If cystoscopic guidance is unsuccessful, recent experience suggests that using a ureteroscope occasionally proves successful. This approach also can result in a resolution of this condition, avoiding major surgery.

Persistent fistulas require surgical repair. Vaginal approaches for vesicovaginal repair are usually indicated. Meticulous technique is required; adequate mobilization of local tissue with a layered closure without tension is successful in the majority of cases. Ureterovaginal fistulas require neoureterocystostomy in most instances.

Irradiated patients with vesicovaginal fistulas should be considered for graft placement to provide a fresh blood supply. Common techniques incorporate the omentum or bulbocavernosus muscle. Recurrent or persistent malignancy must be ruled out in these cases.

Bladder dysfunction is the most common complaint after radical hysterectomy. Unfortunately, just as normal micturition itself is not completely understood, the pathophysiology underlying post–radical hysterectomy voiding disorder

**Table 31-2** Bladder Changes After Radical Hysterectomy

| Author | Total bladder capacity | | Bladder compliance | | Residual volume | |
|---|---|---|---|---|---|---|
| | <9 months | >9 months | <9 months | >9 months | <9 months | >9 months |
| Scotti et al. (1986) | NS | NS | ↓ | ↓ | c | ↑ |
| Westby and Asmussen (1985) | NS | NS | c | c | ↑ | NS |
| Farquharson et al. (1987) | ↑ | c | ↓ | c | ↑ | c |
| Vervest et al. (1989) | ↓ | c | ↓ | c | ↑ | NS |
| Forney (1980)* | ↑ | ↑ | c | c | ↑ | NS |
| Low et al. (1981) | c | c | ↓ | ↓ | c | c |
| Carenza et al. (1982)* | ↑ | c | c | c | c | c |

*NS*, No change; *c*, not examined; ↓, decreased; ↑, increased.
*$CO_2$ cystoscopy.

is even less well understood, although several theories attempt to explain the changes.

Neurologic dysfunction secondary to bladder denervation has been proposed as a cause of bladder dysfunction after radical hysterectomy. Originally, Ramon-Lopez and Barclay (1973) suggested parasympathetic overdominance. Nerve regeneration was proposed to explain the resolution of this problem over time in most patients. However, the use of parasympatholytic agents could not correct the dysfunction, indicating involvement of another mechanism.

Forney (1980) implicated sympathetic denervation in postoperative voiding dysfunction. He demonstrated that with partial resection of the cardinal ligament, less than half the patients developed a voiding disorder, whereas almost all patients with complete transection developed a voiding disorder. To strengthen this theory, Photopulos and Vander Zwaag (1991) reported on 102 patients with radical hysterectomy and 21 with modified radical hysterectomy. Although the patients with less extensive radical surgery had less voiding dysfunction, no statistical difference could be demonstrated.

Edema, hematoma, and scar formation also have been postulated as contributing to bladder dysfunction. Seski and Diokno (1977) suggested that the surgical trauma alone adversely affects the detrusor muscle and paravesical tissue via these mechanisms. Resolution of postsurgical trauma accounted for the return to normal voiding.

In summary, the exact reason for the dysfunction is not known. A combination of the previous theories probably represents the cause. Further studies in this area will elucidate the origin of this difficult problem. Several urodynamic studies have examined bladder parameters after radical hysterectomy; most have been consistent (Table 31-2). Postoperatively, in both the short and long term, bladder compliance is decreased and is associated with bladder instability. Increased residual volume, at least in the short term, is also demonstrated. It is initially surprising that total bladder capacity is usually increased after radical hysterectomy when compliance is decreased. However, most patients have decreased bladder sensation

with resultant overdistention, accounting for the increase in bladder capacity.

Because overdistention results in slower bladder recovery, bladder drainage is used routinely. Many different protocols have been suggested to treat this problem, each with advantages and disadvantages. Currently, we teach self-catheterization when the patient is mobile. Once residual volume is less than 50 ml with two consecutive voids, this is discontinued.

Urethral changes after radical hysterectomy have been documented by several urodynamic studies. Early findings include a decrease in functional length, which appears to resolve with time (Table 31-3); however, urethral pressure is adversely affected for a long time. Scotti et al. (1986) commented on 12 patients, 5 of whom developed genuine stress urinary incontinence as documented by urodynamic evaluation. No relationship was demonstrated between the radicality of the procedure and the degree of urethrovesical dysfunction.

Prehysterectomy patient education regarding possible bladder dysfunction after surgery helps alleviate anxiety. The need for prolonged bladder catheterization after radical pelvic surgery generally should be explained to the patient preoperatively.

## Radical Vulvectomy

Vulvar carcinoma has a predilection for the periurethral area. Approximately 50% of vulvar cancers develop within 2 cm of the urethral orifice. Common sites include the labia majora, labia minora, and clitoris. Because most authorities recommend a 2-cm margin of excision around the malignancy, the urethra is commonly in a vulnerable position. A careful, thorough examination of the vulvar area should be performed with every Pap smear and pelvic examination. The physician should not hesitate to perform vulvar biopsies. Early diagnosis, less radical surgery, and a better prognosis are the rewards of this approach.

Historically, under the tutelage of Taussig (1940) and Way (1982), en bloc radical vulvectomy with groin node dissection has been performed routinely for this disease.

**Table 31-3** Urethral Changes After Radical Hysterectomy

| Author | Functional urethral length | | Maximal urethral pressure | |
|---|---|---|---|---|
| | <9 months | >9 months | <9 months | >9 months |
| Scotti et al. (1986) | NS | NS | ↓ | ↓ |
| Westby and Asmussen (1985) | NS | NS | ↓ | ↓ |
| Farquharson et al. (1987) | ↓ | ↓ | c | c |
| Vervest et al. (1989) | NS | c | NS | c |
| Forney (1980)* | c | c | ↓ | ↓ |
| Low et al. (1981) | ↓ | ↓ | ↓ | ↓ |
| Carenza et al. (1982) | ↓ | c | ↓ | c |
| Sasaki et al. (1982) | NS | NS | ↓ | ↓ |

*NS*, No change; *c*, not examined; ↓, decreased.
*$CO_2$ cystoscopy.

These procedures are colloquially called trapezoid, butterfly, or Texas longhorn incisions. Partial urethral resection has been included as an occasional adjunct to this procedure, thus ensuring adequate tumor margins.

The most commonly encountered urinary complication of radical vulvectomy is urine stream misdirection. Reid et al. (1990) described 41 patients who underwent vulvectomy, 27 (65%) of whom complained of significant urine spray. Similarly, of the 58 patients undergoing radical vulvectomy reported by Culame (1980), 17% developed a spraying urine stream. Few reliable options are available to treat this distressing problem. Surgical correction often is unsuccessful. Different appliances resembling funnels have been placed in the urethra to direct flow, but results have not been encouraging. Self-catheterization is another alternative.

Genuine stress urinary incontinence (GSUI) is another major problem. The incidence varies between 5% to 50% as a sequela to vulvectomy. Cystocele, rectocele, and uterine prolapse accompany GSUI in some cases. Patients with preoperative GSUI are particularly at risk. Distal urethral resection increases the incidence and severity of GSUI. Morley (1976) hypothesized that introital enlargement caused by loss of pelvic support along with cicatrization were attributable causes. Unfortunately, few urodynamic studies have been performed in this area. The report by Reid et al. (1990) appears to be the most exhaustive. They examined 21 patients who underwent major vulvar resection and performed preoperative and postoperative urodynamic studies. Bladder urodynamics were unaffected by the surgery. On the other hand, urethral dynamics were adversely affected. A significant decrease in distal urethral pressure was demonstrated in patients with resected urethral tissue. Overall, urethral length and pressure were decreased.

During the last decade, attention has focused on individualizing therapy for patients with vulvar cancer, including performing less radical vulvar surgery to obtain the same cure rate without the resultant morbidity. Using this technique, Burke et al. (1990) reported no urinary dysfunction in their patients. Further experience will determine whether this technique may be expanded to other situations, thereby decreasing the likelihood of developing these urologic complications.

## Pelvic Exenteration

Pelvic exenteration is a last-ditch effort to eradicate genital malignancy. The major indication is recurrent or persistent cervical cancer following therapeutic irradiation. Selected vulvar carcinomas make up the majority of other indications.

There are three major types of pelvic exenteration: total, anterior, and posterior. Total and anterior pelvic exenteration both result in bladder extirpation; therefore, urinary diversion is an integral portion of this operation. Also associated with these procedures is removal of the urethra. A posterior exenteration is rarely indicated or performed.

Two types of urinary diversion are commonly performed today: incontinent and continent, as revolutionized by Bricker in 1950. The ileal conduit remains the standard. Transverse and sigmoid colon conduits are used in some centers. Proponents of the latter two conduits claim lower complication rates than with the ileal conduit.

Jejunal conduits are to be avoided unless no alternatives are available. They are associated with a high incidence of metabolic abnormalities, which include hyponatremia, hyperkalemia, and hyperchloremic acidosis. The length of the jejunum is associated directly with the severity of the electrolyte imbalance.

Increasing familiarity with conduit formation has decreased the immediate postoperative complication rate to approximately 10%. These complications include fistulas, leaks, infection, and ureteral obstruction. Long-term complications include ureteral obstruction and chronic infection, with resultant deterioration of renal function. Current recommendations include evaluation of renal function tests and urinalysis (including culture) at regular intervals. Renal US should be performed to detect ureteral obstruction once or twice a year and when clinically indicated.

Over the last decade, continent urinary diversions have become more popular. The Koch pouch is derived from 80 cm of ileum that has been detubularized and folded, forming a reservoir. Extensive research has demonstrated that a low-pressure reservoir is thereby created, thus preventing damage to the kidneys by back pressure. Reservoir capacity is between 400 and 600 ml, allowing intermittent catheterization every 4 to 6 hours and obviating a stomal bag. Recently, an orthotopic modification has been described that uses salvaged urethral tissue to connect to the reservoir, obviating an abdominal stoma. Numerous modifications and alternative mechanisms have been used, including the Mainz, Indiana, and Miami pouches. Experience with these alternative reservoirs is increasing.

Current recommendations as to which procedure the patient should undergo vary. Urostomy formation should be tailored to each situation. Expertise and familiarity with each procedure, as well as the patient's preference and mental and physical condition, should weigh in the final decision.

## Vaginectomy

Vaginectomy is rarely performed as the sole procedure. Rubin et al. (1985) reported on 15 patients with vaginal carcinoma who underwent surgery for cure. Only 1 patient underwent radical vaginectomy alone. Treatment for vaginal malignancy located in the upper vagina is usually associated with a radical hysterectomy, whereas in the lower vagina, a vulvar excision is commonly included. Barclay (1979) reported on six patients who underwent vaginectomy (partial or total). The reason for therapy was vaginal cancer following hysterectomy for dysplasia. Preoperative and postoperative cystometric studies revealed no bladder dysfunction secondary to denervation. An effort was made during surgery to preserve 2 cm of vaginal epithelium or to place a split-thickness graft adjacent to the urethrovesical junction.

Experience has revealed that colpocleisis places the patient at high risk for developing GSUI. The resulting scarification apparently straightens the urethrovesical junction, resulting in a "leadpipe urethra." Reconstruction of the vagina, usually with split-thickness skin grafts, may help avoid this complication.

## UROLOGIC COMPLICATIONS OF RADIATION THERAPY

Radiation therapy is an important tool in the treatment of genital cancer. The type of irradiation depends on a multitude of factors, including the location, stage, type, and extent of disease. Most clinical experience with radiation therapy is derived from cervical cancer treatment.

The proximate location of the bladder and ureters to the cervix makes these structures particularly vulnerable to the effects of radiation therapy. The advent of afterloading

tandem and ovoids has reduced the incidence of radiotherapy complications. Afterloading allows time for precise application of the tandem and ovoids because sources are added after checking placement. Location of these vulnerable structures is essential after the placement of radiotherapy guides, before source placement. Once radiation therapy is completed, close follow-up is needed to detect any active disease and complications. Vaginal dilators and local estrogen cream should be used when clinically indicated.

Radiation complications are divided into acute and chronic types. Acute radiation complications usually occur near the end of therapy. Field and fraction size are but two factors that affect the severity and number of acute urinary tract complications. Symptoms include frequency, dysuria, and, rarely, hematuria. Patients receiving pelvic radiation appear to have a predilection for a urinary tract infection. Bacteriologic examination of the urine with appropriate treatment is essential. Occasionally, bladder antispasmodics and analgesics are indicated. If symptoms are extreme, a delay in therapy may be necessary.

Chronic radiation complications are more difficult to treat. The total amount of radiation given and fraction size are positively associated with the level of chronic complications. Bladder constriction secondary to radiation fibrosis is particularly troublesome. Nocturia, frequency, and dysuria are common complaints.

One of the few urodynamic studies evaluating the effect of radiation on the bladder and urethra was conducted by Parkin et al. (1988). Symptoms including urgency and frequency were expressed by half the patients. Bladder capacity and volume required for first bladder sensation were 25% lower than in controls. Detrusor pressure was increased to three times that of controls. Functional urethral length and urethral closing pressure were also lower. Estrogen replacement or use was not discussed. The authors concluded that before attributing symptoms to fibrosis, medical management for detrusor instability may be helpful. Furthermore, urinary tract infections should be evaluated and treated appropriately. In their study of 33 patients, Farquharson et al. (1987) concluded that bladder compliance was dose dependent.

Vesicovaginal fistulas develop in fewer than 5% of patients receiving radiation therapy for cervical cancer. Patients with large-volume disease extending along the anterior vaginal wall are particularly susceptible. Cushing et al. (1968) demonstrated that 50% of these patients have viable tumor at the time of vesicovaginal fistula diagnosis. Therefore, it is prudent to perform a biopsy on any fistula site to rule out persistent or recurrent cancer before surgery. Complete evaluation of the urinary system is also required.

Once malignancy is ruled out, repair may ensue. Meticulous preparation of the involved site includes the use of local vaginal creams and douches to clear necrotic debris and decrease inflammation. Successful repair usually includes providing a new blood supply to the affected area.

Sources include the omentum and bulbocavernosus muscle. Hyperbaric oxygen has been used in this setting as well. Further work will determine whether this approach is truly beneficial. Unfortunately, not all fistulas can be repaired and urinary diversion may be indicated.

Ureteral stricture caused by radiation damage alone is rare. Only five cases were discovered by Slater and Fletcher (1971) among 1416 patients treated at the MD Anderson Hospital. McIntyre et al. (1995) reviewed 1784 patients treated with radiation for stage Ib carcinoma of the cervix. Severe ureteral stricture rates were 1%, 12%, 22%, and 25% at 5, 10, 15, and 20 years, respectively. They concluded that tumor recurrence is the most common cause of ureteral stenosis for the first 5 years; radiation-induced ureteral stricture, although rare, may not manifest for years. The majority of strictures are unilateral and located near the ureterovesical junction. Surgical intervention is required in most cases. Ureterolysis alone is usually unsuccessful. Neoureterocystostomy or, rarely, urinary diversion is required in the majority of cases. Recurrent or persistent disease must be ruled out.

## UROLOGIC COMPLICATIONS OF CHEMOTHERAPY

The number of chemotherapeutic agents continues to increase. Recognition of urinary tract side effects associated with each drug is important.

### Cisplatin

Cisplatin is a widely used drug in gynecologic cancer. Extensive experience has shown that renal failure will develop unless therapy is closely monitored. Cisplatin causes renal insufficiency with electrolyte loss, which can become irreversible with continued use. Hydration with resultant increase in renal blood flow during therapy appears to blunt renal damage. Attention to electrolytes, especially magnesium and calcium, is required. Before each chemotherapy course is begun, renal function tests should be obtained. If creatine clearance is less than 60 ml/min, alternative therapies should be considered. The concurrent use of nephrotoxic drugs (e.g., aminoglycosides) should be avoided.

### Cyclophosphamide

Cyclophosphamide (CTX) is used extensively in the treatment of ovarian cancer. The major toxic side effect of the urinary tract is hemorrhagic cystitis. Acrolein, a metabolite of CTX, is believed to be responsible. Direct irritation of the urothelium results and is localized primarily to the bladder. Generous hydration with frequent bladder emptying decreases the incidence and severity of this complication. The use of N-acetylcysteine sulfonate (Mesna) is warranted in patients receiving high-dose CTX. This agent conjugates with acrolein, thereby preventing urothe-

lial irritation without decreasing CTX efficacy. An antidiuretic hormone-type effect secondary to CTX is rarely seen. Close observation of electrolytes and fluids is recommended during administration.

The risk of bladder tumors increases fourfold with CTX. This risk is further elevated with concomitant radiation therapy. Unexplained hematuria should be investigated completely in these settings to rule out bladder cancer.

### Ifosfamide

Ifosfamide is an alkylating agent structurally similar to CTX. Metabolites formed secondary to its use are extremely toxic to the urothelium. Before the advent of Mesna, these side effects prevented the use of this agent. The mechanism of action is similar to that described for CTX. Additionally, high-dose ifosfamide has been associated with renal damage with resultant elevation of serum urea and creatinine. As with CTX, renal function should be closely monitored.

## GYNECOLOGIC CANCER: HEMORRHAGIC CYSTITIS AND ITS TREATMENT

Hemorrhagic cystitis may arise from a constellation of agents or insults. Interestingly, the treatments of female genital cancer are more likely than the disease itself to cause hemorrhagic cystitis. Immediate causes of hemorrhagic cystitis include radical hysterectomy and extrafascial hysterectomy after radiation therapy. Difficult bladder dissection and rough handling of urogenital tissue compound this problem. Meticulous surgical technique with gentle manipulation is required to lessen the chance of this complication. Fortunately, when this scenario is responsible, this complication is mild and resolves spontaneously in most cases.

Another well-known cause of hemorrhagic cystitis is pelvic radiotherapy. Unlike surgical or chemotherapy-induced hematuria, hemorrhagic cystitis caused by irradiation has a delayed presentation. It can occur without warning 1 to 20 years after therapy. Unfortunately, there is no reliable method to determine which patients will develop this complication. Once infection has been ruled out, a search for active malignancy with radiologic imaging techniques and cystoscopy is essential. Cystoscopy allows the immediate fulguration of any observed active bleeding site. The mechanism explaining this hematuria is well described. It is believed to arise secondary to edema, followed by submucosal hemorrhage of the bladder muscle, which causes the epithelium to become friable, leading to spontaneous hemorrhage. The spectrum of hemorrhagic cystitis extends from subclinical to life-threatening.

Chemotherapeutic agents are often implicated as a cause of hemorrhagic cystitis in gynecologic oncology patients. Two prime causative agents are ifosfamide and cyclophosphamide. As previously discussed, the parent compound does not have a direct toxic effect on the urothelium; certain metabolic by-products (e.g., acrolein) are responsible for the development of hemorrhagic cystitis. Hemorrhage develops during or immediately after administration in most cases. The offending agent should be discontinued until an investigation is complete, which includes patient history, physical examination, and renal function tests. It is imperative to rule out an infective cause.

The treatment and evaluation of hemorrhagic cystitis begins with the removal of any bladder clots. This procedure is facilitated by the placement of a large-bore catheter with generous saline irrigation and evacuation. The use of cold fluid for bladder irrigation enhances efficacy. Occasionally, cystoscopic removal of clots is indicated, which also provides an opportunity for fulguration of observed bleeding points. A regimen that includes the removal of clots, irrigation, and treatment of any urinary tract infection is successful in the majority of cases.

Failure to stop bladder hemorrhage with these techniques requires the use of more intensive therapy. Alum has a variable success rate. A 1% solution instilled continuously usually requires less than 24 hours to correct the hemorrhagic cystitis. If it is unsuccessful, silver nitrate is an alternative. A 1% solution is placed in the bladder for 10 to 20 minutes and then removed. Several instillations may be required.

Other chemical means include the use of phenol, $\epsilon$-aminocaproic acid, and formalin. These treatments are associated with severe side effects, including death. Their use is indicated only in severe cases that do not respond to the previously discussed maneuvers. If a hyperbaric chamber is accessible, this treatment may be effective in some cases.

Selective vascular embolization is very effective. It is particularly indicated in the nonoperative patient. Side effects of this procedure include fever, pain, and renal failure caused by radiographic dye use. Bladder necrosis with pain is a described complication. An experienced interventional radiologist is required for this procedure.

Urinary diversion is used once medical therapy has been exhausted without relief. Removing the bladder from the urinary circuit resolves the condition in the majority of cases. The question whether to create a continent or incontinent urostomy should be individually addressed between the patient and her surgeon. Cystectomy is indicated for intractable cases.

## SUMMARY

The field of gynecologic oncology has made rapid progress over the last century. Education, awareness, and better diagnostic tests have allowed for earlier diagnosis in several genital cancers. Improved surgical techniques, higher-energy radiotherapy units, and increasing experience with chemotherapeutic agents have decreased urologic side effects, both during and after treatment. This trend should continue as more progress is made.

## BIBLIOGRAPHY
### Urologic Complications of Surgical Therapy

Ahlering TE, Kanellos A, Boyd SD, et al: A comparative study of perioperative complications with Koch pouch urinary diversion in highly irradiated versus nonirradiated patients, *J Urol* 139:1201, 1987.

Anthopoulos AP, Manetta A, Larson JE, et al: Pelvic exenteration: a morbidity and mortality analysis of a seven-year experience, *Gynecol Oncol* 35:219, 1989.

Barclay DL, Roman-Lopez JJ: Bladder dysfunction after Schauta hysterectomy, *Am J Obstet Gynecol* 123:519, 1975.

Bricker EM: Bladder substituted after pelvic evisceration, *Surg Clin North Am* 30:1511, 1950.

Bricker EM: Current status of urinary diversion, *Cancer* 45:2986, 1980.

Burke TW, Stringer A, Gershenson DM, et al: Radical wide excision and selective inguinal node dissection for squamous cell carcinoma of the vulva, *Gynecol Oncol* 38:328, 1990.

Carenza L, Nobili F, Giacobini S: Voiding disorders after radical hysterectomy, *Gynecol Oncol* 13:213, 1982.

Culame RJ: Pelvic relaxation as a complication of the radical vulvectomy, *Obstet Gynecol* 55:716, 1980.

Farquharson DI, Shingleton HM, Orr JW, et al: The short-term effect of radical hysterectomy on urethral and bladder function, *Br J Obstet Gynaecol* 94:351, 1987.

Fiorica JV, Roberts WS, Greenberg H, et al: Morbidity and survival patterns in patients after radical hysterectomy and postoperative adjuvant pelvic radiotherapy, *Gynecol Oncol* 36:343, 1990.

Forney JP: The effect of radical hysterectomy on bladder physiology, *Am J Obstet Gynecol* 138:374, 1980.

Green TM, Meigs JV, Ulfelder H, et al: Urologic complications of radical Wertheim hysterectomy: incidence, etiology, management and prevention, *Obstet Gynecol* 20:293, 1962.

Henriet MP, Neyra P, Elman B: Koch pouch procedures: continuing experience and evolution in 135 cases, *J Urol* 145:16, 1991.

Kadar N, Nelson JH: Treatment of urinary incontinence after radical hysterectomy, *Obstet Gynecol* 64:400, 1984.

Langmade CV, Oliver JA Jr: Partial colpocleisis, *Am J Obstet Gynecol* 154:1200, 1986.

Larson DM, Malone JM, Copeland LJ, et al: Ureteral assessment after radical hysterectomy, *Obstet Gynecol* 69:612, 1987.

Lee Y-N, Eang KL, Lin M-H, et al: Radical hysterectomy with pelvic lymph node dissection for treatment of cervical cancer: a clinical review of 954 cases, *Gynecol Oncol* 32:135, 1989.

Low JA, Mauger GM, Carmichael JA: The effect of Wertheim hysterectomy upon bladder and urethral function, *Am J Obstet Gynecol* 139:826, 1981.

Meigs JV: Radical hysterectomy with bilateral pelvic lymph node dissections. A report of 100 patients operated on five or more years ago, *Am J Obstet Gynecol* 62:854, 1951.

Mench H, Garfinkel L, Dodd GD: Preliminary report of the National Cancer Data Base, *CA Cancer J Clin* 41:7, 1991.

Monaghan JM, Ireland D, Mor-Yosef S, et al: Role of centralization of surgery in stage IB carcinoma of the cervix: a review of 498 cases, *Gynecol Oncol* 37:206, 1990.

Morley GW: Infiltrative carcinoma of the vulva: results of surgical treatment, *Am J Obstet Gynecol* 124:874, 1976.

Morley GW, Hopkins MP, Lindenauer SM, et al: Pelvic exenteration, University of Michigan: 100 patients at 5 years, *Obstet Gynecol* 74:935, 1989.

Morley GW, Seski JC: Radical pelvic surgery versus radiation therapy for stage I carcinoma of the cervix (exclusive of microinvasion), *Am J Obstet Gynecol* 126:785, 1976.

Narayan P, Broderick GA, Tanagho EA: Bladder substitution with ileocecal (Mainz) pouch. Clinical performance over 2 years, *Br J Urol* 68:588, 1991.

Parker RT, Wilbanks GD, Yowell RK, et al: Radical hysterectomy and pelvic lymphadenectomy with and without preoperative radiotherapy for cervical cancer, *Am J Obstet Gynecol* 99:933, 1967.

Penalver MA, Bejany DE, Averette HE, et al: Continent urinary diversion in gynecologic oncology, *Gynecol Oncol* 34:274, 1989.

Perez CA, Breaux S, Bedwinek JM, et al: Radiation therapy alone in the treatment of carcinoma of the uterine cervix, *Cancer* 54:235, 1984.

Pettersson F, ed: Annual report of the results of treatment in gynecological cancer, ed 22, Stockholm, 1995, Radiumhemmet.

Photopulos GJ, Vander Zwaag R: Class II radical hysterectomy shows less morbidity and good treatment efficacy compared to class III, *Gynecol Oncol* 40:21, 1991.

Ramon-Lopez JJ, Barclay DL: Bladder dysfunction following Schauta hysterectomy, *Am J Obstet Gynecol* 115:81, 1973.

Reid GC, DeLancey JOL, Hopkins MP, et al: Urinary incontinence following radical vulvectomy, *Obstet Gynecol* 75:852, 1990.

Roberts WS, Cavanagh D, Marsden DE, et al: Urinary tract fistulas following ligation of the internal iliac artery during radical hysterectomy, *Gynecol Oncol* 21:359, 1985.

Rotmensch J, Rubin SJ, Sutton HG, et al: Preoperative radiotherapy followed by radical vulvectomy with inguinal lymphadenectomy for advanced vulvar carcinomas, *Gynecol Oncol* 36:181, 1990.

Rubin SC, Young J, Mikuta JJ: Squamous carcinoma of the vagina: treatment complications and long-term follow-up, *Gynecol Oncol* 20:346, 1985.

Sasaki H, Yoshida T, Noda K, et al: Urethral pressure profiles following radical hysterectomy, *Obstet Gynecol* 59:101, 1982.

Scotti RJ, Bergman A, Bhatia NN, et al: Urodynamic changes in urethrovesical function after radical hysterectomy, *Obstet Gynecol* 68:111, 1986.

Seski JC, Diokno AC: Bladder dysfunction after radical abdominal hysterectomy, *Am J Obstet Gynecol* 128:643, 1977.

Shingleton HM, Fowler WC Jr, Pepper ED, et al: Ureteral strictures following therapy for carcinoma of the cervix, *Cancer* 24:7783, 1969.

Soisson AP, Soper JT, Clarke-Pearson DL, et al: Adjuvant radiotherapy following radical hysterectomy for patients with stage IB and IIA cervical cancer, *Gynecol Oncol* 37:390, 1990.

Tarkington MA, Dejter SW, Bresette JF: Early surgical management of extensive gynecologic ureteral injuries, *Surg Gynecol Obstet* 173:17, 1991.

Underwood PB, Wilson WC, Kreutner A, et al: Radical hysterectomy: a critical review of twenty-two years' experience, *Am J Obstet Gynecol* 134:889, 1979.

Vervest HAM, Barents JW, Haspels AA, et al: Radical hysterectomy and the function of the lower urinary tract, *Acta Obstet Gynecol Scand* 68:331, 1989.

Way S: *Malignant disease of the vulva,* Edinburgh, 1982, Churchill Livingstone.

Wertheim E: The extended abdominal operation for carcinoma uteri, *Am J Obstet Gynecol* 66:169, 1912.

Westby M, Asmussen M: Anatomical and functional changes in the lower urinary tract after radical hysterectomy with lymph node dissection as studied by dynamic urethrocystography and simultaneous urethrocystometry, *Gynecol Oncol* 21:261, 1985.

## Urologic Complications of Genital Cancer

Ball HG, Berman ML: Management of primary vaginal carcinoma, *Gynecol Oncol* 14:154, 1982.

Barclay DL: Carcinoma of the vagina after hysterectomy for severe dysplasia or carcinoma in situ of the cervix, *Obstet Gynecol* 8:1, 1979.

Coia L, Won M, Lanciano R, et al: The patterns of care outcome study for cancer of the uterine cervix, *Cancer* 66:2451, 1990.

Crowley AR, Byrne JC, Vaughan ED Jr, et al: The effect of acute obstruction on ureteral function, *J Urol* 143:596, 1990.

Dudley BS, Gershenson DM, Kavanaugh JV, et al: Percutaneous nephrostomy catheter use in gynecologic malignancy: MD Anderson Hospital experience, *Gynecol Oncol* 24:273, 1986.

Frolich EP, Bex P, Nissenbaum MM, et al: Comparison between renal ultrasonography and excretory urography in cervical cancer, *Int J Gynecol Obstet* 34:49, 1990.

Geisler JP, Perry RW, Ayres GM, et al: Ovarian cancer causes upper and lower urinary tract obstruction, *Eur J Gynaecol Oncol* 15:343, 1994.

Henriksen E: The lymphatic spread of carcinoma of the cervix and of the body of the uterus, *Am J Obstet Gynecol* 58:924, 1949.

Koonings PP, Teitelbaum GP, Finck EJ, et al: Case report. Renal artery laceration secondary to percutaneous nephrostomy catheter placement, *Gynecol Oncol* 40:164, 1991.

Lerner HM, Jones HW III, Hill EC: Radical surgery for the treatment of early invasive cervical carcinoma (stage IB): review of 15 years' experience, *Obstet Gynecol* 54:413, 1980.

McClinton S, Richmond P, Steyn JH: Spontaneous extravasation and urinoma formation secondary to cervical carcinoma, *Br J Urol* 64:100, 1989.

Soper JT, Blaszczyk TM, Oke E, et al: Percutaneous nephrostomy in gynecologic oncology patients, *Am J Obstet Gynecol* 158:1126, 1988.

Taussig FV: Cancer of the vulva: analysis of 155 cases, 1911-40, *Am J Obstet Gynecol* 40:764, 1940.

van Nagell JR Jr, Donaldson ES, Gay ER: Urinary tract involvement by invasive cervical cancer. In Buchsbaum HJ, Schmidt JD, eds: *Gynecologic and obstetric urology,* Philadelphia, 1982, WB Saunders.

Webb JAW, Reznek RH, White FE, et al: Can ultrasound and computerized tomography replace high-dose urography in patients with impaired renal function? *Q J Med* 53:411, 1984.

## Urologic Complications of Radiation Therapy

Antonakopoulos GN, Hicks RM, Berry RJ: The subcellular basis of damage to the human urinary bladder induced by radiation, *J Pathol* 143:103, 1989.

Barton DPJ, Morse SS, Fiorica JV, et al: Percutaneous nephrostomy and ureteral stenting in gynecologic malignancies, *Obstet Gynecol* 80:805, 1992.

Boronow RC, Rutledge FN: Vesicovaginal fistula, radiation and gynecologic cancer, *Am J Obstet Gynecol* 111:85, 1971.

Cushing RM, Tovell HMM, Liegner LM: Major urologic complications following radium and x-ray therapy for carcinoma of the cervix, *Am J Obstet Gynecol* 101:750, 1968.

Farquharson DI, Shingleton HM, Sanford SP, et al: The short-term effect of pelvic irradiation for gynecologic malignancies on bladder function, *Obstet Gynecol* 70:81, 1987.

Graham JB, Abad RS: Ureteral obstruction due to radiation, *Am J Obstet Gynecol* 99:409, 1967.

Hartman P, Diddle AW: Vaginal stenosis following irradiation therapy for carcinoma of the cervix uteri, *Cancer* 30:426, 1972.

Lentz SS, Homesley HD: Radiation-induced vesicosacral fistula: treatment with continent urinary diversion, *Gynecol Oncol* 58:278, 1995.

McIntyre JF, Eifel PJ, Levenback C, et al: Ureteral stricture as a late complication of radiotherapy for stage Ib carcinoma of the uterine cervix, *Cancer* 75:836, 1995.

Parkin DE, Davis JA, Symmonds RP: Urodynamic findings following radiotherapy for cervical carcinoma, *Br J Urol* 61:213, 1988.

Prasad KN, Pradhan S, Datta NR: Urinary tract infection in patients of gynecological malignancies undergoing external pelvic radiotherapy, *Gynecol Oncol* 57:380, 1995.

Rhamy RK, Stander RW: Postradiation ureteral stricture, *Surg Gynecol Obstet* 113:615, 1961.

Sklaroff DM, Gnaneswaran P, Sklaroff PB: Postirradiation ureteric stricture, *Gynecol Oncol* 6:538, 1978.

Slater JM, Fletcher GH: Ureteral strictures after radiation therapy for carcinoma of the uterine cervix, *Am J Radiat Ther Nucl Med* 3:269, 1971.

Stryker JA, Bartholomew M, Velkley DE, et al: Bladder and rectal complications following radiotherapy for cervix cancer, *Gynecol Oncol* 29:1, 1988.

Taylor PM, Johnson RJ, Eddleston B, et al: Radiological changes in the gastrointestinal and genitourinary tract following radiotherapy for carcinoma of the cervix, *Clin Radiol* 41:165, 1990.

## Urologic Complications of Chemotherapy

Kaldor JM, Day NE, Kittleman BJ, et al: Bladder tumours following chemotherapy and radiation therapy for ovarian cancers. A case-control study, *Int J Cancer* 63:1, 1995.

Kline Z, Gang M, Venditti JM: Protection with N-acetylcysteine (NAC) against isophosphamide (ISOPH, NSD-10924) host toxicity and enhancement of therapy in early murine leukaemia L1210, *Proc Am Assoc Cancer Res* 13:29, 1972.

Phillips FS, Sternberg SS, Cronin AP, et al: Cyclophosphamide and urinary bladder toxicity, *Cancer Res* 13:29, 1972.

Safirstein R, Winston J, Goldstein M, et al: Cisplatinum nephrotoxicity, *Am J Kidney Dis* 8:356, 1988.

Sutton GP, Blessing JA, Photopulos G, et al: Gynecologic oncology group experience with ifosfamide, *Semin Oncol* 17: 6, 1990.

## Hemorrhagic Cystitis

deVries CR, Freiha FS: Hemorrhagic cystitis: a review, *J Urol* 143:1, 1990.

Godec CJ, Geich P: Intractable hematuria and formalin, *J Urol* 133:956, 1985.

Goel AK, Rao MS, Bhagwat S, et al: Intravesical irrigation with alum for the control of massive bladder hemorrhage, *J Urol* 133:956, 1985.

Primack A: Amelioration of cyclophosphamide-induced cystitis, *J Natl Cancer Inst* 47:223, 1971.

Rubin JS, Rubin RT: Cyclophosphamide hemorrhagic cystitis, *J Urol* 96:313, 1966.

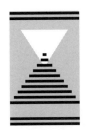

CHAPTER **32**
*The Urinary Tract in Pregnancy*

Edward R. Newton

## ANATOMY AND PHYSIOLOGY OF THE URINARY TRACT IN PREGNANCY

### Anatomy

The kidneys and urinary tract play a major role in maternal adaptation to pregnancy. Consequently, the clinician must understand that observed differences in function cannot be judged by nonpregnant standards (Table 32-1).

The renal system increases in size and capacity during pregnancy. Intravenous pyelograms (IVPs) performed immediately postpartum demonstrate a 1 to 1.5 cm increase in renal length regardless of the size of the individual. Autopsy studies report an average kidney weight of 307 g in pregnant women, compared to 259 g for kidneys in nonpregnant women. The increase in functional demand (a 50% increase in glomerular filtration rate [GFR]) stimulates renal cell hyperplasia and an increase in proximal tube length much like the renal growth that occurs after a unilateral nephrectomy. Additionally, increased water content explains a portion of the increase in the size and weight of the kidney.

The most striking anatomic change in the urinary tract is dilation of the ureters (Fig. 32-1). Bilateral dilation of the calyces, renal pelvis, and ureters can be seen early in the first trimester and is present in 90% of women in the late third trimester or early puerperium. The changes are usually more prominent on the right and may persist for 3 to 4 months. In 11% of women, ureteral dilation persists indefinitely. It is not known whether these patients suffer adverse sequelae, such as persistent asymptomatic bacteriuria from persistent ureteral dilation.

Vesicoureteric reflux is a sporadic, transient occurrence during pregnancy and has been demonstrated radiologically in 7 of 200 (3.5%) pregnant women; the authors felt that this incidence was an underestimate. The enlarging uterus displaces the ureters laterally, and the intravesical ureters are shortened and enter the bladder perpendicularly rather than obliquely. Consequently, the ureterovesical junction is less efficient in preventing reflux. This increased incidence of reflux may explain the high incidence of pyelonephritis during pregnancy; however, only 1 of 23 patients with asymptomatic bacteriuria ($\geq 10^5$ colonies/ml) had reflux. In a population of 321 pregnant and immediate postpartum patients, 24 had a history of pyelonephritis; 15 did not have reflux and 3 of the 9 with reflux had a history of pyelonephritis. In summary, the transitory nature of vesicoureteral reflux and the necessary exposure to x-rays for study purposes hinders adequate evaluation of the problem. Nevertheless, vesicoureteric reflux plays only a small role in symptomatic or asymptomatic urinary tract infection.

The capacity of the urinary tract increases during pregnancy. Bladder volume during pregnancy increases to 450 to 650 ml, compared to 400 ml in nonpregnant controls (see Table 32-1), and the hydronephrotic ureters can hold as much as 200 ml extra urine; however, no changes appear in the contraction patterns on retrograde cystometry. Depending on maternal position, uterine size, and position of the fetus, the functional volume of the bladder and ureters is dynamic in the third trimester. This increased functional volume, coupled with high urine flows (especially with fluid mobilization at night), causes polyuria and nocturia in most pregnant women.

The etiology of ureteral and bladder dilation generates much discussion. Sharp termination of the ureteral dilation at the pelvic brim seen on IVP suggests an obstruction. When a woman is upright or supine, as during the filming of an IVP, the pregnant uterus compresses the ureter against the pelvic rim and its overlying iliac vessels. On the left side, the ureter is somewhat protected by the iliac arteries and sigmoid colon and, as a result, is usually less dilated than the right ureter. Although mechanical obstruction plays a major role in ureteral dilation during pregnancy, the relative infrequency of ureteral obstruction by large ovarian tumors or fibroids in nonpregnant women suggests additional factors. In addition, high urine production, as occurs in diabetes

**Table 32-1** Urologic Symptoms and Measurements in Pregnancy

| | Trimester | | | |
| | First | Second | Third | Postpartum |
| --- | --- | --- | --- | --- |
| Symptom | | | | |
| Frequency | | | | |
| Day ≥7 | 45% | 61% | 96% | 17% |
| Night ≥2 | 22% | 39% | 64% | 6% |
| Incontinence | | | | |
| Stress | 30% | 31% | 85% | 6% |
| Urge | 4% | 13% | 12% | 8% |
| Hesitancy | 24% | 28% | 22% | 9% |
| Measurement | | | | |
| Urine output (ml) | 1917 | 2020 | 1820 | 1475 |
| Bladder capacity (ml) | 410 | 460 | 272 | 410 |
| Functional urethral length (mm) | — | $30.3 \pm 4.6$ | $35.1 \pm 5.1$ | $27.6 \pm 3.7$ |
| Bladder pressure (cm $H_2O$) | — | $9 \pm 3$ | $20 \pm 3$ | $9 \pm 2$ |
| Closure pressure (cm $H_2O$) | — | $61 \pm 14$ | $73 \pm 18$ | $60 \pm 14$ |

Data from Francis WJA: *J Obstet Gynaecol Br Commonw* 1960a, b; Iosif et al: *Am J Obstet Gynecol* 13:696, 1980; Stanton et al: *Br J Obstet Gynaecol* 87:897, 1980.

insipidus or pregnancy, is also associated with urinary tract dilation.

In the past, the elevated progesterone levels that accompany pregnancy were thought to cause smooth muscle relaxation and subsequent hypotonicity and hypomotility of the ureter, defects that would contribute to ureteral dilation. Contrary to the latter observation, the large doses of synthetic progesterone used in cancer chemotherapy do not cause ureteral dilation. Measurements of ureteral tone during pregnancy reveal an increase in ureteral tone and no decrease in frequency or amplitude of ureteral contractions. Histologic study of the ureters of pregnant animals reveals smooth muscle hypertrophy and hyperplasia of the connective tissue. Thus, progesterone probably plays a small role in ureteric dilation during pregnancy.

## Physiology

The kidneys play a fundamental role in adaptation to pregnancy through regulation of body fluids. During pregnancy, the average healthy gravida accretes 6 to 8 liters of total body fluid, 950 mEq sodium, 2350 mEq potassium, and 400 ml red cell volume. Soon after conception, plasma osmolarity and thirst threshold fall to a level 10 mOsm/kg below the mean for nonpregnant women (Table 32-2). In nonpregnant women, this drop would shut off antidiuretic hormone (ADH) secretion, but in pregnancy the lower level of osmolarity is maintained and women dilute and concentrate their urine appropriately. In fact, ADH levels are higher in pregnant than in nonpregnant women.

The blood volume in a normal, singleton pregnancy increases from $2.38 \pm 0.11$ L/M$^2$ (nonpregnant) to $3.44 \pm 0.2$ L/M$^2$ (37 to 40 weeks' gestation). The most pronounced effect of these changes is a 30% to 50% increase in glomerular and effective renal plasma flow (ERPF). Fig. 32-2 depicts the changes in creatinine clearance by trimester. It is not clear whether the change results from a primary renal event or is secondary to peripheral vasodilation. An increase in blood volume occurs within a week or two of conception; however, the normal fall in mean arterial pressure occurs later in the second trimester of pregnancy. Late in pregnancy, a supine or a sitting position is associated with decreased ERPF, GFR, sodium excretion, and urine flow.

On the surface, pregnancy appears to create a natriuretic state by producing a 50% increase in GFR and an additional 5000 to 10,000 mEq of filtered sodium, which must be reabsorbed; increased progesterone values (blood levels are 10 to 100 times higher in pregnancy) that cause natriuresis; increased levels of natriuretic hormones such as ADH; and physical factors such as decreased plasma albumin (decreased plasma oncotic pressure) and decreased vascular resistance (increased ERPF).

These natriuretic influences are opposed and, in fact, exceeded by the accretion of 950 mg of sodium through several mechanisms: increased levels of renin, angiotensin, and aldosterone; increased concentrations of other salt-retaining hormones such as estrogen, cortisol, placental lactogen, and prolactin; and physical factors such as decreased mean arterial pressure (decreases ERPF), increased ureteral pressure, and an exaggerated antinatriuretic response to upright positions in pregnant women.

The elevated concentrations of renin, prorenin, angiotensin I, angiotensin II, and aldosterone seen in pregnancy would create severe hypertension, edema, and hypokalemia in the nonpregnant woman. Fortunately, the normal pregnant woman is highly resistant to the pressor effects of infused angiotensin. This resistance occurs early and seems specific to angiotensin II; response to other pressors remains unaltered.

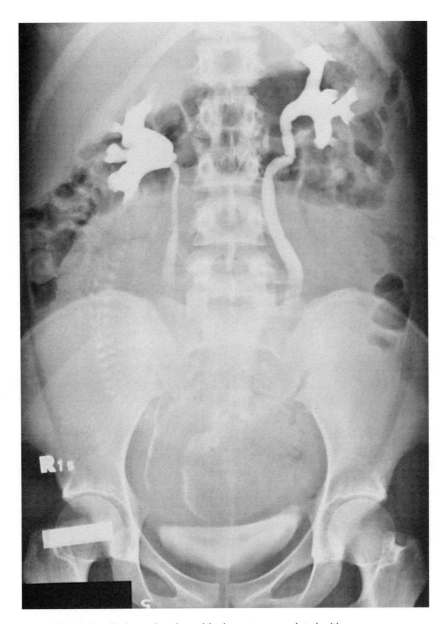

**Fig. 32-1** Hydronephrosis and hydroureter associated with pregnancy.

Interestingly, the decidua produce high concentrations of prorenin and renin, and production of these two hormones is enhanced by progesterone. The physiology of decidual renin is an area of active investigation. It is tempting to associate decidual renin production with the regulation of blood flow to the uterus and fetoplacental unit.

The expansion in blood volume affects the oxygen-carrying capacity of the blood. There is a rapid expansion of the plasma volume (1250 to 1500 ml), with most of the increase occurring before 32 to 34 weeks. On the other hand, red cell mass increases from 1400 (nonpregnant) to 1800 ml (pregnant and receiving iron supplements), with the maximum being reached at 40 weeks. During the second trimester, the increase in plasma volume relative to red cell mass creates a physiologic anemia of pregnancy. During pregnancy, a hemoglobin below 10 g/dl or a hematocrit below 30% is considered abnormal and warrants investigation and intervention.

The kidney is the major source of erythropoietin. Increased levels of erythropoietin are recognized in the first trimester and reach a maximum of 31 ± 16 mU/ml. This response correlates well with the physiologic anemia of pregnancy. Renal disease may limit erythropoietin production, and chronic, unresponsive anemia during pregnancy may be the initial symptom of that disease.

The characteristic increases in blood volume and subsequent increases in GFR result in clinically important laboratory values. These changes can be classified into two basic categories: findings resulting from increased clearance and urinary findings associated with a lowered renal threshold for reabsorption. These changes are included in Table 32-2.

**Table 32-2** Diagnostic Indices* for Renal Disease in Pregnancy: Normal Values

|  | Pregnant | Nonpregnant |
|---|---|---|
| **Blood** | | |
| Bicarbonate (mEq/L) | 17-22 | 24-30 |
| Arterial pH | 7.40-7.45 | 7.38-7.44 |
| BUN (mg/dl) | 4-12 | 10-18 |
| Uric acid (mg/dl) | 2.6-3.4 | 2.6-6.6 |
| Creatinine (mg/dl) | 0.4-0.9 | 0.6-1.2 |
| Creatinine clearance (ml/min) | 89-222 | 46-136 |
| Osmolarity (mOsm/kg) | 275-285 | 275-295 |
| Albumin (g/dl) | 3.0-4.5 | 3.5-5.0 |
| Hematocrit (%) | 32-42 | 37-48 |
| Renal threshold for glucose (mg/dl) | 121-189 | 188-200 |
| **Urine** | | |
| Protein (mg/24 hr) | 0-300 | 0-150 |
| Alanine (μmol/24 hr) | 673-2093† | 101-429 |
| Glycine (μmol/24 hr) | 2216-7560† | 614-2014 |
| Phenylalanine (μmol/24 hr) | 46-152† | 0-77 |

*95% confidence intervals.
†Third trimester.

## URINARY TRACT DISEASES IN PREGNANCY

Diseases of the urinary tract and kidneys constitute a major portion of obstetric complications and may be classified as infection, renal disease, and urologic disease.

### Urinary Tract Infection
#### Pathophysiology

During their lives, 15% to 20% of women will suffer one or more urinary tract infections. The physiologic changes of pregnancy increase the likelihood of symptomatic upper urinary tract disease, resulting in maternal and fetal morbidity and, occasionally, mortality. In fact, urinary tract infections are one of the most common medical complications of pregnancy (Table 32-3). Thus, an understanding of the pathogenesis, clinical presentation, diagnosis, therapy, and prognosis is essential.

Although bloodborne organisms (e.g., staphylococcal bacteremia) may occasionally infect the renal parenchyma, the most common route of infection is ascension up the urinary tract. Female anatomy and behavior set the stage for inoculation of the bladder. The urethra is in close proximity to the vagina and rectum; both are fertile reservoirs for uropathogens. Indeed, the presence of Enterobacteriaceae at the vaginal vestibule is a predictor of asymptomatic bacteriuria. Pumping action by intravaginal coitus or urethral massage allows inoculation of the bladder.

Inoculation of the bladder does not always lead to colonization or symptomatic disease. Host-parasite interactions determine the likelihood of infection. The presence or absence of bacterial virulence factors may explain why some women with asymptomatic urinary tract infection go on to develop symptoms. These factors have been best defined for *Escherichia coli,* the most common uropathogen, and include increased adherence to uroepithelial cells, high quantities of K-antigen, the presence of aerobactin, and hemolysin production. Of these, adhesive properties seem to be the most important. *E. coli* pyelonephritis isolates adhere to uroepithelial cells better than do *E. coli* cystitis isolates, and urinary isolates tend to adhere better than do random fecal *E. coli* isolates. This adhesive capacity is mediated by the presence of adhesions on the bacterial cell surface. Often these adhesions are pili or fimbriae. Pili or fimbriae bind to the β-globoseries glycolipid receptors on the surface of the uroepithelial cells.

In nonpregnant women, 10% to 20% of *E. coli* strains isolated from patients with cystitis or asymptomatic bacteriuria express P-fimbriae. On the other hand, 80% to 90% of strains isolated from acute, nonobstructive, pyelonephritis express P-fimbriae. Recently, the same pattern has been shown in pregnant women.

Usually, the normal urinary tract resists colonization by bacteria and rapidly and efficiently eliminates microorganisms that gain access to the bladder. Urine has antibacterial activity, extremes in osmolarity, high urea concentrations, and low pH levels that inhibit the growth of uropathogens. However, pregnancy makes the urine more suitable for bacterial growth by increasing pH and normalizing osmolarity.

The flushing mechanism of the bladder adds an additional protective effect. The bladder mucosa has an active antiadherence mechanism. A surface mucopolysaccharide, glycosaminoglycan, inhibits bacterial adherence. As a result, the bacteria remain in suspension and are more easily flushed out with urination. The impact of pregnancy on these mechanisms is unclear.

### Diagnosis

The diagnosis of urinary tract infection has been based on the landmark studies by Kass (1956) and Elder et al. (1971) at Boston City Hospital. In a population of asymptomatic pregnant and nonpregnant women, a bacterial colony count of $\geq 10^5$ colony-forming units (cfu) per milliliter in two or more clean-catch midstream urine specimens reliably distinguished infection from contamination. Ten percent to 20% of pregnant women with an initial positive culture have a second negative culture within a week, even without antibiotic therapy. Furthermore, 95% of patients with clinical pyelonephritis have persistent positive cultures at $\geq 10^5$ cfu/ml. Since these studies, most clinicians have used the criterion of $10^5$ cfu/ml on a clean-catch midstream urine specimen to diagnose urinary tract infection. However, this criterion has not proven to be sufficiently predictive in nonpregnant women with acute dysuria or infections with fastidious organisms, or in catheterized patients.

Suprapubic or urethral aspiration of urine has been used to prevent vaginal contamination. In a series of classic articles, Stamm et al. (1982, 1989) demonstrated the

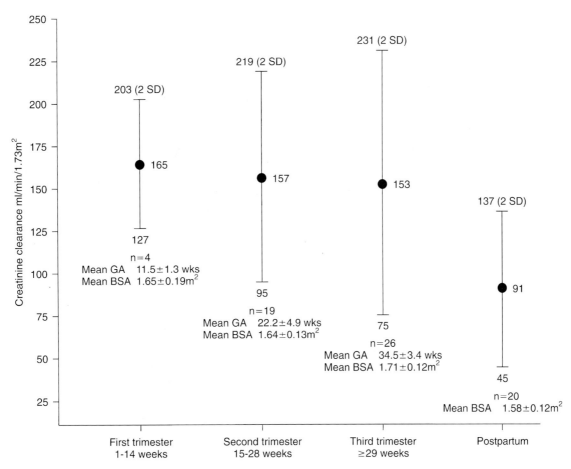

**Fig. 32-2** Changes in creatinine clearance during pregnancy, by trimester. *BSA,* Body surface area; *GA,* gestational age.

**Table 32-3** Incidence of Urinary Tract Infection During Pregnancy

| Infection | Incidence (%) |
|---|---|
| Asymptomatic bacteriuria | 2-11 |
| Acute cystitis | 1-2 |
| Acute pyelonephritis | 1-5 |

following in acutely dysuric nonpregnant women: the correlation between midstream urine (MSU) colony counts and bladder bacteria (by suprapubic or urethral aspiration) was 0.78; in women who were dysuric and whose bladders contained coliform bacteria, approximately 50% have MSU $<10^5$ cfu/ml; and an MSU with $\geq10^2$ cfu/ml predicted most accurately a positive culture by bladder aspiration (sensitivity 0.95 and specificity 0.85). In contrast, an MSU with $\geq10^5$ cfu/ml had a sensitivity of 0.51 and a specificity of 0.99; pyuria ($\geq8$ leukocytes/mm$^3$) on an unspun MSU specimen was highly sensitive (0.91) but not specific (0.5); over one half of women have an MSU culture positive for more than one organism; and 48% of patients with more than one

organism isolated on MSU, "a contaminated urine," have coliform $\geq10^2$ cfu/ml on bladder or urethral aspiration.

Using the criterion of $\geq10^5$ cfu/ml, the urine culture cannot be viewed as a precise quantitative assay. The lack of precision results from several causes, including the following: the type or stage of the disease (e.g., asymptomatic bacteriuria versus clinical pyelonephritis); obstructions or abnormalities of the urinary tract; perinephric abscess; urolithiasis; acidification of the urine; hydration and diuresis; polyuria; collection methods (e.g., MSU versus suprapubic aspiration); transport, storage, or culture methods; and fastidious organisms.

Many women harbor fastidious organisms in their genitourinary tracts, which have been identified only through suprapubic aspiration or specialized microbiologic techniques. Stamm et al. (1982) found that 37% of nonpregnant women with sterile pyuria have *Chlamydia trachomatis* in their genitourinary tracts. Slowly growing fastidious bacteria were isolated from urine obtained by bladder aspiration in 10% to 15% of asymptomatic pregnant women. *Gardnerella vaginalis* and *Ureaplasma urealyticum* are the most common additional bacteria. The isolation of fastidious organisms such as *G. vaginalis* and *U. urealyti-cum* seems to be more common in patients with suspected renal disease (70%) than in normal pregnant women (26%).

Asymptomatic bacteriuria with aerobic organisms has been associated with adverse pregnancy outcome. Many of the preceding fastidious organisms in the vagina or cervix are also associated with adverse pregnancy outcome and, at least with group B streptococcus, a urinary tract infection is more often associated with adverse pregnancy outcome than is vaginal colonization alone. It is tempting to speculate that urinary tract infections with fastidious organisms may also predict adverse pregnancy outcome, but neither the correlation between vaginal and urinary tract colonization nor the correlation between fastidious organisms in the urinary tract and adverse pregnancy outcome has been studied.

The classic criterion of $\geq 10^5$ cfu/ml for diagnosing urinary tract infection is challenged in catheterized women. Stark and Maki (1984) demonstrated that 96% of patients with low levels of coliform bacteriuria ($<10^5$ cfu/ml) progressed to $\geq 10^5$ cfu/ml within 3 days if they did not receive antibiotics and remained catheterized. Although these observations help with the interpretation and management of positive urine cultures in catheterized patients, the questions of who and when to sample the urine in catheterized patients remain unanswered.

Urine cultures delay definitive diagnosis, are expensive ($50 to $70), and require microbiologic technology. Thus, culture-independent diagnostic tools have appeal. The most commonly used tests include microscopic examination of urine, measurement of leukocyte esterase and nitrite, filter isolation of bacteria and white blood cells, and screening for bioluminescence.

For years, the technique for rapid diagnosis has been microscopic examination of the urine. A Gram stain is performed by placing a drop of uncentrifuged urine on a slide. A positive Gram stain is $\geq 3$ bacteria per oil immersion field (1000× magnification). The sensitivity (84% to 94%) and specificity (68% to 97%) of this technique in predicting a culture positive at $10^5$ cfu/ml compare favorably to those of other newer tests. In addition, the Gram stain and examination of unstrained urinary sediment after centrifugation can identify the most probable pathogen (e.g., gram-negative rods) and the presence of upper urinary tract disease (e.g., white cell casts). The test takes about 5 minutes to perform and costs very little ($.20).

The least expensive and least labor-intensive of the other rapid tests is the test for nitrite and leukocyte esterase, Chemstrip LN (Biodynamics; Indianapolis, Indiana). The plastic dipstick contains patches of color-responsive reagents that identify esterase and nitrite. The test takes 2 minutes to perform and costs approximately $.25 per test. At a threshold of $\geq 10^5$ cfu/ml, the leukocyte esterase-nitrite strip has a sensitivity of 60% to 100% and a specificity of 60% to 98%. At a threshold of $\geq 10^3$ cfu/ml, the strip has a sensitivity of 52% to 73% and specificity of 68% to 83%.

**Table 32-4** Culture-Independent Tests for Urinary Tract Infections

| Test | Prevalence of $\geq 10^5$ cfu/ml | | | | | |
|------|------|------|------|------|------|------|
| | 5% | | | 50% | | |
| | PP+ | PP− | FN | PP+ | PP− | FN |
| Gram stain | 14 | 99 | 1 | 76 | 80 | 20 |
| Leukocyte esterase/nitrite | 22 | 99 | 1 | 84 | 81 | 19 |
| Filter test | 14 | 99 | 1 | 75 | 88 | 12 |
| Bioluminescence | 33 | 99 | 1 | 83 | 94 | 6 |

Gram stain: sensitivity 90%, specificity 75%.
Leukocyte esterase/nitrite: sensitivity 80%, specificity 85%.
Filter test: sensitivity 90%, specificity 70%.
Bioluminescence: sensitivity 95%, specificity 90%.
*PP+*, Positive predictive value; *PP−*, negative predictive value; *FN*, false negative.

The filter isolation test, Bac-T-Screen (Marion Laboratories, Inc, Kansas City, Missouri), uses an instrument ($2000) to filter 1 ml of urine. The attached bacteria and sediment (white blood cells) are stained and decolorized. The residual stain is proportional to the amount of bacteria and number of white blood cells in the urine. The test can be performed in 2 to 3 minutes and costs $.85 per test. At a culture threshold of $\geq 10^5$ cfu/ml, the Bac-T-Screen has a sensitivity of 85% to 96% and a specificity of 38% to 81%. At a culture threshold of $\geq 10^3$ cfu/ml, the sensitivity is 74% and specificity is 78%.

The bioluminescence tests (e.g., 3M LUMAC [Biocounter, 3M Company, St Paul, Minnesota]) are based on the principle that bacteria and mammals have distinct adenosine triphosphate (ATP) that can be destroyed selectively. After destruction of mammalian ATP, bacterial ATP can be detected by the bioluminescence produced in the firefly luciferin-luciferase reaction. The test takes about 30 minutes to produce a result, and the instrument costs $9000. The price of the reagents is approximately $1.60 per test. At a culture threshold of $\geq 10^5$ cfu/ml, the test has a sensitivity of 93% to 99% and a specificity of 81% to 96%. At a culture threshold of $\geq 10^4$ cfu/ml, the test has a sensitivity of 88% to 95% and a specificity of 81% to 95%.

The essential question is whether culture-independent tests are sufficiently robust to replace or enhance urine culture in the diagnosis of urinary tract infection. Table 32-4 depicts the efficiency of culture-independent tests at common prevalences of urinary infection at $\geq 10^5$ cfu/ml: 5% to reflect the prevalence of asymptomatic bacteriuria in pregnancy and 50% to reflect the prevalence of positive culture in women with dysuria. A false-negative rate of 6% to 20% with the culture-independent tests does not qualify them to supplant urine culture; however, many clinicians recommend that acutely dysuric nonpregnant women be treated without a culture. In pregnancy, the acutely dysuric women should always have a culture because 10% to 15% of positive cultures have group B streptococcus, an organism that predicts adverse pregnancy outcome.

**Box 32-1**

## CONDITIONS THAT PLACE PATIENTS AT HIGH RISK FOR URINARY TRACT INFECTIONS DURING PREGNANCY

Diabetes
Sickle cell disease or trait
Urinary tract abnormalities
Müllerian duct abnormalities
Renal disease
Urolithiasis
Hypertensive diseases
Chronic analgesic use
Genitourinary group B streptococcus
History of urinary tract infections
Severe ureteral reflux
Urinary infections as a child less than 4 years old

**Table 32-5** Microbiology of Urinary Tract Infections in Pregnancy

| Organism | Percentage |
|---|---|
| *E. coli* | 60-90 |
| *K. pneumoniae-Enterobacter* | 5-15 |
| *Proteus* sp. | 1-10 |
| *Streptococcus faecalis* | 1-4 |
| Group B streptococcus | 1-4 |
| *Staphylococcus saprophyticus* | 1-11 |

At a prevalence of 2% to 10%, as is seen in asymptomatic bacteriuria during pregnancy, the positive predictive values of culture-independent tests drop precipitously in both theory (Table 32-4) and practice and should not be used for diagnosis. On the other hand, the negative predictive value is 98% or more with any of these tests. In a low-risk population, urine testing for leukocyte esterase and nitrite on a clean-catch, first-void midstream specimen can supplant urine culture. In high-risk groups (Box 32-1), a culture should be obtained each trimester.

### Asymptomatic Bacteriuria

A combination of host defense inefficiency, anatomy, behavior, and microbial virulence factors identifies a cohort of women who will have episodes of bacteriuria throughout their lifetimes. Cross-sectional prevalence studies identify 1% to 8% of women with asymptomatic bacteriuria. In longitudinal studies, 30% to 50% of nonpregnant women with bacteriuria have symptomatic lower tract infections during 3 to 5 years of follow-up. Most episodes cluster over a 3- to 4-month period followed by an asymptomatic interval of variable length. Nine to 19-year follow-up studies on 60 asymptomatic bacteriuric schoolgirls (6 to 10 years old) were compared with studies on 38 nonbacteriuric control schoolgirls matched for age, race, and school. Episodes of bacteriuria in the 5-year study period for infected girls and controls were 5 or more episodes, 22% and 3%, and episodes during pregnancy, 64% and 27%, respectively. Interestingly, the children of bacteriuric women were more likely to have urinary tract infections than were the children of controls.

Twenty percent to 30% of women who are bacteriuric during pregnancy will be bacteriuric on long-term follow-up cultures when not pregnant. Radiologic examination at follow-up of women who were bacteriuric during pregnancy

revealed abnormalities in 316 (41%) of 777 women (range, 5% to 75%). Chronic pyelonephritis was the most common radiologic diagnosis (47% of abnormalities). The incidence of bacteriuria during first pregnancies was significantly greater in women with (47%) than without (27%) renal scarring from childhood urinary infections. Similar controls who had not had childhood urinary infections had an incidence of 2%.

The cohort of women with chronic, episodic bacteriuria is identified by routine screening of urine cultures at the first prenatal visit. The prevalence of asymptomatic bacteriuria (two or more cultures at $\geq 10^5$ cfu/ml) is increased by prior renal or urinary tract disease, diabetes, sickle cell trait or disease, poor hygiene, high parity, increased age, and lower socioeconomic status. The overall prevalence varies between 1.9% and 11.8%, with the lowest prevalence in primiparous patients of the upper socioeconomic class and the highest among indigent multiparas. Although most women with asymptomatic bacteriuria are identified shortly after entering prenatal care, approximately 1% to 2% acquire bacteriuria later in pregnancy.

The microbiology of urinary tract infections in pregnancy is summarized in Table 32-5. The predominant organism is *E. coli,* and the identification markers and virulence traits from strains isolated from pregnant women with pyelonephritis do not differ significantly from those found in strains isolated from nonpregnant women with pyelonephritis. The pyelonephritic *E. coli* strains and strains from asymptomatic bacteriuria or cystitis patients differed in resistance to serum antibodies (83% versus 51%, $P < 0.05$) and epithelial adherence (63% versus 19%, $P < .001$).

The isolation and concentration of organisms other than gram-negative rods depend on preparation (cleansing the urethral orifice), collection methods (midstream versus suprapubic aspiration), and selective medium (Todd-Hewitt broth for group B streptococcus). Although *E. coli* and other gram-negative rods are associated with pyelonephritis during pregnancy, other organisms may be important in other adverse pregnancy outcomes. A large study that uses modern, comprehensive microbiologic techniques is needed to relate specific urinary tract pathogens to pregnancy outcome.

Uncomplicated, asymptomatic bacteriuria is a significant health risk for pregnant but not nonpregnant women.

Asymptomatic bacteriuria has been associated with pyelonephritis, preterm birth, growth retardation, hypertension, and fetal neuropathology. The most consistent association is a greater likelihood of pyelonephritis. Sweet (1977) reviewed the relationship between asymptomatic bacteriuria and acute pyelonephritis. In 1699 patients with untreated asymptomatic bacteriuria (18 studies), pyelonephritis developed in 471 (27.8%, range 16% to 65%). In addition, placebo-controlled trials demonstrated a significant reduction (80%) in the frequency of pyelonephritis in asymptomatic bacteriuria that had been treated with antibiotics. The incidence of pyelonephritis in the treated groups ranged from 0 to 5.3%. On the basis of these observations, treatment of asymptomatic bacteriuria in pregnancy is warranted to reduce the incidence of pyelonephritis.

The association between preterm birth and asymptomatic bacteriuria was first identified by Elder, Kass, and others at Boston City Hospital between 1955 and 1960. As is true of many early studies, prematurity was defined as a birthweight of 2500 grams or less, a definition that would include 30% to 50% of growth-retarded term infants. His initial study reported that 32 of 179 (17.8%) bacteriuric patients delivered low-birthweight (LBW) infants, whereas 88 of 1000 (8.8%) nonbacteriuric patients delivered LBW infants. Since that report, many studies of small numbers and heterogenous populations have both supported and rejected this observation. Sweet and Gibbs (1990) reviewed 19 studies that related bacteriuria to LBW infants. In these studies, 3619 bacteriuric pregnant women delivered 400 (11%, range 4.4% to 23%) LBW infants. In these same studies, 31,277 nonbacteriuric women delivered 2725 (8.7%, range 3% to 13.5%) LBW infants. Some cohort studies designed to adjust for socioeconomic demographic variables failed to show a difference in LBW between women with and without asymptomatic bacteriuria. Perhaps asymptomatic bacteriuria is not associated with LBW per se, but is a marker for low socioeconomic status that does predict LBW.

On the other hand, when confounding variables are controlled, a strong relationship between asymptomatic bacteriuria and LBW remains. In 1989, Romero et al. reported on the relationship between asymptomatic bacteriuria and LBW. A meta-analysis was performed to increase the statistical power for primary and secondary outcome variables and to improve estimations of the effect of sample size treatment trials. Previous cohort, case-controlled, and randomized antibiotic trials, many of which were also reviewed by Sweet (1977), were analyzed for comparable and appropriate study design. Seventeen cohort studies met their criteria. The typical relative risk for a nonbacteriuric woman to deliver a LBW infant as compared to a bacteriuric woman was 0.65 (95% confidence interval 0.52, 0.72). One case-controlled study compared the prevalence of bacteriuria in women delivering at less than 36 weeks (33/404, 8.1%) to the prevalence of bacteriuria in women delivering

at 37 or more weeks (15/404, 3.7%; $P = 0.0036$) after matching for maternal race, age, parity, smoking habits, physical dimensions, and sex of the newborn infant. Eight randomized clinical trials of antibiotic therapy showed a significant reduction in the frequency of LBW after antibiotic therapy (typical relative risk of 0.56, with a 95% confidence interval of 0.43, 0.73). These analyses support the hypothesis that untreated asymptomatic bacteriuria is directly associated with a higher incidence of LBW. It is unclear whether the benefit from antibiotics results from a reduction in asymptomatic or symptomatic pyelonephritis or from beneficial changes in abnormal genital tract flora, which are associated with LBW.

The association between asymptomatic bacteriuria and other adverse pregnancy outcomes (hypertension, anemia, chronic renal disease, and fetal neuropathology) is controversial, being both supported and refuted by different cohort studies. Small sample size and heterogenous populations contribute to the conflicting results. Most studies are retrospective and fail to identify and control preexisting risk factors (e.g., prior obstetric or smoking history). Additionally, the portion of the population with prior renal disease or current renal involvement is not identified or controlled.

Renal involvement in urinary tract infections is determined by fever and costovertebral angle tenderness (acute pyelonephritis), elevated C-reactive protein or erythrocyte sedimentation rate, decreased renal concentration capacity, or the identification of renal bacteriuria by ureteral catheterization, bladder washout, or fluorescent antibody tests for antibody-coated bacteria. Between 25% and 50% of pregnant women with asymptomatic bacteriuria have evidence of asymptomatic renal involvement, and these women are twice as likely to relapse within 2 weeks after therapy as women with bladder bacteriuria alone.

Perhaps women with asymptomatic renal parenchymal involvement may be at higher risk for other adverse pregnancy outcomes. Harris et al. (1976) found that 35 of 70 of women with asymptomatic bacteriuria ($\geq 10^5$ cfu/ml) had asymptomatic renal infection caused by antibody-coated bacteria. Asymptomatic renal infection was associated with decreased creatinine clearance, intrauterine growth retardation, and maternal hypertension.

On the other hand, Gilstrap et al. (1981b) failed to note a difference in outcomes between asymptomatic women with and without renal infection, as defined by fluorescent antibody testing (Table 32-6). Two hundred forty-eight women with asymptomatic bacteriuria were compared with patients without bacteriuria who were matched for age, race, parity, and gestational age at enrollment. Forty-six percent of bacteriuric women had renal infections. Complication rates in women with asymptomatic renal infection were similar to those in women without renal infection and matched nonbacteriuric controls.

A variety of antimicrobial agents and treatment regimens have been used to treat asymptomatic bacteriuria during

**Table 32-6**  Consequences of Asymptomatic Renal Infection

| | Renal infection | | Bladder infection | |
|---|---|---|---|---|
| | Bacteriuria $n = 114$ | Control $n = 114$ | Bacteriuria $n = 134$ | Control $n = 134$ |
| Preeclampsia | 12% | 15% | 15% | 14% |
| Hematocrit <30% | 2.6% | 2.6% | 3.7% | 1.5% |
| Delivery <37 wk | 4% | 14% | 13% | 12% |
| Small for gestational age | 8% | 6% | 8% | 10% |

Adapted from Gilstrap LC et al: *Am J Obstet Gynecol* 141:709, 1981.

pregnancy. Most community-acquired pathogens associated with asymptomatic bacteriuria during pregnancy are sensitive to sulfa drugs (sulfisoxazole 1 g qid × 10 days), nitrofurantoin (100 mg qid × 10 days), or cephalosporins (cephalexin 500 mg qid × 10 days). Ampicillin (500 mg qid × 10 days) is a time-honored, safe, and inexpensive therapy; however, there are a growing number of resistant *E. coli* strains. Other antibiotics must be used.

Patient education should accompany any prescription for antibiotics to treat urinary tract infection. The essentials of behavior intervention include the following: Avoid the female superior position during sexual activity; avoid anal intercourse before vaginal intercourse; void within 15 minutes after sexual activity; avoid bubble baths and oils; avoid vaginal douching or deodorant sprays; and always wipe the perineum, urethra, and anus from front to back. These interventions reduce the frequency of recurrent urinary tract infections in high-risk women.

Fihn and Stamm (1985) reviewed 62 treatment trials for uncomplicated urinary tract infections to assess whether methodologic problems compromised the validity of the study. These trials fulfilled an average of 56% of 12 standards necessary for accurate interpretation and comparability. The standards least often met were sufficient power to detect a meaningful difference (21%), double-blind assignment of treatment regimens (37%), and clear definitions of cure and failure (35%). Those deficiencies were especially true when comparing single versus multiple-dose therapy. None of 14 randomized controlled trials had sufficient power to prevent a type II error. In fact, when roughly comparable studies were pooled, single-dose amoxicillin (3 g) was significantly less effective than was conventional multidose therapy (69% versus 84%). Until a larger study is performed, single-dose therapy should not be used in the treatment of urinary tract infections in pregnancy.

Antibiotics sterilize the urine in asymptomatic bacteriuria in 60% to 90% of women. The cure rate depends on compliance, length of regimen, preexisting risk factors, asymptomatic renal infection, and the sensitivity of the organism. A test of cure by culture within 2 weeks after the end of the antibiotic regimen discriminates between relapse and reinfection.

Relapse (a positive test-of-cure culture) has been associated with complicated asymptomatic bacteriuria. These women may have urinary tract abnormalities, asymptomatic renal infection, or silent urolithiasis. Unusual organisms or antibiotic sensitivity patterns alert the clinician to a reservoir of partially protected bacteria, (e.g., renal abnormality, urolithiasis, or noncompliance). A urine pH above 6.0 (*Proteus* sp.) and persistent hematuria are clues for an infection-related stone. During pregnancy, a renal ultrasound will help identify a renal stone as a cause for relapse. A postpartum IVP is warranted in any case of relapse. Relapse should be treated with another 10-day course of antibiotics chosen by the sensitivity pattern from the test-of-cure culture. The therapeutic regimen should be followed by suppressive therapy.

Suppressive antibiotic therapy is effective in reducing recurrent cystitis in nonpregnant women and recurrent pyelonephritis in pregnant women. The prophylactic efficacy depends on nightly bactericidal activity against sensitive reinfecting bacteria entering the bladder urine. Vaginal colonization with uropathogenic Enterobacteriaceae continues unabated, depending on the regimen chosen. The rectal reservoir for potential uropathogens is rarely sterilized by therapeutic or prolonged suppressive regimens. One danger of suppressive therapy is the emergence of antibiotic-resistant strains. High-dose (500 mg qid) cephalexin, but not low-dose cephalexin (250 mg qid), induces resistant *E. coli* strains.

Nitrofurantoin macrocrystals (100 mg qhs) neither reduce the prevalence of Enterobacteriaceae in rectal or periurethral flora nor induce antibiotic resistance. Trimethoprim 40 mg plus sulfamethoxazole 200 mg qhs reduces the incidence of Enterobacteriaceae in rectal and periurethral flora, but it is also not associated with antibiotic resistance, although Lincoln et al. (1970) reported resistant urinary infections resulting from sulfonamide suppression therapy.

In motivated patients, a combination of patient education and urine testing biweekly for leukocyte esterase and nitrite is just as effective as prophylactic antibiotic suppression in reducing the incidence of recurrent pyelonephritis after an initial episode during pregnancy. The incidence of recurrent pyelonephritis in the antibiotic suppression group was 7% versus 8% in the close surveillance group. The latter surveillance regimen may be further enhanced by antibiotic prophylaxis (nitrofurantoin macrocrystals, 100 mg, or cephalexin monohydrate, 500 mg) after each episode of sexual intercourse or masturbation.

### Acute Cystitis

Acute cystitis occurs in 0.3% to 2% of pregnancies. The reported frequency is only minimally greater than the frequency of cystitis in sexually active nonpregnant women. Unfortunately, the diagnosis is more difficult to make during pregnancy. Most pregnant women have urgency, frequency, or suprapubic discomfort. Suprapubic discomfort in pregnancy often results from pressure from the presenting fetal part or early labor. Nevertheless, suprapubic discomfort from cystitis is unique, and most women with a history of acute cystitis can discriminate accurately between cystitis and pregnancy-related discomfort. The most reliable findings are dysuria and hematuria. Acute dysuria may also result from labial or perivaginal irritation from vaginitis, vulvitis, herpes simplex, condylomata acuminatum, or genital ulcers. Because of the separate pregnancy risks encumbered with these factors, an inspection of the vulva and vagina is warranted in patients with acute cystitis during pregnancy.

Preterm labor and threatening second trimester loss often present with signs and symptoms similar to those of acute cystitis. As the lower uterine segment expands and the presenting fetal part descends, hesitancy, urgency, frequency, and suprapubic discomfort occur. A bloody vaginal discharge may contaminate and confuse urine testing and may lead to misdiagnosis of urinary tract infection. Pelvic examination is warranted in patients presenting with signs and symptoms of lower urinary tract infection to rule out preterm labor.

The pathophysiology of acute cystitis is more similar to that of asymptomatic bacteriuria than that of pyelonephritis. Acute cystitis has sociodemographic and behavioral risk factors similar to those of asymptomatic bacteriuria. Enterobacteriaceae, especially *E. coli,* are the most common uropathogens. Acute cystitis is associated with a high prevalence of uropathogens in the periurethral flora. *E. coli* serotypes are associated with more epithelial cell adherence, hence virulence, than are fecal strains. Antibody-coated bacteria, indicative of renal infection, is present in only 5% of acute cystitis, compared to 45% for asymptomatic bacteriuria and 65% for acute pyelonephritis. This difference may result from earlier identification and treatment of the patient in these latter conditions because of the intense discomfort that accompanies cystitis.

Treatment of acute cystitis is similar to that of asymptomatic bacteriuria: nitrofurantoin 100 mg qid × 7 days, a cephalosporin 500 mg qid × 7 days, or a sulfonamide 1 g qid × 7 days. Because these patients are symptomatic, therapy is initiated as soon as a midstream, clean-catch urine culture has been obtained. A test-of-cure culture is obtained within 2 weeks after therapy is complete. Between 10% and 20% have a positive test-of-cure culture, representing a relapse. These women should be retreated with another antibiotic, as determined by bacterial sensitivities. After retreatment, these patients should be placed on suppressive antibiotic therapy. Without suppressive therapy, an additional 20% to 30% of women develop another urinary tract infection—a reinfection—during the remainder of their pregnancies and puerperia. Because of the risk of recurrence, patients with cystitis should be followed intensively with a urine screen biweekly for nitrite and leukocyte esterase.

The delivery process includes a significant risk period for symptomatic urinary tract infections. Trauma to the urethra, periurethra, and labia creates swelling and pain that inhibits frequent and complete voiding. Multiple vaginal examinations and the pumping action of the fetal head in the second stage inoculate the urine with periurethral flora. Urinary retention is exacerbated by epidural anesthesia and perineal trauma. Interventions such as simple in-and-out catheterization to relieve urinary retention pose a 10% to 15% risk of bacteriuria. As a result, 10% to 25% of all pyelonephritis associated with pregnancy occurs in the first 14 days postpartum.

### Acute Pyelonephritis

Acute pyelonephritis is the most common serious medical complication of pregnancy. The modern incidence of pyelonephritis is 1% to 5%. Often these patients present for prenatal care late in pregnancy with the signs and symptoms of pyelonephritis. Only 40% to 67% of pyelonephritis occurs in patients with a known history of asymptomatic bacteriuria. Three fourths of women with pyelonephritis present in the antepartum period, 5% to 10% in labor, and 15% to 20% postpartum. Antepartum pyelonephritis occurs mainly after the first trimester: 10% to 20% during the first trimester, 45% to 70% during the second trimester, and 8% to 45% during the third trimester. The predominance of pyelonephritis in late pregnancy and the puerperium relates to the partial obstruction caused by the growing uterus and to trauma or interventions at birth.

The diagnosis of acute pyelonephritis is based on clinical presentation: temperature ≥38° C, costovertebral angle (CVA) tenderness, and either bacteriuria or pyuria. Among patients meeting these criteria ($n = 656$), 12% had temperatures ≥40° C; CVA tenderness was on the right side in 54%, on the left side in 16%, and bilateral in 27%. Chills and back pain were a presenting complaint in 82% of patients, whereas only 40% had dysuria, frequency, urgency, or hematuria. Twenty-four percent had nausea and vomiting.

Enterobacteriaceae cause a majority of the cases of pyelonephritis: *E. coli,* 72% to 90%; *Klebsiella-enterobacter* spp., 5% to 23%; and *Proteus* sp., 2% to 4%. Blood cultures are positive in 15% of cases. Infection of the kidney has a profound effect on function. About 50% of patients have an endogenous creatinine clearance 100 ml/min/1.73 $M^2$ or less and 20%, 70 ml/min/1.73 $M^2$ or less. Twenty percent have a serum creatinine above 1 mg/dl. This dysfunction is a direct result of endotoxic injury to both kidneys. After appropriate antibiotic treatment, renal function returns to normal by 3 to 8 weeks.

Endotoxins produced by Enterobacteriaceae have adverse consequences on multiple organ systems as well as the kidneys. The injuries include thermoregulatory instability (fever and chills), destruction of blood cells (leukocytopenia, thrombocytopenia, anemia), hypercoagulability (disseminated intravascular coagulation), endothelial injury (adult respiratory distress syndrome), cardiomyopathy (pulmonary edema), and myometrial irritability (preterm labor).

Overt septic shock or adult respiratory distress syndrome occurs in 1% to 2% of pregnant women with acute pyelonephritis. Clinical clues to the development of these life-threatening complications are leukocytopenia (<6000 cells/ml$^2$), hypothermia (≤35° C), elevated respiratory rate, and widened pulse pressure. In the late stages, hypothermia, mental confusion, and symptomatic hyperstimulation of the sympathetic nervous system (cold, clammy extremities) herald a scenario that often leads to maternal or fetal death. In all cases, the mother and fetus should be treated in facilities having the expertise and equipment to handle critically ill mothers and infants.

All pregnant women with pyelonephritis should be hospitalized because of the additional fetal and maternal risks of acute pyelonephritis in pregnancy. Intravenous antibiotics (cefazolin 2 g IV q6h, ampicillin 2 g plus sulbactam 1 g IV q6h, cefamandole 2 g IV q8h, or mezlocillin 4 IV q6h) should be initiated as soon as possible after urine and blood cultures are obtained. Because many patients are dehydrated because of nausea and vomiting, careful rehydration is started. The degree of endothelial damage in the lungs may not be apparent, so careful attention to fluid intake and output and vital signs, especially respiratory rate, is imperative. Respiratory symptoms (e.g., an increased respiratory rate), peripheral cyanosis, or mental confusion prompt an immediate radiographic study and measurement of arterial blood gases. Colloid oncotic pressure and serum albumin measurements are important in the fluid management of these critically ill patients.

Endotoxins stimulate cytokine and prostaglandin production by decidual macrophages and fetal membranes. The ensuing preterm contractions raise concern for preterm birth. Three major problems confront the physician at this point. First, although pyelonephritis is often a clear diagnosis, the presence of lower abdominal pain and contractions raises the possibility of intraamniotic infection, a diagnosis that precludes tocolytic therapy. The presence of white blood cells and bacteria on an unspun Gram stain of amniotic fluid is sufficiently sensitive in the diagnosis of intraamniotic infection to preclude the use of tocolysis. Second, premature contractions do not necessarily indicate labor. Often uterine irritability ceases after hydration and administration of antibiotics. On the other hand, if contractions are of sufficient frequency and strength to change the cervix on serial pelvic examinations (≥2 cm in dilation, ≤1 cm in length and ≥50% effacement), the diagnosis of preterm labor is made. Third, preterm labor must be treated with an appropriate tocolytic agent if no other contraindication to tocolysis is present (e.g., intraamniotic infection, fetal lung maturity, fetal abnormalities, or rupture of membranes). Ritodrine hydrochloride, the only tocolytic approved by the Food and Drug Administration, exacerbates the cardiovascular effects of endotoxemia. The risk of

pulmonary edema, cardiac toxicity, and adult respiratory distress is increased. Magnesium sulfate (4 g IV slow bolus, followed by 2 to 4 g/hr) is the tocolytic of choice. However, serum magnesium levels (≤10 mEq/L) and physical signs of toxicity (loss of deep tendon reflexes) are especially important to follow because one half of patients with acute pyelonephritis have renal dysfunction.

Maternal hyperthermia (≥38.3° C) should be aggressively treated with antipyretics such as acetaminophen. Maternal hyperthermia, hence fetal hyperthermia (an additional 0.5° C), increases the metabolic demand of the fetus. Glucocorticoids should not be used to enhance fetal lung maturity because they may exacerbate maternal infection.

Eighty percent to 90% of patients become afebrile within 48 hours, an additional 5% to 15% by 72 hours, and 5% to 10% are classified as initial treatment failures. In patients with a significant deterioration of their condition after the first 18 hours of therapy or in patients with temperatures above 38° C at 48 hours of therapy, gentamicin, 1.5 mg/kg every 8 hours, should be added. The dosing frequency is lengthened for serum creatinine above 1.0 mg/dl (8 × serum creatinine). Antibiotic therapy should be continued until the patient is afebrile (<37° C) for more than 24 hours. The patient should finish a 14-day course of antibiotics with oral medication (nitrofurantoin, 100 mg qid or cephalosporin, 500 mg qid). A test-of-cure urine culture should be performed 2 weeks after therapy. Reinfection is common in these patients; 20% have asymptomatic bacteriuria and 23% have recurrent pyelonephritis. Frequent surveillance (nitrite/leukocyte esterase testing biweekly) or suppressive antibiotic therapy (nitrofurantoin, 100 mg qhs) is warranted. With either regimen the risk of recurrent pyelonephritis is less than 10%.

The differential diagnosis in patients with persistent fever and CVA tenderness at 72 hours of therapy includes a resistant organism, urolithiasis, renal abscess, complete ureteral obstruction, or another source of infection (e.g., appendicitis or intraamniotic infection). A radiologic evaluation of the urinary tract is warranted after reexamination of the patient and review of culture and sensitivity reports. Many radiologists have undue concern regarding the fetal dangers of IVPs during pregnancy and advocate renal ultrasound. A renal ultrasound is useful for evaluating renal abscess, but not for evaluating function or ureteral abnormalities, the more common issues associated with antibiotic failure. A "one-shot" IVP (no plain film and one 20-minute film) is appropriate (Fig. 32-3).

## Renal Disease in Pregnancy

A wide variety of diseases and injuries can occur in the kidneys and urinary tract during pregnancy. The diagnosis and management of renal disease is unchanged, except for the recognition of four principles of medical care during pregnancy.

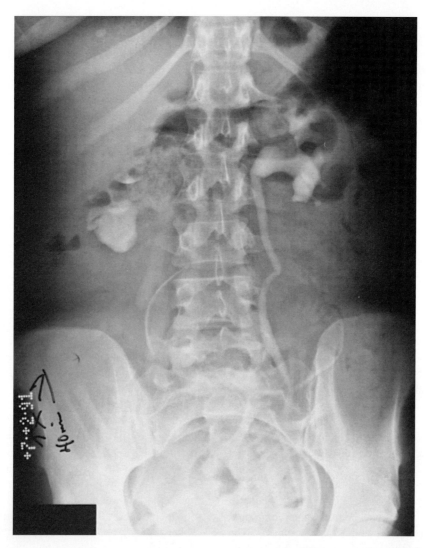

**Fig. 32-3** One-shot IVP can be used to examine the kidneys and ureters in pregnant women with pyelonephritis who do not respond to appropriate antibiotic therapy.

- No ordinarily performed radiologic examination should be withheld if the results will change management and if less invasive techniques (e.g., ultrasound) will not give the clinician as reliable or valid information. A delay in radiologic study until after 13 weeks' gestation and limited use of fluoroscopy are prudent.
- The clinician must remember the fetus is his or her patient. Any disease or procedure has the potential for fetal compromise or early delivery. If delivery occurs at a medical center with certified maternal-fetal medicine and neonatal specialists, intact survival is common (>50%) after 25 weeks or at least 750 g birthweight. Consultation with a maternal-fetal medicine specialist is usually prudent.
- The fetus is remarkably tolerant to noxious drugs after the first trimester; however, each medication should be scrutinized for fetal effects and risk must be weighed against the benefits to the mother.

- Hypertension is a major manifestation of renal parenchymal disease, especially in pregnancies in which antecedent renal disease increases the risk of pre-eclampsia, abruptio placentae, fetal growth retardation, and fetal death.

## Urologic Disease

Five areas of urologic disease deserve closer scrutiny: urolithiasis during pregnancy, delivery in patients who have had previous urologic surgery, complete obstruction by a gravid uterus, renal transplant, and urologic injuries during delivery.

### Urolithiasis

Urolithiasis occurs in 0.03% to 0.5% of pregnancies, usually in the last two trimesters. Between 30% and 60% of women with urolithiasis during pregnancy have a history of urolithiasis. Although pregnancy does not appear to increase the risk of urolithiasis over any 9-month period in susceptible persons, recurrent urolithiasis may indicate primary renal disease (medullary sponge kidney), transport diseases (renal tubular acidosis), or metabolic diseases (hyperparathyroidism). The fetal or maternal risk may reflect these systemic diseases rather than urolithiasis alone.

Most stones (70%) pass in the second or third trimester, with equal distribution between the right and left sides. The presentation is more obscure during pregnancy, the most common signs being severe flank pain, nausea, and vomiting. Renal colic is less common after the first trimester because of ureteral dilation. Likewise, gross hematuria is less common, but microscopic hematuria occurs in 60% to 90% of cases.

The differential diagnosis includes premature labor, appendicitis, and, most commonly, pyelonephritis. Premature labor is diagnosed by contractions and cervical dilation. Urolithiasis is more likely than appendicitis when the patient has no fever, the abdominal pain is not localized to the right lower quadrant, and no peritoneal signs are present. The most difficult differentiation is between pyelonephritis and urolithiasis. Indeed, they may coexist.

IVP is the diagnostic technique of choice. In pregnancy, the protocol and frequency of IVP are curtailed. The IVP should be limited to a 20-minute film and, if there is delayed excretion, a 60-minute film. Fluoroscopy is used only in very exceptional circumstances. An IVP is indicated when the patient has renal colic and gross hematuria, persistent fever or a positive culture after 48 hours of parenteral antibiotic therapy, persistent nausea and vomiting after 48 hours of conservative therapy, or evidence of a complete obstruction (e.g., increasing levels of blood urea nitrogen and serum creatinine).

Transabdominal or transvaginal ultrasound often is the first diagnostic choice of radiologists. Their concern is the 0.4 to 1 rad of radiation the fetus would receive with a limited IVP. There is concern that doses this low may double childhood cancer rates. Although ultrasound is a good diagnostic tool for renal abnormalities and ureteral dilation, its sensitivity is 34%, with an 86% specificity for the detection of an abnormality in the presence of a stone in a symptomatic patient. IVP is clearly more efficacious for diagnosis of distal stone.

Urolithiasis in pregnancy is treated conservatively with bed rest, hydration, and analgesics. Seventy percent of patients pass the stone spontaneously. Urolithiasis during pregnancy does not increase the likelihood of abortion, prematurity, or hypertension, but the incidence of symptomatic urinary tract disease is higher in pregnancies complicated by a history of urolithiasis (20% to 65%). Parenteral antibiotics (cefazolin 2 g IV q6h) are added to conservative management when infection is likely.

When conservative management is unsuccessful (complete obstruction, persistent pain, or sepsis), surgical intervention is indicated. The choice of procedure depends on the size and location of the stone. The usual procedures include basket extraction or retrograde stent placement at cystoscopy. Percutaneous nephrostomy under ultrasound guidance also has been used as a temporizing procedure. Rarely and with considerably more fetal and maternal morbidity, ureterolithotomy, pyelolithotomy/pyelotomy, or partial nephrectomy can be performed. Extracorporeal lithotripsy has gained popularity in the management of renal calculi outside pregnancy, but its safety during pregnancy has not been established. This technique should not be used in pregnancy until more information is available.

## Previous Urologic Surgery

An increasing number of women are becoming pregnant who were born with urinary tract abnormalities that were corrected surgically. These operations include urinary diversion procedures (ileal conduit and ureterosigmoidostomy), augmentation cystoplasty, and ureteral reimplantation for vesicoureteral reflux. The changes in pelvic anatomy caused by the enlarging uterus create the potential for infection, obstruction, and trauma at cesarean section.

Pregnancy in patients with a urinary diversion is complicated by premature delivery, 20% to 50%; symptomatic urinary tract infections, 15%; urinary obstruction, 10%; and intestinal obstruction, 10%. Cesarean delivery should be reserved for obstetric indications, except for ureterosigmoidostomy. In this case, the integrity of the anal sphincter must be preserved and cesarean delivery is indicated.

In the past 20 years, the treatment of patients with abnormal urinary tracts has changed from cutaneous diversion to continent internal diversion with the popularization of intermittent catheterization and augmentation cystoplasty. These operations include vesical neck reconstruction or artificial sphincter placement and may place the patient at risk for the development of incontinence after vaginal delivery.

Hill et al. (1990) reviewed 15 pregnancies in 15 women after augmentation cystoplasty. Eight of 13 were continent before, during, and after pregnancy. One patient who was continent before delivery became incontinent after vaginal delivery. Four patients became incontinent during the last trimester, but regained continence postpartum. The pregnancies were complicated by urinary tract infections (60%), preterm labor (20%), and urinary obstruction (7%). Five cesarean deliveries were performed, three electively for vesical neck or artificial sphincter construction. One cesarean operation was complicated by extensive anterior uterine adhesions. Although stretching of the mesentery by the enlarging uterus has the potential risk of vascular compromise, this complication was not seen among the 15 patients.

Ureteral reimplantation has been performed routinely for severe primary vesicoureteral reflux for many years. Austenfeld and Snow (1988) reviewed 64 pregnancies in 34 women after ureteroneocystostomy for primary reflux. The overall infection rate before pregnancy was 48%. During pregnancy, 57% experienced a urinary tract infection.

Pyelonephritis was more common during pregnancy (17%) than before pregnancy (4%). Eight of the 64 pregnancies were lost between 9 and 21 weeks, and six were associated with a urinary tract infection. The authors did not report the route of delivery and the difficulty of cesarean section.

The latter reviews of pregnancies in women with urinary tract surgery suggest the following obstetric management: close monitoring for preterm labor (patient education, frequent office visits, frequent pelvic examinations); suppressive antibiotic therapy (nitrofurantoin 100 mg qhs); monthly blood urea nitrogen and serum creatinine evaluation; vigilance for ureteral obstruction; vaginal delivery except for obstetric indications and patients with urinary diversion to the sigmoid and bladder neck/sphincter surgery; and urologic consultation at cesarean section for patients with a history of complex urologic surgery, especially augmentation cystoplasty.

### Urinary Tract Obstruction by Gravid Uterus

Occasionally, the enlarging uterus completely obstructs both ureters and causes azotemia. Risk factors for obstruction include previous urologic surgery, unilateral absence of a kidney, polyhydramnios, multiple gestation, and ovarian or uterine neoplasia. Patients usually present in the third trimester with flank pain and minimal signs of infection. The differential diagnosis includes pyelonephritis, renal calculi, or papillary necrosis. Serum creatinine is elevated (3.8 to 11.6 ml/dl) but urinary sediment does not indicate intrinsic renal disease or prerenal azotemia. The diagnosis is confirmed by IVP or renal ultrasound.

Ultimately, delivery relieves the obstruction and postpartum recovery is complete. In cases remote from term, fetal risk from preterm delivery outweighs the risks of urologic management. In one case, conservative management with decubitus positioning and bed rest resulted in an immediate increase in urine output (36 ml/hr to 200 ml/hr) and a fall in serum creatinine (from 6.6 mg/dl to 2.0 mg/dl) after 60 hours of hospitalization. Conservative management for 12 to 24 hours is warranted before more aggressive therapy is initiated, including amniocentesis (in cases with polyhydramnios), cystoscopically placed ureteral stents, or percutaneous nephrostomy under ultrasound guidance.

### Pregnancy and Chronic Renal Disease

Pregnancy occurs in 1 in 200 women of reproductive age on dialysis and 1 in 50 women of childbearing age after renal transplantation. This high incidence is secondary to the increased risk of pregnancy after correction of the woman's metabolic disorders. There is progressive loss of ovulatory function as chronic renal failure progresses. Once the serum creatinine rises above 2.0 mg/dl, serum prolactin increases and ovulation frequency drops progressively. Irregular bleeding and prolonged amenorrhea become more common. Pregnancy rarely occurs in patients who have a creatinine above 3.5 mg/dl. Once dialysis or renal transplantation

occurs, menstrual function returns in 4 to 6 months. Often, the need for contraception is not recognized by the nephrologist or patient, and the pregnancy comes as a surprise. This is reflected in the high incidence of therapeutic abortion (30%) in pregnancies after correction of their metabolic dysfunction. The surprise pregnancy places enormous strain on the woman. Misinformation and faulty opinion are provided by friends, family, co-workers, medical office support people, and, often, physicians. A key role of care providers is to realistically present the risks of dialysis or renal transplantation for mother and baby.

All women of childbearing age need specific counseling regarding family planning as they progress through the late stages of renal failure. Pregnancy should be planned because the risks are high. The most optimal results occur when pregnancy occurs 2 to 5 years after transplantation; it is not complicated by hypertension, diabetes, or lupus nephropathy; there is no pelvicaliceal distention on recent abdominal or pelvic ultrasound or intravenous urogram; renal function is stable, with serum creatinine below 1.5 mg/dl; proteinuria is below 300 mg/24 hours; there is no evidence of rejection; and stable doses of immunosuppressive drugs (prednisone, <15 mg/day; azathioprine, <2 mg/kg body weight; cyclosporine A, 5 mg/kg/day) are given.

Both hemodialysis and peritoneal dialysis have been used in pregnancy. There is greater experience with hemodialysis because it lends itself to easier long-term use. Peritoneal dialysis is useful as a temporary intervention (e.g., as therapy for a drug overdose, acute renal failure during pregnancy, end-stage renal failure during pregnancy, or kidney rejection during pregnancy). Chronic ambulatory peritoneal dialysis has significant advantages over hemodialysis: a more constant biochemical and extracellular environment for the fetus, less need for heparinization, higher maternal hematocrits, and less frequent hypotensive episodes.

During pregnancy all patients on dialysis require a 50% increase in the hours and frequency. Dialysis management during pregnancy has several goals: maintain plasma urea levels below 17 mmol/L to prevent polyhydramnios and fetal death, hypotension during dialysis (supine hypotension of pregnancy exaggerates this risk), and rapid fluctuations of intravascular volume by limiting the interdialysis weight gain to 1 kg; allow rigid control of hypertension; and allow careful control of calcium levels.

Anemia is an invariable problem with chronic renal failure and dialysis. Thirty-five percent of pregnant patients on dialysis require blood transfusion because they have an subnormal physiologic response to red cell volume expansion during pregnancy. The goal is to maintain the hematocrit above 30%. Erythropoietin therapy may be a useful adjunct.

Despite more frequent dialysis, uncontrolled dietary intake should be discouraged. The recommended daily oral intake includes 70 g protein, 1500 mg calcium, 50 mmol potassium, and 80 mmol sodium. Prenatal vitamins with at least 800 µg folic acid should be started 2 months preconceptually. Vitamin D and calcium supplementation is problematic in patients with secondary hyperthyroidism or after thyroidectomy. A consult with a nutritional specialist is helpful.

Patients with renal disease are at risk (30% to 50%) for preeclampsia/eclampsia; preexisting hypertension exacerbates that risk. The diagnosis of preeclampsia may be very difficult in a woman with chronic renal failure and dialysis. Preexisting hypertension is common, and frequent dialysis controls the blood pressure temporarily. Preeclampsia should be suspected when systolic and diastolic blood pressures are consistently more than 30 mm Hg and more than 15 mm Hg above baseline, respectively. Increasing proteinuria is to be expected with the normal increases in renal blood flow during pregnancy (40%), but rapidly progressive and massive increases in protein on 24-hour urine collections raise the possibility of preeclampsia. Thrombocytopenia or elevated liver function tests may be the result of superimposed preeclampsia and should be investigated aggressively.

Despite the outward appearance of deteriorating function (hypertension and worsening proteinuria), pregnancy does not change the progression of renal disease. The fetal risks of dialysis during pregnancy are affected by the underlying cause of the renal failure (i.e., diabetes or lupus, pregnancy history, and prepregnancy hypertension). Overall, the fetal prognosis is poor. There is an excessive risk of spontaneous abortion and perinatal death. When elective abortion is excluded, the live birth outcome is less than 20%. Of fetuses that survive past 20 weeks' gestation, fetal growth restriction complicates 50%, especially in the presence of hypertension or preeclampsia.

Since 1958, renal transplantation has become increasingly more common among women of childbearing age. The current rate of pregnancy among women of childbearing age is about 1 in 50, and the incidence may be increasing. Contraception and family planning are critically important in the pretreatment discussion of dialysis or renal transplantation. Among pregnancies complicated by renal transplantation, 40% do not go beyond the first trimester through elective abortion (20%) and spontaneous abortion (20%). Although immunosuppressive drugs would be expected to increase the risk, there does not seem to be a clinically significant increase in ectopic pregnancy or spontaneous abortion when superimposed risks (i.e., diabetes or lupus) are controlled. On the basis of survey data of 2309 pregnancies among renal transplant recipients who had reached at least 28 weeks' gestation, 49% had major complications and 92% had a successful obstetric outcome (71% if complications developed before 28 weeks); 12% had infants with long-term problems.

The major maternal issues related to pregnancy after renal transplantation include renal dysfunction, anemia,

hypertension or preeclampsia, maternal infection, osteodystrophy, and surgical issues. Despite the trauma of transplantation, the kidney responds to pregnancy, with an increase in GFR proportional to the degree and speed of immediate posttransplant recovery of function. Although transient decreases in GFR often occur in the third trimester in these patients, 85% of women have return of function to baseline status. This 15% decline in function over a 1-year period is related more to the natural history of renal transplants than to pregnancy itself. Some degree of chronic rejection occurs in all allograft transplants. Transient proteinuria occurs in 40% of renal transplant recipients during pregnancy. Renal function is measured throughout pregnancy with monthly renal chemistries and 24-hour urine collection for protein and creatinine clearance.

During pregnancy and the first 3 months after delivery, acute rejection occurs in 9% to 11%, an incidence no greater than the incidence in nonpregnant transplant recipients followed for a year. Rejection is heralded by fever, oliguria, elevated renal function tests, renal enlargement, and tenderness. Because many complications of pregnancy can mimic allograft rejection (preeclampsia, pyelonephritis, intraamniotic infection), the differential diagnosis must include these diagnoses. Although it is associated with greater risk during pregnancy (increased blood flow), a renal biopsy may be necessary. Serial renal ultrasounds may add diagnostic sensitivity. Clinical circumstances may require nephrectomy, but usually hemodialysis or peritoneal dialysis can be used until the pregnancy ends and the patient is prepared for transplantation.

Anemia (hematocrit less than 30%) is a coexistent problem and is difficult to manage. The primary renal disease and chronic failure result in anemia of chronic disease. Initially, the usual conservative methods are used to correct the problem (through dietary correction or oral iron therapy), with a goal of keeping the hematocrit above 30%. Selective transfusion of packed red blood cells or erythropoietin therapy is commonly used because conservative therapy often is inadequate.

Chronic hypertension complicates the pregnancies of many renal transplant recipients. The common antihypertensives are nifedipine and labetalol. Both of these agents have been used successfully and safely in pregnancy; the obstetrician must resist changing the patient's therapy from these effective agents to alpha-methyldopa. Angiotensin-converting enzyme inhibitors and diuretics should not be used because of potential fetal effects. Superimposed preeclampsia is a serious maternal threat in 30% of renal transplant recipients, and it is often the reason for early delivery. Sudden increases in blood pressure or proteinuria, falling platelet counts, elevated liver function tests, or symptoms of severity (headache, scotomata, or epigastric pain) are usually caused by preeclampsia. Delivery is the cure of the disease, but the risk of major maternal morbidity is weighed against the risks of preterm delivery. Magnesium

**Table 32-7** Maternal Outcomes in 197 Pregnancies After Renal Transplantation and Cyclosporine Therapy

| Maternal characteristics and complications | Incidence (%) |
|---|---|
| Hypertension | 107 (56%) |
| Preeclampsia | 40 (29%) |
| Diabetes | 21 (11%) |
| Infection | 42 (22%) |
| Rejection during pregnancy and first 3 months postpartum | 53 (11%) |
| Delivery for medical indications | 81 (60%) |
| Cesarean section | 67 (64%) |

Data from Armenti V, Ahlswede K, Ahlswede B, et al: *Transplantation* 59:476, 1995.

**Table 32-8** Fetal Outcomes in 197 Pregnancies After Renal Transplantation and Cyclosporine Therapy

| Outcome | Incidence (%) |
|---|---|
| Therapeutic abortion | 25 (12%) |
| Miscarriage or ectopic pregnancy | 34 (17%) |
| Fetal death | 5 (3.6%) |
| Live birth | 137 (68%) |
| Premature delivery | 75 (54%) |
| Fetal growth restriction | 68 (50%) |
| Perinatal death | 6 (45/1000 births) |

Data from Armenti V, Ahlswede K, Ahlswede B, et al: *Transplantation* 59:476, 1995.

sulfate is the agent of choice in preventing seizures (eclampsia). It has been shown to be superior to Dilantin in two comparative trials. Close monitoring of serum magnesium levels (therapeutic range 4 to 7 mEq/L) is necessary because toxicity (including death) occurs more often as the result of reduced renal excretion.

Infection is a major risk in immunocompromised pregnant women. A series of 201 pregnancies in which cyclosporine was used in addition to other immunosuppressive medications showed infectious complications in 22%. The incidence of bloodborne infection (hepatitis B and C, human immunodeficiency virus, and cytomegalovirus) is a risk to both the fetus and the mother. Bacterial infections, as manifested by tuberculosis, pyelonephritis, pneumonia, intraamniotic infection, postpartum endometritis, or wound infection, occur more often in transplant recipients. Often infections with unusual or opportunistic organisms such as *Aspergillus* species are managed as in normal pregnant women, but with concern for drug toxicity because of reduced renal excretion.

Secondary hyperparathyroidism and osteodystrophy with hypercalcemia and hypophosphatemia are present during dialysis and after renal transplantation. This condition results from the exaggerated normal physiologic changes of pregnancy, increased bone resorption, and the limitations to mineralization through the effects of steroid therapy. There is a 20% incidence of aseptic necrosis of the femoral head or compression fractures of the spine after renal transplantation. Of women with successful renal transplantation, 10% to 15% require parathyroidectomy for tertiary hyperparathyroidism. Both complications can occur during pregnancy. Calcium and phosphate levels are measured monthly and adequate supplements of calcium and vitamin D administered if hypocalcemia is identified. Supplemental calcium appears to have a secondary beneficial effect on blood pressure and preterm labor. Pregnancy is not a contraindication for parathyroid surgery if it would be indicated in a similar nonpregnant renal transplant recipient.

Most allograft kidneys are placed in the false pelvis above the pelvic rim, and obstructed labor or mechanical trauma rarely occurs. Operative reports for transplantation can reveal the location of the transplant. If a question arises during labor, an ultrasound easily delineates the location of acute ureteral distention (obstruction). More often than expected, the surgical approach to the lower uterine segment for cesarean section is complex and difficult, so a classic uterine incision may be the safest choice. Unless the obstetrician is experienced in the repair of complex urinary tract injury, a urology consult should be attained preoperatively.

The fetal complications associated with maternal renal transplantation include medication effects, developmental or congenital birth defects, fetal growth restriction, and preterm birth. Currently, most immunosuppressive regimens include cyclosporine. Armenti et al. (1995) reviewed 197 pregnancies in renal transplant recipients whose regimens included cyclosporine. This study gives the scope of maternal and fetal complications associated with current management of pregnancy in the presence of an allograft renal transplantation. Tables 32-7 and 32-8 give the results of the descriptive study.

When logistic regression was used to identify predictors of poor outcomes, the following adjusted associations were made: for low birthweight, preconceptual creatinine above 1.5 mg/dl, rising creatinine during pregnancy, graft dysfunction, and hypertension; for rejection, infection. The mean gestational age at delivery for patients with poor graft function was 33.9 weeks, and for those with good graft function it was 36 weeks.

Fetal growth restriction is a significant, complex problem. Suboptimal fetal growth may be the result of three different processes: uteroplacental insufficiency, effects of chemotherapeutic agents, or nutritional issues. Each has different implications as they relate to fetal prognosis and management. The most important is uteroplacental insufficiency because it may result in early delivery or fetal death. Uteroplacental insufficiency is predicted by the degree and complications of hypertension (preeclampsia). In the extreme, hypertension can lead to severe maternal bleeding or coagulopathy, tender uterus, and a hypertonic uterus (abruptio placentae). The incidence of abruptio placentae in hypertensive renal transplant recipients is 5% to 10%. The pregnancy is monitored with obstetric ultrasounds every 4 weeks, daily fetal kick counts (>4 movements within 2 hours after each meal), and biophysical testing every week (nonstress test and amniotic fluid index). In the presence of fetal growth restriction, doppler velocimetry of the umbilical cord is appropriate.

Generally, the risks of chemotherapy for immunosuppression are minimal. Azathioprine at dosages less than 2 mg/kg is not associated with increased congenital defects. When it is used in conjunction with prednisone, the incidence of fetal growth restriction is 20%. Animal studies suggest that the elevated risk of growth restriction is caused in part by a primary effect of the drug rather than the disease process (hypertension). Case reports suggest a self-limited reduction of leukocyte and platelet counts in newborns exposed in utero to azathioprine at higher dosages than are currently recommended. There are minimal data concerning the use of azathioprine in breast-feeding. When the mother received 25 mg/day azathioprine, the maximum level in the breast milk was 18 ng/ml. Azathioprine has 60% bioavailability. The minimal absorbed infant dose from breast-feeding is likely to be of little clinical significance.

There has been extensive use of prednisone during pregnancy in asthma or autoimmune disease. In studies in which high dosages (>20 mg/day) of prednisone were used to ameliorate the complications of lupus anticoagulant syndrome, there was a significant increase in the incidence of prematurely ruptured membranes. The incidence of premature rupture of membranes is 20% to 40% in patients with a renal allograft. There appears to be no increased risk of congenital defects of fetuses exposed to prednisone in the first trimester. Although it is a theoretical possibility, immunosuppression of the breast-fed newborn is very rare. The American Academy of Pediatrics (AAP) considers maternal prednisone therapy to be compatible with breast-feeding.

Cyclosporine A has a principal maternal dose-related toxicity: nephrotoxicity. Because nephrotoxicity may be very difficult to distinguish from rejection, the monitoring of serum cyclosporine levels is essential to the appropriate management of these patients. Cyclosporine A readily crosses the placenta with a cord blood:maternal serum ratio of 0.30 to 0.60. There has been no consistent pattern of animal or human birth defects after exposure to cyclosporine. Immunologic function of neonates after in utero exposure reveals a few subclinical differences in the newborn immune functions. The use of cyclosporine is considered safe in pregnancy. The breast milk:maternal serum cyclosporine ratio is 0.17 to 0.4. Despite the lack of demonstrated clinical effect on the breast-feeding infant, the AAP considers cyclosporine A to be contraindicated in breast-feeding. A recent study of simultaneous cyclosporine levels in maternal serum, breast milk, and neonatal serum observed that breast-fed infants whose mothers were treated with cyclosporine A received less than 300 µg/day and serum levels in the newborn were undetectable (<30 ng/ml).

There were no simultaneous changes in the infants' serum creatinine levels. This study raises questions about the AAP recommendation. If there is a strong desire to breast-feed and the patient has been informed of the controversy, breast-feeding could be supported.

### Lower Urinary Tract Injuries During Delivery

Injury to the urethra or bladder trigone from prolonged, obstructed labor or difficult operative deliveries is rare in modern obstetrics. On the other hand, the dramatic increase in cesarean deliveries from 5% to 25% in the last 20 years has increased the rates of bladder dome and ureteral injury. Recently, a large, descriptive study reported injury to the bladder in 0.19% of primary and 0.6% of repeat cesarean deliveries. Most bladder injuries are associated with post-surgical (cesarean) adhesions between the bladder and the lower uterine segment. The risk of bladder injury is increased among patients with four or more uterine incisions (1.5%) and cesarean hysterectomy (1.7%).

Ureteral injury occurs in 0.09% to 0.6% of cesarean operations and usually occurs in association with late second-stage dystocia; deep uterine, cervical, or vaginal lacerations; or cesarean hysterectomy. Two thirds of urinary tract injuries are identified at the time of surgery. In difficult cases, evaluation for injury should be routine. Bladder injury can be identified by the instillation of sterile infant formula into the bladder through a three-way Foley catheter. Ureteral function is documented by the efflux of blue-green urine from the ureters after intravenous injection of indigo carmine. The technique and management of bladder and ureteral injury repair are described in Chapter 30.

## BIBLIOGRAPHY
### Anatomy and Physiology of the Urinary Tract in Pregnancy
Bailey RR, Rolleston GL: Kidney length and ureteric dilatation in the puerperium, *J Obstet Gynaecol Br Commonw* 78:55, 1971.

Beguin Y, Lipscei G, Oris R, et al: Serum immunoreactive erythropoietin during pregnancy and in the early postpartum, *Br J Haematol* 70:545, 1990.

Davison JM, Hytten FE: Glomerular filtration during and after pregnancy, *Am J Obstet Gynecol* 81:588, 1974.

Davison JM, Shiells EA, Phillips PR, et al: Influence of humoral and volume factors on altered osmoregulation of normal human pregnancy, *Am J Physiol* 258:F900, 1990.

Dure-Smith P: Pregnancy dilatation of the urinary tract: the iliac sign and its significance, *Radiology* 96:545, 1970.

Fainstat T: Ureteral dilatation in pregnancy: a review, *Obstet Gynecol Surv* 18:845, 1963.

Francis WJA: Disturbances in bladder function in relation to pregnancy, *J Obstet Gynaecol Br Commonw* 67:353, 1960a.

Francis WJA: The onset of stress incontinence, *J Obstet Gynaecol Br Commonw* 67:89, 1960b.

Gant NF, Daley GL, Chand S, et al: A study of angiotensin II pressor response throughout primigravid pregnancy, *J Clin Invest* 52:2682, 1973.

Hedrick WP, Mattingly RF, Amberg JR: Vesicoureteral reflux in pregnancy, *Obstet Gynecol* 29:571, 1967.

Iosif S, Ingermarsson I, Ulmsten U: Urodynamic studies in normal pregnancy and puerperium, *Am J Obstet Gynecol* 137:696, 1980.

Lindheimer MD, Katz AI: The kidney in pregnancy, *N Engl J Med* 283:1095, 1970.

Marchant DJ: Alterations in anatomy and function of the urinary tract during pregnancy, *Clin Obstet Gynecol* 21:855, 1978.

Mattingly RF, Borkouf HI: Clinical implications of ureteral reflux in pregnancy, *Clin Obstet Gynecol* 21:863, 1978.

Rubi RA, Sala NL: Ureteral function in pregnant women. III. Effect of different position and fetal delivery upon ureteral tone, *Am J Obstet Gynecol* 101:230, 1968.

Sala NL, Rubi RA: Ureteral function in pregnant women. II. Ureteral contractibility during normal pregnancy, *Am J Obstet Gynecol* 99:228, 1967.

Shah DM, Higuchi K, Inagama T, et al: Effect of progesterone on renin secretion in endometrial stromal, chorionic trophoblast, and mesenchymal monolayer cultures, *Am J Obstet Gynecol* 164:1145, 1991.

Sheehan HL, Lynch JB: *Pathology of toxemia of pregnancy,* New York, 1973, Churchill-Livingstone.

Stanton SL, Kerr-Wilson R, Harris VG: The incidence of urological symptoms in normal pregnancy, *Br J Obstet Gynaecol* 87:897, 1980.

van Geelen JM, Lemmens WA, Eskes TK, et al: The urethral pressure profile in pregnancy and after delivery in healthy nulliparous women, *Am J Obstet Gynecol* 144:636, 1982.

Weinberger MH, Kramer NJ, Grim CE, et al: The effect of posture and saline loading on plasma renin activity and aldosterone concentration in pregnant, nonpregnant and estrogen-treated women, *J Clin Endocrinol Metab* 44:69, 1977.

Weir RJ, Doig A, Fraser R, et al: Studies in the renin angiotensin aldosterone system, cortisol, DOC and ADH in normal and hypertensive pregnancy. In Lindheimer AI, Katz MS, Zuspan FP, eds: *Hypertension in pregnancy,* New York, 1976, Wiley.

Zuspan FP, Nelson GH, Ahlquist RP: Epinephrine infusion in normal and toxemic pregnancy, *Am J Obstet Gynecol* 90:88, 1964.

## Urinary Tract Disease in Pregnancy

Andriole VT, Patterson TF: Epidemiology, natural history and management of urinary tract infections in pregnancy, *Med Clin North Am* 75:359, 1991.

Armenti V, Ahlswede K, Ahlswede B, et al: Variables affecting birth weight and graft survival in 197 pregnancies in cyclosporine-treated female kidney transplant recipients, *Transplantation* 59:476, 1995.

Austenfeld MS, Snow BW: Complication of pregnancy in women after reimplantation for vesicoureteral reflux, *J Urol* 140:1103, 1988.

Bran JL, Levison ME, Kaye D: Entrance of bacteria into the female urinary bladder, *N Engl J Med* 286:626, 1972.

Buckley RM, McGuckin M, MacGregor RR: Urine bacterial counts after sexual intercourse, *N Engl J Med* 298:321, 1978.

Bukowski T, Betrus G, Aquilina J, et al: Urinary tract infections and pregnancy in women who underwent antireflux surgery in childhood, *J Urol* 159:1286, 1998.

Campbell-Brown M, McFadyen IR, Seal DV, et al: Is screening for bacteriuria in pregnancy worthwhile? *BMJ* 294:1579, 1987.

Coe FL, Parks JH, Lundheimer MD: Nephrolithiasis during pregnancy, *N Engl J Med* 298:324, 1978.

Coulam C, Moyer T, Jiang N-S, et al: Breast-feeding after renal transplantation, *Transplant Proc* 14:605, 1982.

Cox CE, Hinman F: Experiments with induced bacteriuria, vesical emptying and bacterial growth on the mechanism of bladder defense to infection, *J Urol* 86:739, 1961.

Cunningham FG, Morris GB, Mickal A: Acute pyelonephritis of pregnancy: a clinical review, *Obstet Gynecol* 42:112, 1973.

Davison J: Dialysis, transplantation, and pregnancy, *Am J Kidney Dis* 17:127, 1991.

Eisenkop SM, Richman R, Platt LD, et al: Urinary tract injury during cesarean section, *Obstet Gynecol* 60:591, 1982.

Elder HA, Santamarine BAG, Smith S, et al: The natural history of asymptomatic bacteriuria during pregnancy: the effect of tetracycline on the clinical course and the outcome of pregnancy, *Am J Obstet Gynecol* 111:44, 1971.

Ersay A, Oygür N, Coskun M, et al: Immunologic evaluation of a neonate born to an immunosuppressed kidney transplant recipient, *Am J Perinatol* 12:413, 1995.

Fihn ST, Stamm WE: Interpretation and comparison of treatment studies for uncomplicated urinary tract infections in women, *Rev Infect Dis* 7:468, 1985.

First M, Combs C, Weiskittel P, et al: Lack of effect of pregnancy on renal allograft survival or function, *Transplantation* 59:472, 1995.

Flechner S, Katz A, Rogers A, et al: The presence of cyclosporine in body tissues and fluids during pregnancy, *Am J Kidney Dis* 5:60, 1985.

Gaudier F, Santiago-Delpin E, Rivera J, et al: Pregnancy after renal transplantation, *Surg Gynecol Obstet* 167:533, 1988.

Gilbert GL, Garland SM, Fairley KF, et al: Bacteriuria due to ureaplasmas and other fastidious organisms during pregnancy: prevalence and significance, *Pediatr Infect Dis* 5:239, 1986.

Gillenwater JY, Harrison RB, Kunin CM: Natural history of bacteriuria in schoolgirls, *N Engl J Med* 301:396, 1979.

Gilstrap LC, Cunningham FG, Whalley PJ: Acute pyelonephritis in pregnancy: an anterospective study, *Obstet Gynecol* 57:409, 1981a.

Gilstrap LC, Leveno KJ, Cunningham FG, et al: Renal infection and pregnancy outcome, *Am J Obstet Gynecol* 141:709, 1981b.

Grekas D, Tourkantonis A: Serum and human milk IgA and zinc concentration after successful renal transplantation, *Biol Res Pregnancy Perinatol* 7:118, 1986.

Harris RE: The significance of eradication of bacteriuria during pregnancy, *Obstet Gynecol* 53:71, 1979.

Harris RE: Correlation of postpartum intravenous pyelograms with clinical localization of antepartum pyelonephritis, *Am J Obstet Gynecol* 141:105, 1981.

Harris RE, Gilstrap LC: Cystitis during pregnancy: a distinct clinical entity, *Obstet Gynecol* 57:578, 1981.

Harris RE, Thomas VL, Shelokov A: Asymptomatic bacteriuria in pregnancy: antibody-coated bacteria, renal function, and intrauterine growth retardation, *Am J Obstet Gynecol* 126:20, 1976.

Hedegarrd CK, Wallace D: Percutaneous nephrostomy: current indications and potential uses in obstetrics and gynecology, *Obstet Gynecol Surv* 42:671, 1987.

Hill DE, Chantigian PM, Kramer SA: Pregnancy after augmentation cystoplasty, *Surg Gynecol Obstet* 170:485, 1990.

Hill DE, Kramer SA: Management of pregnancy after augmentation cystoplasty, *J Urol* 140:457, 1990.

Holland D, Bliss K, Allen C: A comparison of chemical dipsticks read visually or by photometry in the routine screening of urine specimens in the clinical microbiology laboratory, *Pathology* 27:91, 1995.

Homans DC, Blake GD, Harrington JT, et al: Acute renal failure caused by ureteral obstruction by a gravid uterus, *JAMA* 246:1230, 1981.

Horowitz E, Schmidt JD: Renal calculi in pregnancy, *Clin Obstet Gynecol* 28:324, 1985.

Jarrard D, Gerber G, Lyon E: Management of acute ureteral obstruction in pregnancy utilizing ultrasound-guided placement of ureteral stents, *Urology* 42:263, 1993.

Johnson JR, Moseley SL, Roberts PL, et al: Aerobactin and other virulence factor genes among strains of *Escherichia coli* causing urosepsis: association with patient characteristics, *Infect Immun* 56:405, 1988.

Jungers P, Chauveau D: Pregnancy in renal disease, *Kidney Int* 52:871, 1997.

Kass EH: Asymptomatic infections of the urinary tract, *Trans Assoc Am Physicians* 69:56, 1956.

Kellogg JA, Manzella JP, Shaffer SN, et al: Clinical relevance of culture versus screens for the detection of microbial pathogens in urine specimens, *Am J Med* 83:739, 1987.

Komaroff AL: Acute dysuria in women, *N Engl J Med* 310:368, 1984.

Latham RH, Wong ES, Larson A, et al: Laboratory diagnosis of urinary tract infection in ambulatory women, *JAMA* 254:3333, 1985.

Lattan ZI, Cook WA: Urinary calculi in pregnancy, *Obstet Gynecol* 56:462, 1980.

Leigh DA, Gruneberg RN, Brumfit W: Long-term follow-up of bacteriuria in pregnancy, *Lancet* 1:603, 1968.

Lenke RR, van Dorsten JP, Schifin BS: Pyelonephritis in pregnancy: a prospective randomized trial to prevent recurrent disease evaluating suppressive therapy with nitrofurantoin and close surveillance, *Am J Obstet Gynecol* 146:953, 1983.

Leveno KJ, Harris RE, Gilstrap LC, et al: Bladder versus renal bacteriuria during pregnancy: recurrence after treatment, *Am J Obstet Gynecol* 139:403, 1981.

Levine D, Filly R, Graber M: The sonographic appearance of renal transplants during pregnancy, *J Ultrasound Med* 14:291, 1995.

Lincoln K, Lidin-Janson G, Winberg J: Resistant urinary infections resulting from changes in resistance pattern of fecal flora induced by sulphonamide and hospital environment, *BMJ* 3:305, 1970.

Lindheimer MD, Katz AI: The kidney in pregnancy, *N Engl J Med* 283:1095, 1970.

Little PJ, McPherson DR, Wardener HE: The appearance of the intravenous pyelogram during and after acute pyelonephritis, *Lancet* 1:186, 1965.

Lomberg H, Hellstrom M, Jodal U: Properties of *Escherichia coli* in patients with renal scarring, *J Infect Dis* 159:579, 1989.

Loughlin K: Management of urologic problems during pregnancy, *Urology* 44:159, 1994.

Lumsden L, Hyner GC: Effects of an educational intervention on the rate of recurrent urinary tract infections in selected female outpatients, *Women Health* 310:79, 1985.

Man PD, Jodal U, Svanborg C: Dependence among host response parameters used to diagnose urinary tract infection, *J Infect Dis* 163:331, 1991.

Mansfield J, Snow B, Cartwright P, et al: Complications of pregnancy in women after childhood reimplantation for vesicoureteral reflux: an update with 25 years of follow-up, *J Urol* 154:787, 1995.

Martinell J, Jodal U, Lidin-Janson G: Pregnancies in women with and without renal scarring after urinary infection in childhood, *BMJ* 300:840, 1990.

McDowall DRM, Buchanan JD, Fairley KF, et al: Anaerobic and other fastidious microorganisms in asymptomatic bacteriuria in pregnant women, *J Infect Dis* 144:114, 1981.

McNeeley SG, Baselski VS, Ryan GM: An evaluation of two rapid bacteriuria screening procedures, *Obstet Gynecol* 69:550, 1987.

McNeeley SG: Treatment of urinary tract infections during pregnancy, *Clin Obstet Gynecol* 31:480, 1988.

Meijer-Severs GJ, Aarnoudse JG, Mensing WFA, et al: The presence of antibody-coated anaerobic bacteria in asymptomatic bacteriuria during pregnancy, *J Infect Dis* 140:653, 1979.

Mikhail MS, Anyaegbunam A: Lower urinary tract dysfunction in pregnancy: a review, *Obstet Gynecol Surv* 50:675, 1995.

Miller RD, Kakkis J: Prognosis, management and outcome of obstructive renal disease in pregnancy, *J Reprod Med* 27:199, 1982.

Needham CA: Rapid detection methods in microbiology: are they right for your office? *Med Clin North Am* 71:591, 1987.

Nyberg G, Haljamae U, Frisenette-Fich C, et al: Breast-feeding during treatment with cyclosporine, *Transplantation* 65:253, 1998.

Ojerskog B, Kock NG, Philipson BM, et al: Pregnancy and delivery in patients with a continent ileostomy, *Surg Gynecol Obstet* 167:61, 1988.

Romero R, Oyarzun E, Mazor M, et al: Meta-analysis of the relationship between asymptomatic bacteriuria and preterm delivery/low birthweight, *Obstet Gynecol* 73:576, 1989.

Ronald AR, Cutler RE, Turck M: Effect of bacteriuria on renal concentrating mechanisms, *Ann Intern Med* 70:723, 1969.

Sandberg T, Kaijser B, Lidin-Janson G, et al: Virulence of *Escherichia coli* in relation to host factors in women with symptomatic urinary tract infection, *J Clin Microbiol* 26:1471, 1988.

Schumann GB, Greenberg NF: Usefulness of macroscopic urinalysis as a screening procedure, *Am J Clin Pathol* 452, 1977.

Smith LH: The medical aspects of urolithiasis: an overview, *J Urol* 141:707, 1988.

Soisson AP, Watson WJ, Benson WL, et al: Value of a screening urinalysis in pregnancy, *Obstet Gynecol* 30:586, 1985.

Stamey T: Recurrent urinary tract infections in female patients: an overview of management and treatment, *Rev Infect Dis* 9:195, 1987.

Stamm WE, Counts GW, Running KR, et al: Diagnosis of coliform infection in acutely dysuric women, *N Engl J Med* 307:463, 1982.

Stamm WE, Hooton TM, Johnson JR, et al: Urinary tract infections: from pathogenesis to treatment, *J Infect Dis* 159:400, 1989.

Stark RP, Maki DG: Bacteriuria in the catheterized patient, *N Engl J Med* 311:559, 1984.

Stenqvist K, Dahlen-Nillson I, Lidin-Janson G, et al: Bacteriuria in pregnancy, *Am J Epidemiol* 129:372, 1989.

Stenqvist K, Sandberg T, Lidin-Janson G, et al: Virulence factors of *Escherichia coli* in urinary isolates from pregnant women, *J Infect Dis* 156:870, 1987.

Stothers L, Lee L: Renal colic in pregnancy, *J Urol* 148:1383, 1992.

Strom BL, Collins M, West SL, et al: Sexual activity, contraceptive use, and other risk factors for symptomatic and asymptomatic bacteriuria, *Ann Intern Med* 107:816, 1987.

Sturgiss S, Davidson M: Perinatal outcome in renal allograft recipients: prognostic significance of hypertension and renal function before and during pregnancy, *Obstet Gynecol* 78:573, 1991.

Sweet RL: Bacteriuria and pyelonephritis during pregnancy, *Semin Perinatol* 1:25, 1977.

Sweet RL, Gibbs RS: Urinary tract infections. In *Infectious diseases of the female genital tract*, Baltimore, 1990, Williams & Wilkins.

Thomsen AC, Morup L, Brogaard Hansen K: Antibiotic elimination of group B streptococci in prevention of preterm labor, *Lancet* 1:591, 1987.

Tincello D, Richmond D: Evaluation of reagent strips in detecting asymptomatic bacteriuria in early pregnancy: prospective case series, *BMJ* 316:435, 1998.

Turck M, Anderson KN, Petersdorf RG: Relapse and reinfection in chronic bacteriuria, *N Engl J Med* 275:70, 1966.

Turck M, Goffe B, Petersdorf RG: The urethral catheter and urinary tract infection, *J Urol* 88:834, 1962.

Vosti KL: Recurrent urinary tract infection: prevention by prophylactic antibiotics after sexual intercourse, *JAMA* 231:934, 1975.

Whalley PJ, Cunningham FG, Martin FG: Transient renal dysfunction associated with acute pyelonephritis of pregnancy, *Obstet Gynecol* 46:1747, 1975.

Wong ES, McKevitt M, Running K, et al: Management of recurrent urinary tract infections with patient-administered single-dose therapy, *Ann Intern Med* 102:302, 1985.

Zinner SH, Kass EH: Long-term (10 to 14 years) follow-up of bacteriuria of pregnancy, *N Engl J Med* 235:820, 1971.

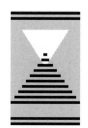

CHAPTER **33**
# Bladder Drainage and Urinary Protective Methods

Carmen J. Sultana

Short- or long-term bladder drainage is required in a variety of situations. Postoperatively, a patient may require catheterization for retention for a period of days to weeks. Patients with areflexic bladders, voiding dysfunction, or intractable incontinence may require intermittent or indwelling catheterization for long-term management. Three catheterization methods—transurethral, suprapubic, and intermittent self-catheterization—can be used.

In incontinent patients who fail or decline treatment, protective products and urinary loss appliances are helpful. They may be preferable when treatment is too risky or more objectionable to the patient than continued incontinence. This chapter will discuss catheterization as well as various protective products and incontinence collecting devices.

## BLADDER DRAINAGE

The gynecologist most often encounters the need for bladder drainage in patients after surgery for genuine stress incontinence or pelvic organ prolapse. These procedures commonly increase urethral resistance to flow and place the patient at risk for postoperative retention requiring prolonged bladder drainage. The risk of this complication after vaginal and retropubic procedures ranges from 3% to 25% and may be higher for suburethral sling procedures. Adequate postoperative bladder drainage is important because overdistension may lead to postoperative infection and difficulty in resuming normal voiding. Bladder drainage can be accomplished by transurethral and suprapubic catheters and by intermittent self-catheterization.

## Transurethral Catheterization

The first self-retaining transurethral catheter was described in 1937 by Foley. A saline-inflated intravesical balloon holds the catheter in place. The ease of insertion of the Foley catheter has led to its use in a variety of situations in which bladder drainage or monitoring of urine output is required. It is commonly used after many gynecologic procedures.

The major difficulty with use of transurethral drainage is the potential for infection. The risk of infection after a single catheterization is 1% to 5%. The risk rises to 20% of patients maintained on closed drainage systems. Bacterial colonization of a closed system is unavoidable, with a rate of 5% to 10% per day. Prophylactic antibiotics do not prevent bacteriuria or cystitis in the presence of a catheter, although they may postpone their onset. Other problems with prolonged use of transurethral catheters include periurethral discomfort and irritation of the trigone, against which the balloon rests. Once the catheter is removed, repeated catheterization is needed if the patient does not void spontaneously. These drawbacks have led to the widespread use of alternatives, such as suprapubic catheters, after incontinence procedures.

The major gynecologic indication for use of a transurethral Foley catheter is bladder drainage after operative procedures with little or no dissection around the urethra (such as a vaginal hysterectomy). It can also be used when the need for drainage is expected to be less than 5 days or for a short time before beginning intermittent self-catheterization.

The minicatheter, as advocated by O'Leary and O'Leary (1970), is a variation on transurethral drainage that has not been widely used. It is an 8- to 10-French plastic catheter that is sutured to the urethral meatus. The small diameter permits voiding around the catheter and causes less urethral irritation.

## Suprapubic Catheterization

Hodgkinson and Hodari (1966) demonstrated a lower incidence of bacteriuria and shorter time to reestablish normal voiding with suprapubic bladder drainage, compared to transurethral drainage, after surgical procedures for

**Table 33-1**   Types of Suprapubic and Self-Catheterization Catheters

| Name | Catheter type and size | Insertion method | Manufacturer |
|---|---|---|---|
| Bonanno | Pigtail loop; 7 French (F) | Over a needle | Beckton Dickinson, Rutherford, New Jersey |
| Argyle-Ingram | Balloon; 12, 16 F | Over a needle | Sherwood Med Co, St. Louis, Missouri |
| Supraflex | Pigtail with or without balloon; silicone 12, 18 F | Over a needle | Rusch Inc, Duluth, Georgia |
| Simplastic | Balloon; PVC plastic 10, 12, 16 F | Over a needle | Rusch Inc, Duluth, Georgia |
| Stamey | Malecot; 8, 10, 12, 14, 16 F Loop; 10, 12, 14 F polyethylene | Over a needle | Cook Urological Inc, Spencer, Indiana |
| Sof-Flex | Loop; polyurethane 8, 10, 12, 14 F | Over a needle | Cook Urological Inc, Spencer, Indiana |
| Rutner | Balloon; polyurethane 10, 12, 16 F | Over a needle | Cook Urological Inc, Spencer, Indiana |
| Pigtail | Pigtail; polyurethane 7 F | Through a needle/cannula | Cook Urological Inc, Spencer, Indiana |
| Cook Cystostomy | Silicone loop | Through steel sheath with stylet | Cook Urological Inc, Spencer, Indiana |
| Cook-Cope Loop | Loop; polyurethane 8.2, 10, 12, 14 F | Through dilators with trocar and wire guides | Cook Urological Inc, Spencer, Indiana |
| Supra Foley inserter | Plastic trocar and sheath; 8, 10, 12, 16 F | Allows Foley insertion through peel-away sheath | Rusch Inc, Duluth, Georgia |
| Trocha Fix | Steel trocar and sheath; 8, 12, 14 F | Allows Foley insertion through pull-away sheath | Rusch Inc. Duluth, Georgia |
| Suprapubic introducer | Steel stylet with TFE sheath; 15, 16 F | Allows Foley insertion through peel-away sheath | Cook Urological Inc, Spencer, Indiana |
| Suprapubic introducer/Foley set | Needle introducer; 14 F | Allows Foley insertion | Bard, Covington, Georgia |
| Self-Cath | Plastic; 5 to 18 F | — | Mentor Corp, Santa Barbara, California |
| Icath | Steel curve with mirror; 12 F | — | Cook Urological Inc, Spencer, Georgia |

incontinence. Other studies have supported these findings. Suprapubic catheters also improve patient comfort and ease of nursing care. They allow patients to control voiding trials, and they obviate repeated transurethral catheterizations to check postvoid residual urine volumes.

The main disadvantage of suprapubic catheterization is infection. No controlled clinical trials prove a lower infection rate when compared to transurethral drainage. When used for long-term drainage in patients with spinal cord injuries, 51% developed infections and 100% had asymptomatic bacteriuria. Urinary deposits and blood clots may obstruct the smaller-caliber catheters, necessitating frequent irrigation. Leakage around the catheter may also be a problem. The invasive nature of insertion can lead to rare complications such as hematuria, cellulitis, bowel injury, urine extravasation, and catheter fracture. Despite these potential problems, suprapubic catheters are preferred to transurethral catheters when prolonged drainage is anticipated or when significant dissection around the urethra has been performed.

The major catheter types available are listed in Table 33-1 and shown in Fig. 33-1. All are refinements of the original catheter used by Hodgkinson and Hodari (1966) and are inserted through a sharp trocar cannula or over a needle obturator.

Suprapubic catheters can be inserted using an open or closed technique. Cystotomy into the bladder dome under direct visualization at the end of a retropubic procedure is the safest method. It is preferred when distention of the bladder is difficult, when gross hematuria is present, when there has been a recent cystotomy, or in the presence of malignancy. Any of the catheter types listed in Table 33-1, as well as a Foley catheter, can be used for open cystotomy. To perform this procedure, the bladder is filled with saline. A stab incision is made through the skin above or below the surgical incision with a scalpel. The catheter and introducer are placed into the incision and inserted through the skin, muscle and fascia. The bladder is then punctured through the dome, taking care to avoid large vessels. The catheter is advanced through the sheath or over the needle guide, which is simultaneously withdrawn. Efflux of urine or saline should be ensured. If the catheter has a balloon, it is inflated. The catheter is sutured in place on the skin.

Closed insertion can be performed using a variety of

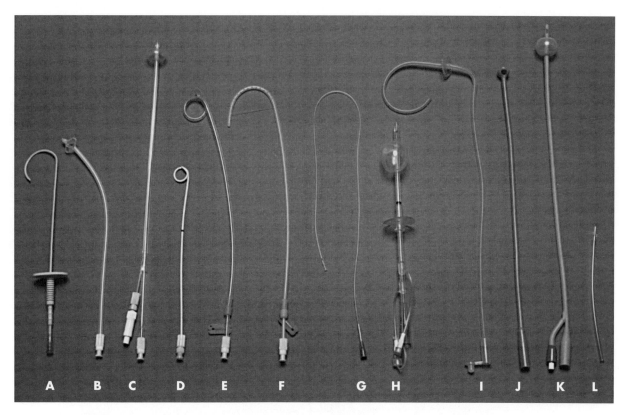

**Fig. 33-1** Suprapubic and self-catheterization bladder drainage catheters. **A,** Bonanno, 7 French (F). **B,** Stamey Malecot, 12 or 14 F. **C,** Rutner balloon, 16 F. **D,** Pigtail, 7 F. **E,** Sof-flex loop, 14 F. **F,** Stamey loop, 12 F. **G,** Cystocath, 8 F. **H,** Argyle-Ingram, 12 or 16 F. **I,** Robertson, 15 F. **J,** Malecot. **K,** Foley. **L,** Mentor Self-Cath, 14 F.
From Hurt WG: *Obstet Gynecol Rep* 2:307, 1990.

catheters when there is no abdominal incision. To insert a catheter, the surgeon should place the patient in the Trendelenburg position and fill the bladder through a transurethral catheter with at least 500 ml sterile saline or water until the bladder is easily palpable abdominally. This positioning helps ensure that no bowel lies between the bladder and the anterior abdominal wall. After the usual skin prepping, the needle or trocar should be inserted through the skin and fascia into the bladder, at a point no more than 3 cm above the pubic symphysis and at an angle, directed downward toward the pubic symphysis (Fig. 33-2, *A*). The trocar or needle is removed (Fig. 33-2, *B*), and the catheter secured. The transurethral catheter is then removed.

A third method of suprapubic insertion of a Foley or Malecot catheter is to insert a perforated urethral sound or Lowsley retractor transurethrally into the bladder. The tip of the sound is directed anteriorly, and the bladder dome and abdominal wall are tented upward by the sound (Fig. 33-3, *A*). An abdominal incision is made into the bladder at this site. The catheter is sutured to the sound and pulled backward to the urethral meatus, where the suture is removed (Fig. 33-3, *B*). The balloon is then inflated after the catheter is withdrawn into the bladder.

## Intermittent Self-Catheterization

The technique of clean, intermittent self-catheterization (ISC) was evaluated initially by Lapides et al. (1972) in patients with incontinence or voiding dysfunction because of neurogenic bladder disease. ISC allows the patient to insert a short plastic catheter into the urethra as needed to empty the bladder. Table 33-1 lists some available brands. There have been studies on newer hydrophilic low-friction catheters (Lofric, Astra Tech, Mö Indel, Sweden) that may be more comfortable than standard plastic catheters.

The rationale for nonsterile, clean ISC is based on the theory that functional abnormalities of the lower urinary tract lead to infection. Decreased blood flow, resulting from overdistention, is cited as one of the most common causes. The benefits of eliminating overdistention outweigh the disadvantages of intermittent insertion of a nonsterile catheter. Although Kass and Schneiderman (1957) have stated that each catheterization event carries a 3% to 4% infection rate, clinical studies of ISC have shown its safety with long-term follow-up of 255 children with neurogenic bladder dysfunction. Ninety percent of these children were free of major kidney infection after 10 years, despite a 56% rate of intermittent bacteriuria. Since then, ISC has been

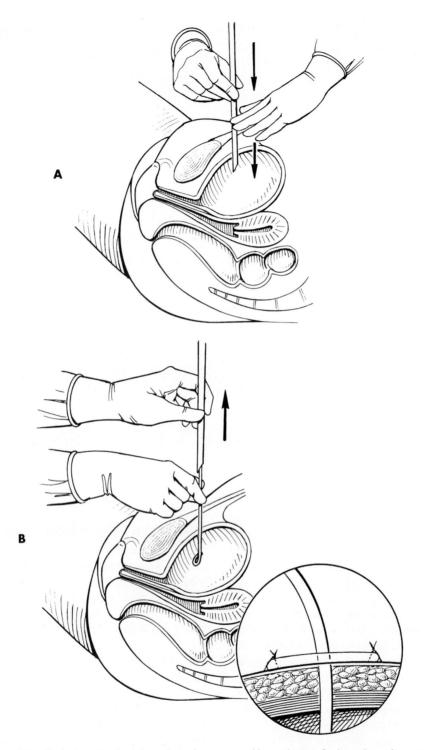

**Fig. 33-2** Typical method of insertion of a suprapubic catheter. **A,** Insertion of suprapubic Cystocath catheter via trocar. **B,** Withdrawal of trocar. *Inset,* Catheter sutured to skin.

evaluated in patients with spinal cord injury and multiple sclerosis. Elderly persons have experienced low infection rates (one per 8 months) with ISC. The complication rate for postoperative use of ISC should be even lower because it is seldom used longer than 6 weeks.

ISC can be started in the immediate postoperative period, usually the first postoperative day. A Foley catheter can be used for the first 24 hours. To use ISC the patient must have the manual dexterity and mental ability to perform catheterization. The bladder capacity should be at least 100 ml.

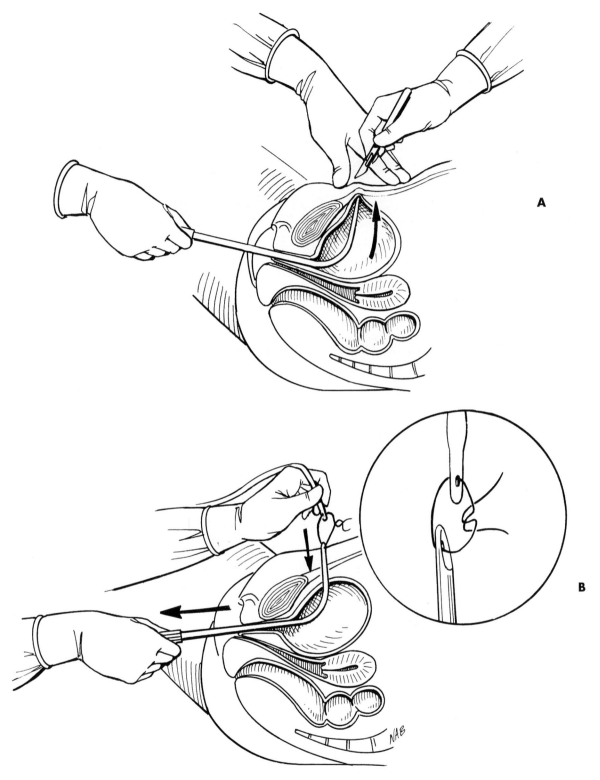

**Fig. 33-3**    Alternative method of insertion of a suprapubic catheter using a transurethral sound. **A,** Tenting of abdominal wall in preparation for incision. **B,** Pulling catheter into bladder. *Inset,* Demonstration of temporary suture.

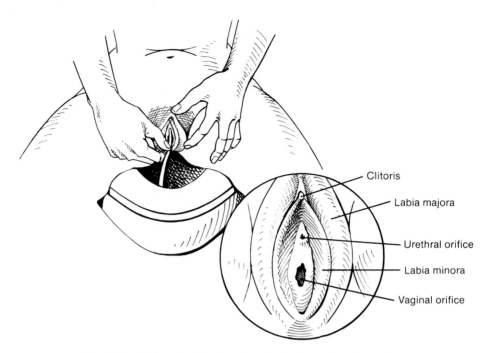

Clitoris
Labia majora
Urethral orifice
Labia minora
Vaginal orifice

**Fig. 33-4**   Illustration of self-catheterization for patient instruction.

**Box 33-1**

## INSTRUCTIONS TO PATIENT ON INTERMITTENT SELF-CATHETERIZATION

1. Wash your hands with soap and water.
2. Use a clean (soap and water) catheter, with water-soluble lubricant if needed.
3. Attempt to empty your bladder before catheterization.
4. Position yourself lying in bed or straddling a toilet.
5. Spread the labia with the fourth and index fingers of one hand and use the middle finger to locate the urethra.
6. Insert the catheter 1 to 2 inches and drain until all urine flow stops.
7. Measure and record the amount of urine ("residual") obtained.

Complications other than infection are rare; they include retention of the catheter and perforation of the urethra to create a false passage.

The technique of ISC can be taught to patients preoperatively or postoperatively by direct demonstration (Fig. 33-4 and Box 33-1). The patient should be supplied with a device to measure urine and with short plastic or rubber catheters. She should be instructed to carry them with her at all times, with separate containers for clean and used catheters. Sterile catheters are not required. Home sterilization with a microwave oven has been described, but whether this technique is of any clinical significance

in preventing bacteriuria and infection remains to be shown. Two studies have suggested no differences in infection rate when comparing clean and sterile catheters. Catheterization can be performed anywhere, and the importance of emptying the bladder often enough to keep the urine volumes obtained less than 300 ml should be stressed to the patient.

Most patients catheterize every 3 to 4 hours and then as needed during the night. The need to catheterize should take priority over the availability of soap and water. The urethra does not need to be cleansed before catheterization. Voiding should be attempted before every catheterization, and the residual urine volume measured and recorded, if possible. When residual volumes are consistently less than 20% of the total voided volume, ISC can be stopped. Prophylactic antibiotics can be given, if desired, for short periods of ISC, although equivocal benefit has been shown in patients using ISC for a long time.

## General Catheter Care

A Foley catheter inserted transurethrally after uncomplicated surgical procedures can be removed on the first postoperative day. If the patient has difficulty voiding, intermittent catheterization can be used until normal voiding is established. Bladder training (i.e., intermittent clamping and unclamping of the catheter without voiding attempts) does not decrease the time required to reestablish normal voiding.

When a suprapubic catheter is used, the patient should drink at least 2 liters of fluid per day. Some hematuria on the first day is common. Narrow-diameter catheters may require periodic irrigation to remove blood clots. The catheter is left to straight drainage until the first or second postoperative day. It should be clamped in the morning and the patient allowed to void with the catheter clamped at least once every 2 to 4 hours. If the patient cannot void, the clamp is opened, the bladder drained, and the catheter reclamped until the next voiding trial. If the patient seems to be voiding well, a postvoid residual urine volume can be obtained by unclamping the tube for 15 minutes after a voiding episode and measuring the amount of urine obtained. The catheter can be left open overnight for convenience. When the residual volume is less than 20% of the total voided volume, the catheter can be removed. There are no trials of prophylaxis against infection at the time of catheter removal. If voiding trials are unsuccessful, the patient should be discharged with the catheter and given written instructions and diary forms to continue the voiding trials at home. She should follow up in the office a few days to 1 week later, or call every 2 days and report progress.

## Catheter and Drainage Bag Management

In general, care of the drainage bag is similar for both suprapubic and transurethral catheters. To prevent ascending infection, disconnection of the catheter and bag should be avoided. A bag with a urometer helps to break the urine column between the bag and catheter. The bag should be below the level of the bladder at all times, and the drainage port should be kept clean. Prophylactic antibiotics are of no benefit in preventing colonization of the system.

## URINE LOSS APPLIANCES
### Absorptive Products

Patients whose incontinence is not correctable with bladder training, medical therapy, or surgical therapy or patients who simply would rather use protective undergarments have a variety of choices. These options range from shields resembling ordinary sanitary pads to disposable briefs to washable garments designed to hold pads. The selection of products should be based on the individual patient fit, skin condition, patient's ability to use the product independently, convenience to caregivers, volume of leakage, living situation, and financial considerations (Box 33-2). Depending on laundry costs, for example, disposable products may be more or less cost-effective for a particular nursing home. The products should not replace toileting or attempts at diagnosis and treatment of incontinence.

Several different brands of disposable shields have become available. These are shaped like sanitary pads but contain a powder (such as sodium polyacrylate) that absorbs liquid to form a gel, thus preventing clothing wetness. They are available in different absorbencies and are ideal for patients who experience small amounts of urine loss (e.g., only with exercise). Specially made, reusable panties that hold disposable pads or shields snugly against the perineum are available.

**Box 33-2**
### CRITERIA FOR SELECTION OF INCONTINENCE PRODUCTS

The ideal product should meet the following criteria:
- It contains urine (and stool) completely and prevents leakage onto clothing, bedding, and furniture.
- It is comfortable to wear and protects vulnerable skin from maceration, chafing, and pressure sores.
- It is easy for the incontinent person to use. If this is not feasible because of physical or mental disability, it should be easy for a caregiver to use.
- It disguises or contains odor.
- It is inconspicuous under clothing, without bulk or noise.
- It is easy to dispose of or clean, as required.
- It is reasonably priced and readily available.

From Jeter KF: In Jeter KF, Faller N, Norton C, eds: *Nursing for continence*, Philadelphia, 1990, WB Saunders, p 210.

Disposable fitted briefs are suitable for moderate to heavy leaking and are available in a variety of absorbencies. Undergarments are less bulky than fitted briefs because they do not wrap around the hips. They are held in place with front-to-back reusable elastic straps. For severe incontinence, rubber and vinyl underpants to wear over regular underpants, as well as reusable, washable absorbent underpants with waterproof outer barriers are available.

Consideration should also be given to use of products to clean, moisturize, and protect skin from urine. Barrier lotions can contain petroleum jelly or silicone. Finally, deodorizers are also available. Oral chlorophyllin copper complex tablets may be helpful in decreasing odor. The National Association for Continence (Spartanburg, South Carolina; 1-800-BLADDER) publishes a *Resource Guide of Continence Products and Services*. This publication is cross-referenced by product categories and manufacturers and contains an index of mail and phone order information.

Indwelling urethral catheters are generally contraindicated for long-term control of urinary incontinence in women. The Omnibus Reconciliation Act of 1987 list three acceptable indications:
- Retention (leading to problems) that cannot be surgically corrected or managed with intermittent self-catheterization
- Prevention of contamination of skin wounds with urine
- The care of impaired or terminally ill patients for whom bedding and clothing changes are disruptive

The risks of urethral catheterization include chronic urinary tract infection, urethral abscess and fistula, bladder stones, bladder spasms, bladder carcinoma, leakage around the catheter, and blockage caused by calcium encrustation. For this reason, there have been attempts at creating devices to control female incontinence that could be worn like a male condom catheter. In 1981, the British Science Research Council concluded that there were no satisfactory commercially available external urinary incontinence devices for women. Female anatomy poses many problems that must be solved to create such a device. These problems include securing the device against the vulva with minimal skin irritation, making application and cleaning easy, fitting for different body types, and minimizing leaking.

## External Collecting Devices

In a review by Pieper et al. (1989), the following attempts at creating external collecting devices were noted. In 1971, Crowley et al. described a vestibulovaginal device that used a suction developed by the drainage of urine. A device introduced in 1975 used a wide, rubber-necked funnel held by straps. During the same year, Fielding and Wells (1975) described a cup with a vaginal locator that was held in place by a special panty. Unfortunately, pressure on and erosion of the vulvar soft tissue was noted.

The Misstique device (Shield Health Care Center, Inc, South Gate, California) was introduced in 1982 and consists of a cup held over the urethra with stoma adhesives. It had a valve to prevent urine backflow. The Femex device was similarly held with an adhesive and marketed for a short time in 1982.

In 1986, Hollister marketed an external device held in place over the urethra by a form-fitting pericup with a vaginal portion to help retain it in place (Hollister, Inc, Libertyville, Illinois). The company also makes an adhesive urinary pouch that fits over the vulva. In nursing tests by Johnson et al. (1990), the device kept 9% of patients dry for 48 hours, with 14% requiring replacement for unacceptable leakage.

## BIBLIOGRAPHY

Bergman A, Matthews L, Ballard CA, et al: Suprapubic vs. transurethral bladder drainage after surgery for stress urinary incontinence, *Obstet Gynecol* 69:546, 1987.

Britt MR, Garibaldi RA, Miller WA, et al: Antimicrobial prophylaxis for catheter associated bacteriuria, *Antimicrob Agents Chemother* 11:240, 1977.

Bump RC: Prevention and management of complications following continence surgery. In Ostergard DR, Bent AE, eds: *Urogynecology and urodynamics,* ed 3, Baltimore, 1991, Wilkins & Wilkins.

Cottenden AM, Stocking B, Jones NB, et al: Biomedical engineering priorities for research in external aids, *J Biomed Eng* 3:325, 1981.

Crowley IP, Cardozo LJ, Lawrence LC: Female incontinence: a new approach, *Br J Urol* 43:492, 1971.

Diokno AC, Mitchell BA, Nash AJ, et al: Patient satisfaction and the Lofric catheter for clean intermittent catheterization, *J Urol* 153:349, 1995.

Faller N, Jeter KF: The ABC's of product selection, *Urol Nurs* 12:52, 1992.

Fielding P, Wells T: Urinary collecting device: a clinical trial among female geriatric patients, *Nurs Times* 71:136, 1975.

Foley FEB: A self-retaining bag catheter, *J Urol* 38:140, 1937.

Garibaldi RA, Burke JP, Dickman ML, et al: Factors predisposing to bacteriuria during indwelling urethral catheterization, *N Engl J Med* 291:215, 1974.

Harlass FE, Magelssen DJ: Benefits of posturethropexy bladder conditioning: fact or fiction? *J Reprod Med* 33:961, 1988.

Hodgkinson CP, Hodari AA: Trocar suprapubic cystotomy for postoperative bladder drainage in the female, *Am J Obstet Gynecol* 96:773, 1966.

Hu TW, Kaltreider DL, Igov J: Incontinence products: which is best? *Geriatr Nurs* 10:184, 1989.

Hurt WG: Bladder drainage after incontinence surgery, *Obstet Gynecol Rep* 2:307, 1990.

Jeter KF, Faller N, Norton C, eds: *Nursing for continence,* Philadelphia, 1990, WB Saunders.

Johnson DE, Muncie HL, O'Reilly JL, et al: An external urine collection device for incontinent women: evaluation of long-term use, *J Am Geriatr Soc* 38:1016, 1990.

Kass EH, Schneiderman LJ: Entry of bacteria into the urinary tracts of patients with inlying catheters, *N Engl J Med* 256:556, 1957.

Kass EJ, Koff SA, Diokno AC, et al: The significance of bacilluria in children on long-term intermittent catheterization, *J Urol* 126:223, 1981.

King RB, Carlson CE, Mervine J, et al: Clean and sterile intermittent catheterization methods in hospitalized patients with SCI, *Arch Phys Med Rehabil* 73:798, 1992.

Lapides J, Diokno AC, Silber SJ, et al: Clean, intermittent self-catheterization in the treatment of urinary tract disease, *J Urol* 107:458, 1972.

Lian CJ, Bracken RB: Urinary catheter sterilization with microwave oven, *Int Urogynecol J* 2:94, 1991.

MacDiarmid SA, Arnold EP, Palmer NB, et al: Management of spinal cord injured patients by indwelling suprapubic catheterization, *J Urol* 154:492, 1995.

Maynard FM, Diokno AC: Urinary infection and complications during clean intermittent catheterization following spinal cord injury, *J Urol* 132:943, 1984.

Moore KN, Kelm M, Sinclair O, et al: Bacteriuria in intermittent catheterization users: the effect of sterile versus clean reused catheters, *Rehab Nurs* 18:306, 1993.

O'Brien WM: Percutaneous placement of a suprapubic tube with peel away sheath introducer, *J Urol* 145:1015, 1991.

O'Leary JR, O'Leary JA: The mini-catheter, a reliable in-dwelling catheter substitute, *Obstet Gynecol* 36:141, 1970.

Pieper B, Cleland V, Johnson DE, et al: Inventing urine incontinence devices for women, *Image* 21:205, 1989.

Pierson CA: Pad testing, nursing interventions, and urine loss appliances. In Ostergard DR, Bent AE, eds: *Urogynecology and urodynamics,* ed 3, Baltimore, 1991, Wilkins & Wilkins.

Segal AI, Corlett RC: Postoperative bladder training, *Am J Obstet Gynecol* 133:366, 1979.

Stickler DJ, Zimakoff J: Complications of urinary tract infections associated with devices used for long-term bladder management, *J Hosp Infect* 28:177, 1994.

Terpenning MS, Allada RA, Kauffman CA: Intermittent urethral catheterization in the elderly, *J Am Geriatr Soc* 37:411, 1989.

Waller L, Johnsson O, Norlen L, et al: Clean intermittent catheterization in spinal cord injury patients: long-term follow-up of a hydrophilic low friction technique, *J Urol* 153:345, 1995.

Wanick CK, Reilly NJ: Incontinence care products: non-surgical management of urinary incontinence, *Ostomy Wound Management* 34:43, 1991.

Warren JW: Catheter-associated urinary tract infections, *Infect Dis Clin North Am* 1:823, 1987.

Webb RJ, Lawson AL, Neal DE: Clean intermittent self-catheterization in 172 adults, *Br J Urol* 65:20, 1990.

Wong ES, Hooton TM, and Working Group: *Guidelines for prevention of catheter-associated urinary tract infections,* Washington, DC, US Department of Health & Human Services, October 1997.

Wyndaele JJ, Maes D: Clean intermittent self-catheterization: a 12-year follow-up, *J Urol* 143:906, 1990.

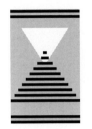

PART VI
*Case Presentations With Expert Discussions*

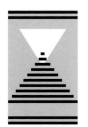

CHAPTER **34**
*Case Presentations With Expert Discussions*

Andrew C. Steele and Mickey M. Karram

---

## CASE 1
### Procidentia and Uterine Preservation

*CASE:* The patient is a 35-year-old para 4 with severe pelvic pressure and mild stress incontinence. She has had a tubal ligation. On examination, there was complete uterine procidentia with eversion of the anterior vaginal wall (Fig. 34-1). Subtracted urodynamics revealed mild anatomic genuine stress incontinence, without evidence of intrinsic sphincter deficiency. She is not interested in using a pessary and insists on uterine preservation.

DISCUSSANT: **W. Allen Addison**

There was a time when I would not have operated on this patient, in compliance with her wishes. Had she not been sterilized, I would have done my best to secure the uterus in an anatomic position to preserve fertility, in conjunction with whatever other reconstructive surgery was indicated. Faced with such a patient who had been sterilized, I would have insisted on hysterectomy as a component of the surgery, only to end up with an unhappy patient. Currently, assuming that the uterus is free of intrinsic disease, I would accede to the patient's wishes for uterine preservation in the course of reconstructive pelvic surgery even though she has been sterilized. I hasten to add that in most situations like this, I would strongly advise a hysterectomy and that most patients find this highly acceptable and experience no untoward sequelae.

To accommodate the wishes of the patient presented here, I would recommend abdominal sacral uteropexy with Mersilene mesh (Ethicon, Somerville, NJ) used as a suspensory bridge.[1] Inferiorly, I would attach this mesh to the origin of the uterosacral ligaments and the lower uterine segment, and superiorly, I would attach it to the anterior surface of the sacrum retroperitoneally. The mesh would be placed over a meticulously performed culdeplasty, and permanent sutures, used to perform the culdeplasty, would be brought out through the mesh and tied to secure it. If there was significant thinning of the posterior vaginal wall or if there were discrete breaks in the fascia of the posterior wall, I would extend the mesh down the posterior vaginal wall to the point where good fascia contiguous with the perineal body could be engaged. This could mean extending the mesh all the way to the perineal body.[2] Anteriorly, I would recommend performance of a Burch urethropexy and paravaginal defect repairs. I would also shorten the round ligaments and, if indicated, would go below and perform a perineorrhaphy.

I do not believe satisfactory data exist on which to base a convincing assessment of success rate. Such patients are rare, but we have had success in treating them as indicated in the preceding text. In addition, we have had fertile patients undergo successful pregnancies after surgery like that just described for total uterine procidentia with associated support defects. I would recommend for such a patient that delivery be accomplished by cesarean section.

### REFERENCES
1. Addison WA, Timmons MC: Abdominal approach to vaginal eversion, *Clin Obstet Gynecol* 36:995, 1993.
2. Cundiff GW, Harris RL, Coates K, et al: Abdominal sacral colpoperineopexy: a new approach for correction of posterior compartment defects and perineal descent associated with vaginal vault prolapse, *Am J Obstet Gynecol* 177:1345, 1998.

DISCUSSANT: **G. Rodney Meeks**

I would agree to perform corrective surgery for this patient and accept the conditions that she has stipulated. Had the patient not completed childbearing, I would have some reservations. I personally have not seen corrective surgery survive a subsequent pregnancy. However, there is literature documenting that delivery can occur with the repair remaining intact.

The patient's complaints of pelvic pressure, urinary incontinence, and uterovaginal prolapse must be addressed. Before surgery, I would reduce the uterine prolapse to accurately assess all sites of prolapse in the vagina. I would determine if the anterior vaginal wall had a central defect or a lateral detachment. Certainly, some lateral detachment is likely with complete prolapse, and an enterocele is often present. I would assess the posterior wall for detachment at the perineal body and at the vaginal apex, as well as for site-specific defects in the rectovaginal fascia.

After clearly defining the defects, one must decide on the surgical approach—vaginal, abdominal, or a combination. Correction of the defects should eliminate the uterine prolapse and pressure symptoms. A specific incontinence procedure will be needed for the genuine stress incontinence.

Four approaches have been described for treating prolapse with uterine preservation. The first is the Manchester procedure: vaginal shortening of the uterosacral and cardinal ligaments with cervical amputation. The Manchester procedure has a recurrent prolapse rate in excess of 20% in the first few months. Chances for subsequent pregnancy are severely compromised, and pregnancy wastage has been reported to range from 20% to 50% if conception occurs. Not amputating the cervix eliminates some of the pregnancy complications.

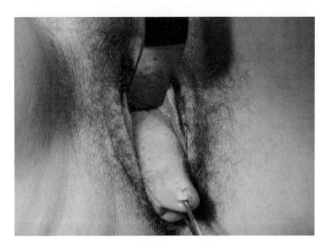

**Fig. 34-1** A patient with complete procidentia and eversion of the anterior vaginal wall.

The second approach is fixation of pelvic structures to the anterior abdominal wall, but this procedure has fallen into disfavor because the rate of enterocele formation is unacceptably high.

The third approach involves anchoring the uterus, cervix, or both to the sacrum with either natural or synthetic materials. Very good success has been reported with this procedure. Complications include hemorrhage from the sacrum and intestinal obstruction. A recent video publication details this technique.[1]

The fourth approach is to anchor the cervix to the sacrospinous ligaments. Richardson et al. described a transvaginal approach in which the uterosacral ligaments were attached to the sacrospinous ligaments.[2] This technique has a high degree of success. Also, subsequent pregnancies have been reported without recurrence of the prolapse. The authors described the inclusion of a needle procedure to treat incontinence.

In this patient, the presence of stress urinary incontinence requires the addition of a specific antiincontinence procedure. Three options for this include retropubic urethropexy, needle procedure, or anterior colporrhaphy.

I remain a proponent of the vaginal approach to prolapse repair and would recommend such an approach for this patient. I would use the technique described by Richardson et al. to suspend the uterus. I would also repair the enterocele, reattach the pubocervical fascia to its lateral attachments, and add a Kelly-Kennedy plication to stabilize the urethrovesical angle.

**REFERENCES**

1. Cholhan HJ: *Transabdominal uterovaginal suspension: an alternative to hysterectomy for uterovaginal prolapse,* Washington, DC, 1998, ACOG Audiovisual Library.
2. Richardson DA, Scotti RJ, Ostergard DR: Surgical management of uterine prolapse in young women, *J Reprod Med* 34:388, 1989.

**EDITORS' COMMENTS**

Both discussants express some concern over the patient's insistence on uterine preservation, although both would honor the patient's wishes in this regard. Despite the lack of consensus as to the route of prolapse correction, careful attention to all anatomic locations of prolapse is essential to obtain an optimal outcome.

## CASE 2
## Mixed Incontinence

*CASE:* The patient is a 48-year-old para 3 with a 9-year history of gradually worsening urinary incontinence. Her incontinence began after the birth of her last child and can occur both with an uncontrollable urge to void and with a cough or sneeze. Physical examination revealed a hypermobile urethra, first- to second-degree cystocele, and first-degree uterine prolapse. Findings from a directed neurologic examination were normal. During multichannel urodynamics, genuine stress incontinence was demonstrated with a cough when the prolapse was reduced, with a leak point pressure (LPP) of 65 cm $H_2O$ and a maximum urethral closure pressure of 42 cm $H_2O$. At maximum bladder capacity of 230 ml, she had a detrusor contraction of 20 cm $H_2O$ following provocative stimulus. She desires definitive therapy of her incontinence.

**DISCUSSANT: Alfred E. Bent**

This patient has mixed urinary incontinence in the presence of borderline pelvic organ prolapse (demonstrable cystocele and first-degree uterine prolapse). The cystocele is not further described with respect to bilateral or central defects. The prolapse does not appear symptomatic, and we are not informed of any menstrual irregularity. The stress component of her incontinence is associated with a hypermobile urethra, and urodynamic evaluation showed borderline sphincter function with LPP of 65 cm $H_2O$. Motor urge incontinence (detrusor instability) is demonstrated at bladder capacity, which is less than normal. The clinical and urodynamic evaluations reproduce the patient's urinary tract complaints.

The initial management for her incontinence should be conservative therapy with pelvic muscle rehabilitation[1] by using pelvic muscle exercises and bladder inhibition augmented by biofeedback therapy.[2] The key to this program is patient compliance, and if adequately followed, she has a cure or improved rate of 54% to 87%. The improvement in pelvic muscle control may possibly stabilize the pelvic organ prolapse. If the patient is unable to comply with this plan, then pelvic muscle rehabilitation could be attempted with vaginal cone therapy or functional electrical stimulation. The urge component could be addressed by a program of bladder retraining, functional electrical stimulation, or pharmacologic intervention.

Upon failure of the above programs or by patient request, surgical intervention may be offered. All anatomic defects should be considered in preparation for surgery. The primary repair for stress incontinence with bladder neck hypermobility is a retropubic urethropexy. This would be accompanied by a paravaginal defect repair, if the cystocele is at least grade 2 and is a lateral defect. Because the uterus already has a grade 1 prolapse and the operative procedures just described alter apical and posterior support, then an internal cul-de-sac and uterosacral ligament plication or Halban procedure should be considered. These procedures may be performed laparoscopically or by open technique. If a decision is made to remove the uterus and most likely the ovaries, then vault support to the uterosacral ligaments should be ensured. At the end of the procedure, bladder and ureteral integrity should be demonstrated. A vaginal and rectal examination should be performed to ensure there is no residual midline cystocele defect or posterior defect.

If the patient states that her incontinence is quite severe or that she leaks with coughing or sneezing immediately after emptying her bladder, or if she has severe allergic rhinitis, chronic bronchitis, or asthma, one could also make a case for a primary sling procedure. This alters the apical support mechanism minimally, and other repairs may not be required.

The surgical cure rates for either procedure are 85% to 90% for the stress incontinence component and 60% for the urge incontinence. Extensive preoperative counseling is required with respect to persistent urge incontinence, benefits and risks of concomitant hysterectomy and bilateral salpingo-oophorectomy, and potential for other pelvic support defects depending on the type of surgery performed.

For this specific patient, using only the information given, unless extremely skilled at laparoscopy, I would suggest an open Burch retropubic urethropexy. If there is moderate or more severe cystocele, then a paravaginal defect repair should be performed and consideration given to performing cul-de-sac and uterosacral ligament plication. If there is an indication for hysterectomy, this should be performed by a preferred technique, and vault support ensured. All possibilities must to be discussed in detail with the patient preoperatively and recorded in the chart.

### REFERENCES

1. Committee on Quality Assessment: *ACOG criteria set: surgery for genuine stress incontinence due to urethral hypermobility*, American College of Obstetricians and Gynecologists, No 4, 1995.
2. Fantl JA, Newman DK, Colling J, et al: Urinary incontinence in adults: acute and chronic management, Clinical Practice Guideline No 2, 1996 update, Rockville, Md: US Department of Health and Human Services. Public Health Service, Agency for Health Care Policy and Research, AHCPR Pub No 96-0682, March 1996.

### DISCUSSANT: **Michael P. Aronson**

This 48-year-old para 3 has a 9-year history consistent with worsening mixed incontinence. Her graded pelvic examination reveals grade 1 to 2 descent of the urethra and anterior vaginal wall with grade 1 descent of the uterus. Her posterior compartment appears well supported. During multichannel urodynamics, she demonstrated genuine stress urinary incontinence (SUI) with borderline urethral function measured both by leak point pressure (LPP) and maximal urethral closure pressure (MUCP). She also demonstrated a diminished bladder capacity with unprovoked bladder contractions that, combined with urethral relaxation, resulted in leakage consistent with detrusor instability (DI). She "desires definitive therapy of her incontinence."

Although this patient suffers from mixed incontinence (i.e., both SUI and DI), she most likely feels that she has just one problem: leaking urine. She may think that it comes from one cause and may come to the physician for "definitive" treatment. Patient education is the crucial first step in treating patients with mixed incontinence. To the patient, her leaking urine appears as one problem, so it is important that the physician take the time to explain the two different causes of her incontinence problem, their different mechanisms, and the different treatment strategies for each cause. The patient's compliance with her treatment regimen and her overall expectations of therapy will be more realistic.

Treatment of the patient with mixed incontinence must be individualized. The patient who suffers predominantly from DI and has only occasional loss of urine with stress differs greatly from the patient with daily SUI and only occasional episodes of DI. The former patient can be treated for her DI first with discontinuation of bladder irritants, some form of anticholinergic medication, and bladder retraining and urge suppression drills. In the current patient, imipramine would be a good pharmacologic choice because in addition to its anticholinergic properties, it also exerts an alpha-adrenergic agonist effect at the bladder neck to help with her SUI component. Functional electrical stimulation may also be useful.[1]

Many patients with predominant DI whose DI component resolves with therapy may opt for no further treatment or conservative therapy only for their minor SUI component.

The patient with mixed incontinence that is predominantly SUI is different. This patient may come seeking surgical repair and think this will definitively address her total leakage problem. A conservative regimen as stated previously, augmented with pelvic floor rehabilitation, may be a valuable initial step. If surgical treatment is contemplated, the physician must explain that surgery will only address the SUI component of her problem and that 50% to 65% of patients will be left with residual DI or perhaps even worsened DI.[2] Depending on the patient, the DI component can be addressed preoperatively or, if it persists postoperatively, after surgery.

If surgery were contemplated in the current patient, an operation should be chosen that would elevate and stabilize her proximal urethra to address her SUI, with the least amount of obstruction that might exacerbate her DI. While her urethral function is borderline, her LPP is greater than 60 cm $H_2O$ and her MUCP is greater than 20 cm $H_2O$, excluding her from the classification of intrinsic sphincter deficiency by either criteria. Because of this, one might avoid a suburethral sling procedure, which is more obstructive, and recommend a Burch retropubic urethropexy, combined with a bilateral paravaginal support defect repair as needed, to treat her urethral hypermobility and cystocele. To address all of this patient's support defects under the same anesthesia, her coexisting apical support defect could be treated with total abdominal hysterectomy with uterosacral suspension of the apex and cul-de-sac ablation. Her posterior compartment support was normal.

Treatment of the patient with mixed urinary incontinence requires communication skills along with excellent clinical skills and judgment. Individualization of treatment strategy is important for a good outcome.

### REFERENCES

1. Brubaker L, Benson JT, Bart A, et al: Transvaginal electrical stimulation for female urinary incontinence, *Am J Obstet Gynecol* 177:536, 1997.
2. Bent AE: Etiology and management of detrusor instability and mixed incontinence, *Obstet Gynecol Clin North Am* 16:853, 1989.

### EDITORS' COMMENTS

The discussants point out the important role of an individual patient's desires and expectations in the management of mixed incontinence. Both discussants support the value of initial conservative management, and both stress that the move from conservative to surgical therapy must be individualized and patient driven. The potential for detrusor instability to persist or even worsen after surgery for stress incontinence must be fully understood by the patient.

## CASE 3
### Cystocele and Potential Stress Incontinence

*CASE:* A 49-year-old para 5 complains of pelvic pressure and the feeling that she does not empty her bladder completely. She had an anterior colporrhaphy (without hysterectomy) 7 years ago. On examination, she had recurrent anterior vaginal wall prolapse that descended beyond the hymen with straining in the supine position (Fig. 34-2). The cervix descended to the hymen, and a small enterocele and rectocele were also noted. On spontaneous uroflowmetry, the patient voided 240 ml with a 10-ml postvoid residual urine volume. Time to void was 42 seconds with a maximum flow rate of 12 ml/sec. Filling subtracted cystometry showed a stable cystometrogram to maximum capacity of 440 ml. Despite numerous provocative maneuvers in the standing position, no stress incontinence could be demonstrated. A static maximum urethral closure pressure with prolapse unreduced was 53 cm $H_2O$. The prolapse was then gently reduced using a Sims' speculum (Fig. 34-3), and leakage was demonstrated with coughing and straining, with a Valsalva LPP of 45 cm $H_2O$ and MUCP of 30 cm $H_2O$. The patient desires surgical correction of her prolapse.

DISCUSSANT: **Richard C. Bump**
*Potential Stress Incontinence*

It is well recognized that women with advanced stages of pelvic organ prolapse rarely, if ever, complain of the symptom of stress incontinence. Advanced anterior segment prolapse, when accentuated by stress, descends and obstructs the urethra, preventing vesical pressure from exceeding urethral pressure and preventing the occurrence of genuine stress incontinence (GSI).[1] Preoperative reduction of the prolapse, by using pessaries, packs, or a Sims' speculum as a barrier, prevents this stress-activated urethral obstruction and reveals so-called potential stress incontinence in

36% to 80% of women with advanced prolapse.[2] Although barrier testing has been suggested for determining which women should have a suspending urethropexy or pubovaginal sling procedure performed concurrently with prolapse correction surgery, the clinical predictive value of these barrier tests is highly questionable. Despite predicting GSI in up to 80% of these women, clinical series demonstrate a much lower risk of 10% or less.[2] In a recent, randomized prospective comparison of needle urethropexy versus bladder neck endopelvic fascia plication for the prevention of GSI in women undergoing vaginal reconstruction for stage III or IV prolapse, preoperative prolapse reduction testing predicted GSI in 67% (10 of 15) undergoing the latter procedure; however, GSI was observed in only 7% (1 of 15) at 6 months.[2] In the entire study population, intrinsic sphincteric deficiency (ISD) was predicted in 25% (8 of 32) but was observed in only two subjects (6%), one of whom had been predicted preoperatively (although no prophylactic slings were performed). In this study, the positive predictive value of barrier testing was 20% for GSI and 12.5% for ISD. To put the risk of potential incontinence into some perspective, one should remember that the risk of de novo GSI after vaginal prolapse surgery (7% to 10%) is lower than the risk of persistent GSI after a Burch colposuspension performed to cure GSI (8% to 15%). I am always aware that severe prolapse may mask potential GSI; one major goal of my prolapse surgery is for the patient to leave the operating room with durable and preferential support to the bladder neck. However, I have abandoned the notion that preoperative barrier testing determines the route or type of surgery.

*Route of Prolapse Correction Surgery*

Several considerations have an impact on my choice of surgical route for reconstructive surgery, including the precise defects responsible for prolapse, the cause of the defects, whether the inciting and promoting events are continuing processes, and the patient's desires and expectations. About 60% of women I see with prolapse have discrete endopelvic fascia defects and low-risk profiles for recurrence; in this situation, I perform a vaginal route anatomic repair that corrects all defects (inferior, lateral, superior, and midline) of the indigenous tissues. However, there are

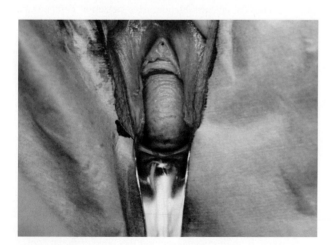

**Fig. 34-2**  Anterior vaginal wall prolapse (unreduced).

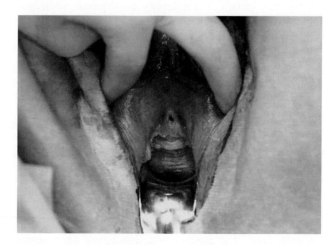

**Fig. 34-3**  The same patient after the prolapse is reduced with a Sims' speculum. The aim of this reductive maneuver is to determine if underlying "occult" or "potential" stress incontinence is present.

circumstances that I think compromise the longevity of these repairs, which are intended to realign the pelvic organs over a relatively normal pelvic floor and to withstand normal physical stresses. Vaginal approaches depend on normal pelvic floor muscle support, and I avoid them in women with poor muscle function following attempts at pelvic floor rehabilitation or in women with overwhelming neuromuscular dysfunction such as spinal cord injuries. Extreme attenuation of native tissues may also compromise the success of these repairs, and I will use mesh or fascial substitutions for the endopelvic fascia in these situations, via either abdominal or vaginal approaches. Finally, women with rapidly recurrent prolapse, extremely active lifestyles, significant perineal descent, or chronic ongoing causes for prolapse (e.g., obesity, refractory constipation, chronic obstructive pulmonary disease) require a repair with more strength than is offered by my anatomic vaginal repair. Under these circumstances, I perform a compensatory repair that will include an abdominal sacral colpoperineopexy, combined usually with a Halban culdeplasty, retropubic paravaginal repair and bladder neck suspension, and often with a perineal reconstruction and distal posterior fascial repair and reattachment.

## REFERENCES

1. Bump RC, Fantl JA, Hurt WG: The mechanism of urinary continence in women with severe uterovaginal prolapse: results of barrier studies, *Obstet Gynecol* 72:291, 1988.
2. Bump RC, Hurt WG, Theofrastous JP, et al: Randomized prospective comparison of needle colposuspension versus endopelvic fascia plication for potential stress incontinence prophylaxis in women undergoing vaginal reconstruction for stage III or IV pelvic organ prolapse, *Am J Obstet Gynecol* 175:326, 1996.

**DISCUSSANT: R. Edward Varner**

This relatively young patient desires surgical correction for her symptomatic pelvic relaxation and stress incontinence that is concealed by the mechanical effect of the prolapse on the urethra or bladder neck. Her anterior vaginal wall descends beyond the hymen as a result of (1) descent of the cervix, (2) opening of the genital hiatus, and (3) probable attenuation or laceration of the anterior vaginal connective tissue and muscularis.

Assuming that the patient has reasonable anterior lateral vaginal support, I would start with a vaginal hysterectomy by using the Heaney technique. I would perform an anterior colporrhaphy with dissection and plication of the pubocervical connective tissues from the point of the bladder neck suspension to the level of the vaginal cuff. After trimming and closing the anterior vaginal mucosa, I would then perform a procedure to approximate the pubocervical to posterior paravaginal tissues at the cuff, repair the enterocele, and suspend the paravaginal fascia of the vaginal cuff to the uterosacral ligaments when they can be identified in the posterior pelvis. Cystoscopy would be performed at the completion of all procedures.

When the uterosacral ligaments are not adequate for suspension, a sacrospinous ligament suspension would be performed with a modified Nichols' technique, with care taken to avoid excess traction on the anterior vaginal wall. Before securing the sacrospinous suspension sutures, the paravaginal fascia on the left side of the vaginal cuff would be approximated to the superior pararectal fascia with sutures.

After dissection of the rectovaginal space and, when indicated, sacrospinous suspension, specific defects in the rectal wall and

pararectal fascia would be repaired. Rectal examination during the procedure facilitates delineation of these defects. The repairs would produce an intact connective tissue plate attached to the perineal tissues inferiorly, to the pelvic side walls laterally, and to the paravaginal tissue of the suspended cuff. The perineal body would be reconstructed to produce a good posterior vaginal angle. Plication of the levator muscles across the midline is sometimes necessary to produce this; however, it should be avoided if adequate vaginal caliber cannot be maintained.

The management of this patient's stress incontinence is more of a challenge. Her urethral incompetence, despite a lack of symptoms, is relatively severe as evidenced by a low Valsalva leak point pressure and a marginally low resting urethral closure pressure with the prolapse reduced. The change in urethral dynamics afforded by the Sims' speculum has been well documented in patients with large anterior defects, as well as posterior wall defects.[1] Urethral dysfunction may be even more pronounced when the cervix or vaginal cuff is supported with greater tension with ring forceps or some type of suspension procedure.

Based on our outcome data, I agree with those who report relatively low long-term success rates with pubourethral ligament plication techniques and with long-needle suspension procedures.[2] I also think that Burch suspensions and paravaginal suspensions have relatively poor success rates in patients with evidence of more severe intrinsic urethral defects. The procedures that create a greater obstructive effect, such as Marshall-Marchetti-Krantz procedures, Burch procedures with excessive elevation, and tightly placed slings, may have a higher likelihood of producing long-term voiding dysfunction; this patient is at risk for this result.

For the reasons mentioned, I would choose a relatively unique bladder neck suspension using a 1½- to 2-cm wide strip of cadaveric fascia lata. The procedure requires a transvaginal dissection into the space of Retzius immediately adjacent to the bladder neck to expose the obturator fascia. This dissection can be performed as an extension of the anterior colporrhaphy. The ends of the strip are sutured to the obturator fascia immediately adjacent to the pubic rami on each side and attached with small absorbable sutures to the adventitia proximal and distal to the urethrovesical junction. The strip can be tightened by adjusting its length to produce preferential, but not excessive, elevation of the bladder neck. Although we do not yet have long-term follow-up on this procedure or experience with a large number of patients, it has subjectively and objectively cured stress incontinence while maintaining adequate micturition function in four of four patients similar to this one who had intrinsic sphincter deficiency and bladder support defects combined with severe pelvic prolapse.

## REFERENCES

1. Bump RC, Fantl JA, Hurt WG: The mechanism of urinary continence in women with severe uterovaginal prolapse: results of barrier studies, *Obstet Gynecol* 72:291, 1988.
2. Leach GE, Dmochowski RR, Appell RA, et al: Female stress urinary incontinence clinical guidelines: panel summary report on surgical management of female stress urinary incontinence, *J Urol* 158:875, 1997.

## EDITORS' COMMENTS

The challenge of addressing a potential problem (i.e., the unmasking of stress incontinence) with a potentially morbid prophylactic procedure is well addressed by the discussants. Both discussants favor the use of mesh or fascia to bolster the patient's weakened tissue, suggesting an expanded role for these materials in future corrective prolapse surgery.

## CASE 4
### Recurrent Urethrovaginal Fistula

*CASE:* The patient is a 24-year-old para 4 who initially had a large symptomatic urethral diverticulum. Urethral diverticulectomy resulted in a urethrovaginal fistula, and initial repair resulted in recurrence of the fistula. On examination, a fistulous tract with granulation tissue was noted at the urethrovesical crease of the anterior vaginal wall. Urethroscopy noted the urethral opening of the fistula to be approximately 0.5 cm distal to the urethrovesical junction. A bridge of scar tissue was found in the proximal urethra.

DISCUSSANT: **Rodney A. Appell**

Basic surgical tenets for repair of fistulas depend on adequate vascularization, the ability to perform tension-free and nonoverlapping closure of all suture lines, and watertight anastomosis without distal obstruction. Preoperative evaluation would include cystourethroscopy, pelvic examination, and vaginoscopy to evaluate the extent of the defect, the possibility of unrecognized secondary fistulas, and the pliability of local tissue. Urodynamics are indicated if the patient is incontinent, to help delineate the pathophysiology. For example, in the case where the fistula is 0.5 cm distal to the urethrovesical junction, there should be no incontinence unless the proximal urethra or bladder neck is damaged. Concomitant urethral damage and incontinence, when corrected in the same setting, generally require construction of a fascial pubovaginal sling[1] with an interposed Martius labial fat pad flap[2] between the sling and the reconstructed urethra. In this case where there is no incontinence, I would incise or laser coagulate the proximal urethral scar, repair the fistula in layers, cover the repair with a Martius labial fat pad flap between the urethral and vaginal closures, and provide urinary drainage via a 16-French silicone Foley catheter for 10 days. Postoperative stress incontinence, if it should occur, can be handled with injectable collagen.

The technique for repair of a vesicovaginal fistula follows these basic surgical tenets and has been described in detail elsewhere.[3] A weighted vaginal speculum and 16-French Foley catheter are placed, and the anterior vaginal wall is exposed. The area of the fistula is incised circumferentially, and the anterior vaginal epithelium is mobilized for more than 1 cm around the fistula. The urethral mucosa is closed with fine No. 4-0 chromic catgut suture, avoiding tension by undermining the vaginal flaps laterally. The overlying tissue (periurethral fascia) is closed with a continuous No. 3-0 polyglycolic acid (PGA) suture. At this point, the labial fat pad is mobilized. A vertical skin incision is made in one of the labia majora. The fat pad is grasped and kept on its posterolateral pedicle (to be in alignment with its blood supply from branches of the pudendal artery). A length of 6 to 10 cm is usually necessary to cover the defect completely. A tunnel is created from the pedicle base to the vaginal incision, and the labial fat pad flap is delivered into the vaginal wound and sutured over the defect with No. 3-0 PGA suture. The labium is closed in two layers with No. 3-0 PGA suture, with a small Penrose drain placed out the most inferior end of the incision

for 48 hours. The vaginal epithelium is then closed with No. 2-0 PGA suture. A vaginal packing covered with conjugated estrogen cream is left in the vagina for 24 hours.

**REFERENCES**
1. Zimmern P, Schmidbauer C, Leach G, et al: Vesicovaginal and urethrovaginal fistulae, *Semin Urol* 4:24, 1986.
2. Patil U, Waterhouse K, Laungani G: Management of 18 difficult vesicovaginal and urethrovaginal fistulae with modified Ingelman-Sundberg and Martius operations, *J Urol* 123:653, 1982.
3. Appell RA: Urethral diverticulum and fistula. In Glenn JF, ed: *Urologic surgery,* Philadelphia, 1991, JB Lippincott, pp 755-762.

DISCUSSANT: **Donald R. Ostergard**

This 24-year-old patient has a recurrent urethrovaginal fistula after a urethral diverticulectomy, with the fistula located approximately 0.5 cm distal to the urethrovesical junction. This problem is best managed surgically. Because the patient has had two surgical procedures in this area, she most likely has denervation, devascularization, and fibrosis in and around the recurrent fistula. No further preoperative testing is necessary in this individual.

The surgical repair begins with the placement of a transurethral Foley catheter followed by distention of the urethrovaginal septum with a diluted vasopressin (Pitressin) solution (one unit in 30 ml of saline). This distends the surrounding scar tissue, provides better planes for dissection, and decreases bleeding at the surgical site. The area surrounding the fistula should be mobilized widely, such that the anticipated closure will be totally without tension. The intraurethral scar tissue should be lysed. After adequate mobilization is achieved, closure is begun using a "vest-over pants" technique by layering tissue derived from the peripheral dissection, taking care not to overlap suture lines.[1] Because this area is relatively devascularized, a bulbocavernosus fat pad graft should be used to improve the vascularity to the area. To accomplish this, an incision is made in either labium majus and the bulbocavernosus graft mobilized, leaving the posterior vascular end of the pedicle intact. A tunnel is then created under the vaginal mucosa from the labium majus so that the graft may be brought into the operative field and placed over the repaired fistula site without tension. The tunnel for the graft must be wide enough so that strangulation of the graft does not occur. The graft should be attached to the periurethral tissue on the opposite side of the closed fistula, at least 2 cm away from the fistulous site, covering the entire fistula closure site completely. Subsequent to this, the vaginal mucosa is closed, and a Foley catheter is left to drain the bladder for 7 days.

Regarding concomitant stress incontinence repair, we are not provided with any information regarding the presence or absence of urethral hypermobility or demonstrable stress incontinence. In the absence of demonstrable stress incontinence even in the presence of urethral hypermobility, I would not perform a concomitant sling procedure. Should urodynamic evaluation reveal genuine stress incontinence, then a suburethral sling procedure would be indicated.

**REFERENCE**
1. Ostergard DR, Bent AE, eds: *Urogynecology and urodynamics: theory and practice,* ed 4, Baltimore, 1996, Williams & Wilkins.

## EDITORS' COMMENTS

Both discussants give very practical advice on the surgical management of patients with recurrent urethrovaginal fistulas. There is agreement on the need for a fat pad flap to improve vascularity of the area. Should urinary incontinence also be present, both discussants agree that a suburethral sling should be added to the repair.

## CASE 5

### Evaluation and Management of Complete Vaginal Eversion

*CASE:* The patient is a 56-year-old with severe pelvic pressure. She had an abdominal hysterectomy and retropubic repair 20 years ago. She had a history of recurrent stress incontinence; however, over the last 2 years, this resolved, and she currently has to reduce her prolapse to empty her bladder. Complete vaginal eversion was found on examination (Fig. 34-4). Filling cystometry revealed an uninhibited detrusor contraction at maximum capacity, which was less than 200 ml.

DISCUSSANT: **Jeffrey L. Cornella**

The management of patients with symptomatic vaginal vault prolapse must always include historical and physical assessment of the bladder. The historical bladder assessment includes questions regarding voiding dysfunction and urinary incontinence. The physical examination includes assessment of vaginal support defects, degree of urethrovesical junction descent, and the impact of the posterior compartment on the bladder.

Prolapse and incontinence have a shared genesis, as patients with pelvic denervation and reenervation are predisposed to weakness and dysfunction in both areas. Pudendal neuropathy, connective tissue defects, and loss of elasticity with aging may impact both incontinence and prolapse.

A percentage of patients with vaginal prolapse may sustain urinary retention secondary to obstruction from prolapse. Similarly, some patients who demonstrate stress urinary incontinence early in their history may have resolution of symptoms as the prolapse enlarges and subsequently obstructs the urethra. If these patients do not receive a concomitant urethropexy at the time of

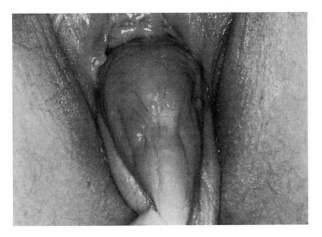

**Fig. 34-4**   Complete vaginal eversion.

prolapse repair, they will most likely exhibit significant urinary incontinence postoperatively.

As reported by Wall et al., simple office bladder filling has a high positive predictive value when compared with multichannel urodynamic testing.[1] We perform residual urine determination, simple bladder filling, and stress testing with a full bladder in prolapse patients. The patient is asked to perform serial coughing in both the standing and supine positions. Observation includes the presence or absence of immediate, nonsustained urine leakage. We then use a rectal pledget, which gently reduces the prolapse to straighten the urethra. Care is taken not to press on the anterior wall and induce artifact. The presence or absence of leakage is again noted in both the supine and standing positions. A standing rectovaginal examination may be considered to assess for enterocele descent. If the patient demonstrates projectile, immediate, and nonsustained leakage with cough, we perform a urethropexy at the time of vaginal vault surgery.

The suggestion of detrusor contractions at a capacity of less than 200 ml would be an indication for multichannel urodynamic testing. Mixed incontinent patients who demonstrate uninhibited contractions at high volumes (>250 ml) are candidates for surgery without multichannel testing. We counsel the patient that bladder instability may not respond to surgery and that there is a small risk of increased bladder instability.

If the patient has a history of obstructed defecation or severe constipation, gastrointestinal consultation is considered, with review of bowel motility and rectal outlet assessment with defecating proctography. The patient must reach a point before surgery at which she can empty her rectum without excessive straining.

The surgical approach to prolapse depends on the patient's history of prolapse surgery, tissue integrity, and presence or absence of stress urinary incontinence. Patients with urinary retention are counseled that bladder emptying after the operation is not completely predictable.

If the patient has a history of multiple prolapse operations or poor tissues, we may perform a fascia lata sacrocolpopexy. If the patient has good tissue integrity, we would perform a miniincision paravaginal defect repair, concomitant Burch urethropexy, and vaginal repair of the high bladder prolapse and enterocele. Our vaginal enterocele repair consists of a modified McCall culdeplasty performed with two delayed absorbable sutures. Postmenopausal patients receive a third permanent McCall suture placed internally.

Sacrocolpopexy has a high success rate for enterocele. The vaginal area with the greatest risk of recurrence is along the high bladder. The incontinent patient would receive a paravaginal defect repair and Burch urethropexy at the time of the sacrocolpopexy. The sacrocolpopexy procedure has multiple points of suture attachment to the vagina, including a significant portion of the posterior vaginal wall. It also attaches to the anterior apex of the vault. If possible, we would reapproximate the break in endopelvic fascia before suture placement for the sacrocolpopexy graft material. The fascia lata is sutured to the midline of the sacrum at S1-S2. The patient's legs are repositioned after the abdominal aspect of the operation to allow a vaginal approach to residual cystocele and rectocele.

Sacrospinous ligament procedures have limitations. Unless a graft material is used for bridging between the ligament and vagina, there are usually only one or two points of suture attachment to the vagina. In addition, this procedure creates a deviation of the vagina and may predispose to a higher incidence of recurrent cystoceles than other prolapse operations.

**REFERENCE**

1. Wall LL, Wiskind AK, Taylor PA: Simple bladder filling with cough stress test compared with subtracted cystometry for the diagnosis of urinary incontinence, *Am J Obstet Gynecol* 171:1477, 1994.

**DISCUSSANT: Lester A. Ballard**

In this patient with massive eversion of the vagina, it is interesting that she had a previous retropubic repair, which can pull the vagina anteriorly and produce an enterocele. Also of interest is that she developed recurrent stress urinary incontinence but the symptoms had subsided over the past 2 years, and she has to reduce the prolapse to empty her bladder. This suggests that as the vaginal vault descended, kinking of the urethra protected the patient from incontinence. I would perform urodynamic testing after reduction of the prolapse with a pessary to study for the type of incontinence. In addition to the detrusor instability, she may have genuine stress urinary incontinence (GSUI) with urethral hypermobility or intrinsic sphincter deficiency (ISD). If GSUI or ISD is found, then a bladder neck suspension or suburethral sling will need to be done. One might also do a pelvic or renal ultrasound to evaluate the ovaries and to look for any partial renal obstruction or hydronephrosis.

At surgery, I grasp the two vaginal dimples at the apex with long Allis clamps and identify the strongest tissue in the uterosacral cardinal complex. I then open posteriorly from the perineum up the posterior wall, over the apex, and up the anterior wall. Once I am sure that I am over the bladder base, I check for an enterocele, open the enterocele sac (if found), and dissect the bladder off anteriorly and laterally. I then close the sac with two sutures of No. 0 Prolene on an M0-6 needle and try to include both uterosacral-cardinal ligaments in the closure. If the patient had no GSUI with prolapse reduction on preoperative testing, then I do a high suburethral plication with No. 0 PDS suture. If she was found to have GSUI (with or without ISD), then our urogynecologist would perform an in-situ vaginal wall or fascial patch sling.

After the suburethral plication or sling has been done but not tied, the cystocele repair is then performed by suturing No. 0 PDS on a CT-1 needle through the dissected anterior vaginal wall fascia to the obturator fascia. These are tied, redundant vaginal mucosa is excised, and the vagina is closed with a running locking No. 2-0 delayed absorbable suture. Following this, the sling sutures are tied.

I then perform an iliococcygeus vaginal vault suspension using No. 0 PDS suture on a CT-1 or CT-2 needle. Previously I had done sacrospinous ligament fixation in 243 cases but was concerned about the recurrent anterior wall defects.[1] I have been performing the iliococcygeus fascia suspension since 1991, and I believe it gives good vault support; however, it remains to be determined if there is a difference in the occurrence of anterior defects with this procedure. Last, a posterior colporrhaphy is done using multiple, close, horizontal mattress sutures to give good posterior wall support without banding the upper vagina. A perineorrhaphy is performed routinely.

**REFERENCE**

1. Paraiso MF, Ballard LA, Walters MD, et al: Pelvic support defects and visceral and sexual function in women treated with sacrospinous ligament suspension and pelvic reconstruction, *Am J Obstet Gynecol* 175:1423, 1996.

**EDITORS' COMMENTS**

The discussants stress the need for urodynamic evaluation with the prolapse reduced, although they differ as to the reduction maneuver. In mapping out their surgical repairs, it is interesting that both discussants specifically recommended against a sacrospinous fixation in favor of other techniques to support the vaginal vault.

## CASE 6
### Intractable Detrusor Instability

*CASE:* The patient is a 42-year-old para 1 with a 1-year history of mixed incontinence. She initially complained of urine loss both with cough and sneeze, as well as with a strong urge to void. She has enuresis and daytime frequency with voiding up to every 15 minutes. Her medical history was remarkable for psychosis and seizure disorders; her medications include multiple antipsychotic and antiepileptic drugs, oxybutynin for neuroleptic-induced ptyalism, and DDAVP that was begun by her psychiatrist in an attempt to control her enuresis. Subtracted cystometry (Fig. 34-5) revealed a detrusor contraction at a volume of 135 ml that measured 40 cm $H_2O$ and was associated with leakage. Genuine stress incontinence was demonstrated at a volume of 150 ml with a Valsalva leak point pressure of approximately 70 cm $H_2O$. Maximum cystometric capacity was 287 ml. Given her mixed incontinence picture, the patient was counseled, and she desired surgical therapy for her stress incontinence fully understanding that the postoperative course of her detrusor instability was unpredictable. She underwent a laparoscopic Burch urethropexy that was successful in correcting her stress incontinence; however, she continued to have profound urge incontinence 3 months after surgery. Repeat urodynamics (Fig. 34-6) revealed a first sensation at 251 ml and a strong desire to void at 269 ml. This was followed immediately by an insuppressible detrusor contraction rising to 40 cm $H_2O$ above baseline

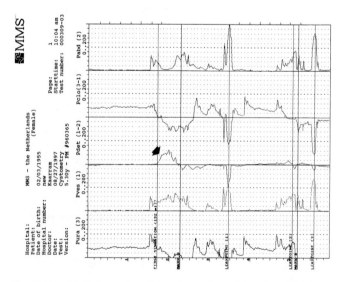

**Fig. 34-5** Multichannel urodynamic tracing of a patient with intractable detrusor instability and concomitant stress incontinence.

vesical pressure. No stress incontinence could be elicited. Postoperative cystoscopy revealed no suture penetration or other intravesical pathology. Attempts were made as part of a multidisciplinary team to adjust her medications to optimize her bladder control; this was unsuccessful. The patient is still voiding every 15 to 30 minutes during the day and saturating four to six large pads a day.

### DISCUSSANT: David R. Staskin

#### Clinical Presentation

A patient previously diagnosed with mixed genuine stress and urge urinary incontinence presents with persistent urge incontinence following surgical correction of her stress incontinence. Although this clinical presentation is not unusual, this particular case is complicated by the patient's expectations before and after her surgical intervention, her psychiatric and neurologic diagnoses, and multiple medications. Before planning further intervention for her incontinence, the treating physician must consider the continuing limitations presented by her coexisting medical conditions.

#### Initial Impression

A patient's expectations before surgery are often based on the information that she has received before surgery. Preoperative counseling should specifically mention the probability of persistent urinary urge incontinence (UUI). If the patient's stress symptoms are significant, surgical intervention may be appropriate. Symptomatic UUI may improve in 35% to 50% of patients with mixed symptoms after a procedure for GSI. This number decreases significantly when the detrusor instability is greater than 40 cm $H_2O$; improvement should not be expected when the cause of the overactive bladder is secondary to a neurologic lesion (detrusor hyperreflexia). In patients with pure GSI treated with surgery, de novo urge symptoms may be seen in 18% to 33% of patients. In this patient, the "surgical complication" of persistent urge may have been prevented by deferring surgery, unless the urge incontinence responded to therapy.

#### Clinical Evaluations

The patient should fill out a voiding diary. An accurate assessment of fluid intake and output is helpful in many patients.

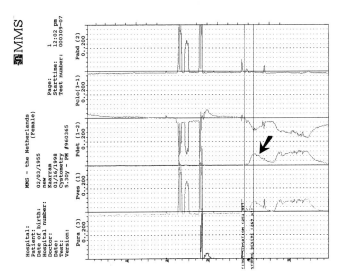

**Fig. 34-6** Multichannel urodynamic evaluation of the same patient in Fig. 34-5 after a retropubic urethropexy. The patient continues to have high pressure detrusor instability.

In patients with conditions such as peripheral edema and diabetes, nocturnal diuresis secondary to fluid balance and osmotic diuresis may be contributing to symptoms. A diary is critical in evaluating patients with psychiatric disorders who may have psychogenic polydipsia or lithium-induced diabetes insipidus.

The character of the enuresis should be elicited. Adult patients who wet the bed without awakening usually have a sleep disorder with or without lower urinary tract pathology. Sedative medications may be causing some of the problems at night.

Is the patient compliant with medications? Patients may misunderstand the dosage or timing of medications or fail to take them at all. Patients with psychiatric disease may have an accessory gain associated with noncompliance.

#### Urodynamic Evaluation

*Uroflowmetry:* If the patient has poor flow or increased postvoid residual urine, a pressure flow test should be considered to rule out obstruction contributing to instability. Urethrolysis is indicated if obstruction is present, although it may not change the patient's symptoms. In this patient, an underlying neurologic component is suspected as the cause of persistent bladder overactivity. If further surgery for bladder overactivity is contemplated, efficient bladder emptying should be confirmed.

*Postvoiding residual (PVR):* Patients with overflow incontinence who require intermittent catheterization will often mimic the symptoms of UUI. A patient with profound diuresis may fill rapidly following voiding and should be tested immediately after the uroflow.

*Cystometrogram (CMG):* This patient has demonstrated the clinical symptoms and the urodynamic findings associated with UUI. A dilemma may arise in patients with symptomatic UUI with a negative CMG (although the presumptive diagnosis is UUI) or in patients who demonstrate a positive CMG without the symptoms of UUI (subclinical bladder instability, which does not require treatment).

#### Conservative Measures

With continuing evaluation of pharmacologic therapy, behavioral interventions and pelvic muscle physiotherapy with exercises alone or with electrical stimulation should be considered. There is no literature on the value of this therapy in the subgroup of patients with psychiatric or neurologic disease.

#### Surgical Intervention

*Bladder denervation procedures:* Bladder denervation and subtrigonal phenol injection are not recommended because of their poor risk/benefit ratio.

*Sacral root modulation:* The use of sacral root modulation with an implantable stimulator may be considered.

*Bladder augmentation:* The use of small or large bowel to augment bladder capacity and decrease the degree of bladder overactivity should be considered in patients with intractable symptoms. The specific issues surrounding postoperative self-catheterization must be addressed. Patients with voluntary pelvic floor activity may learn to relax and perform the Credé maneuver following cystoplasty and therefore void to completion. Patients with complete neurologic lesions, decreased voluntary pelvic floor control, or bladder outlet obstruction should expect to catheterize.

### DISCUSSANT: Jerry G. Blaivas

This woman had urinary frequency, urgency, urge incontinence, and enuresis (in addition to stress incontinence) preoperatively and continues to have the same symptoms postoperatively—minus the stress incontinence.

Historically, her symptoms began only 1 year before a laparoscopic Burch colposuspension at the age of 41. The symptoms were very severe; she voided up to every 15 minutes and also had enuresis. The severity of her symptoms and the presence of enuresis are causes for concern and require a careful evaluation to exclude previously undiagnosed neurologic disease, urethral obstruction, and urinary retention with overflow incontinence. The latter could be caused by the oxybutynin that she was taking for ptyalism. She could have diabetes insipidus from an underlying neurologic condition or she could be an obsessive-compulsive water drinker as a manifestation of her psychiatric condition.

Before embarking on further treatment, it is important to attain an accurate diagnosis. To begin with, she should have a focused neurologic history and examination, urinalysis, and urine culture. Assuming these are unremarkable, urinary cytology should be done to screen for in-situ bladder cancer. A voiding diary will rule out polyuria (and diabetes insipidus). Uroflow and postvoid residual urine volume will screen for urethral obstruction and incomplete bladder emptying, but a definitive diagnosis can only be made by synchronous detrusor pressure and uroflow studies.

Assuming that the diagnostic evaluation did not disclose any remediable factors, there are few therapeutic alternatives for detrusor instability that is refractory to behavioral and pharmacologic treatment. Intravesical instillation of oxybutynin has been reported to work well in some patients, although it has not worked well in my patients. In the hands of Dr. Ed McGuire, an Ingelman-Sundberg procedure is effective in about 60% of patients,[1] but that does not seem to work very well in my hands either. Neuromodulation is a new technique that has a reported success rate of about 60% in selected patients, but it requires specialized expertise that is not widely available at present.

I would recommend augmentation enterocystoplasty for this woman. It is almost always effective in patients with refractory detrusor instability but usually requires a lifetime of intermittent self-catheterization, which, for most, is a small price to pay for control of an otherwise disabling condition. The general principles of augmentation cystoplasty are well known. The surgery is intended to create a low-pressure urinary reservoir. Almost any segment of bowel except jejunum may be used, but in practice almost all surgeons use either ileum or right colon. It is necessary to divide the antimesenteric border of the bowel and reconfigure it from a tubular to a spherical shape. This accomplishes two purposes—it increases the volume and impairs bowel contractions. The reconfigured intestine (the upper half of the sphere) is then anastomosed to the bladder that has been reconfigured to form the lower half of the sphere.

Finally, I doubt very much that I would have recommended colposuspension or any other operation for stress incontinence, but things are always clearer in hindsight.

### REFERENCE

1. Cespides RO, Cross CA, McGuire EJ: Modified Ingelman-Sundberg bladder denervation procedure for intractable urge incontinence, *J Urol* 156:1744, 1996.

### EDITORS' COMMENTS

The discussants clearly demonstrate that such difficult patient management problems require a thorough and multifaceted approach. All aspects of this patient's status, including medication use and fluid intake, should be scrutinized carefully. Nonsurgical options may provide rewarding results in many patients with severe detrusor instability. The discussants agree on the use of an augmentation cystoplasty should surgical treatment finally be entertained.

## CASE 7
## Evaluation and Management of Fecal Incontinence

*CASE:* The patient is a 59-year-old para 7 who had a vaginal hysterectomy and anterior and posterior colporrhaphy 2 years ago for pelvic organ prolapse. She had a long history of incontinence to flatus and, over the last 2 to 3 years, has noticed incontinence of stool, which has become socially debilitating. Her obstetric history with reference to perineal lacerations was unknown; she had a hemorrhoidectomy 10 years ago. On physical examination, the perineal body appeared somewhat attenuated despite the previous colporrhaphy. A grossly noticeable defect in the external anal sphincter was found on rectovaginal examination that extended from the 10 o'clock to 2 o'clock position. No obvious rectovaginal fistula was identified. Rectovaginal examination revealed a diminished tone of the anal sphincter, and a directed neurologic examination revealed diminished anal wink and bulbocavernosus reflex bilaterally.

DISCUSSANT: **Janice F. Rafferty**

Additional history should be obtained, including personal or family history of inflammatory bowel disease or presence of increased risk for colorectal cancer. In addition, direct questions should be asked about difficult bowel movements, straining, prolapse of tissue from the anus, need for transvaginal or transanal digital maneuvers to accomplish a bowel movement, and presence of mucus or blood. Important historical information would include prolonged second stage of labor, use of obstetric forceps, or a history of pelvic irradiation.

Physical examination begins with observation of the perineum. Noting the contour of the perineum is the first step; a flattened perineum is suggestive of generalized pelvic floor abnormality and pudendal nerve injury. The presence and location of scarring should be noted. Next, digital rectal examination will reveal resting tone as well as palpable abnormalities such as mucosal defects, masses, and rectocele. The ability to generate a "squeeze" with the anal sphincter should be determined. Proctoscopic examination is next performed to assess the anorectal mucosa, looking for erythema suggestive of intussusception, ulceration, mucosal discoloration, mass, or fistula. Finally, having the patient strain on the commode will show prolapse or pelvic descent.

Useful physiologic tests include anal manometry to quantify rest and squeeze pressures, length of the high-pressure zone (anal sphincter length), anorectal sensation, and rectal compliance. Finally, the extent of the neurologic deficit must be established through neuromuscular testing. Commonly this is performed by transanal stimulation of the pudendal nerve at the ischial spine[1] but anal evoked potentials, needle electromyography (EMG), and transcutaneous spinal stimulation are also used to determine integrity of the innervation of the anal sphincter.[2]

Transrectal ultrasound will define anatomy of the anal canal, showing defects in the internal and external anal sphincters. Clear delineation of anatomic sphincter injury must be made in this patient because she has not only a potential obstetric injury but also a history of perineal surgery including posterior colporrhaphy and hemorrhoidectomy.

After complete testing, surgical and nonsurgical therapies can be discussed. If transrectal ultrasound demonstrates a clear disruption of the anal sphincter and physiology testing supports inadequate sphincter pressures, she may benefit from an anal sphincter reconstruction. Prediction of successful outcome can be made through assessment of the pudendal nerves as well as general patient status. Less successful outcomes are associated with pudendal neuropathy (either unilateral or bilateral) and patient comorbid conditions such as obesity.

On the other hand, if no clear anatomic defect is identified on ultrasound examination or if bilateral pudendal neuropathy is found, pelvic floor physical therapy and biofeedback would be a reasonable first step in this patient's management.

## REFERENCES

1. Kiffe E, Swash M: Slowed conduction in the pudendal nerves in idiopathic (neurogenic) fecal incontinence, *Br J Surg* 74:614, 1984.
2. Emsellen HA, Bergsrud DW: Anal evoked potentials. In Smith LE, ed: *Practical guide to anorectal testing*, New York, 1990, Igaku-Shoin Ltd.

### Discussant: J. Thomas Benson

### *Evaluation*

It is a mistake to assume that a patient with a defect in the external anal sphincter who has fecal incontinence has the incontinence because of the defect. Therefore, other causes of fecal incontinence must be sought. First, liquid stool may occur as a result of infection, inflammatory bowel disease, rapid colon transit, or small bowel dysfunction such as lactase deficiency. Second, an inadequate rectal reservoir is seen in inflammatory bowel disease, cancer, pelvic masses or adhesions, and scleroderma. Third, inadequate rectal sensation may cause fecal incontinence and is usually a result of neuropathy or sustained fecal impaction. Fourth, defects in neuromuscular function must be considered, including traumatic sphincter injury (likely in this case from obstetric and surgical causes), pudendal nerve injury, pelvic plexus injury, and cauda equina or central nervous system disorders.

Evaluation of these causes is performed using a diverse array of tests. Sigmoidoscopy or colonoscopy may detect intrinsic intestinal disorders. Lactase levels and colon transit study (ingestion of "markers" followed by flat plate of abdomen 5 days later) aid in diagnosing transit disorders. Defecography would be useful for evaluating abnormalities of rectal storage and emptying, such as intussusception and rectocele. Anal manometry evaluates resting anal pressure (80% due to internal anal sphincter), "squeeze" pressure (due to external anal sphincter), rectal distention perception (an index of rectal sensation), and presence of rectoanal inhibitory reflex (decrease in anal canal pressure secondary to rectal distention). Anal ultrasound delineates the internal and external anal sphincter anatomy. Finally, pelvic and lower limb clinical neurophysiologic studies, including EMG, may help to localize potential neuropathy. These studies provide the ability to evaluate duration and activity of any denervating or reinnervating processes and aid in selection of neurologically "healthier" muscle (e.g., puborectalis, which has a different nerve supply than the external anal sphincter) to use in surgical repair. In the case described, the minimal workup would include sigmoidoscopy, anal manometry, anal ultrasound, and clinical neurophysiologic studies.

### *Management*

Treatment of fecal incontinence involves dietary and behavioral changes, pharmaceuticals, sensory and motor biofeedback, electrical stimulation, pelvic physical therapy, and surgery. Surgical management includes sphincteroplasty, retrorectal levatorplasty, gracilis or other muscle transplant (preferably with neurostimulation),[1] and diversion.

In this case, if sigmoidoscopy indicates specific intracolonic disease, that would be specifically treated. If anal manometry (and history) indicate a sensory disorder, treatment would be with sensory biofeedback. If the manometry suggests a motor disorder, anal ultrasound would be used to determine the extent of anatomic defects in the external and internal anal sphincters. The clinical neurophysiologic studies will assist in determining the presence and extent of neuropathy (which affects prognosis) and, in the case of neuromuscularly damaged external anal sphincter and healthier puborectalis, the choice of muscle for the repair.

If the determination is made that the incontinence is caused by a sphincter defect, therapy would still begin with a high-fiber diet. Motor biofeedback (perineal reeducation) would be instituted. Constipating agents and daily enemas may be suggested. If conservative treatment fails, internal and external anal sphincteroplasty, possibly augmented by puborectalis levatorplasty, would be performed. The patient would be counseled to follow conservative measures first, regardless of expected success rate. If surgery is elected, continence restoration should be excellent or good in 80% if there is no nerve damage. If there is nerve damage, only 10% may have excellent restoration, but improvement over preoperative status may be present in 80%.[2,3]

## REFERENCES

1. Baeten C, Geerdes BP, Adong EM, et al: Anal dynamic graciloplasty in the treatment of intractable fecal incontinence, *N Engl J Med* 332:1600, 1995.
2. Laurberg S, Swash M, Henry MM: Delayed external sphincter repair for obstetric tear, *Br J Surg* 75:786, 1988.
3. Engel AF, Kamm MA, Sultan AH, et al: Anterior anal sphincter repair in patients with obstetric trauma, *Br J Surg* 81:1231, 1994.

## EDITORS' COMMENTS

Both discussants warn of the dangers of attributing functional impairment in fecal storage and evacuation to sphincter injury alone. A significant differential diagnosis must be considered in the evaluation of these patients. In addition, the value of conservative measures including pelvic floor physical therapy cannot be understated, even in a patient with obvious anatomic abnormalities.

## CASE 8

## Complete Procidentia in the Elderly

*CASE:* The patient is an 86-year-old para 2 with a long history of prolapse that was visible, palpable, and caused her difficulty in sitting. She denied urinary incontinence; she was not sexually active. Her medical history was remarkable for hypertension and mild congestive heart failure. Physical examination revealed complete procidentia with large areas of erosion (Figs. 34-7 and 34-8). When the prolapse was reduced with a full bladder,

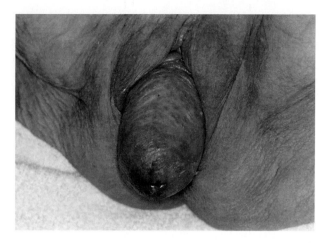

**Fig. 34-7**    Complete procidentia in an elderly patient.

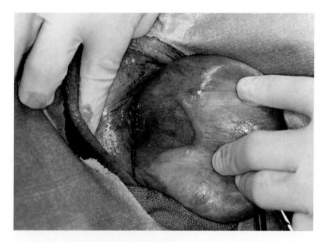

**Fig. 34-8**    A large ulceration noted in a patient with prolonged procidentia and hypoestrogenism.

coughing in the supine position demonstrated the sign of stress incontinence. The patient failed numerous attempts at pessary therapy and desires definitive surgical therapy.

**DISCUSSANT: David H. Nichols†**

This elderly woman with some obvious cardiac problems is clearly a candidate for restoration of quality of life, insofar as it applies to her pelvis, even though her life expectancy is unknown and therefore unpredictable. She requires preoperative medical stabilization, control, and documented medical clearance for surgery. Her age, per se, is not a contraindication, but one must have a clear understanding, as must the patient and her family, of the risk/benefit ratio. The ulceration described is probably of deficient circulatory origin, although a malignant neoplasm should be ruled out by cytologic smear or biopsy. If the lesion is not grossly purulent, I would ignore it at surgery. However, if the lesion is purulent, the exudate should be cultured and the vagina packed daily around-the-clock preoperatively to reduce the pro-

†Deceased.

lapse. The packing material should be saturated with cod liver oil, povidone-iodine (Betadine), and on alternate days, estrogen cream; this routine is continued until the purulence is gone.

Initially and again preoperatively, the patient and her family must be given a thoughtful informed consent describing the options to be considered and which ones might be recommended for this particular patient, along with an explanation of the risks and prognosis and some statement of the experience of the operator in dealing with similar cases in the past.

Urinary incontinence that is demonstrated only when the prolapse is reduced suggests an underlying low urethral closure pressure, which is to be expected in about 50% of postmenopausal patients with total procidentia. This should be proven by urodynamic assessment, with the prolapse reduced by rectal swabs during the laboratory study,[1] and a coincident urinalysis done to exclude chronic cystitis. Because one wishes not to exchange the unwelcome symptom of the prolapse for an equally unwelcome symptom of postoperative urinary incontinence, specific steps must be taken to lessen this risk. Complete uterovaginal procidentia includes hypermobility of the vesicourethral junction and requires addition of a vesicourethral sling procedure to achieve postoperative continence.[2] If, following recovery from the initial surgery, the patient is not completely dry, future transurethral collagen injections will probably provide relief.

Presuming that medical stabilization and clearance have been obtained, my choice for surgery would be among the following four options:

1. A LeFort colpocleisis could be done, even under local anesthesia if general anesthesia is precluded. Although treatment of any postoperative urinary incontinence may be difficult, transurethral collagen injections are possible. This would be the easiest and fastest surgical procedure to perform, with attention given to transvaginal support of the vesicourethral junction, and would be considered if the preoperative medical clearance was only conditional.

2. Vaginal hysterectomy with colpectomy is an operation that is a bit more formidable than the preceding procedure. To it, one should add an appropriate colporrhaphy with attention to the vesicourethral junction and, if postoperative incontinence should supervene, postoperative transurethral collagen injections could be a consideration.

3. Transvaginal hysterectomy with sacrospinous colpopexy (probably bilateral), with colporrhaphy and a vesicourethral sling procedure, is another option. This is an operation for the experienced reconstructive surgeon who has good surgical assistance available and who can work efficiently so that completion of the entire operative procedure, preferably under spinal anesthesia, could be accomplished in 2½ to 3 hours.

4. Transabdominal sacrocervicopexy with retropubic colposuspension would be a consideration, or if the surgeon should wish to remove the uterus, a transabdominal total hysterectomy with sacrocolpopexy and retropubic vesicourethral colposuspension would be a consideration. This is the most formidable choice among this group, and there are increased risks for various severe and life-threatening complications, including ileus, embolism, and wound hernia, to name but a few.

If I were the surgeon, and adequate medical clearance had been obtained, my first choice and recommendation to the patient would be the third option listed: vaginal hysterectomy with bilateral sacrospinous colpopexy, colporrhaphy, and vesicourethral sling procedure. We have followed this recommendation in the past, and our results have been most favorable and without complication. If limited medical clearance were obtained, the first option listed would be a good choice because of the speed with which it can be accomplished and because it can be done under a local anesthetic if general anesthesia is precluded; however, some problems with postoperative urinary continence should be anticipated.

## REFERENCES

1. Veronikis DK, Nichols DH, Wakamatsu MM: The incidence of low pressure urethra as a function of prolapse-reducing technique in patients with massive pelvic organ prolapse (maximum descent at all vaginal sites), *Am J Obstet Gynecol* 177:1305, 1997.
2. Nichols DH, Randall CL: *Vaginal surgery,* ed 4, Baltimore, 1996, Williams & Wilkins.

DISCUSSANT: **Marvin H. Terry Grody**

Subjecting a woman of this age with major defects of the extent described to any further testing will be a waste of time and money. The history and physical examination in themselves are adequate enough for an appropriate determination of surgical approach.

Objectively, especially with emphasis on the patient's age, medical problems, vaginal erosion, and extent of deteriorated connective tissue, I would opt primarily for an obliterative procedure. This decision is easily fortified if the patient is a widow who has not been engaging in coitus and who volunteers that she has no prospects for future coitus. No matter what we may assume, or how redundant it may seem, the patient must absolutely understand and agree to the asexual consequences of obliteration.

Estrogen priming preoperatively followed by continued oral estrogen replacement postoperatively is critical in prophylaxis against surgical breakdown, regardless of the operative method that is chosen. The eroded and ulcerated areas of vagina are never a problem and can be totally ignored. They are generally sterile, nothing will make them heal, and they can always be stripped out summarily in the course of vaginal denudation. The priming estrogen will thicken and vascularize the connective tissue under the erosions.

At Temple University, we consider the LeFort procedure of partial colpocleisis inappropriate for a case such as this. With modern medical adjuncts, this patient may be destined to live several more years. In this kind of case, partial colpocleisis has a reasonable probability of deteriorating with recurrence of massive prolapse within 1 to 3 years. We have been confronted many times with such situations in cases referred to our pelvic reconstructive center.

Our specific choice for surgery in this kind of case, considering current sophisticated anesthesia techniques, current antibiotics, and blood replacement availability, would be total colpocleisis. The photographs accompanying the case history reveal an obvious prolapsed uterus leading the severe panpelvic procidentia. Were this case simply one of posthysterectomy massive vaginal eversion, assuming skilled surgeons were in charge, we would not tolerate for a moment an argument in favor of a LeFort over total colpocleisis, especially since local anesthesia could be a consideration. Practically speaking, any discussion regarding choice of operation would revolve around time. A LeFort operation, with or without a uterus present, should take at most 30 minutes, adding 10 minutes more in efforts made to correct rotational descent of the urethrovesical junction. A total colpocleisis, including our usual paravaginal stitches (three on each side) and also our usual two to three perineorrhaphy stitches, takes an average of 80 to 90 minutes to complete. The additional time is not that great and is well worth it, considering the much greater guarantee of permanence.

In this case, we would perform a vaginal hysterectomy first and then go ahead with the total colpocleisis. We feel that the additional time of 20 more minutes adds minimal risk and, all things considered, is well worth the effort in removing a central lodestone and a source of estrogen-stimulated endometrium.

A full reconstructive procedure, which would necessarily include a hysterectomy, to give the best possibility of lasting correction in tissues presumably extremely poor in texture from the aging effects of wear and tear alone, would involve meticulous work through the full extent of both the anterior and posterior pelvic compartments. Certainly the time element would be doubled, the exposure of raw surfaces would be doubled, and the risks would certainly be reckoned as significantly increased from all points of view. In addition, one would have to think that despite the best surgical efforts, a full sophisticated reconstruction might be more apt to break down than the total colpocleisis simply because we would be asking for too much from the poor tissue.

In these cases, we consider urodynamic testing to be unnecessary and redundant. These tests will not help us. We already know that masked or potential urinary incontinence has been demonstrated. Our experience has shown surprisingly pleasant postoperative results from the inclusion of our urethrovesical paravaginal stitches with our total colpocleisis, and patients have thus demonstrated reasonable continence. In those situations when incontinence persists or is unmasked, we then resort to periurethral collagen injections, which are almost always accompanied by significant improvement.

## EDITORS' COMMENTS

Obliterative procedures for pelvic organ prolapse are useful options to have available in the reconstructive pelvic surgeon's armamentarium. The discussants differ somewhat on their approach to the evaluation of the patient's incontinence. However, both agree that periurethral bulking agents (such as glutaraldehyde cross-linked collagen) are very useful in those women who postoperatively develop stress incontinence.

## CASE 9
## Surgical Management of Enterocele Following Burch Colposuspension

*CASE:* The patient is a 65-year-old para 2 receiving hormone replacement therapy who had a vaginal hysterectomy for fibroids with anterior and posterior colporrhaphy 20 years ago. Five years ago, she underwent a Burch colposuspension for stress incontinence. Over the last 2 to 3 years, she has noticed increasing pelvic pressure and vaginal protrusion that is worse by the end of the day. On examination, the posterior vaginal wall descended 5 cm outside the hymen with straining in a supine position. The defect was felt to be a large enterocele. The anterior vaginal wall was somewhat scarred with the bladder neck well supported. The patient denied any lower urinary tract dysfunction; however, when the prolapse was reduced in a posterior direction, coughing in the supine position with a full bladder easily demonstrated the sign of stress incontinence. The patient desires definitive therapy for her prolapse.

DISCUSSANT: **Fred Miyazaki**

The problems of this patient, although closely interrelated, will be discussed separately.

***Problem 1: Recurrent Stress Incontinence After Burch Colposuspension***

From the data given, the patient's occult stress incontinence is probably caused by intrinsic sphincter deficiency. Evaluation would include urinalysis, culture, postvoid residual urine volume, filling cystometry (a single channel would suffice), and triple cough stress test with the enterocele reduced by a pessary, cotton swabs, or retractor. The cough stress test would visually confirm a large urine leakage per urethra simultaneous with the cough. Repeating the same stress test during a Miyazaki-Bonney test (Miya-Bonney)[1] would result in persistent stress incontinence, thereby ruling out anatomic support defects as the cause of her incontinence. By default, the urethra would be incriminated. A Q-tip test would show normal support at rest and minimal mobility with stress. A Valsalva leak point pressure would be less than 60 cm $H_2O$ (optional). Urethrocystoscopy and a minineurologic examination complete the evaluation. The diagnosis is recurrent stress incontinence caused by intrinsic sphincter deficiency without hypermobility. The treatment is intraurethral collagen injections. If hypermobility were present, a suburethral sling would be in order.

***Problem 2: Large Enterocele After Burch Colposuspension***

Evaluation should include a complete quantitation of pelvic organ prolapse; however, only those aspects pertinent to this case will be discussed. While in 45-degree dorsolithotomy position, the patient is encouraged to perform a maximal Valsalva maneuver to display her pathology at its worst. The lengths of the anterior and posterior vagina are measured with the prolapse out. The apical dimples of the cuff are identified, usually near the level of the hymenal ring. An enterocele of this size would usually cause traction descent of the upper vagina. The patient then relaxes, and the enterocele is manually reduced. The left middle and index fingers are inserted into the vagina, and the right index finger, middle finger, or both are inserted into the rectum. When the patient again Valsalvas, the contents of the enterocele may be felt as they pass between the apposing fingers. This may be small bowel, large bowel, omentum, and rarely, rectum (sigmoidocele). On rectal examination, the extent of anterior rectal wall involvement is assessed. The diagnosis is large enterocele with traction prolapse of the upper vagina. The treatment is (1) vaginal resection of enterocele, (2) excision of redundant vaginal wall to construct a three-fingers-breadth caliber vagina, and (3) abdominal colposacropexy with Mersilene mesh to correct the apical prolapse.

This author's technique of Mersilene mesh colposacropexy provides strong apical support and positions the cuff and upper vagina posteriorly over the levator plate with a modified Moschcowitz closure of the cul-de-sac. In brief, a two-layer mesh is sutured to the cuff, one layer anteriorly and the other posteriorly over a 5 × 3 cm area. This provides strong, even support to both walls. The sacral sutures are placed down to the hollow of the sacrum (S2, S3). The mesh tension is relaxed so that the vaginal cuff can be pushed almost to the coccyx. A modified Moschcowitz closure of the cul-de-sac is performed by several pursestring sutures of No. 2-0 nylon that incorporates the anterior rectal wall and adjacent peritoneum with the posterior cuff and attached mesh.

DeLancey[2] has succinctly described alternative techniques for the prevention and treatment of enteroceles.

**REFERENCES**

1. Miyazaki FS: The Bonney test: a reassessment, *Am J Obstet Gynecol* 177:1322, 1997.
2. DeLancey JOL: Treatment and prevention of enterocele not associated with vaginal or uterine prolapse, *Operative Techniques in Gynecologic Surgery* 1:86, 1996.

DISCUSSANT: **Nicolette S. Horbach**

Given the patient's history of prior pelvic surgery, my preoperative assessment of this patient would include postvoid residual urine determination, cystoscopy to evaluate ureteral patency and the pliability of the urethra, and urodynamics. Although bladder capacity, compliance, and the presence of abnormal detrusor activity are important, with her demonstration of leakage with the prolapse reduced, I would be most interested in the status of her intrinsic urethral sphincter function by leak point pressure and maximum urethral closure pressure.

My surgical approach would depend on the patient's level of physical activity, her desire for future sexual activity, the anatomic location of her vaginal apex (defined as the Pelvic Organ Prolapse Quantitation System's [POP-Q] point C) relative to the maximum descent of her enterocele, the status of her intrinsic urethral sphincter, and her overall medical condition. If the patient were both physically and sexually active and the enterocele were associated with significant descent of the vaginal apex (point C ranging from −4 cm up to prolapse of the total vaginal length), I would perform an abdominal sacrocolpopexy using Mersilene mesh and a Halban's culdeplasty with permanent sutures. The mesh would be used to reinforce the posterior vaginal wall and would be sutured inferiorly into the substance of the perineal body. This technique would obliterate the enterocele and prevent a subsequent rectocele. If the vaginal apex were well supported (point C ranging from −6 cm to full support of the total vaginal length) and the enterocele had simply dissected down the rectovaginal septum, I would consider a transvaginal enterocele repair with extensive culdeplasty. However, unless the patient is medically unstable or very inactive, my preferred approach for treating an enterocele with any moderate degree of apical descent is a transabdominal route.

The patient's occult incontinence is of concern. Assuming a truly well-supported urethra and occult incontinence, I would expect evidence of ISD. If her urethral function were still normal (Valsalva LPPs greater than 60 to 65 cm $H_2O$ and MUCPs greater than 20 cm $H_2O$), I would postpone any treatment of her "occult" incontinence. Our ability to predict postoperative incontinence in women with severe pelvic prolapse is often imprecise. The contributions of the posterior vaginal wall and reflex pelvic muscle contraction to the patient's continence mechanism are inadequately assessed during barrier reduction urodynamics. If the patient complained of postoperative incontinence, a transurethral collagen injection could be performed.

If the ISD were severe, I would consider a simultaneous transurethral collagen injection at the time of her prolapse repair. Alternatively, if a vaginal approach were planned, I would consider urethrolysis and a fascia lata suburethral sling.

**EDITORS' COMMENTS**

Both authors recognize the distinct possibility that this patient's occult incontinence is caused by intrinsic sphincter deficiency, and both suggest a thorough evaluation of the urethral continence mechanism preoperatively. Interestingly, both discussants would perform an abdominal sacral colpopexy for this patient's prolapse.

# CASE 10
## Chronic Constipation

*CASE:* The patient is a 37-year-old para 3 with a 15-year history of chronic constipation. She has bowel movements every 3 weeks only after using magnesium citrate. She attempts defecation by straining several times daily because of a sense of rectal fullness with associated pelvic pressure. Stools are flat and soft. She has used perineal splinting and digital evacuation in the past without much benefit. She has also used enemas and is currently using 30 g of dietary fiber daily, but she usually needs laxatives to achieve evacuation.

In addition to constipation, she complains of low back pain, vaginal bulging, and recent onset of fecal staining. The vaginal bulging has limited her sexual relations because of a sense of obstruction during coitus. The fecal staining is primarily passage of mucus. She denies urinary incontinence, urgency, and voiding dysfunction.

### DISCUSSANT: Geoffrey W. Cundiff

The initial evaluation of this patient should focus on eliminating metabolic and endocrinologic causes of constipation from the differential diagnosis. These include diabetes, amyloidosis, hypocalcemia, hypokalemia, hypothyroidism, hyperparathyroidism, and panhypopituitarism. A thorough history and physical examination combined with serum electrolytes, glucose, and indicated hormone assays are usually sufficient. Neurologic causes, such as multiple sclerosis, Parkinson's disease, cerebral vascular disease, and autonomic neuropathy should also be considered and ruled out through history and neurologic examination. The use of common medications that cause constipation, including antidepressants, anticholinergics, antacids, beta blockers, calcium channel blockers, cholestyramine, diuretics, nonsteroidal antiinflammatory agents, and narcotics, should be sought as well. If the diagnosis remains inconclusive after excluding these potential causes, then the patient has idiopathic constipation.[1]

Idiopathic constipation has traditionally been subdivided into disorders of colonic motility and outlet obstruction, although this classification is somewhat artificial as both conditions may coexist. Outlet obstruction can occur as a result of pelvic organ prolapse, including rectoceles and enteroceles, although both can exist without compromising defecatory function. Usually vaginal support defects can be detected by a careful pelvic examination that assesses support of the vault and integrity of the rectovaginal fascia. Women with constipation caused by a dissecting enterocele will often have perineal descent as well, which may result in pudendal neuropathy and fecal incontinence if neglected. Defecography provides a fluoroscopic evaluation of the pelvic organ relationships and often reveals enteroceles missed at pelvic examination. It also provides an objective measure of perineal descent. Rectal prolapse and rectal intussusception can also result in outlet obstruction and are often detected at defecography. Finally, a nonrelaxing pelvic floor (puborectalis or external anal sphincter), also know as anismus, can also cause outlet obstruction.

This condition may be detected on defecography. If rectal prolapse or anismus is suspected, anorectal evaluation with manometry, surface EMG, and proctoscopy are indicated for confirmation.

The presence of outlet obstruction does not preclude a colonic motility disorder. In fact, a woman with long-standing constipation resulting from colonic inertia often will develop pelvic organ prolapse caused by chronic straining. Colonic motility disorders include megarectum, megacolon, irritable bowel syndrome, colonic inertia, and Hirschsprung's disease, although the latter is rare in women. The colonic transit study is the diagnostic modality for investigating motility disorders. Patients are given 24 radiopaque markers that are taken orally. In the patient with normal colonic motility, 80% of the markers should be passed by 72 hours.

Initial therapy for women with idiopathic constipation should focus on maximizing medical management. At least 30 g of dietary fiber with adequate fluid intake is indicated. If unsuccessful, surgical management may be appropriate, although anismus should not be treated surgically, as it responds to biofeedback in 80% to 90% of patients. Women with isolated rectoceles may be adequately treated with a discrete defect rectocele repair; this has been reported to improve constipation in 84% of women, tenesmus in 66%, and splinting in 44%.[2] Posterior colporrhaphy with levator plication should be avoided, as it has been shown to increase defecatory dysfunction.[3] In the presence of perineal descent and a dissecting enterocele, I will use an abdominal sacral colpoperineopexy to reestablish the integrity of the rectovaginal fascia and perineal support. An initial evaluation of this procedure suggests that it relieves bowel-related symptoms in 66% of women.[4] A suture rectopexy or Ripstein rectopexy should be used in women with rectal prolapse and can be combined with other pelvic support surgery. A colectomy may be curative in the patient with colonic inertia, although it is imperative that before surgery, she has failed medical management and has demonstrated normal upper intestinal motility and an intact anal sphincter. In these circumstances, reported success rates range from 70% to 90%, but the patient should recognize the potential for postoperative cramping, bloating, diarrhea, and fecal incontinence. Postoperative bowel obstruction requiring laparotomy has also been reported in about 30% of patients.

Collaboration with colorectal surgeons, both in diagnosis and treatment of these complicated patients, should help to eliminate misdiagnosis and inappropriate treatment.

### REFERENCES

1. Kumar D, Bartolo DCC, Deroaede G, et al: Symposium on constipation, *Int J Colorectal Dis* 7:47, 1992.
2. Cundiff GW, Weidner AC, Visco AG, et al: An anatomical and functional assessment of the discrete defect rectocele repair, *Am J Obstet Gynecol* 179:1451, 1998.
3. Kahn MA, Stanton SL: Posterior colporrhaphy: its effects on bowel and sexual function, *Br J Obstet Gynaecol* 104:882, 1997.
4. Cundiff GW, Harris RL, Coates KW, et al: Abdominal sacral colpoperineopexy: a new approach for correction of posterior compartment defects and perineal descent associated with vaginal vault prolapse, *Am J Obstet Gynecol* 177:1345, 1997.

### EDITORS' COMMENTS

Chronic constipation is often neglected by physicians, although this problem may be both a marker for and contributor to pelvic floor dysfunction. The importance of a thorough evaluation and the value of conservative measures in the treatment of this disorder have been well reviewed by the discussant.

## CASE 11

### Coexistent Anatomic Stress Incontinence and a Vesicovaginal Fistula

*CASE:* The patient is a 56-year-old para 3 who is not receiving hormone replacement therapy and who underwent laparoscopic-assisted vaginal hysterectomy 1 year ago. Two weeks after her surgery, she noted an increase in watery discharge from her vagina. On speculum examination, an area of friable granulation tissue was noted on the anterior aspect of the vaginal cuff. Cystourethroscopy revealed a 2-mm vesicovaginal fistula approximately 2 cm cephalad to the right ureteral orifice. Use of a lacrimal duct probe revealed the fistulous tract to be contiguous with the area of granulation tissue at the vaginal apex. When the patient coughs in the supine position, an obvious loss of urine from the urethra is noted. The patient gives a history of stress incontinence dating back at least 2 years before her hysterectomy.

DISCUSSANT: **W. Glenn Hurt**

Findings suggest the coexistence of a vesicovaginal fistula located in the vaginal apex above the trigone and stress urinary incontinence. Both have been present for more than 1 year.

I would start oral estrogen replacement therapy for this patient, if there is no contraindication to its use. If there is vaginal atrophy or significant vaginal scarring, I would consider the placement of an estrogen-containing vaginal pessary. Any urinary tract or vaginal infection must be eradicated.

It is important to know if the patient has urethral hypermobility (anatomic) or ISD stress incontinence. Q-tip testing and urethral pressure studies would help differentiate the two. If any question exists about the condition of the tissues around the fistula, cystoscopy should be repeated to determine the optimum time for repair.

If the patient has hypermobility (anatomic) stress incontinence and a posthysterectomy vesicovaginal fistula located in the apex of the vagina, my choice would be to perform a Latzko procedure and a Burch retropubic colposuspension. This combination of procedures would require a vagina of adequate length to allow a partial apical colpocleisis and slight shortening of the anterior vaginal wall.

If the patient has an immobile urethrovesical junction, I might choose to perform a layered repair of the vesicovaginal fistula and the placement of a suburethral sling. Should I use this combination of procedures, I would have more concern about the healing of the vesicovaginal fistula because of the more extensive dissection between the urethra, bladder, and vagina. In either case, I would insert a Malecot suprapubic catheter of at least 18-French size and leave it to straight drainage for 12 to 14 days before attempting voiding trials. Voiding trials must be monitored closely to be sure that there is no overdistention of the bladder that might jeopardize healing of the vesicovaginal repair.

DISCUSSANT: **Robert L. Summitt, Jr.**

Although the literature is replete with descriptions of how to surgically treat stress incontinence and how to repair vesicovaginal fistulas, there are no accounts describing how to approach the

patient with both entities, as described in this case. The surgeon must approach each functional or anatomic defect independently and then derive a treatment plan that ensures a successful outcome for both problems. For this case, I would evaluate and treat both defects together.

Two weeks after a hysterectomy, physical examination and cystourethroscopy confirmed the presence and location of the vesicovaginal fistula. I would add an intravenous pyelogram to confirm the integrity of both ureters despite the fistula being 2 cm above the right orifice. Because the patient lost urine in the supine position with coughing, she is at a slightly higher risk of exhibiting intrinsic sphincter deficiency. Therefore urodynamic studies, including urethral pressure profilometry and measurement of leak point pressures, should be performed. Occasionally, difficulty with performing a cystometrogram may be encountered in a patient with a vesicovaginal fistula as the fluid will leak out very quickly through the tract, or local irritation may induce involuntary detrusor activity. In either case, performing leak point pressure measurements may be difficult, thereby leaving urethral profilometry as the only method to evaluate urethral sphincter function in the face of genuine stress incontinence. To complete the evaluation, some measure of urethral mobility, such as a cotton-swab test, should be performed.

Although descriptions of repairing bladder neck fistulas and stress incontinence in two stages exist,[1] the current patient can be treated in one combined operation. The operative approach, transvaginal or transabdominal, would depend on whether intrinsic sphincter deficiency is diagnosed. This approach may seem contrary to principles of directing surgery to the most severe problem when using combined operations, but the surgical outcomes for treating stress incontinence can vary greatly depending on the operation selected. In addition, the vesicovaginal fistula is amenable to repair by either route with a relatively high correction rate.

If urodynamic testing revealed stress incontinence without intrinsic sphincter deficiency, I would perform a Burch retropubic urethropexy combined with a transabdominal repair of the vesicovaginal fistula. If intrinsic sphincter deficiency were diagnosed, a transvaginal approach using a cadaver fascia suburethral sling combined with a Latzko repair of the fistula would be performed. In either case, I would wait at least 8 weeks before performing surgery to maximize resolution of inflammation around the fistula site. However, in some situations, the abdominal approach can be undertaken at a much earlier time.

For postoperative bladder drainage, I would use a suprapubic catheter in either operative approach. This provides more comfortable and sterile bladder drainage for 7 to 10 days, when compared with transurethral drainage. After 7 to 10 days, voiding protocols may be started with minimal trauma to the repairs. Once voiding well for 24 hours, with postvoid residual volumes consistently less than 100 ml per void, the suprapubic catheter can simply be removed.

**REFERENCE**

1. Tancer ML: A report of thirty-four instances of urethrovaginal and bladder neck fistulas, *Surg Gynecol Obstet* 177:77, 1993.

**EDITORS' COMMENTS**

Careful preparation for the repair of vesicovaginal fistulas is mandatory. The discussants agree that the procedure used to correct this patient's incontinence should be unrelated to the presence of the vesicovaginal fistula.

# CASE 12
# Mesh Erosion After Abdominal Sacrocolpopexy

*CASE:* The patient is a 57-year-old para 4 who is currently not receiving hormone replacement therapy because of a stage I breast cancer treated 5 years ago. Ten years ago, she had a vaginal hysterectomy and anterior and posterior colporrhaphy for prolapse. Six months ago, she complained of recurrent prolapse and underwent an abdominal sacrocolpopexy with synthetic mesh material used. She now complains of dyspareunia and vaginal spotting. On examination, a $1 \times 2$ cm defect was noted at the vaginal cuff with granulation tissue surrounding mesh material.

### DISCUSSANT: Ingrid Nygaard

This case brings up several salient issues: What is the role of estrogen in women with breast cancer who require pelvic reconstructive surgery? What is the incidence of postoperative mesh complication after sacrocolpopexy? Can this incidence be reduced through perioperative care? When erosion does occur, how should this be managed?

The erosion rate following abdominal sacrocolpopexy is approximately 3%,[1] although some authors report no erosions in a large, well-followed population.[2] Few data are available about the remaining issues previously mentioned, and thus, management must be based on experience and thoughtful consideration.

Although estrogen has long been considered contraband in women with breast cancer, some clinicians and researchers disagree with this dictum. Once the vagina is cornified, minimal amounts of estrogen are absorbed into the systemic circulation. Because estrogen does tend to thicken vaginal mucosa, which may play a role in preventing mesh erosion, its use should be considered pre- and postoperatively, even in women with breast cancer.

In the earlier phases of sacrocolpopexy, mesh was attached directly to the apex of the vagina with a couple of sutures. As the technique has evolved, it has become apparent that a broad attachment over the anterior and posterior vagina, at least to the upper one third, is important to ensure success. Avoiding a heap of mesh at the apex may also help to prevent future erosion. Many surgeons recommend imbricating the apex of the vagina, such that mesh is only exposed to a thicker layer. Finally, great care should be taken to ensure sterile technique intraoperatively.

There is no accepted practice or correct method to treat mesh erosion. Options include (1) expectant management only, (2) vaginal estrogen cream, (3) excision of protruding mesh in the office, (4) opening the vaginal apex vaginally and excising the accessible mesh, and (5) removing the entire mesh segment via an intraabdominal approach.

It is my belief that patients rarely improve with expectant management or estrogen cream alone. Colleagues have shared success stories in which mesh was excised in the office and the women were treated concurrently with estrogen cream. Generally, this was a long process, requiring four to eight visits over several months. We recently consulted on a patient who had repeated visits for excision of mesh and granulation tissue; after 2 years, the mesh had eroded into her rectum and was diagnosed during an evaluation for rectal bleeding. Because of the concern about mesh erosion into viscera, some experienced surgeons recommend removing the strip of mesh in toto via an abdominal approach. This is generally a very difficult dissection, and significant blood loss may ensue when removing the mesh from the sacrum.

Because the risk of erosion into viscera is small and the risk of presacral bleeding with attempts to remove the mesh in toto is large, we have turned instead to a middle ground in which the vaginal apex is opened and the mesh is removed as far back into the pelvis as possible. The vaginal apex is then left open to close by secondary intention. In four women for whom this procedure was done with follow-up of 1 to 5 years, none had recurrence of prolapse or continued erosion of mesh. Of interest is that in the removal of mesh in each case, the mesh was quite firm initially, as one would expect, but when it was tracked 3 to 4 cm back, it suddenly gave way, such that the segment was removed in one piece. The remaining mesh could still be felt attached to the sacrum. We counsel women who have a history of mesh erosion to report any hematochezia or hematuria promptly.

### REFERENCES

1. Iglesia CB, Fenner DE, Brubaker L: The use of mesh in gynecologic surgery, *Int Urogynecol J* 8:105, 1997.
2. Timmons MC, Addison WA, Addison SB, et al: Abdominal sacral colpopexy in 163 women with posthysterectomy vaginal vault prolapse and enterocele, *J Reprod Med* 37: 323, 1992.

### DISCUSSANT: Neeraj Kohli

The abdominal sacrocolpopexy procedure has been associated with good long-term surgical outcomes in the cure of vaginal vault prolapse. Unfortunately, postoperative complications including sacral osteomyelitis, pelvic abscess, and mesh or suture erosion can occur following this procedure. The timing of mesh or suture erosion can be highly variable and has been reported to occur as early as 6 weeks or as late as 6 years after surgery.[1,2] Similar to the patient just presented, most patients have symptoms of vaginal bleeding, abnormal discharge, or dyspareunia. Erosion of synthetic materials into the vagina should be suspected in such patients. To date, there is limited data regarding the optimal management of mesh erosion following abdominal sacrocolpopexy.

In patients with erosion of permanent suture into the vagina following abdominal sacrocolpopexy, Burch colposuspension, or other reconstructive vaginal procedures, conservative therapy consisting of rest, vaginal estrogen cream, and intermittent observation usually results in reepithelialization of the vaginal mucosa over the eroded suture within 6 to 8 weeks. In patients with persistent suture erosion, transvaginal removal of the suture is recommended. Recent data suggest that mesh erosion into the vagina following sacrocolpopexy usually requires surgical correction and does not respond to nonsurgical therapy.[2]

In my opinion, the surgical procedure of choice for the correction of post-sacrocolpopexy mesh erosion is excision of the mesh at the vaginal apex. Simple mobilization of the surrounding granulation tissue and vaginal mucosa with approximation of the vaginal edges over the eroded mesh (vaginal advancement) has been associated with a high rate of recurrent erosion. Although mesh excision has been described abdominally and laparoscopically,[3,4] transvaginal excision of the mesh with vaginal advancement is an effective, minimally invasive procedure. Vaginal retractors are used to expose the eroded mesh, and the surrounding granulation tissue is excised and the mesh mobilized. Downward traction exposes as much mesh as possible, and the mesh is then cut at its highest visible margin. The residual mesh then retracts into the abdominal cavity beyond visibility. The surrounding vaginal mucosa and its underlying fascia are mobilized circumferentially and then closed in layers using interrupted, delayed absorbable suture. This results in detachment of the permanent mesh material from the reapproximated vaginal apex, thereby preventing recurrent erosion.[2]

Abdominal excision of the eroded mesh has also been reported, but it may be associated with increased morbidity because of the laparotomy incision and difficult surgery resulting from postoperative adhesions. When excising the eroded mesh abdominally, the gynecologic surgeon should only remove the distal portion of the mesh attached to the vaginal apex. Attempts to remove the entire mesh have been associated with life-threatening hemorrhage from the blood vessels in the presacral space. Although laparoscopic excision of the mesh has been reported, this technique should only be used by the experienced laparoscopic surgeon, as hemorrhage and visceral injury are potential complications.[4]

Based on my experience, I have not found the rate of recurrent vault prolapse to be increased following excision of the eroded mesh. This probably is due to subsequent fibrosis and scarring of the surgical repair to the vaginal apex around the permanent mesh material. However, the rate of recurrent prolapse may be related to the timing of mesh removal following the sacrocolpopexy. Given the short time between the surgery and the postoperative mesh erosion in this case, the patient should be counseled that there may be an increased risk of recurrent prolapse following mesh excision, but this factor should not delay the surgical correction of this postoperative complication.

Strategies to prevent mesh erosion have been advocated by several authors.[2,3,5] The use of autologous or homologous materials, such as rectus fascia, dermal grafts, and dura mater, as the suspensory graft material has been reported and found to have cure rates comparable to those using synthetic material. For clinicians continuing to use synthetic materials as the suspensory graft, single-thickness mesh with anterior and posterior flaps, as opposed to double-thickness mesh attached circumferentially to the vaginal vault, will reduce the amount of foreign body at the vaginal apex. The use of monofilament suture as opposed to braided suture may also reduce the risk of mesh/suture erosion. Finally, care should be given to avoid full-thickness stitches into the vagina because these may serve as a precursor to full mesh erosion.

**REFERENCES**

1. Timmons MC, Addison WB, Addison SB, et al: Abdominal sacral colpopexy in 163 women with posthysterectomy vaginal vault prolapse and enterocele: evolution of operative techniques, *J Reprod Med* 37:323, 1992.
2. Kohli N, Walsh PM, Roat TW, et al: Mesh erosion after abdominal sacrocolpopexy, *Obstet Gynecol* 92:999, 1998.
3. Timmons MC, Addison WA: Mesh erosion after abdominal sacrocolpopexy, *J Pelvic Surg* 3:75, 1997.
4. Atlas I, Hallum AV, Hatch K: Laparoscopic repair of vaginal Gore-tex erosion after sacral colpopexy, *J Gynecol Surg* 11:177, 1995.
5. Iglesia CB, Fenner DE, Brubaker L: The use of mesh in gynecologic surgery, *Int Urogynecol J* 8:105, 1997.

**EDITORS' COMMENTS**

The discussants have clearly identified the difficult choices that have to be made when faced with erosion of synthetic mesh after

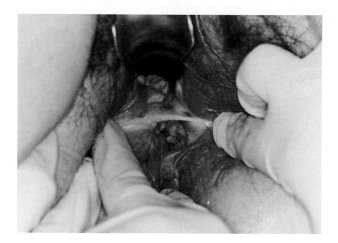

**Fig. 34-9**   A recurrent rectovaginal fistula. Note the markedly attenuated perineal body.

sacrocolpopexy. Both discussants have balanced the surgical morbidity associated with total excision of the mesh via laparotomy with the relatively poor success of conservative therapy and have both arrived at partial excision done transvaginally as the treatment of choice.

## CASE 13
## Recurrent Rectovaginal Fistula

*CASE:* The patient is a 30-year-old para 1 whose delivery 6 months ago was complicated by a fourth-degree perineal laceration and postpartum endomyometritis. Approximately 3 months after delivery, the patient underwent surgical repair of a rectovaginal fistula. She presents now, approximately 1 year after her initial repair, with complaints of recurrent fecal soilage from the vagina. On physical examination, there is a fistulous tract extending 2 cm proximal to the anal verge and opening approximately 1 cm distal to the hymenal ring (Fig. 34-9). The anal sphincter and perineal body appear attenuated. The patient is unclear about her future childbearing desires.

DISCUSSANT: **Raymond A. Lee**

Patients with recurrent rectovaginal fistula must undergo careful evaluation before consideration of reoperation. We present an overview of our plan to the patient so that she better understands the reason for each examination and testing device. We must be able to rule out primary inflammatory disease of the bowel, which frequently leads to failure if operative repair is undertaken. Thus, our first examination consists of colonoscopy; if this is negative, upper gastrointestinal barium studies are necessary to evaluate the small intestine to rule out inflammatory disease. If the results are normal, one could consider possible reasons for failure of previous operative repairs, with the understanding that failure can occur even in the best of surgical hands.

*Possible Reasons for Failure*

The following are possible causes of failure: (1) inadequate mobilization of the fistula site, resulting in tension to the closed suture line; (2) failure to excise sufficient scar tissue around the fistula; (3) failure to accurately approximate and invert the initial suture line of the repair; (4) infection or hematoma formation in the repair; (5) inaccurate approximation of the submucosa; and (6) passage of a hard stool (with disruption of the suture line) after what should have been a successful repair.

### Preoperative Evaluation

The history must be reviewed to accurately assess the conditions that led to identification of a rectovaginal fistula. Had there been a change in the patient's bowel habits? Had there been any evidence of perianal disease suggesting primary inflammatory disease? After operative repair, when did the patient first experience symptoms consistent with or suggestive of failure?

Physical examination should be performed carefully to identify the location and number of rectovaginal fistulas and their proximity to the anal sphincter. Is there evidence of contractile external anal sphincter? Is a contracting puborectalis muscle present? One needs to assess the presence of muscle in the sphincter mechanism that will respond when appropriately stimulated and thus provide continence. The location of the fistula suggests whether the operative repair will require incision of the remaining sphincter to accurately excise the scar tissue and permit an accurate tension-free closure of the suture line.

### Preoperative Preparation

The patient is placed on a low-residue diet 48 hours before the operation. She has liquids the afternoon before her operation and GOLYTELY bowel preparation that evening.

### Operative Technique

The repair is begun by making a circular incision about the anus beginning in the 8 to 9 o'clock position on the patient's right side to the 12 o'clock position and continuing around to the 3 to 4 o'clock position on the patient's left side. The skin and subcutaneous tissues are then freed from the underlying external anal sphincter. When indicated, it will be necessary to incise the bridge of sphincter and scar to permit accurate excision and mobilization of the scarred fistula tract. The incision is made around the fistula to include the scar tissue and also to provide a rim around the fistula tract to apply countertraction for later mobilization of the vagina from the rectal wall. With traction on the vaginal wall and countertraction applied to the edge of the fistula tract, the vagina is separated from the underlying rectal wall with sharp dissection that proceeds circumferentially; this mobilization permits later approximation of the fresh injury free of tension.

Once the vaginal walls are widely mobilized from the underlying rectum, the entire fistula tract is excised, including a small rim of rectal mucosa, to convert the fistula to a fresh injury. With the surgeon's left index finger lifting the rectum, the initial sutures are placed extramucosally, including a portion of the muscularis and submucosa, with No. 3-0 delayed absorbable sutures. The initial suture line is extended a full 5 mm above and below the site of the fistulous tract. A second layer of inverting sutures begins 5 mm above the previously closed suture line, extends 5 mm distal to the fistulous closure, and inverts the initial suture line into the rectum, with no sutures located within the rectal lumen. With the surgeon's left index finger in the anal canal, the surgeon uses a muscle stimulator to identify the contractile muscles of the external anal sphincter bilaterally. Once these are identified, the surgeon begins at the apex with the deep placement of No. 0 delayed absorbable monofilament sutures in the most superior border of the external anal sphincter on the patient's left side. The sutures are continued, including small portions of the anterior rectal wall, to the patient's right side, where a deep bite is placed in the most superior border of the external anal sphincter. This is continued from the superior position toward the lowest portion

of the anal canal over an area of approximately 5 to 6 cm with approximately six to seven interrupted sutures. The surgeon changes gloves and then ties the sutures in the order in which they were placed. This suture line results in a narrowing of the anal canal, which will be snug to the insertion of a lubricated little finger. The initial suture line is covered by a second layer of No. 2-0 delayed absorbable sutures, and the skin is closed with No. 4-0 sutures. Infrequently, the blood supply is insufficient (e.g., postradiation), or there is tension on the vaginal closure that will require a Martius flap from the perineum. Postoperatively, the patient is prescribed a liquid diet the first 48 hours, then gradually receives a soft diet, and generally is dismissed from the hospital on the fourth postoperative day. I recommend that the patient continue receiving stool softeners and a soft diet for the initial 2 weeks following the operation and that she receive a stool softener for the next 8 weeks.

For pregnancies after rectovaginal fistula repair, the final decision regarding the route of delivery must be made by the obstetrician. I favor elective cesarean section.

### EDITORS' COMMENTS

Certain preoperative conditions must be excluded and postoperative care must be optimized in the patient with a recurrent rectovaginal fistula. The discussant carefully describes the importance of meticulous closure of these recurrent defects.

---

## CASE 14
### Vaginal Stenosis After Radiation Therapy

*CASE:* The patient is a 54-year-old para 2 who is not receiving hormone replacement therapy. Three years ago, she was treated with brachytherapy for stage II vaginal carcinoma, and she is apparently free of disease at this point. She complains of apareunia caused by extreme narrowing of her vagina. She had not resumed intercourse for several months following her radiation treatment and was not compliant with vaginal dilators that were given to her. She was otherwise medically stable. On physical examination, the external epithelium appeared healthy. Approximately 3 to 4 cm proximal to the hymen, there was a vaginal constriction ring that barely admitted one finger. The patient is willing to undergo nonsurgical or surgical therapy to correct this problem.

**DISCUSSANT: Neil D. Jackson**

As is the case so many times, the best treatment for many conditions rests in anticipation of the potential outcome and institution of preventive measures to avoid the consequential outcome. Postbrachytherapy stenosis and constriction of the vaginal canal can often be prevented by the use of a vaginal obturator following therapy. The obturator can maintain length and circumference of the vagina during the period of time when scar tissue formation and shrinkage may occur. Frequently, couples refrain from intercourse following radiation therapy initially because of pain and later for fear of cancer contagion and misunderstanding concerning radiation effects. As a result, there is nothing introduced into the vagina to help maintain its adequacy of dimension.

After the fact, as in this case, one should begin with major efforts toward empathetic understanding, building trust and confidence with the patient. Although this patient was noncompliant with vaginal dilators, perhaps she could be encouraged to start with her own finger as the first dilator. If the finger is well-lubricated and she is sitting in the comfort of a warm bath, she is less likely to have pain. A major degree of success can be obtained with dilators of progressive length and circumference in the hands of a motivated patient, particularly when encouraged by a fully supportive therapist.[1]

A simple constriction ring in the mid-vagina can be addressed surgically with longitudinal lateral relaxing incisions at the 3 and 9 o'clock positions at the site of the constraint.[2] The vaginal incisions should be undermined in all directions to the point where two fingers are easily admitted at the site of narrowing. These incisions will epithelialize, but during that time, a stent must be worn to maintain adequate vaginal caliber and to prevent reformation of the stricture. The stent may be removed during toileting but should be worn at all other times until healing has occurred. If there is no contraindication to its use dependent on the original pathology, local application of estrogen cream to the vagina can aid in the healing process.

### REFERENCES

1. Evans TN, Polland ML, Boving RL: Vaginal malformations, *Am J Obstet Gynecol* 141:910, 1989.
2. Nichols DH: The small and painful vagina. In Nichols DH, Clarke-Pearson DL, eds: *Obstetric, gynecologic and related surgery,* ed 2, St Louis, 1999, Mosby.

### EDITORS' COMMENTS

The use of vaginal dilators should always be attempted in cases of vaginal constriction before surgical correction. The discussant prefers to use bilateral relaxing incisions with postoperative placement of a vaginal stent until the vagina has reepithelialized.

## CASE 15
### Ureteral Obstruction After Vaginal Repair of Advanced Prolapse

*CASE:* The patient is an 81-year-old with vaginal vault eversion (Pelvic Organ Prolapse Quantitation System's stage IV) who underwent an anterior and posterior colporrhaphy and enterocele repair with uterosacral ligament vault suspension. The surgery was uncomplicated. Near the completion of the procedure, the patient was given 5 ml of IV indigo carmine, and a cystoscopy was performed. After 15 minutes of continuous observation, no dye could be seen to efflux from either ureteral orifice.

DISCUSSANT: **Mark D. Walters**

This is a situation that can create substantial anxiety for the surgeon. My main rule in this case is to not leave the operating room unless verification of kidney and ureteral function is accomplished. In an older woman, renal function may be somewhat delayed, or the anesthesiologist may be overly cautious about volume replacement. Before taking further action, I would wait at least 45 more minutes; during this time I would give another 5 ml of IV indigo carmine and 5 ml of IV furosemide. I would also call for ureteral stents to be brought to the operating room. At this point, consideration can be given to obtaining an intraoperative urology consult, depending on the operator's comfort with the management of this condition. I would use this time to recheck the chart to make sure that the blood urea nitrogen (BUN) and creatinine levels were normal. Were a previous renal

ultrasound or intravenous pyelogram (IVP) obtained, I would review these results again at this time; however, I do not routinely obtain these radiologic studies, even in patients with total vaginal prolapse. I would also confirm that the patient has not had a previous nephrectomy.

After about 1 hour, if blue dye has still not passed through one or both ureteral orifices, then I would try to pass retrograde ureteral stents. If they pass easily, I would remove them and follow the patient closely postoperatively. If they do not pass, as is frequently the case, I would then obtain a one-shot IVP in the operating room. This is to confirm that both kidneys are present and functioning and also to look for early hydronephrosis. By now, I would also start removing the culdeplasty and vaginal vault suspension sutures, which are the likely source of the obstruction if one or both ureters have been ligated or kinked. If the IVP shows that both kidneys are functional, there is no efflux of urine from one or both ureters despite removal of the culdeplasty sutures, and I am still unable to pass a ureteral stent, the next decision is more difficult. I would then have to decide whether to perform a laparotomy with ureteral reimplantation or to place nephrostomy tubes to temporarily divert the urine. If it is felt that the patient is able to tolerate the additional time of surgery with its morbidity, I would prefer to proceed with laparotomy. If not, nephrostomy tubes could be placed, and the antegrade passage of a stent into the bladder could be attempted. If this cannot be accomplished, then the patient would remain with nephrostomy tubes until she is able to tolerate reimplantation.

### EDITORS' COMMENTS

Intraoperative recognition of ureteral injuries is of vital importance in gynecologic surgery. The discussant makes it clear that any question of ureteral patency should set into motion a progressively more complex series of actions that will result in either reassurance for the surgeon or management of the ureteral injury. Even the most skilled gynecologic surgeon may defer definitive correction of a ureteral injury with the use of a nephrostomy if the patient's condition will not allow more aggressive surgical measures.

## CASE 16
### Management of Retention After Retropubic Urethropexy

*CASE:* The patient is a 52-year-old para 2 who had a total abdominal hysterectomy and Marshall-Marchetti-Krantz procedure 4 weeks ago. She has been unable to void since surgery. She is currently performing intermittent self-catheterization every 1 to 2 hours because of severe urgency. She also complains of suprapubic pain. Her urine culture was negative, and recent cystoscopy revealed no sutures in the bladder or other intravesical pathology. Examination of the anterior vaginal wall showed the bladder neck was fixed in a high retropubic position. The patient is upset that she has to perform self-catheterization.

DISCUSSANT: **Mickey M. Karram**

It would seem at a glance that this case represents an overzealous retropubic repair for stress incontinence. It is important to ensure that this patient is neurologically intact, and it would be helpful to know if she had any voiding dysfunction or had a high postvoid residual volume before her retropubic repair.

Certain questions need to be addressed when one is dealing with postoperative retention and voiding dysfunction. First and foremost, the patient's perceptions regarding her current state must be firmly understood. Some women have very little difficulty performing intermittent self-catheterization and have no problems continuing this mode of therapy as long as they are cured of their stress incontinence. Other women, as in the case presented, are extremely distressed by the idea of having to perform intermittent self-catheterization and will go to great lengths to have the issue resolved. Second, the patient should never feel that the physician is overly concerned about this being a prolonged phenomenon, as this will instill fear and create much anxiety. Simply stated, if the patient thinks she is never going to be able to void normally again, then she never will. So reassurance and positive thinking are of extreme importance.

I would initially attempt to rule out any complicating factors that could be ongoing. As mentioned, cystourethroscopy is important to rule out any injury, stitch penetration, or coexisting conditions. A pelvic examination and directed neurologic examination should be performed to rule out the development or persistence of a large prolapse, a pelvic mass, or the presence of an underlying neurologic condition.

Nonsurgical or conservative methods have been used in the hope of either improving detrusor contraction strength or decreasing outlet resistance. I am unaware of any pharmacologic agent that has consistently been shown to improve detrusor contraction strength and decrease the time to resumption of normal voiding. Bethanechol has been and continues to be used, although numerous trials have shown that it is no more effective than a placebo. Agents used to decrease urethral resistance have also been used. Some data suggest that diazepam may be beneficial in this setting. I also think it is important to clinically address the pelvic floor muscles and to note whether the patient is able to relax and contract her pelvic muscles appropriately. If she is unable to relax her muscles, pelvic floor rehabilitation in the form of physical therapy and biofeedback may be beneficial. I feel urethral dilation only creates discomfort to the patient; it has not been shown to effectively initiate or accelerate the time to resumption of normal voiding.

Ultimately, assuming nonsurgical techniques are unsuccessful, one is left with determining with the highest probability whether the patient's voiding dysfunction is due to some form of outlet obstruction, and thus, surgically relieving this obstruction would lead to a resumption of normal voiding. It must be kept in mind that bladder denervation or undiagnosed neurologic dysfunction could certainly contribute to the problem and would not be effected by a takedown surgery. I would not consider a takedown until at least 6 weeks after the bladder suspension. The most objective way of determining whether the patient is truly obstructed versus a problem with denervation or neurologic dysfunction would be to perform a filling and voiding cystometrogram. If the patient is able to void small amounts of urine around the catheter during a pressure flow study and is able to generate bladder contractions exceeding 20 cm $H_2O$, one can be assured that a fair amount of outlet obstruction exists. This would be a patient that has a high potential for success of a takedown procedure. Unfortunately, as in this case, many patients are in complete retention. In my opinion, filling cystometry is extremely helpful in identifying whether normal motor and sensory function is present. If the patient has normal or hypersensitive parameters with many involuntary detrusor contractions, she would be more likely to be obstructed.

However, if filling CMG is performed and the patient has very little sensation with accommodation of huge amounts of urine, one must be concerned that sensory and motor deficits may be present.

Once the decision to take down the repair has been made, it is somewhat controversial whether it is best performed vaginally or abdominally. It has been our experience that cases initially done retropubically are best taken down retropubically. If I were to do this, I would put a Foley catheter with a 30-ml Foley balloon into the bladder. I would make a transverse muscle-cutting (Cherney) incision to facilitate exposure into the retropubic space. The bladder is then taken down sharply off the back of the symphysis pubis all the way down to the proximal urethra. It is best to make an advertent high cystotomy to help in this dissection. It is important to completely mobilize the bladder as well as the proximal urethra from the back of the symphysis. There is always a concern for rescarification in this area, and on two occasions, we have made a small window in the peritoneum and brought in a piece of omentum to be placed between the back of the symphysis and the proximal urethra. I would not advocate resuspension unless obvious prolapse is present, which is usually secondary to a paravaginal defect. If this were the case, then I would certainly advocate stabilization of the base of the bladder by a paravaginal defect repair and possibly a midline cystocele repair via the transvaginal route. The patient must fully understand that there is no guarantee her voiding dysfunction will be completely normal after such a takedown and that there is always a potential for redevelopment of stress incontinence. In a small series of approximately 12 cases, we have had good success with this technique.

There are those who advocate a vaginal takedown in such a situation. This is best accomplished by again placing a Foley catheter with a 30-ml balloon, then performing either an inverted "U" or a midline incision in the anterior vaginal wall. The goal is to create mobility of the bladder neck by dissecting toward the inferior pubic ramus on either side. This may involve perforating the urogenital diaphragm. Urethral mobility is subjectively assessed via traction on the Foley catheter. Some also advocate the placement of a labial fat pad around the urethra to prevent rescarification. I would again discourage any attempts at resuspension.

## EDITORS' COMMENTS

Urinary retention and voiding dysfunction are very frustrating problems that can occur after any antiincontinence procedure. Reassurance and a thorough evaluation are very important before considering surgical takedown. The discussant prefers a retropubic approach to takedown in contrast to vaginal urethrolysis.

## CASE 17

### Incontinence With an Areflexic Bladder

*CASE:* The patient is a 38-year-old para 2 with a 2-year history of worsening urinary incontinence. Over the past year, she has been leaking with most activities and seems to leak at multiple times during the day without any other associated symptoms. She also has noticed that she tends to void small amounts of urine multiple times during the day and is unsure if she is completely emptying her bladder. She has no significant past medical history and takes no medications. She had two spontaneous vaginal deliveries and a postpartum tubal ligation. On physical examination, she has no significant vaginal or uterine support abnormalities, and a Q-tip test notes a rotation of 40 degrees with straining. She does leak urine with coughing in the supine position. Simple bladder filling in the office revealed no sensation to filling until 950 ml. The filling was stopped at 1100 ml, even though the patient did not feel particularly full. She voided 300 ml and had a postvoid residual urine volume of 820 ml.

**DISCUSSANTS: Edward J. McGuire and O. Lenaine Westney**

In constructing a list of differential diagnosis for this patient, the explanation for the areflexia and incontinence may require a combination of conditions. The need for multiple diagnosis results from a physical examination, fluorodynamic evaluation, and additional imaging studies, which do not unify satisfactorily to a single entity. This situation commonly occurs when neurologic and anatomic abnormalities coexist. Explanations for poor emptying include overdistention, afferent decentralization, or a sacral root or cord lesion, and rarely a posterior spinal cord lesion. The latter, associated with bladder dysfunction only, would be distinctly unusual. Motor decentralization does not usually produce this picture (i.e., absent sensation with a large-capacity bladder). Afferent lesions result in lack of brain stem reflex center activation for voiding and dominance of the inhibitory system as occurs with anesthesia, tabes dorsalis, or a spinal cord lesion. Overdistention injuries, if prolonged, appear to produce an afferent neural injury, not an efferent one. The combination of a large-capacity, low-pressure bladder and stress incontinence is unusual. Causes of loss of reflex detrusor contractility and stress incontinence include sacral root injury or lesions and peripheral neural injury. An example would be what may occur after an abdominal perineal resection or a radical hysterectomy. Peripheral lesions are characterized by poor detrusor storage function associated with high detrusor pressure at mean volumes (as in this example, at 800 ml) and an open nonfunctional bladder neck.

To determine if this is present, which would then suggest a pelvic malignancy, one would need a cystometrogram, measurement of pressure at her average residual urine volume, and an upright cystogram or video study to evaluate proximal sphincter function.

A sacral lesion that produced a large and poorly compliant bladder (e.g., sacral stenosis or a large intervertebral disk) would not affect internal sphincter function but could be associated with pelvic floor muscular dysfunction and resultant stress urinary incontinence related to hypermobility. To test this hypothesis, a careful neurologic examination with perineal sensation testing and rectal sphincter examination should be combined with a video study. A sacral lesion could produce a poorly compliant bladder that, when filled, would drive urine into the proximal urethra and create Type III stress incontinence. That theory would best be tested with a video-urodynamic study.

A demyelinating disease such as multiple sclerosis (MS) occasionally is associated with a large, low-pressure bladder that gradually becomes hyperreflexic, although this is not generally associated with stress incontinence. Anatomic stress incontinence might coexist with a neurologic lesion such as MS. To test this hypothesis, simple urodynamics can be done and the bladder pressure proven to be low. A final possibility that should be entertained after all more serious entities have been eliminated

would be an unrecognized postpartum distention injury that led to long-term overflow incontinence in combination with anatomic stress incontinence. Again, that diagnosis should only be considered after all the more ominous possibilities have been excluded.

With all the aforementioned conditions taken into account, the first diagnostic step is a focused neurologic examination to discern rectal tone, perineal sensation, and presence of bulbocavernosus and anal wink reflexes. Any abnormalities in this portion of the examination will indicate the need for formal neurologic evaluation. The next logical step to clearly examine bladder and urethral function would be fluorourodynamics to evaluate compliance, detrusor, and Valsalva leak point pressures; competence of the bladder neck; and bladder–external urethral sphincter synergy. Fluorourodynamics are key to defining the bladder and urethral components of the patient's voiding dysfunction. The patient should be filled at least to first sensation unless poor compliance is exhibited or reflux occurs before that volume. After filling, upright Valsalva maneuvers should be performed and the degree of cystocele, urethral mobility, and leak pressure noted. During voiding, vesical pressure and external urethral pressures should be monitored. Regardless of the result of the screening neurologic examination, magnetic resonance imaging (MRI) of the spinal cord should be ordered to rule out any spinal lesions, including multiple sclerosis. Naturally, positive findings on imaging would necessitate a neurology consult.

Primary management of her incontinence is centered around intermittent catheterization on a round-the-clock basis. If her Valsalva leak point pressure is not extremely low, which is supported by her pattern of leakage, regular bladder emptying should relieve her incontinence. If this approach is not immediately successful, no incontinence procedures should be planned until formal neurologic evaluation is complete. The patient should be instructed to catheterize for postvoid residuals and record the volumes. Reevaluation should take place 3 to 4 weeks after initiating intermittent catheterization. At that time, the voiding record should be reviewed and repeat urodynamics performed if the patient has not resumed normal emptying. In cases where leakage has occurred between catheterizations and primary intrinsic sphincter deficiency is identified, treatment must be postponed until after the postvoid residuals have stabilized. It is best to allow detrusor function to improve maximally before increasing the outlet resistance. When a postvoid nadir has been reached, either periurethral or intraurethral collagen injections or a pubovaginal sling may be performed to improve coaptation. Finally, the patient should be counseled that whether the cause of her areflexia is primarily neurologic or secondary to an initial distention injury that intermittent catheterization might be necessary indefinitely.

**EDITORS' COMMENTS**

Bladder areflexia may be a marker for more severe underlying conditions such as demyelinating disorders. The postvoid residual determination therefore becomes a critical portion of the workup of every incontinent woman. Because many antiincontinence procedures can lead to urinary retention, this patient appears stuck "between a rock and a hard place." The discussants provide a logical approach to the evaluation and treatment of two seemingly contradictory conditions.

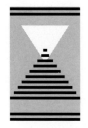

*Appendixes*

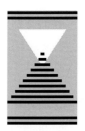

APPENDIX **A**

# *The Standardisation of Terminology of Lower Urinary Tract Function Recommended by the International Continence Society*

## CONTENTS

## 1. INTRODUCTION

The International Continence Society (ICS) established a committee for the standardisation of terminology of lower urinary tract function in 1973. Five of the six reports from this committee, approved by the Society, have been published.[1-5] The fifth report on "Quantification of urine loss" was an internal ICS document but appears, in part, in this document.

These reports are revised, extended and collated in this monograph. The standards are recommended to facilitate comparison of results by investigators who use urodynamic methods. These standards are recommended not only for urodynamic investigations carried out on humans but also during animal studies. When using urodynamic studies in animals the type of any anesthesia used should be stated. It is suggested that acknowledgement of these standards in written publications be indicated by a footnote to the section "Methods and Materials" or its equivalent, to read as follows: "Methods, definitions and units conform to the standards recommended by the International Continence Society, except where specifically noted."

*Urodynamic studies* involve the assessment of the function and dysfunction of the urinary tract by any appropriate method. Aspects of urinary tract morphology, physiology, biochemistry and hydrodynamics affect urine transport and storage. Other methods of investigation such as the radiographic visualisation of the lower urinary tract are a useful adjunct to conventional urodynamics. This monograph concerns the urodynamics of the lower urinary tract.

## 2. CLINICAL ASSESSMENT

The clinical assessment of patients with lower urinary tract dysfunction should consist of a detailed history, a frequency/volume chart and a physical examination. In urinary incontinence, leakage should be demonstrated objectively.

### 2.1 History

The general history should include questions relevant to neurological and congenital abnormalities as well as information on previous urinary infections and relevant surgery. Information must be obtained on medication with known or possible effects on the lower urinary tract. The general history should also include assessment of menstrual, sexual and bowel function and obstetric history.

The urinary history must consist of symptoms related to both the storage and the evacuation functions of the lower urinary tract.

### 2.2 Frequency/Volume Chart

The frequency/volume chart is a specific urodynamic investigation recording fluid intake and urine output

From Abrams P, Blaivas JG, Stanton SL, et al: *Int Urogynecol J* 1:45, 1990.

per 24-hour period. The chart gives objective information on the number of voidings, the distribution of voidings between daytime and nighttime and each voided volume. The chart can also be used to record episodes of urgency and leakage and the number of incontinence pads used. The frequency/volume chart is very useful in the assessment of voiding disorders, and in the follow-up of treatment.

## 2.3 Physical Examination

Besides a general urological and, when appropriate, gynecological examination, the physical examination should include the assessment of perineal sensation, the perineal reflexes supplied by the sacral segments S2-S4, and anal sphincter tone and control.

## 3. PROCEDURES RELATED TO THE EVALUATION OF URINE STORAGE
## 3.1 Cystometry

Cystometry is the method by which the pressure/volume relationship of the bladder is measured. All systems are zeroed at atmospheric pressure. For external transducers the reference point is the level of the superior edge of the symphysis pubis. For catheter mounted transducers the reference point is the transducer itself. Cystometry is used to assess detrusor activity, sensation, capacity and compliance.

Before starting to fill the bladder the residual urine may be measured. However, the removal of a large volume of residual urine may alter detrusor function especially in neuropathic disorders. Certain cystometric parameters may be significantly altered by the speed of bladder filling (see Compliance, 6.2.1).

During cystometry it is taken for granted that the patient is aware, unanesthetized and neither sedated nor taking drugs that affect bladder function. Any variations should be specified.

*3.1.1. General Information.* The following details should be given:
1. Access (transurethral or percutaneous).
2. Fluid medium (liquid or gas).
3. Temperature of fluid (state in degrees Celsius).
4. Position of patient (e.g., supine, sitting, or standing).
5. Filling method—may be by diuresis or catheter. Filling by catheter may be continuous or incremental; the precise filling rate should be stated. When the incremental method is used the volume increment should be stated. For general discussion, the following terms for the range of filling rate may be used:
   a. Up to 10 ml per minute is *slow fill cystometry* ("physiological" filling).
   b. 10-100 ml per minute is *medium fill cystometry.*
   c. Over 100 ml per minute is *rapid fill cystometry.*
*3.1.2. Technical Information.* The following details should be given:
1. Fluid-filled catheter—specify number of catheters,

single or multiple lumens, type of catheter (manufacturer), size of catheter.
2. Catheter tip transducer—list specifications.
3. Other catheters—list specifications.
4. Measuring equipment.
*3.1.3. Definitions.* Cystometric terminology is defined as follows:
*Intravesical pressure* is the pressure within the bladder.
*Abdominal pressure* is taken to be the pressure surrounding the bladder. In current practice it is estimated from rectal or, less commonly, extraperitoneal pressure.
*Detrusor pressure* is that component of intravesical pressure that is created by forces in the bladder wall (passive or active). It is estimated by subtracting abdominal pressure from intravesical pressure. The simultaneous measurement of abdominal pressure is essential for the interpretation of the intravesical pressure trace. However, artifacts on the detrusor pressure trace may be produced by intrinsic rectal contractions.
*Bladder sensation.* Sensation is difficult to evaluate because of its subjective nature. It is usually assessed by questioning the patient in relation to the fullness of the bladder during cystometry.
Commonly used descriptive terms include:
*First desire to void.*
*Normal desire to void*—defined as the feeling that leads the patient to pass urine at the next convenient moment, but voiding can be delayed if necessary.
*Strong desire to void*—defined as a persistent desire to void without the fear of leakage.
*Urgency*—defined as a strong desire to void accompanied by fear of leakage or fear of pain.
*Pain* (the site and character of which should be specified). Pain during bladder filling or micturition is abnormal.
The use of objective or semi-objective tests for sensory function, such as electrical threshold studies (sensory testing), is discussed under Sensory Testing (see 5.6).
The term "capacity" must be qualified as follows:
*Maximum cystometric capacity,* in patients with normal sensation, is the volume at which the patient feels he/she can no longer delay micturition. In the absence of sensation the maximum cystometric capacity cannot be defined in the same terms and is the volume at which the clinician decides to terminate filling. In the presence of sphincter incompetence the maximum cystometric capacity may be significantly increased by occlusion of the urethra, e.g., by Foley catheter.
The *functional bladder capacity,* or voided volume, is more relevant and is assessed from a frequency/volume chart (urinary diary).
The *maximum (anesthetic) bladder capacity* is the volume measured after filling during a deep general or spinal/epidural anaesthetic, specifying fluid temperature, filling pressure and filling time.

*Compliance* indicates the change in volume for a change in pressure. Compliance is calculated by dividing the volume change ($\Delta V$) by the change in detrusor pressure ($\Delta P_{det}$) during that change in bladder volume ($C = \Delta V / \Delta P_{det}$). Compliance is expressed as milliliters per centimeters of water pressure. (See also Compliance, 6.2.1.)

## 3.2 Urethral Pressure Measurement

It should be noted that the urethral pressure and the urethral closure pressure are idealised concepts which represent the ability of the urethra to prevent leakage (see Urinary Incontinence, 6.2.3). In current urodynamic practice the urethral pressure is measured by a number of different techniques which do not always yield consistent values. Not only do the values differ with the method of measurement but there is often lack of consistency for a single method (e.g., the effect of catheter rotation when urethral pressure is measured by a catheter mounted transducer).

*Intraluminal urethral pressure* may be measured:

At rest, with the bladder at any given volume.

During coughing or straining.

During the process of voiding (see section on voiding urethral pressure profile, 4.4).

Measurements may be made of one point in the urethra over a period of time, or at several points along the urethra consecutively forming a *urethral pressure profile* (UPP).

Two types of UPP may be measured in the *storage phase:*

1. Resting urethral pressure profile—with the bladder and subject at rest.
2. Stress urethral pressure profile—with a defined applied stress (e.g., cough, strain, Valsalva).

In the storage phase the *urethral pressure profile* denotes the intraluminal pressure along the length of the urethra. All systems are zeroed at atmospheric pressure. For external transducers the reference point is the superior edge of the symphysis pubis. For catheter mounted transducers the reference point is the transducer itself. Intravesical pressure should be measured to exclude a simultaneous detrusor contraction. The subtraction of intravesical pressure from urethral pressure produces the *urethral closure pressure profile.*

The simultaneous recording of both intravesical and intra-urethral pressures is essential during stress urethral profilometry.

*3.2.1 General Information.* The following details should be given:

1. Infusion medium (liquid or gas).
2. Rate of infusion.
3. Stationary, continuous or intermittent withdrawal.
4. Rate of withdrawal.
5. Bladder volume.
6. Position of patient (supine, sitting or standing).

*3.2.2. Technical Information.* The following details should be given:

1. Open catheter—specify type (manufacturer), size, number, position and orientation of side or end hole.

2. Catheter mounted transducers—specify manufacturer, number of transducers, spacing of transducers along the catheter, orientation with respect to one another; transducer design, e.g., transducer face depressed or flush with catheter surface; catheter diameter and material. The orientation of the transducer(s) in the urethra should be stated.
3. Other catheters, e.g., membrane, fiberoptic—specify type (manufacturer), size, and number of channels as for microtransducer catheter.
4. Measurement technique: For stress profiles the particular stress employed should be stated, e.g., cough or Valsalva.
5. Recording apparatus: Describe type of recording apparatus. The frequency response of the total system should be stated. The frequency response of the catheter in the perfusion method can be assessed by blocking the eyeholes and recording the consequent rate of change of pressure.

*3.2.3. Definitions.* Terminology referring to profiles measured in storage phase (see Fig. A-1) is defined as follows:

*Maximum urethral pressure* is the maximum pressure of the measured profile.

*Maximum urethral closure pressure* is the maximum difference, between the urethral pressure and the intravesical pressure.

*Functional profile length* is the length of the urethra along which the urethral pressure exceeds intravesical pressure.

*Functional profile length (on stress)* is the length over which the urethral pressure exceeds the intravesical pressure on stress.

*Pressure "transmission" ratio* is the increment in urethral pressure on stress as a percentage of the simultaneously recorded increment in intravesical pressure. For stress

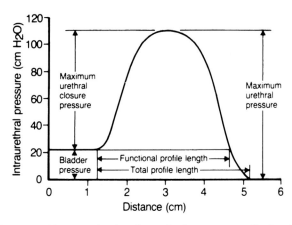

**Fig. A-1** Diagram of a female urethral pressure profile (static) with ICS recommended nomenclature.

profiles obtained during coughing, pressure transmission ratios can be obtained at any point along the urethra. If single values are given the position in the urethra should be stated. If several pressure transmission ratios are defined at different points along the urethra a pressure "transmission" profile is obtained. During "cough profiles" the amplitude of the cough should be stated if possible. NOTE: The term "transmission" is in common usage and cannot be changed. However, transmission implies a completely passive process. Such an assumption is not yet justified by scientific evidence. A role for muscular activity cannot be excluded.

*Total profile length* is not generally regarded as a useful parameter.

The information gained from urethral pressure measurements in the storage phase is of limited value in the assessment of voiding disorders.

## 3.3 Quantification of Urine Loss

Subjective grading of incontinence may not indicate reliably the degree of abnormality. However, it is important to relate the management of the individual patients to their complaints and personal circumstances, as well as to objective measurements.

In order to assess and compare the results of the treatment of different types of incontinence in different centres, a simple standard test can be used to measure urine loss objectively in any subject. In order to obtain a representative result, especially in subjects with variable or intermittent urinary incontinence, the test should occupy as long a period as possible; yet it must be practical. The circumstances should approximate to those of everyday life, yet be similar for all subjects to allow meaningful comparison. On the basis of pilot studies performed in various centres, an internal report of the ICS (5th) recommended a test occupying a 1-hour period during which a series of standard activities was carried out. This test *can* be extended by further 1-hour periods if the result of the first 1-hour test was not considered representative by either the patient or the investigator. Alternatively the test can be repeated having filled the bladder to a defined volume.

The total amount of urine lost during the test period is determined by weighing a collecting device such as a nappy, absorbent pad or condom appliance. A nappy or pad should be worn inside waterproof underpants or should have a waterproof backing. Care should be taken to use a collecting device of adequate capacity. Immediately before the test begins the collecting device is weighed to the nearest gram.

### 3.3.1. Typical Test Schedule
1. Test is started without the patient voiding.
2. Preweighed collecting device is put on and first 1-hour test period begins.
3. Subject drinks 500 ml sodium-free liquid within a short period (max. 15 min), then sits or rests.
4. Half-hour period: Subject walks, including stair climbing equivalent to one flight up and down.

5. During the remaining period the subject performs the following activities:
   a. Standing up from sitting, 10 times.
   b. Coughing vigorously, 10 times.
   c. Running on the spot for 1 min.
   d. Bending to pick up small object from floor, 5 times.
   e. Wash hands in running water for 1 min.
6. At the end of the 1-hour test the collecting device is removed and weighed.
7. If the test is regarded as representative the subject voids and the volume is recorded.
8. Otherwise the test is repeated preferably without voiding.

If the collecting device becomes saturated or filled during the test it should be removed and weighed and replaced by a fresh device. The total weight of urine lost during the test period is taken to be equal to the gain in weight of the collecting device(s). In interpreting the results of the test it should be born in mind that a weight gain of up to 1 gram may be due to weighing errors, sweating or vaginal discharge.

The activity program may be modified according to the subject's physical ability. If substantial variations from the usual test schedule occur, this should be recorded so that the same schedule can be used on subsequent occasions.

In principle the subject should not void during the test period. If the patient experiences urgency, then he/she should be persuaded to postpone voiding and to perform as many of the activities in section 3.3.1 (5a-e) as possible in order to detect leakage. Before voiding the collection device is removed for weighing. If inevitable voiding cannot be postponed then the test is terminated. The voided volume and the duration of the test should be recorded. For subjects not completing the full test the results may require separate analysis, or the test may be repeated after rehydration.

The test result is given as grams urine lost in the 1-hour test period in which the greatest urine loss is recorded.

### 3.3.2. Additional Procedures. 
Provided that there is no interference with the basic test, additional procedures intended to give information of diagnostic value are permissible. For example, additional changes and weighing of the collecting device can give information about the timing of urine loss; the absorbent nappy may be an electronic recording nappy so that the timing is recorded directly.

### 3.3.3. Presentation of Results. 
The following details should be given:
1. Collecting device.
2. Physical condition of subject (ambulant, chairbound, bedridden).
3. Relevant medical conditions of subject.
4. Relevant drug treatments.
5. Test schedule.

In some situations the timing of the test (e.g., in relation to the menstrual cycle) may be relevant.

*Findings.* Record weight of urine lost during the test (in the case of repeated tests, greatest weight in any stated period). A loss of less than 1 gram is within experimental error, and the patients should be regarded as essentially dry. Urine loss should be measured and recorded in grams.

*Statistics.* When performing statistical analysis of urine loss in a group of subjects, non-parametric statistics should be employed, since the values are not normally distributed.

## 4. PROCEDURES RELATED TO THE EVALUATION OF MICTURITION

### 4.1. Measurement of Urinary Flow

*Urinary flow* may be described in terms of *rate* and *pattern* and may be *continuous* or *intermittent*. *Flow rate* is defined as the volume of fluid expelled via the urethra per unit time. It is expressed in ml/s.

*4.1.1. General Information.* The following details should be given:

1. Voided volume.
2. Patient environment and position (supine, sitting, or standing).
3. Filling:
   a. By diuresis (spontaneous or forced: specify regimen).
   b. By catheter (transurethral or suprapubic).
4. Type of fluid.

*4.1.2. Technical Information.* The following details should be given:

1. Measuring equipment.
2. Solitary procedure or combined with other measurements.

*4.1.3. Definitions.* The terminology referring to urinary flow is defined as follows:

1. *Continuous flow* (Fig. A-2):
   *Voided volume* is the total volume expelled via the urethra.

*Maximum flow rate* is the maximum measured value of the flow rate.

*Average flow rate* is voided volume divided by flow time. The calculation of average flow rate is only meaningful if flow is continuous and without terminal dribbling.

*Flow time* is the time over which measurable flow actually occurs.

*Time to maximum flow* is the elapsed time from onset of flow to maximum flow.

The flow pattern must be described when flow time and average flow rate are measured.

2. *Intermittent flow* (Fig. A-3):
   The same parameters used to characterise continuous flow may be applicable if care is exercised in patients with intermittent flow. In measuring flow time the time intervals between flow episodes are disregarded.

*Voiding time* is total duration of micturition, i.e., includes interruptions. When voiding is completed without interruption, voiding time is equal to flow time.

### 4.2. Bladder Pressure Measurements During Micturition

The specifications of patient position, access for pressure measurement, catheter type and measuring equipment are as for cystometry (see 3.1).

*4.2.1. Definitions.* The terminology referring to bladder pressure during micturition is defined as follows (Fig. A-4):

*Opening time* is the elapsed time from initial rise in detrusor pressure to onset of flow. This is the initial isovolumetric contraction period of micturition. Time lags should be taken into account. In most urodynamic systems a time lag occurs equal to the time taken for the urine to pass from the point of pressure measurement to the uroflow transducer.

The following parameters are applicable to measurements of each of the pressure curves: intravesical, abdominal and detrusor pressure.

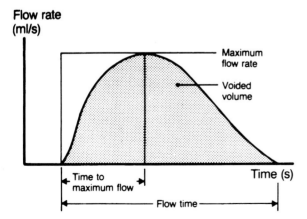

**Fig. A-2** Diagram of a continuous urine flow recording with ICS recommended nomenclature.

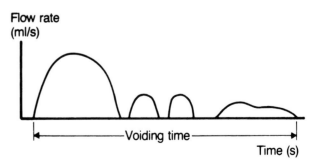

**Fig. A-3** Diagram of an interrupted urine flow recording with ICS recommended nomenclature.

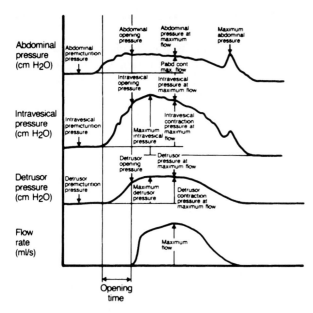

**Fig. A-4** Diagram of a pressure-flow recording of micturition with ICS recommended nomenclature.

*Premicturition pressure* is the pressure recorded immediately before the initial isovolumetric contraction.

*Opening pressure* is the pressure recorded at the onset of measured flow.

*Maximum pressure* is the maximum value of the measured pressure.

*Pressure at maximum flow* is the pressure recorded at maximum measured flow rate.

*Contraction pressure at maximum flow* is the difference between pressure at maximum flow and premicturition pressure.

Postmicturition events (e.g., after contraction) are not well understood and so cannot be defined as yet.

## 4.3 Pressure-Flow Relationships

In the early days of urodynamics the flow rate and voiding pressure were related as a "urethral resistance factor." The concept of a resistance factor originates from rigid tube hydrodynamics. The urethra does not generally behave as a rigid tube as it is an irregular and distensible conduit whose walls and surroundings have active and passive elements and hence, influence the flow through it. Therefore a resistance factor cannot provide a valid comparison between patients.

There are many ways of displaying the relationships between flow and pressure during micturition; an example is suggested in the ICS Third Report[4] (Fig. A-5). As yet available data do not permit a standard presentation of pressure/flow parameters.

When data from a group of patients are presented, pressure-flow relationships may be shown on a graph as illustrated in Fig. A-5. This form of presentation allows lines of demarcation to be drawn on the graph to separate the results according to the problem being studied. The points

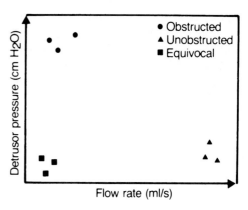

**Fig. A-5** Diagram illustrating the presentation of pressure flow data on individual patients in three groups of three patients: obstructed, equivocal, and unobstructed.

shown in Fig. A-5 are purely illustrative to indicate how the data might fall into groups. The group of equivocal results might include either an unrepresentative micturition in an obstructed or an unobstructed patient, or underactive detrusor function with or without obstruction. This is the group which invalidates the use of "urethral resistance factors."

## 4.4 Urethral Pressure Measurements During Voiding

The voiding urethral pressure profile (VUPP) is used to determine the pressure and site of urethral obstruction. Pressure is recorded in the urethra during voiding. The technique is similar to that used in the UPP measured during storage (the resting and stress profiles; see 3.2).

General and technical information should be recorded as for UPP during storage (see 3.2).

Accurate interpretation of the VUPP depends on the simultaneous measurement of intravesical pressure and the measurement of pressure at a precisely localised point in the urethra. Localisation may be achieved by radio-opaque marker on the catheter which allows the pressure measurements to be related to a visualised point in the urethra. This technique is not fully developed, and a number of technical as well as clinical problems need to be solved before the VUPP is widely used.

## 4.5 Residual Urine

Residual urine is defined as the volume of fluid remaining in the bladder immediately following the completion of micturition. The measurement of residual urine forms an integral part of the study of micturition. However, voiding in unfamiliar surroundings may lead to unrepresentative results, as may voiding on command with a partially filled or overfilled bladder. Residual urine is commonly estimated by the following methods:

1. Catheter or cystoscope (transurethral, suprapubic).
2. Radiography (excretion urography, micturition cystography).

3. Ultrasonics.

4. Radioisotopes (clearance, gamma camera).

When estimating residual urine the measurement of voided volume and the time interval between voiding and residual urine estimation should be recorded; this is particularly important if the patient is in a diuretic phase. In the condition of vesicoureteric reflux, urine may re-enter the bladder after micturition and may falsely be interpreted as residual urine. The presence of urine in bladder diverticula following micturition presents special problems of interpretation, since a diverticulum may be regarded either as part of the bladder cavity or as outside the functioning bladder.

The various methods of measurement each have limitations as to their applicability and accuracy in the various conditions associated with residual urine. Therefore it is necessary to choose a method appropriate to the clinical problems. The absence of residual urine is usually an observation of clinical value but does not exclude infravesical obstruction or bladder dysfunction. An isolated finding of residual urine requires confirmation before being considered significant.

## 5. PROCEDURES RELATED TO NEUROPHYSIOLOGICAL EVALUATION OF THE URINARY TRACT DURING FILLING AND VOIDING

### 5.1 Electromyography

Electromyography (EMG) is the study of electrical potentials generated by the depolarization of muscle. The following refers to striated muscle EMG. The functional unit in EMG is the motor unit. This is comprised of a single motor neurone and the muscle fibers it innervates. A motor unit action potential is the recorded depolarization of muscle fibres which results from activation of a single anterior horn cell. Muscle action potentials may be detected either by needle electrodes or by surface electrodes.

Needle electrodes are placed directly into the muscle mass and permit visualization of the individual motor unit action potentials.

Surface electrodes are applied to an epithelial surface as close to the muscle under study as possible. Surface electrodes detect the action potentials from groups of adjacent motor units underlying the recording surface.

EMG potentials may be displayed on an oscilloscope screen or played through audio amplifiers. A permanent record of EMG potentials can only be made using a chart recorder with a high frequency response (in the range of 10 kHz).

EMG should be interpreted in the light of the patient's symptoms, physical findings and urological and urodynamic investigations.

*5.1.1. General Information.* The following details should be given:

1. EMG (solitary procedure, part of urodynamic or other electrophysiological investigation).

2. Patient position (supine, standing, sitting or other).

3. Electrode placement:

   a. Sampling site (intrinsic striated muscle of the urethra, periurethral striated muscle, bulbocavernosus muscle, external anal sphincter, pubococcygeus or other). State whether sites are single or multiple, unilateral or bilateral. Also state number of samples per site.

   b. Recording electrode: Define the precise anatomical location of the electrode. For needle electrodes, include site of needle entry, angle of entry and needle depth. For vaginal or urethral surface electrodes state method of determining position of electrode.

   c. Reference electrode position. NOTE: Ensure that there is no electrical interference with any other machines, e.g., x-ray apparatus.

*5.1.2. Technical Information.* The following details should be given:

1. Electrodes:

   a. Needle electrodes—design (concentric, bipolar, monopolar, single fibre, other); dimensions (length, diameter, recording area); electrode material (e.g., platinum).

   b. Surface electrodes—type (skin, plug, catheter, other); size and shape; electrode material; mode of fixation to recording surface; conducting medium (e.g., saline, jelly).

2. Amplifier (make and specifications).

3. Signal processing (data: raw, averaged, integrated, or other).

4. Display equipment (make and specifications to include method of calibration, time base, full scale deflection in microvolts and polarity).

   a. Oscilloscope.

   b. Chart recorder.

   c. Loudspeaker.

   d. Other.

5. Storage (make and specifications).

   a. Paper.

   b. Magnetic tape recorder.

   c. Microprocessor.

   d. Other.

6. Hard copy production (make and specifications).

   a. Chart recorder.

   b. Photographic/video reproduction of oscilloscope screen.

   c. Other.

### 5.2 EMG Findings

*5.2.1. Individual Motor Unit Action Potentials.* Normal motor unit potentials have a characteristic configuration, amplitude and duration. Abnormalities of the motor unit may include an increase in the amplitude, duration and complexity of waveform (polyphasicity) of the potentials. A polyphasic potential is defined as one having more than 5 deflections. The EMG findings of fibrillations, positive sharp waves and bizarre high frequency potentials are thought to be abnormal.

*5.2.2. Recruitment Patterns.* In normal subjects there is a gradual increase in "pelvic floor" and "sphincter" EMG activity during bladder filling. At the onset of micturition there is complete absence of activity. Any sphincter EMG activity during voiding is abnormal unless the patient is attempting to inhibit micturition. The finding of increased sphincter EMG activity, during voiding, accompanied by characteristic simultaneous detrusor pressure and flow changes is described by the term *detrusor-sphincter dyssynergia.* In this condition detrusor contraction occurs concurrently with an inappropriate contraction of the urethral and or periurethral striated muscle.

## 5.3 Nerve Conduction Studies

Nerve conduction studies involve stimulation of a peripheral nerve and recording the time taken for a response to occur in muscle, innervated by the nerve under study. The time taken from stimulation of the nerve to the response in the muscle is called the "latency." Motor latency is the time taken by the fastest motor fibres in the nerve to conduct impulses to the muscle and depends on conduction distance and the conduction velocity of the fastest fibers.

*5.3.1. General Information.* Also applicable to reflex latencies and evoked potentials (see 5.4 and 5.5). The following details should be given:
1. Type of investigation:
   a. Nerve conduction study (e.g., pudendal nerve).
   b. Reflex latency determination (e.g., bulbocavernosus).
   c. Spinal evoked potential.
   d. Cortical evoked potential.
   e. Other.
2. Is the study a solitary procedure or part of urodynamic or neurophysiological investigations?
3. Patient position and environmental temperature, noise level and illumination.
4. Electrode placement: Define electrode placement in precise anatomical terms. The exact interelectrode distance is required for nerve conduction velocity calculations.
   a. Stimulation site (penis, clitoris, urethra, bladder neck, bladder or other).
   b. Recording sites (external anal sphincter, periurethral striated muscle, bulbocavernosus muscle, spinal cord, cerebral cortex or other).
   When recording spinal evoked responses, the sites of the recording electrodes should be specified according to the bony landmarks (e.g., L4). In cortical evoked responses the sites of the recording electrodes should be specified as in the International 10-20 system.[6] The sampling techniques should be specified (single or multiple, unilateral or bilateral, ipsilateral or contralateral, or other).

   c. Reference electrode position.
   d. Grounding electrode site. Ideally this should be between the stimulation and recording sites to reduce stimulus artifact.

*5.3.2. Technical Information.* Also applicable to reflex latencies and evoked potential (see 5.4 and 5.5). The following details should be given:
1. Electrodes (make and specifications). Describe separately stimulus and recording electrodes as below:
   a. Design (e.g., needle, plate, ring, and configuration of anode and cathode where applicable).
   b. Dimensions.
   c. Electrode material (e.g., platinum).
   d. Contact medium.
2. Stimulator (make and specifications):
   a. Stimulus parameters (pulse width, frequency, pattern, current density, electrode impedance in kOhms). Also define in terms of threshold (e.g., in case of supramaximal stimulation).
3. Amplifier (make and specifications):
   a. Sensitivity (mV-μV).
   b. Filters—low pass (Hz) or high pass (kHz).
   c. Sampling time (ms).
4. Averager (make and specifications):
   a. Number of stimuli sampled.
5. Display equipment (make and specifications to include method of calibration, time base, full scale deflection in microvolts and polarity):
   a. Oscilloscope.
6. Storage (make and specifications):
   a. Paper.
   b. Magnetic tape recorder.
   c. Microprocessor.
   d. Other.
7. Hard copy production (make and specification):
   a. Chart recorder.
   b. Photographic/video reproduction of oscilloscope screen.
   c. XY recorder.
   d. Other.

*5.3.3. Description of Nerve Conduction Studies.* Recordings are made from muscle and latency of response of the muscle is measured. The latency is taken as the time to onset, of the earliest response.

To ensure that response time can be precisely measured, the gain should be increased to give a clearly defined takeoff point. (Gain setting at least 100 μV/div and using a short time base, e.g., 1-2 ms/div.)

Additional information may be obtained from nerve conduction studies, if, when using surface electrodes to record a compound muscle action potential, the amplitude is measured. The gain setting must be reduced so that the whole response is displayed and a longer time base is recommended (e.g., 1 mV/div and 5 ms/div). Since the amplitude is proportional to the number of motor unit potentials within the vicinity of the recording electrodes, a reduction in amplitude indicates loss of motor units and therefore denervation. (NOTE: A prolongation of latency is not necessarily indicative of denervation.)

## 5.4 Reflex Latencies

Reflex latencies require stimulation of sensory fields and recordings from the muscle which contracts reflexly in response to the stimulation. Such responses are a test of reflex arcs which are comprised of both afferent and efferent limbs and a synaptic region within the central nervous system. The reflex latency expresses the nerve conduction velocity in both limbs of the are and the integrity of the central nervous system at the level of the synapse(s). Increased reflex latency may occur as a result of slowed afferent or efferent nerve conduction or due to central nervous system conduction delays.

*5.4.1. General Information and Technical Information.* The same technical and general details apply as discussed above under Nerve Conduction Studies.

*5.4.2. Description of Reflex Latency Measurements.* Recordings are made from muscle and the latency of response of the muscle is measured. The latency is taken as the time to onset, of the earliest response.

To ensure that response time can be precisely measured, the gain should be increased to give a clearly defined take-off point (gain setting at least 100 µV/div and using a short time base, e.g., 1-2 ms/div).

## 5.5 Evoked Responses

Evoked responses are potential changes in central nervous system neurones resulting from distant stimulation, usually electrical. They are recorded using averaging techniques. Evoked responses may be used to test the integrity of peripheral, spinal and central nervous pathways. As with nerve conduction studies, the conduction time (latency) may be measured. In addition, information may be gained from the amplitude and configuration of these responses.

*5.5.1. General Information and Technical Information.* See above Nerve Conduction Studies (5.3).

*5.5.2. Description of Evoked Responses.* When describing the presence or absence of stimulus evoked responses and their configuration the following details should be given:

1. Single or multiphasic response.
2. Onset of response—defined as the start of the first reproducible potential. Since the onset of the response may be difficult to ascertain precisely, the criteria used should be stated.
3. Latency to onset—defined as the time (ms) from the onset of stimulus to the onset of response. The central conduction time relates to cortical evoked potentials and is defined as the difference between the latencies of the cortical and the spinal evoked potentials. This parameter may be used to test the integrity of the corticospinal neuraxis.
4. Latencies to peaks of positive and negative deflections

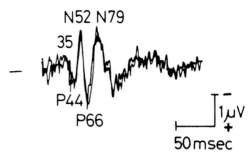

**Fig. A-6** Multiphasic evoked response recorded from the cerebral cortex after stimulation of the dorsal aspect of the penis. The recording shows the conventional labelling of negative (N) and positive (P) deflections with the latency of each deflection from the point of stimulation in milliseconds.

in multiphasic responses (Fig. A-6). *P* denotes positive deflections, *N* denotes negative deflections. In multiphasic responses, the peaks are numbered consecutively (e.g., P1, N1, P2, N2 . . . ) or according to the latencies to peaks in milliseconds (e.g., P44, N52, P66 . . . ).

5. The amplitude of the responses is measured in microvolts.

## 5.6 Sensory Testing

Limited information, of a subjective nature, may be obtained during cystometry by recording such parameters as the first desire to micturate, urgency or pain. However, sensory function in the lower urinary tract can be assessed by semi-objective tests by the measurement of urethral and/or vesical sensory thresholds to a standard applied stimulus such as a known electrical current.

*5.6.1. General Information.* The following details should be given:

1. Patient's position (supine, sitting, standing, other).
2. Bladder volume at time of testing.
3. Site of applied stimulus (intravesical, intraurethral).
4. Number of times the stimulus was applied and the response recorded. Define the sensation recorded, e.g., the first sensation or the sensation of pulsing.
5. Type of applied stimulus:
   a. Electrical current—is usual to use a constant current stimulator in urethral sensory measurement. State electrode characteristics and placement as in section on EMG (5.1); electrode contact area and distance between electrodes if applicable; impedance characteristics of the system; type of conductive medium used for electrode/epithelial contact. NOTE: *Topical anesthetic agents should not be used.* Also state stimulator make and specifications and stimulation parameters (pulse width, frequency, pattern, duration, current density).
   b. Other (e.g, mechanical, chemical).

*5.6.2. Definition of Sensory Thresholds.* The vesical/urethral sensory threshold is defined as the least current which consistently produces a sensation perceived by the subject during stimulation at the site under investigation. However, the absolute values will vary in relation to the site of the stimulus, the characteristics of the equipment and the stimulation parameters. Normal values should be established for each system.

# 6. CLASSIFICATION OF LOWER URINARY TRACT DYSFUNCTION

The lower urinary tract is composed of the *bladder* and *urethra*. They form a functional unit and their interaction cannot be ignored. Each has two functions, the bladder to store and void, the urethra to control and convey. When a reference is made to the hydrodynamic function or to the whole anatomical unit as a storage organ—the vesica urinaria—the correct term is the *bladder*. When the smooth muscle structure known as the m. detrusor urinae is being discussed, the correct term is *detrusor*. For simplicity the bladder/detrusor and the urethra will be considered separately so that a classification based on a combination of functional anomalies can be reached. Sensation cannot be precisely evaluated but must be assessed. This classification depends on the results of various objective urodynamic investigations. A complete urodynamic assessment is not necessary in all patients. However, studies of the filling and voiding phases are essential for each patient. As the bladder and urethra may behave differently during the storage and micturition phases of bladder function, it is most useful to examine bladder and urethral activity separately in each phase.

Terms used should be objective and definable and ideally should be applicable to the whole range of abnormality. When authors disagree with the classification presented below, or use terms which have not been defined here, their meaning should be made clear.

Assuming the absence of inflammation, infection and neoplasm, *lower urinary tract dysfunction* may be caused by:

1. Disturbance of the pertinent nervous or psychological control system.
2. Disorders of muscle function.
3. Structural abnormalities.

Urodynamic diagnoses based on this classification should correlate with the patient's symptoms and signs. For example, the presence of an unstable contraction in an asymptomatic continent patient does not warrant a diagnosis of detrusor overactivity during storage.

## 6.1 The Storage Phase

*6.1.1. Bladder Function During Storage.* This may be described according to:

1. Detrusor activity.
2. Bladder sensation.
3. Bladder capacity.
4. Compliance.

*6.1.1.1. Detrusor Activity.* In this context detrusor activity is interpreted from the measurement of detrusor pressure ($P_{det}$). Detrusor activity may be:

Normal.

Overactive.

In *normal detrusor function* the bladder volume increases without a significant rise in pressure (accommodation). No involuntary contractions occur despite provocation. A normal detrusor so defined may be described as "stable."

*Overactive detrusor function* is characterised by involuntary detrusor contractions during the filling phase, which may be spontaneous or provoked and which the patient cannot completely suppress. Involuntary detrusor contractions may be provoked by rapid filling, alterations of posture, coughing, walking, jumping and other triggering procedures. Various terms have been used to describe these features and they are defined as follows:

The *unstable detrusor* is one that is shown objectively to contract, spontaneously or on provocation, during the filling phase while the patient is attempting to inhibit micturition. Unstable detrusor contractions may be asymptomatic or may be interpreted as a normal desire to void. The presence of these contractions does not necessarily imply a neurological disorder. Unstable contractions are usually phasic in type (Fig. A-7, *A*). A gradual increase in detrusor pressure without subsequent decrease is best regarded as a change of compliance (Fig. A-7, *B*).

*Detrusor hyperreflexia* is defined as overactivity due to disturbance of the nervous control mechanisms. The term *detrusor hyperreflexia* should only be used when there is objective evidence of a relevant neurological disorder. The use of conceptual and undefined terms such as *hypertonic, systolic, uninhibited, spastic* and *automatic* should be avoided.

*6.1.1.2. Bladder Sensation.* During filling bladder sensation can be classified in qualitative terms (see 3.1) and by objective measurement (see Sensory Testing, 5.6). Sensation can be classified broadly as follows:

Normal.

Increased (hypersensitive).

Reduced (hyposensitive).

Absent.

*6.1.1.3. Bladder Capacity* (see Cystometry, 3.1)

*6.1.1.4. Compliance.* This is defined as: $\Delta V / \Delta p$ (see 3.1).

Compliance may change during the cystometric examination and is variably dependent upon a number of factors including:

1. Rate of filling.
2. The part of the cystometrogram curve used for compliance calculation.

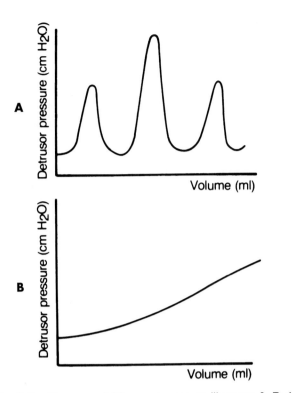

**Fig. A-7** Diagrams of filling cystometry to illustrate: **A,** Typical phasic unstable detrusor contraction; **B,** the gradual increase of detrusor pressure with filling characteristic of reduced bladder compliance.

From Abrams P, Blaivas JG, Stanton SL, et al: *Int Urogynecol J* 1:45, 1990.

3. The volume interval over which compliance is calculated.
4. The geometry (shape) of the bladder.
5. The thickness of the bladder wall.
6. The mechanical properties of the bladder wall.
7. The contractile/relaxant properties of the detrusor.

During normal bladder filling little or no pressure change occurs and this is termed "normal compliance." However, at the present time there is insufficient data to define normal, high and low compliance. When reporting compliance, specify:

1. The rate of bladder filling.
2. The bladder volume at which compliance is calculated.
3. The volume increment over which compliance is calculated.
4. The part of the cystometrogram curve used for the calculation of compliance.

*6.1.2. Urethral Function During Storage.* The urethral closure mechanism during storage may be:

Normal.

Incompetent.

The *normal urethra closure mechanism* maintains a positive urethral closure pressure during filling even in the presence of increased abdominal pressure. Immediately prior to micturition the normal closure pressure decreases to allow flow.

An *incompetent urethral closure mechanism* is defined as one which allows leakage of urine in the absence of a detrusor contraction. Leakage may occur whenever intravesical pressure exceeds intraurethral pressure (genuine stress incontinence) or when there is an involuntary fall in urethral pressure. Terms such as "the unstable urethra" await further data and precise definition.

*6.1.3. Urinary Incontinence.* This is defined as involuntary loss of urine which is objectively demonstrable and a social or hygienic problem. Loss of urine through channels other than the urethra is extraurethral incontinence.

*Urinary incontinence* denotes:

1. A symptom.
2. A sign.
3. A condition.

The symptom indicates the patient's statement of involuntary urine loss, the sign is the objective demonstration of urine loss, and the condition is the urodynamic demonstration of urine loss.

*6.1.3.1. Symptoms.* These can be defined as follows:

*Urge incontinence*—the involuntary loss of urine associated with a strong desire to void (urgency). *Urgency* may be associated with two types of dysfunction:

Overactive detrusor function *(motor urgency).*

Hypersensitivity *(sensory urgency).*

*Stress incontinence*—the symptom indicates the patient's statement of involuntary loss of urine during physical exertion.

*"Unconscious" incontinence*—Incontinence may occur in the absence of urge and without conscious recognition of the urinary loss.

*Enuresis*—any involuntary loss of urine. If the term is used to denote incontinence during sleep, it should always be qualified with the adjective "nocturnal."

*Post-micturition dribble* and *continuous leakage*—denote other symptomatic forms of incontinence.

*6.1.3.2. Signs.* The sign stress incontinence denotes the observation of loss of urine from the urethra synchronous with physical exertion (e.g., coughing). Incontinence may also be observed without physical exercise. Post-micturition dribble and continuous leakage denote other signs of incontinence. Symptoms and signs alone may not disclose the cause of urinary incontinence. Accurate diagnosis often requires urodynamic investigation in addition to careful history and physical examination.

*6.1.3.3. Conditions.* These can be defined as follows:

*Genuine stress incontinence*—the involuntary loss of urine occurring when, in the absence of a detrusor contraction, the intravesical pressure exceeds the maximum urethral pressure.

*Reflex incontinence*—loss of urine due to detrusor hyperreflexia and/or involuntary urethral relaxation in the absence of the sensation usually associated with the desire to micturate. This condition is only seen in patients with neuropathic bladder/urethral disorders.

*Overflow incontinence*—any involuntary loss of urine associated with over-distension of the bladder.

## 6.2 The Voiding Phase

*6.2.1. The Detrusor During Voiding.* During micturition the detrusor may be:

Acontractile.

Underactive.

Normal.

*The acontractile detrusor* is one that cannot be demonstrated to contract during urodynamic studies. *Detrusor areflexia* is defined as acontractility due to an abnormality of nervous control and denotes the complete absence of centrally coordinated contraction. In detrusor areflexia due to a lesion of the conus medullaris or sacral nerve outflow, the detrusor should be described as *decentralised,* not denervated, since the peripheral neurones remain. In such bladders pressure fluctuations of low amplitude, sometimes known as "autonomous" waves, may occasionally occur. The use of terms such as "atonic," "hypotonic," "autonomic," and "flaccid" should be avoided.

*Detrusor underactivity* is defined as a detrusor contraction of inadequate magnitude and/or duration to effect bladder emptying with a normal time span. Patients may have underactivity during micturition and detrusor overactivity during filling.

*Normal detrusor contractility.* Normal voiding is achieved by a voluntarily initiated detrusor contraction that is sustained and can usually be suppressed voluntarily. A normal detrusor contraction will effect complete bladder emptying in the absence of obstruction. For a given detrusor contraction, the magnitude of the recorded pressure rise will depend on the degree of outlet resistance.

*6.2.2. Urethral Function During Micturition.* During voiding urethral function may be:

Normal.

Obstructive.

Overactivity.

Mechanical.

*Normal.* The normal urethra opens to allow the bladder to be emptied.

*Obstruction.* This occurs when the urethral closure mechanism contracts against a detrusor contraction or fails to open at attempted micturition.

Synchronous detrusor and urethral contraction is *detrusor/urethral dyssynergia.* This diagnosis should be qualified by stating the location and type of the urethral muscles (striated or smooth) which are involved. Despite the confusion surrounding "sphincter" terminology the use of certain terms is so widespread that they are retained and defined here. The term *detrusor/external sphincter dyssynergia or detrusor-sphincter dyssynergia (DSD)* describes a detrusor contraction concurrent with an involuntary contraction of the urethral and/or periurethral striated muscle. In the adult, detrusor-sphincter dyssynergia is a feature of neurological voiding disorders. In the absence of neurological features the validity of this diagnosis should be questioned. The term *detrusor/bladder neck dyssynergia* is used to denote a detrusor contraction concurrent with an objectively demonstrated failure of bladder neck opening. No parallel term has been elaborated for possible detrusor/distal urethral (smooth muscle) dyssynergia.

Overactivity of the striated urethral sphincter may occur in the absence of detrusor contraction, and may prevent voiding. This is not detrusor/sphincter dyssynergia.

Overactivity of the urethral sphincter may occur during voiding in the absence of neurological disease and is termed *dysfunctional voiding.* The use of terms such as "nonneurogenic" or "occult neuropathic" should be avoided.

*Mechanical obstruction.* This is most commonly anatomical, e.g., urethral stricture.

## Summary

Using the characteristics of detrusor and urethral function during storage and micturition, an accurate definition of lower urinary tract behavior in each patient becomes possible.

## 7. UNITS OF MEASUREMENT

In the urodynamic literature pressure is measured in cm $H_2O$ and *not* in millimeters of mercury. When Laplace's law is used to calculate tension in the bladder wall, it is often found that pressure is then measured in dyne $cm^{-2}$. This lack of uniformity in the systems used leads to confusion when other parameters, which are a function of pressure, are computed (for instance, "compliance," contraction force, velocity, etc.). From these few examples it is evident that standardisation is essential for meaningful communication. Many journals now require that the results be given in SI units. This section is designed to give guidance in the application of the SI system to urodynamics and defines the units involved. The principal units to be used are listed in Table A-l.

**Table A-1**  Recommended Units of Measurement

| Quantity | Acceptable unit | Symbol |
|---|---|---|
| Volume | Milliliter | ml |
| Time | Second | s |
| Flow rate | Milliliters/second | ml/s |
| Pressure | Centimeters of water[a] | cm $H_2O$ |
| Length | Meters or submultiples | m, cm, mm |
| Velocity | Meters/second or submultiples | m/s, cm/s |
| Temperature | Degrees Celsius | ° C |

[a]The SI unit is the pascal (Pa), but it is only practical at present to calibrate our instruments in cm $H_2O$. One centimetre of water pressure is approximately equal to 100 pascals (1 cm $H_2O$ = 98.07 Pa = 0.098 kPa).

## 8. SYMBOLS

It is often helpful to use symbols in a communication. The system in Table A-2 has been devised to standardise a code of symbols for use in urodynamics. The rationale of the system is to have a basic symbol representing the physical quantity with qualifying subscripts. The list of basic symbols largely conforms to international usage. The

qualifying subscripts relate to the basic symbols to commonly used urodynamic parameters.

**Table A-2**  List of Symbols

| Basic symbols | | Urologic qualifiers | | Value | |
|---|---|---|---|---|---|
| Pressure | P | Bladder | ves | Maximum | max |
| Volume | V | Urethra | ura | Minimum | min |
| Flow rate | Q | Ureter | ure | Average | ave |
| Velocity | v | Detrusor | det | Isovolumetric | isv |
| Time | t | Abdomen | abd | Isotonic | ist |
| Temperature | T | External | | Isobaric | isb |
| Length | l | stream | ext | Isometric | ism |
| Area | A | | | | |
| Diameter | d | | | | |
| Force | F | | | | |
| Energy | E | | | | |
| Power | P | | | | |
| Compliance | C | | | | |
| Work | W | | | | |
| Energy per unit volume | e | | | | |

$P_{det,max}$ = maximum detrusor pressure
$e_{ext}$ = kinetic energy per unit volume in the external stream

## REFERENCES

1. Abrams P, Blaivas JG, Stanton SL, et al: Sixth report on the standardisation of terminology of lower urinary tract function. Procedures related to neurophysiological investigations: Electromyography, nerve conduction studies, reflex latencies, evoked potentials and sensory testing, *World J Urol* 1986; 4:2-5; *Scand J Urol Nephrol* 1986; 20:161-164; *Br J Urol* 1987; 59:300-307.
2. Bates P, Bradley WE, Glen E, et al: First report on the standardisation of terminology of lower urinary tract function. Urinary incontinence. Procedures related to the evaluation of urine storage—cystometry, urethral closure pressure profile, units of measurement, *Br J Urol* 1976; 48:39-42; *Eur Urol* 1976; 2:274-276; *Scand J Urol Nephrol* 1976; 11:193-196; *Urol Int* 1976; 32:81-87.
3. Bates P, Glen E, Griffiths D, et al: Second report on the standardisation of terminology of lower urinary tract function. Procedures related to the evaluation of micturition: Flow rate, pressure measurement, symbols, *Acta Urol Jpn* 1977; 27:1563-1566; *Br J Urol* 1977; 49:207-210; *Eur Urol* 1977; 3:168-170; *Scand J Urol Nephrol* 1977; 11:197-199.
4. Bates P, Bradley WE, Glen E, et al: Third report on the standardisation of terminology of lower urinary tract function. Procedures related to the evaluation of micturition: Pressure flow relationships, residual urine, *Br J Urol* 1980; 52:348-350; *Eur Urol* 1980; 6:170-171; *Acta Urol Jpn* 1980; 27:1566-1568; *Scand J Urol Nephrol* 1980; 12:191-193.
5. Bates P, Bradley WE, Glen E, et al: Fourth report on the standardisation of terminology of lower urinary tract function. Terminology related to neuromuscular dysfunction of lower urinary tract, *Br J Urol* 1981; 52:333-335; *Urology* 1981; 17:618-620; *Scand J Urol Nephrol* 1981; 15:169-171; *Acta Urol Jpn* 1981; 26:1568-1571.
6. Jasper HH: Report to the committee on the methods of clinical examination in electroencephalography, *Electroencephalogr Clin Neurophysiol* 1958; 10:370-375.

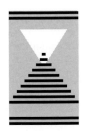

APPENDIX B

# *Lower Urinary Tract Rehabilitation Techniques*

## Seventh Report on the Standardization of Terminology of Lower Urinary Tract Function

## CONTENTS

## 1. INTRODUCTION

Lower urinary tract rehabilitation comprises non-surgical, non-pharmacological treatment for lower urinary tract dysfunction. The specific techniques defined in this report are listed in the contents above.

Most of the conditions for which rehabilitation techniques are employed have both a subjective and an objective component. In many instances, treatment is only capable of relieving symptoms, not curing the underlying disease. Therefore, symptoms should be quantified before and after treatment, and the means by which the physiology is altered should be clearly stated.

From Andersen JT, Blaivas JG, Cardozo L, et al: *Int Urogynecol J* 3:75, 1992.

The applications of the individual types of treatment cited here are taken from the scientific literature and from current clinical practice. It is not within the scope of this committee to endorse specific recommendations for treatment, nor to restrict the use of these treatments to the examples given.

The standards set in this report are recommended to ensure the reproducibility of methods of treatment and to facilitate the comparison of results obtained by different investigators and therapists. It is suggested that acknowledgement of these standards, in written publications, should be indicated by a footnote to the section "Methods and Materials" or its equivalent, to read as follows:

> Methods, definitions and units conform to the standards recommended by the International Continence Society, except where specifically noted.

## 2. PELVIC FLOOR TRAINING
### 2.1 Definition

Pelvic floor training is defined as repetitive selective voluntary contraction and relaxation of specific pelvic floor muscles. This necessitates muscle awareness in order to be sure that the correct muscles are being utilized and to avoid unwanted contractions of adjacent muscle groups.

### 2.2 Techniques

*2.2.1. Standard of Diagnosis and Implementation.* The professional status of the individual who establishes the diagnosis must be stated as well as the diagnostic techniques employed. Also the professional status of the person who institutes, supervises and assesses treatment must be specified.

*2.2.2. Muscle Awareness.* The technique used for obtaining selective pelvic floor contractions and relaxations should be stated. Registration of electromyographic (EMG) activity in the muscles of the pelvic floor, urethral or anal sphincter, or the anterior abdominal wall may be necessary to obtain this muscle awareness. Alternatively or additionally, registration of abdominal, vaginal, urethral or anal pressure may be used for the same purpose.

*2.2.3. Muscle Training.* It should be specified as to

whether treatment is given on an inpatient or outpatient basis. Specific details of training must be stated:

1. Patient position.
2. Duration of each contraction.
3. Interval between contractions.
4. Number of contractions per exercise.
5. Number of exercises per day.
6. Length of treatment program (weeks, months).

*2.2.4. Adjunctive Equipment.* Adjunctive equipment may be employed to enhance muscle awareness or muscle training. The following should be specified:

1. Type of equipment.
2. Mechanism of action.
3. Duration of use.
4. Therapeutic goals.

Examples of equipment in current use are:

Perineometers and other pressure-recording devices.
EMG equipment.
Ultrasound equipment.
Faradic stimulators.
Interferential current equipment.
Vaginal cones.

*2.2.5. Compliance.* Patient compliance has three major components:

1. Appropriate comprehension of the instructions and the technique.
2. Ability to perform the exercises.
3. Completion of the training programme.

Objective documentation of both the patient's ability to perform the exercises and the result of the training programme is mandatory. The parameters employed for objective documentation during training should be the same as those used for teaching muscle awareness.

## 2.3 Applications

Pelvic floor training can be used as treatment on its own, or as an adjunctive therapy, or for prophylaxis. The indications, mode of action and therapeutic goals must be specified. Examples of indications for therapeutic pelvic floor training are incontinence and descent of the pelvic viscera (prolapse). Examples of indications for prophylactic pelvic floor training are postpartum and following pelvic surgery.

## 3. BIOFEEDBACK
### 3.1 Definition

Biofeedback is a technique by which information about a normally unconscious physiological process is presented to the patient and the therapist as a visual, auditory or tactile signal. The signal is derived from a measurable physiological parameter, which is subsequently used in an educational process to accomplish a specific therapeutic result. The signal is displayed in a quantitative way and the patient is taught how to alter it and thus control the basic physiological process.

## 3.2 Techniques

The physiological parameter (e.g., pressure, flow, EMG) which is being monitored, the method of measurement and the mode by which it is displayed as a signal (e.g., light, sound, electric stimulus) should all be specified. Further, the specific instructions to the patient by which he/she is to alter the signal must be stated. The following details of biofeedback treatment must also be stated:

1. Patient position.
2. Duration of each session.
3. Interval between sessions.
4. Number of sessions per day/week/month and intervals between.
5. Length of treatment program (weeks, months).

## 3.3 Applications

The indications, the intended mode of action and the therapeutic goals must be specified. The aim of biofeedback is to improve a specific lower urinary tract dysfunction by increasing patient awareness, and by alteration of a measurable physiological parameter. Biofeedback can be applied in functional voiding disorders where the underlying pathophysiology can be monitored and subsequently altered by the patient. The following are examples of indications and techniques for biofeedback treatment:

Motor urgency and urge incontinence—display of detrusor pressure and control of detrusor contractions.
Dysfunctional voiding—display of sphincter EMG and relaxation of the external sphincter.
Pelvic floor relaxation—display of pelvic floor EMG and pelvic floor training.

## 4. BEHAVIORAL MODIFICATION
### 4.1 Definition

Behavioral modification comprises analysis and alteration of the relationship between the patient's symptoms and his/her environment for the treatment of maladaptive voiding patterns. This may be achieved by modification of the behaviour and/or environment of the patient.

### 4.2 Techniques

When behavioral modification is considered, a thorough analysis of possible interactions between the patient's symptoms, her general condition and her environment is essential. The following should be specified:

1. Micturition complaints; assessment and quantification:
   a. Symptom analysis.
   b. Visual analogue score.
   c. Fluid intake chart.
   d. Frequency/volume chart (voiding diary).
   e. Pad-weighing test.
   f. Urodynamic studies (when applicable).

2. General patient assessment:
   a. General performance status (e.g., Kurtzke disability scale[1]).
   b. Mobility (e.g., chairbound).
   c. Concurrent medical disorders (e.g., constipation, congestive heart failure, diabetes mellitus, chronic bronchitis, hemiplegia).
   d. Current medication (e.g., diuretics).
   e. Psychological state (e.g., psychoanalysis).
   f. Psychiatric disorders.
   g. Mental state (e.g., dementia, confusion).
3. Environmental assessment:
   a. Toilet facilities (access).
   b. Living conditions.
   c. Working conditions.
   d. Social relations.
   e. Availability of suitable incontinence aids.
   f. Access to health care.

For behavioral modification, various therapeutic concepts and techniques may be employed. The following should be specified:

1. Conditioning techniques:
   a. Timed voiding (e.g., hyposensitive bladder).
   b. Double/triple voiding (e.g., residual urine due to bladder diverticulum).
   c. Increase of intervoiding intervals/bladder drill (e.g., sensory urgency).
   d. Biofeedback (see above).
   e. Enuresis alarm.
2. Fluid intake regulation (e.g., restriction).
3. Measures to improve patient mobility (e.g., physiotherapy, wheelchair).
4. Change of medication (e.g., diuretics, anticholinergics).
5. Treatment of concurrent medical/psychiatric disorders.
6. Psychoanalysis/hypnotherapy (e.g., idiopathic detrusor instability).
7. Environmental changes (e.g., provision of incontinence pads, condom urinals, commode, furniture protection etc.).

Treatment is often empirical and may require a combination of the above-mentioned concepts and techniques. The results of treatment should be objectively documented using the same techniques as used for the initial assessment of micturition complaints.

## 4.3 Applications

Behavioral modification may be used for the treatment of maladaptive voiding patterns in patients when:

The etiology and pathophysiology of their symptoms cannot be identified (e.g., sensory urgency).

The symptoms are caused by a psychological problem.

The symptoms have failed to respond to conventional therapy.

They are unfit for definitive treatment of their condition.

Behavioral modification may be employed alone or as an adjunct to any other form of treatment for lower urinary tract dysfunction.

## 5. ELECTRICAL STIMULATION
## 5.1 Definition

Electrical stimulation is the application of electrical current to stimulate the pelvic viscera or their nerve supply. The aim of electrical stimulation may be to directly induce a therapeutic response or to modulate lower urinary tract, bowel or sexual dysfunction.

## 5.2 Techniques

The following should be specified:
1. Access:
   a. Surface electrodes (e.g., anal plug, vaginal electrode).
   b. Percutaneous electrodes (e.g., needle electrodes, wire electrodes).
   c. Implants.
2. Approach:
   a. Temporary stimulation.
   b. Permanent stimulation.
3. Stimulation site:
   a. Effector organ.
   b. Peripheral nerve.
   c. Spinal nerves (intradural or extradural).
   d. Spinal cord.
4. Stimulation parameters:
   a. Frequency.
   b. Voltage.
   c. Current.
   d. Pulse width.
   e. Pulse shape (e.g., rectangular, biphasic, capacitatively coupled).
   f. With monopolar stimulation, state whether the active electrode is anodic or cathodic.
   g. Duration of pulse trains.
   h. Shape of pulse trains (e.g., surging trains).
5. Mode of stimulation:
   a. Continuous.
   b. Phasic (regular automatic on/off).
   c. Intermittent (variable duration and time intervals).
   d. Single sessions: number and duration of, and intervals between, periods of stimulation.
   e. Multiple sessions: number and duration of, and intervals between sessions.
6. Design of electronic equipment, electrodes and related electrical stimulation characteristics:
   a. Electrodes (monopolar or bipolar).
   b. Surface area of electrodes.
   c. Maximum charge density per pulse at active electrode surface.

**Table B-1**  Parameters for Electrical Stimulation

| Quantity | Unit | Symbol | Definition |
|---|---|---|---|
| Electric current | Ampere | A | 1 A of electric current is the transfer of 1 C of electric charge per second. |
| Direct (D.C.) | | | Steady unidirectional electric current. |
| Galvanic | | | Unidirectional electric current derived from a chemical battery. |
| Alternating (A.C.) | | | Electric current that phasically changes direction of flow in a sinusoidal manner. |
| Faradic | | | Intermittent oscillatory current similar to alternating current (A.C.), e.g., as produced by an induction coil. |
| Voltage (potential difference) | Volt | V | 1 V of potential difference between two points requires 1 J of energy to transfer 1 C of charge from one point to the other. |
| Resistance | Ohm | $\Omega$ | 1 $\Omega$ of resistance between two points allows 1 V of potential difference to cause a flow of 1 A of direct current (D.C.) between them. |
| Impedance (Z) | Ohm | $\Omega$ | Analogue of resistance for alternating current (A.C.); vector sum of ohmic resistance and reactance (inductive and/or capacitative resistance). |
| Charge | Coulomb | C | 1 C of electric charge is transferred through a conductor in 1 s by 1 A of electric current. |
| Capacity | Farad | F | A condensor (capacitor) has 1 F of electric capactiy (capacitance) if transfer of 1 C of electric charge causes 1 V of potential difference between its elements. |
| Frequency | Hertz | $Hz(s^{-1})$ | Number of cycles (phases) of a periodically repeating oscillation per second. |
| Pulse width | Time | ms | Duration of 1 pulse (phase) of a phasic electric current or voltage. |
| Electrode surface area | Area | $mm^2$ | Active area of electrode surface. |
| Charge density per pulse | Coulomb/area/time | $uC\ mm^{-2}ms^{-1}$ | Electric charge delivered to a given electrode surface area in a given time (one pulse width). |

    d. Impedance of the implanted system.
    e. Power source (implants):
       1) Active, self-powered.
       2) Passive, inductive current.
7. For transurethral intravesical stimulation:
    a. Filling medium.
    b. Filling volume.
    c. Number of intravesical electrodes.

## 5.3 Units of Measurement and Symbols

Parameters related to electrical stimulation, units of measurement and the corresponding symbols are listed in Table B-1.

## 5.4 Applications

The aims of treatment should be clearly stated. These may include control of voiding, continence, defecation, erection, ejaculation or relief of pain. Specify whether electrical stimulation aims at:

A functional result completely dependent on the continuous use of electrical current.

Modulation, reflex facilitation, reflex inhibition, reeducation or conditioning with a sustained functional result even after withdrawal of stimulation.

Electrical stimulation is applicable in neurogenic or non-neurogenic lower urinary tract, bowel or sexual dysfunction. Techniques and equipment vary widely with the type of dysfunction and the goal of electrical stimulation. If electrical stimulation is employed for control of a neuropathic dysfunction, and the chosen site of stimulation is the reflex arc (peripheral nerves, spinal nerves or spinal cord), this reflex arc must be intact. Consequently electrical stimulation is not applicable for complete lower motor neuron lesions except when the direct stimulation of the effector organ is chosen.

When ablative surgery is performed (e.g., dorsal rhizotomy, ganglionectomy, sphincterotomy or levatorotomy) in conjunction with an implant to achieve the desired functional effect, the following should be specified.
1. Techniques used to reduce pain or mass reflexes during stimulation:
    a. Number and spinal level of interrupted afferents.
    b. Site of interruption of afferents.
       1) Dorsal rhizotomy (intradural or extradural).
       2) Ganglionectomy.
2. Techniques to reduce stimulated sphincter dyssynergia:
    a. Pudendal block (unilateral or bilateral).
    b. Pudendal neurectomy (unilateral or bilateral).
    c. Levatorotomy (unilateral or bilateral).
    d. Electrically induced sphincter fatigue.
    e. External sphincterectomy.

If electrical stimulation is combined with ablative surgery, other functions (e.g., erection or continence) may be impaired.

*5.4.1. Voiding.* When the aim of electrical stimulation is to achieve voiding, state whether this is obtained by:

Stimulation of the afferent fibres to induce bladder sensation and thus facilitate voiding (transurethral intravesical stimulation).

Stimulation of efferent fibres or detrusor muscle to induce a bladder contraction (electromicturition).

*5.4.2. Continence.* Electrical stimulation may aim to inhibit overactive detrusor function or to improve urethral closure. State whether overactive detrusor function is abolished/reduced by reflex inhibition (pudendal to pelvic nerve) or by blockade of nerve conduction. When electrical stimulation is applied to improve urethral closure, state whether this is by:

A direct effect on the urethra during stimulation.

Reeducation and conditioning to restore pelvic floor tone.

*5.4.3. Pelvic Pain.* If electrical stimulation is applied to control pelvic pain, the nature and etiology of the pain should be stated. When pelvic pain is caused by pelvic floor spasticity, electrical stimulation may be effective by relaxing the pelvic floor muscles.

*5.4.4. Erection and Ejaculation.* If electrical stimulation is applied for the treatment of erectile dysfunction or ejaculatory failure, the etiology should be stated. Electrically induced erection requires an intact arterial supply and cavernous tissue, and a competent venous closure mechanism of the corpora cavernosa. Electroejaculation requires an intact reproductive system.

*5.4.5. Defecation.* Defecation may be obtained by electrical stimulation, either intentionally or as a side-effect of electromicturition.

At present, the mechanism of action of electrically induced control of pelvic pain, erection, ejaculation and defecation are not fully understood. The clinical applications of these techniques have not yet been fully established.

# 6. VOIDING MANEUVERS

Voiding maneuvers are employed to obtain/facilitate bladder emptying. For lower urinary tract rehabilitation, voiding maneuvers may be used alone or in combination with other techniques such as biofeedback or behavioral modification. The aim is to achieve complete bladder emptying at low intravesical pressures. The techniques employed may be invasive (e.g., catheters) or non-invasive (e.g., triggering reflex detrusor contractions, increasing intra-abdominal pressure).

When reporting on voiding maneuvers, the professional status of the individual(s) who establishes the diagnosis must be stated as well as the diagnostic techniques employed. Also the professional status of the person(s) who institutes, supervises and assesses treatment should be specified.

## 6.1 Catheterization

*6.1.1. Definition.* Catheterization is a technique for bladder emptying employing a catheter to drain the bladder or a urinary reservoir. Catheter use may be intermittent or indwelling (temporary or permanent).

*6.1.2. Intermittent (In/Out) Catheterization.* Intermittent (in/out) catheterization is defined as draining or aspiration of the bladder or a urinary reservoir with subsequent removal of the catheter. The following types of intermittent catheterization are defined:

1. Intermittent self-catheterization: performed by the patient himself/herself.
2. Intermittent catheterization by an attendant (e.g., doctor, nurse or relative).
3. Clean intermittent catheterization: use of a clean technique. This implies ordinary washing techniques and use of disposable or cleansed reusable catheters.
4. Aseptic intermittent catheterization: use of a sterile technique. This implies genital disinfection and the use of sterile catheters and instruments/gloves.

*6.1.2.1. Techniques.* The following should be specified:
1. Preparation used for genital disinfection.
2. Preparation and volume of lubricant.
3. Catheter specifications: type, size, material and surface coating.
4. Number of catheterizations per day/week.
5. Length of treatment (e.g., weeks, months, permanent).

*6.1.2.2. Applications.* Specify the indications and the therapeutic goals. Typical examples for the use of intermittent catheterization are: neurogenic bladder with impaired bladder emptying, postoperative urinary retention and transstomal catheterization of continent reservoirs.

*6.1.3. Indwelling Catheter.* An indwelling catheter remains in the bladder, urinary reservoir or urinary conduit for a period of time longer than one emptying. The following routes of access are employed:

Transurethral.

Suprapubic.

*6.1.3.1. Techniques.* The following should be specified:
1. Catheter specifications: type, size, material.
2. Preparation and volume of lubricant.
3. Catheter fixation: e.g., balloon (state filling volume), skin suture.
4. Mode of drainage: continuous/intermittent. For intermittent drainage specify clamping periods.
5. Intervals between catheter change.
6. Duration of catheterization (days, weeks, years).

*6.1.3.2. Applications.* The indications and the therapeutic goals should be specified. Examples of the use of temporary indwelling catheters are:

Suprapubic catheter—after major pelvic surgery.

Transurethral catheter—in order to monitor urine output in a severely ill patient.

Examples of the use of permanent indwelling catheters are:

Suprapubic: candidates for urinary diversion unfit for surgery.

Transurethral: severe bladder symptoms from untreatable bladder cancer.

## 6.2 Bladder Reflex Triggering

*6.2.1. Definition.* Bladder reflex triggering comprises various maneuvers performed by the patient or the therapist in order to elicit reflex detrusor contractions by exteroceptive stimuli. The most commonly used maneuvers are: suprapubic tapping, thigh scratching and anal/rectal manipulation.

*6.2.2. Techniques.* For each maneuver the following should be specified:

1. Details of maneuver.
2. Frequency, intervals and duration (weeks, months, years) of practice.

*6.2.3. Applications.* When using bladder reflex triggering maneuvers, the etiology of the dysfunction and the goals of treatment should be stated. Bladder reflex triggering maneuvers are indicated only in patients with an intact sacral reflex arc (suprasacral spinal cord lesions).

## 6.3. Bladder Expression

*6.3.1. Definition.* Bladder expression comprises various maneuvers aimed at increasing intravesical pressure in order to facilitate bladder emptying. The most commonly used

maneuvers are abdominal straining, Valsalva's maneuver and Credé's maneuver.

*6.3.2. Techniques.* For each maneuver, the following should be specified:

Details of the maneuver.

Frequency, intervals and duration of practice (weeks, months, years).

*6.3.3. Applications.* When using bladder expression, the etiology of the underlying disorder and the goals of treatment should be stated. Bladder expression may be used in patients where the urethral closure mechanism can be easily overcome.

## REFERENCE

1. Kurtzke JF: Rating neurological impairment in multiple sclerosis: An expanded disability status scale (EDSS). *Neurology* 33:1444, 1983.

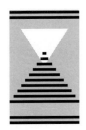

APPENDIX **C**

*The Standardization of Terminology of Female Pelvic Organ Prolapse and Pelvic Floor Dysfunction and the Standardization of Terminology and Assessment of Functional Characteristics of Intestinal Urinary Reservoirs*

## The Standardization of Terminology of Female Pelvic Organ Prolapse and Pelvic Floor Dysfunction

### CONTENTS

From Bump RC, Mattiasson A, Bø K, et al: *Am J Obstet Gynecol* 175:10, 1996.

## Standardization of Terminology and Assessment of Functional Characteristics of Intestinal Urinary Reservoirs

### CONTENTS

From: Thüroff JW, Mattiasson A, Andersen JT, et al: *Neurourol Urodyn* 15:499, 1996.

EDITOR'S NOTE: The two documents mentioned in this appendix were produced by the International Continence Society Committee on Standardization of Terminology and published in 1996. The other documents from this Committee have been published verbatim in Appendixes A, B, and D. The editors have chosen not to publish the entire text of these two documents. The Standardization of Terminology of Female Pelvic Organ Prolapse and Pelvic Floor Dysfunction is summarized, with pertinent figures, in Chapter 4. The Standardization of Terminology and Assessment of Functional Characteristics of Intestinal Urinary Reservoirs is beyond the scope of this text. However, we are printing the Contents of each of these documents and the references for the information of our readers.

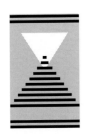

## APPENDIX D
## *The Standardization of Terminology of Lower Urinary Tract Function*
Pressure-Flow Studies of Voiding, Urethral Resistance, and Urethral Obstruction

## CONTENTS

1. Introduction
2. Evaluation of micturition
3. Additional symbols

## 1. INTRODUCTION

This report has been produced at the request of the International Continence Society. It was approved at the twenty-fifth annual meeting of the Society in Sydney, Australia.

The 1988 version of the collated reports on standardization of terminology, which appeared in *Neurourology and Urodynamics* 7:403-427, contains material relevant to pressure-flow studies in many different sections. This report is a revision and expansion of sections 4.2 and 4.3 and parts of sections 6.2 and 7 of the 1988 report. It contains a recommendation for a provisional standard method for defining obstruction on the basis of pressure-flow data.

From Griffiths D, Höfner K, van Mastrigt R, et al: *Neurourol Urodyn* 16:1, 1997.

## 2. EVALUATION OF MICTURITION
## 2.1 Pressure-Flow Studies

At present, the best method of analyzing voiding function quantitatively is the pressure-flow study of micturition, with simultaneous recording of abdominal, intravesical, and detrusor pressures and flow rate (Fig. D-1).

Direct inspection of the raw pressure and flow data before, during, and at the end of micturition is essential because it allows artifacts and untrustworthy data to be recognized and eliminated. More detailed analyses of pressure-flow relationships, described below, are advisable to aid diagnosis and to quantify data for research studies.

The flow pattern in a pressure-flow study should be representative of free-flow studies in the same patient. It is important to eliminate artifacts and unrepresentative studies before applying more detailed analyses.

Pressure-flow studies contain information about the behavior of the urethra and the behavior of the detrusor. Section 2.2 deals with the urethra. Detrusor function is considered in section 2.3.

*2.1.1. Pressure and Flow Rate Parameters*
*Definitions.* See Fig. D-1 and Table D-2; see also Table II in the 1988 version of the collated standardization reports.

*Maximum flow rate* is the maximum measured value of the flow rate. Symbol: $Q_{max}$.

*Maximum pressure* is the maximum value of the pressure measured during a pressure-flow study. Note that this may be attained at a moment when the flow rate is zero. Symbols: $p_{abd.max}$, $p_{ves.max}$, $p_{det.max}$.

*Pressure at maximum flow* is the pressure recorded at maximum measured flow rate. If the same maximum value is attained more than once or if it is sustained for a period of time, then the point of maximum flow is taken to be where the detrusor pressure has its lowest value for this flow rate; abdominal, intravesical, and detrusor pressures at maximum flow are all read at the same point. Flow delay (see 2.1.2) may have a significant influence and should be considered. Symbols: $p_{abd.Qmax}$, $p_{ves.Qmax}$, $p_{det.Qmax}$.

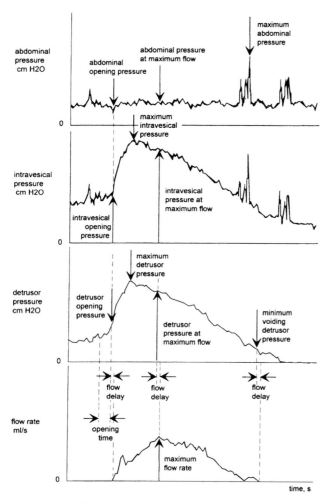

**Fig. D-1** Diagram of a pressure-flow study with nomenclature recommended in this report.

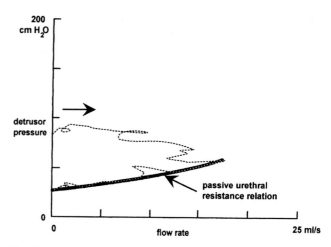

**Fig. D-2** Plot of detrusor pressure against flow rate during voiding *(broken curve)*, providing an indication of the urethral resistance relation (URR). The continuous smooth curve is an estimate of the passive urethral resistance relation.

*Opening pressure* is the pressure recorded at the onset of measured flow. Flow delay should be considered. Symbols: $p_{abd.open}$, $p_{ves.open}$, $p_{det.open}$.

*Closing pressure* is the pressure recorded at the end of measured flow. Flow delay should be considered. Symbols: $p_{abd.clos}$, $p_{ves.clos}$, $p_{det.clos}$.

*Minimum voiding pressure* is the minimum pressure during measurable flow (see Fig. D-1). It may be, but is not necessarily, equal to the opening pressure or the closing pressure. For example, the symbol for minimum voiding detrusor pressure is $p_{det.min.void}$.

*2.1.2. Flow Delay.* When a pressure-flow study is performed, the flow rate is measured at a location downstream of the bladder pressure measurement, so the flow rate measurement is delayed. The delay is partly physiological, but it also depends on the equipment. It may depend on the flow rate.

When considering pressure-flow relationships, it may be important to take this delay into account, especially if there are rapid changes in pressure and flow rate. In current practice an average value is estimated by each investigator from observations of the delay between corresponding pressure and flow rate changes in a number of actual studies. Values from 0.5 to 1.0 s are typical.

*Definition. Flow delay* is the time delay between a change in bladder pressure and the corresponding change in measured flow rate.

*2.1.3. Presentation of Results.* Pressure-flow plots and the nomograms used for analysis should be presented with the flow rate plotted along the X-axis and the detrusor pressure along the Y-axis (Fig. D-2).

*Specify.* The value of the flow delay that is used.

## 2.2 Urethral Resistance and Bladder Outlet Obstruction

*2.2.1. Urethral Function During Voiding.* During voiding, urethral function may be
1. Normal.
2. Obstructive, as a result of:
   a. Overactivity.
   b. Abnormal structure.

Obstruction due to urethral overactivity occurs when the urethral closure mechanism contracts involuntarily or fails to relax during attempted micturition in spite of an ongoing detrusor contraction. Obstruction due to abnormal structure has an anatomical basis, e.g., urethral stricture or prostatic enlargement.

*2.2.2. Urethral Resistance.* Urethral resistance is represented by a relation between pressure and flow rate, describing the pressure required to propel any given flow rate through the urethra. The relation is called the *urethral resistance relation* (URR).

An indication of the urethral resistance relation is obtained by plotting detrusor pressure against flow rate. The most accurate procedure, which requires a computer or an

**Table D-1** Methods of Analyzing Pressure-Flow Plots

| Method | Aim | Number of $p/Q$ points | Assumed shape of URR | Number of parameters | Number of classes or continuous |
|---|---|---|---|---|---|
| Abrams/Griffiths nomogram[1] | Diagnosis | 1 | n/a | n/a | 3 |
| Spångberg nomogram[10] | Diagnosis | 1 | n/a | n/a | 3 |
| URA[2,6] | Resistance | 1 | Curved | 1 | Continuous |
| linPURR[8] | Resistance | 1* | Linear | 1 | 7 |
| Schäfer PURR[7] | Resistance | Many | Curved | 2 | Continuous |
| CHESS[3] | Resistance | Many | Curved | 2 | 16 |
| OBI[4] | Resistance | Many | Linear | 1 | Continuous |
| Spångberg et al.[10] | Resistance | Many | Linear or curved | 3 | Continuous +3 categories |
| DAMPF[9] | Resistance | 2 | Linear | 1 | Continuous |
| A/G number[5] | Resistance | 1 | Linear | 1 | Continuous |

*Schäfer uses 2 points to draw a linear relation, but the point at maximum flow determines the resistance grade.

x/y recorder, is a quasi-continuous plot showing many pairs of corresponding pressure and flow rate values (see Fig. D-2). A simpler procedure, which can be performed by hand, is to plot only 2 or 3 pressure-flow points connected by straight lines; e.g., the points of minimum voiding pressure and of maximum flow may be selected. No matter how the plot is made, flow delay should be considered.

A further simplification is to plot just one point showing the maximum flow rate and the detrusor pressure at maximum flow. Flow delay should be considered.

Methods of analyzing pressure-flow plots are further discussed below.

*2.2.3. Urethral Activity.* Ideally, the urethra is fully relaxed during voiding. The urethral resistance is then at its lowest and the detrusor pressure has its lowest value for any given flow rate. Under these circumstances the urethral resistance relation is defined by the inherent mechanical and morphological properties of the urethra and is called the *passive urethral resistance relation* (see Fig. D-2).

Urethral activity can only increase the detrusor pressure above the value defined by the passive urethral resistance relation. Therefore, any deviation of the pressure-flow plot from the passive urethral resistance relation toward higher pressures are considered to be a result of activity of the urethral or periurethral muscles, striated or smooth.

*2.2.4. Bladder Outlet Obstruction.* Obstruction is a physical concept that is assessed from measurements of pressure and flow rate made during voiding. Whether due to urethral overactivity or to abnormal structure, obstruction implies that the urethral resistance to flow is abnormally elevated. Because of natural variation from subject to subject, there cannot be a sharp boundary between normal and abnormal. Therefore, the definition of abnormality requires further elaboration.

*2.2.5. Methods of Analyzing Pressure-Flow Plots.* The results of pressure-flow studies may be used for various purposes—for example, for objective diagnosis of urethral obstruction or for statistical testing of differences in urethral resistance between groups of patients. For these purposes, methods have been developed to quantify pressure-flow plots in terms of one or more numerical parameters. The parameters are based on aspects such as the position, slope, and curvature of the plot. Some of these methods are intended primarily for use in adult males with possible prostatic hypertrophy.

Some methods of analysis are shown in Table D-1.

*Quantification of urethral resistance.* In all current methods, urethral resistance is derived from the relationship between pressure and flow rate. A commonly used method of demonstrating this relationship is the pressure-flow plot. The lower pressure part of this plot is taken to represent the passive urethral resistance relation (see Fig. D-2). In general, the higher the pressure for a given flow rate, and/or the steeper or more sharply curved upward this part of the plot, the higher the urethral resistance. The various methods differ in how position, slope, and/or curvature of the plot are quantified and how and whether they are combined. Some methods grade urethral resistance on a continuous scale; others grade it in a small number of classes (see Table D-1). If there are few classes, small changes in resistance may not be detected. Conversely, a small change on a continuous scale may not be clinically relevant.

Some methods result in a single parameter; others result in two or more parameters (see Table D-1). A single parameter makes it easy to compare different measurements. A larger number of parameters makes comparison more difficult but potentially gives higher accuracy and validity. If there are too many parameters, however, accuracy may be compromised by poor reproducibility.

*Choice of method.* Some methods in Table D-1 are intended primarily to quantify urethral resistance. Others are intended only for the diagnosis of obstruction. Methods that quantify urethral resistance on a scale can also be used to aid diagnosis of obstruction by comparison with cut-off values. In every case an equivocal zone may be included.

Because of their underlying similarity, all the above methods classify clearly obstructed and clearly unobstructed pressure-flow studies consistently, but there is some lack of agreement in a minority of cases with intermediate urethral resistance.

One method of analyzing pressure-flow studies may be more useful for a particular purpose. In selecting a method, investigators should consider carefully what their aims are and which method is best suited to their purpose.

*Identification of optimum methods.* For a subsequent report, the International Continence Society will compare the above methods with each other and may also develop new methods, with the aim of reaching a consensus on their use. The Society will continue to seek better ways of clinically validating these methods. The following procedure has been chosen.

Making use of good-quality data stored in digital format, the following databases will be examined:

1. Pressure-flow studies in untreated men with lower urinary tract symptoms and signs suggestive of benign prostatic obstruction.
2. Pressure-flow studies repeated after a time interval with no intervention.
3. Pressure-flow studies before and after TURP.
4. Pressure-flow studies before and after alternative therapeutic intervention that causes a small change in urethral resistance.

Database 1 will be used to determine which existing or new methods adequately described the actual pressure-flow plots of male patients with lower urinary tract symptoms. Database 2 will be used to determine the reproducibility of the various methods. Database 3 will be used to determine which groups of patients TURP significantly reduces urethral resistance, and hence which patients are indeed obstructed. Database 4 will be used to test the various methods' sensitivity to small changes of urethral resistance.

On the basis of analyses, the International Continence Society will attempt to identify:

1. A simple and reproducible method with high validity of diagnosing obstruction.
2. A sensitive and reproducible method with high validity of measuring urethral resistance and changes in resistance.

*Provisional recommendation.* Pending the results of these procedures, it is recommended that investigators reporting pressure-flow studies in adult males, particularly subjects with benign prostatic hyperplasia, use one simple standard method of analysis in addition to any other method that they have selected, so that results from different centers can be compared. For this provisional method it is recommended that urethral resistance be specified by the maximum flow rate and the detrusor pressure at maximum flow, i.e., by the pair of values $(Q_{max}, p_{det.Qmax})$. A provisional

diagnostic classification may be derived from these values as follows:

1. If $(p_{det.Qmax} - 2*Qmax) > 40$, the pressure-flow study is obstructed.
2. If $(p_{det.Qmax} - 2*Qmax) < 20$, the pressure-flow study is unobstructed.
3. Otherwise, the study is equivocal.

In these formulas, pressure and flow rate are expressed in cm $H_2O$ and ml/s respectively. This method is illustrated graphically in Fig. D-3. It may be referred to as the *provisional ICS method for definition of obstruction.*

The equivocal zone of the provisional method (Fig. D-3) is similar but not identical to those of the Abrams-Griffiths and Spångberg nomograms and to the region defining linPURR grade II. For micturitions with low to moderate flow rates it is consistent with cut-off values used to define obstruction in the URA and CHESS methods.

## 2.3 Detrusor Contractility During Micturition

During micturition the detrusor may be:

1. Acontractile.
2. Underactive.
3. Normal.

An *acontractile detrusor* is one that cannot be demonstrated to contract during urodynamic studies.

An *underactive detrusor* produces a contraction of inadequate magnitude and/or duration to effect complete bladder emptying in the absence of urethral obstruction. (Concerning the elderly, see below.) Both magnitude and duration should be considered in the evaluation of detrusor contractility.

A *normal detrusor,* in the absence of obstruction, produces a contraction that will effect complete bladder emptying. Detrusor contractility in the elderly may need special consideration.

For a given detrusor contraction, the magnitude of the recorded pressure rise will depend on the outlet resistance.

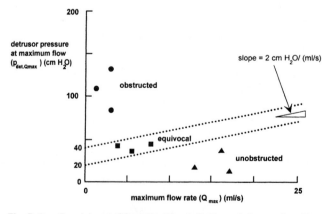

**Fig. D-3** Provisional ICS method for definition of obstruction. The points represent schematically the values of maximum flow rate and detrusor pressure at maximum flow for 9 different voids, 3 in each class.

In general, the higher the detrusor pressure and/or the higher the flow rate, the stronger the detrusor contraction. The magnitude of the detrusor contraction may be quantified approximately by means of a nomogram applied to the pressure-flow plot or by calculation.

## 3. ADDITIONAL SYMBOLS

Qualifiers that can be used to form symbols for variables relevant to voiding are shown in Table D-2. These are additions to those in Table II of the 1988 standardization report.

**Table D-2**   Qualifiers That Can Be Used to Indicate Pressure and Flow Variables Relevant to Voiding*

**Qualifiers**

| | |
|---|---|
| At maximum flow | Qmax |
| During voiding | void |
| Opening | open |
| Closing | clos |

**Examples**

| | |
|---|---|
| $p_{det.Qmax}$ | = detrusor pressure at maximum flow |
| $p_{det.min.void}$ | = minimum voiding detrusor pressure |
| $p_{ves.open}$ | = intravesical opening pressure |
| $p_{ves.clos}$ | = intravesical closing pressure |

*When possible, qualifiers should be printed as subscripts (see above). Note that the preferred symbol for pressure is lowercase $p$, while the symbol for flow rate is uppercase Q.

## REFERENCES

1. Abrams PH, Griffiths DJ: The assessment of prostatic obstruction from urodynamic measurements and from residual urine, *Br J Urol* 51:129-134, 1979.
2. Griffiths D, van Mastrigt R, Bosch R: Quantification of urethral resistance and bladder function during voiding, with special reference to the effects of prostate size reduction on urethral obstruction due to benign prostatic hypertrophy, *Neurourol Urodyn* 8:17-27, 1989.
3. Höfner K, Kramer AEJL, Tan HK, Krah H, Jonas U: CHESS classification of bladder outflow obstruction: a consequence in the discussion of current concepts, *World J Urol* 13:59-64, 1995.
4. Kranse M, Van Mastrigt R: The derivation of an obstruction index from a three-parameter model fitted to the lowest part of the pressure flow plot, *J Urol* 145:261A, 1991.
5. Lim CS, Abrams P: The Abrams-Griffiths nomogram, *World J Urol* 13:34-39, 1995.
6. Rollema HJ, Van Mastrigt R: Improved indication and follow-up in transurethral resection of the prostate (TUR) using the computer program CLIM, *J Urol* 148:111-116, 1992.
7. Schäfer W: The contribution of the bladder outlet to the relation between pressure and flow rate during micturition. In Hinmann F Jr, ed, *Benign prostatic hypertrophy*. New York, 1983, Springer-Verlag, pp. 470-496.
8. Schäfer W: Basic principles and clinical application of advanced analysis of bladder voiding function, *Urol Clin North Am* 17:553-566, 1990.
9. Schäfer W: Analysis of bladder-outlet function with the linearized passive urethral resistance relation, linPURR, and a disease-specific approach for grading obstruction: from complex to simple, *World J Urol* 13:47-58, 1995.
10. Spångberg A, Teriö H, Ask P, Engberg A: Pressure/flow studies preoperatively and postoperatively in patients with benign prostatic hypertrophy: estimation of the urethral pressure/flow relation and urethral elasticity, *Neurourol Urodyn* 10:139-167, 1991.

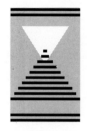

*Index*